Ashok Pandey, PhD
Editor

# Concise Encyclopedia
# of Bioresource Technology

*Pre-publication*
*REVIEWS,*
*COMMENTARIES,*
*EVALUATIONS . . .*

"The broad spectrum of contributors, most of them from Africa, Asia, Australia, Europe, and Latin America, distinguishes this encyclopedia from similar works, giving a fresh view on many topics. The sections on environmental biotechnology, food biotechnology, and solid substrate fermentation are most valuable, since they contain information not readily available in other similar publications."

**Robert P. Tengerdy, PhD**
*Professor Emeritus,*
*Department of Microbiology,*
*Colorado State University*

"This encyclopedia contains, without a doubt, some outstanding short reviews of topics of immediate relevance to the immense field of biotechnology. Current views on environmental, food, and industrial biotechnology are exposed and discussed. The use of microorganisms for wastewater treatment is considered. In addition, extensive fermentation systems are described for a wide variety of uses including enzyme, alcohol, or secondary metabolite production. This book represents an attractive source of information for researchers and students involved in the area of biotechnology."

**Christopher Augur, PhD**
*Research Director,*
*Institute for Research*
*and Development, France*

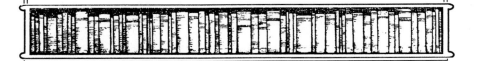

# Concise Encyclopedia
# of Bioresource Technology

# FOOD PRODUCTS PRESS®
## Crop Science
## Amarjit S. Basra, PhD
## Senior Editor

*Heterosis and Hybrid Seed Production in Agronomic Crops* edited by Amarjit S. Basra

*Intensive Cropping: Efficient Use of Water, Nutrients, and Tillage* by S. S. Prihar, P. R. Gajri, D. K. Benbi, and V. K. Arora

*Physiological Bases for Maize Improvement* edited by María E. Otegui and Gustavo A. Slafer

*Plant Growth Regulators in Agriculture and Horticulture: Their Role and Commercial Uses* edited by Amarjit S. Basra

*Crop Responses and Adaptations to Temperature Stress* edited by Amarjit S. Basra

*Plant Viruses As Molecular Pathogens* by Jawaid A. Khan and Jeanne Dijkstra

*In Vitro Plant Breeding* by Acram Taji, Prakash P. Kumar, and Prakash Lakshmanan

*Crop Improvement: Challenges in the Twenty-First Century* edited by Manjit S. Kang

*Barley Science: Recent Advances from Molecular Biology to Agronomy of Yield and Quality* edited by Gustavo A. Slafer, José Luis Molina-Cano, Roxana Savin, José Luis Araus, and Ignacio Romagosa

*Tillage for Sustainable Cropping* by P. R. Gajri, V. K. Arora, and S. S. Prihar

*Bacterial Disease Resistance in Plants: Molecular Biology and Biotechnological Applications* by P. Vidhyasekaran

*Handbook of Formulas and Software for Plant Geneticists and Breeders* edited by Manjit S. Kang

*Postharvest Oxidative Stress in Horticultural Crops* edited by D. M. Hodges

*Encyclopedic Dictionary of Plant Breeding and Related Subjects* by Rolf H. G. Schlegel

*Handbook of Processes and Modeling in the Soil-Plant System* edited by D. K. Benbi and R. Nieder

*The Lowland Maya Area: Three Millennia at the Human-Wildland Interface* edited by A. Gómez-Pompa, M. F. Allen, S. Fedick, and J. J. Jiménez-Osornio

*Biodiversity and Pest Management in Agroecosystems, Second Edition* by Miguel A. Altieri and Clara I. Nicholls

*Plant-Derived Antimycotics: Current Trends and Future Prospects* edited by Mahendra Rai and Donatella Mares

*Concise Encyclopedia of Temperate Tree Fruit* edited by Tara Auxt Baugher and Suman Singha

*Landscape Agroecology* by Paul A Wojkowski

*Molecular Genetics and Breeding of Forest Trees* edited by Sandeep Kumar and Matthias Fladung

*Concise Encylcopedia of Plant Pathology* by P. Vidhyasekaran

*Testing of Genetically Modified Organisms in Foods* edited by Farid E. Ahmed

*Concise Encyclopedia of Bioresource Technology* edited by Ashok Pandey

*Agrometeorology: Principles and Applications of Climate Studies in Agriculture* by Aarpal S. Mavi and Graeme J. Tupper

# Concise Encyclopedia of Bioresource Technology

Ashok Pandey, PhD
Editor

Food Products Press®
The Haworth Reference Press
Imprints of The Haworth Press, Inc.
New York • London • Oxford

Published by

Food Products Press®, The Haworth Reference Press, imprints of The Haworth Press, Inc., 10 Alice Street, Binghamton, NY 13904-1580.

Cover design by Jennifer M. Gaska.

**Library of Congress Cataloging-in-Publication Data**

Concise encyclopedia of bioresource technology / Ashok Pandey, editor.
      p.  cm.
   ISBN 1-56022-980-2 (hard : alk. paper)
   1. Biotechnology—Encyclopedias. I. Pandey, Ashok.

   TP248.16.C65 2004
   660.6'03—dc21

                                                                                                         2003011486

# CONTENTS

# PART II: FOOD BIOTECHNOLOGY

# FIGURES

## Part I: Environmental Biotechnology

## Part II: Food Biotechnology

## Part III: Industrial Biotechnology

# TABLES

# ABOUT THE EDITOR

**Ashok Pandey, PhD,** is head of the biotechnology division of the Regional Research Laboratory, Council of Scientific and Industrial Research, in Trivandrum, India. He serves as Food and Health Chair of the International Society of Food, Environment, and Agriculture; president of biotech Research society of India; president and a life member of the Association of Microbiologists of India (Trivandrum Chapter); and is vice-chairman (Kerala) of the All India Biotech Association-SC. Dr. Pandey is a life member of the National Academy of Sciences, the Society of Biological Chemists, and the Association of Food Scientists and Technologists, and has received many national and international awards and fellowships, including a United Nations Educational, Scientific, and Cultural Organization (UNESCO) professorship in 2000 and a Raman Research Fellowship award from the Council of Scientific and Industrial Research in 1995. His research has been published in more than 300 resources.

# CONTRIBUTORS

**Wan Azlina Ahmad, PhD,** is Associate Professor, Department of Chemistry, Faculty of Science, Universiti Teknologi Malaysia. She has been actively involved in the area of metal-microbe interactions for the past seventeen years and is currently the technical advisor on biotechnology and biodiversity for the state of Johor.

**A. D. Agate, PhD,** is ex-Director, Agharkar Research Institute, Pune, India, and one of several experts for the United Nations Environment Program and the United Nations Development Program. He has worked in the United States and Australia for six years, published 120 papers, edited three books, and guided twenty-two students for MSc/PhD. His research interests include geo-microbiology and environmental microbiology.

**Eduardo Agosin, PhD,** is Professor of Biotechnology at the College of Engineering, Catholic University of Chile, Santiago. His main research interests are quantitative microbial physiology and process biotechnology. Recently, he has worked on the modelling, automation, and scale up of solid substrate cultivation, metabolic engineering of industrial microorganisms, and bioprocess optimization. He has published forty-eight papers in Institute of Scientific Information (ISI) journals and twenty book chapters.

**Cristóbal Noe Aguilar, PhD,** has been working on solid-state cultures (SSC) for the past five years. His research is focused on enzyme production profiles and metabolism for tannin-degrading enzymes and nutraceutical products. He participates in a food science team at the Universidad Autónoma de Coahuila, Mexico, working on production of enzymes for food industries and characterizing native fungal strains for its future use at industrial level.

**R. Ben Aim, PhD,** Institut National des Sciences Appliquées, Toulouse, France.

**Luis Jiménez Alcaide,** Departamento de Ingeniería Química, Universidad de Córdoba, Spain.

**D. Arulneyam, PhD,** Department of Chemical Engineering, Indian Institute of Technology, Madras, Chennai, India.

**Devender Attri** is a doctoral student, Department of Postharvest Technology, Dr. Y. S. Parmar University of Horticulture and Forestry, Nauni, Solan, India.

**Ufuk Bakir** has BS and PhD degrees in chemical engineering and a MS degree in food engineering. Currently, she is working as a faculty member in the Chemical Engineering Department of Middle East Technical University, Ankara, Turkey. Her research interests include production, downstream processing, and characterization of industrial enzymes, especially xylanases and polyphenol oxidases.

**Ibrahim M. Banat, PhD,** is a senior lecturer at the School of Biological and Environmental Sciences, University of Ulster, United Kingdom. He completed his PhD in 1982 and has since worked in both research and academia. To date, he has published more than 100 papers and review articles in international refereed journals in the areas of environmental microbiology, biotechnology, and food science.

**Rintu Banerjee, PhD,** is Professor in the Microbial Biotechnology Laboratory, Department of Agricultural and Food Engineering, Indian Institute of Technology, Kharagpur, India. Enzyme technology has been the area of her main interest. She has published a large number of papers in reputable international journals, has several patents to her credit, and has developed a process for commercial production of protease. She has been guest-editor for a special issue of *Applied Biochemistry and Biotechnology.*

**Javier Barrios-Gonzáles** earned his MSc from the University of Strathclyde, Glasgow, Scotland, and his PhD from the National University of Mexico. He has worked in the fermentations (antibiotics) industry. Since 1982 he has taught and conducted research in the Department of Biotechnology of the Metropolitan University in Mexico City. His research has focused on microbial secondary metabolite production.

**V. K. Batish, PhD,** is presently the Chairman of Dairy Microbiology Division and Officer In-Charge, Process Biotechnology Centre at National Dairy Research Institute, Karnal, India. He has twenty-seven years research and teaching experience and has published more than 100 research publications and a book titled *A Comprehensive Dairy Microbiology*.

**Argyro Becatorou, PhD,** Food Biotechnology Group, Department of Chemistry, University of Patras, Greece.

**Angus J. Beck, PhD,** Department of Agricultural Sciences, Imperial College at Wye, University of London, Wye, Ashford, Kent, United Kingdom.

**Shashi Bhushan** is a doctoral student, Department of Postharvest Technology, Dr. Y. S. Parmar University of Horticulture and Forestry, Nauni, Solan, India.

**Rodolfo Canet-Castello, PhD,** Instituto Valenciano de Investigaciones Agrarias (IVIA), Departamento de Recursos Naturales, Moncado, Valencia, Spain.

**K. Chandraraj** is a doctoral student, Department of Microbial Technology, Centre for Advanced Studies in Genomics, School of Biological Sciences, Madurai Kamaraj University, Madurai, India.

**Bhushan L. Chaudhari, PhD,** Department of Microbiology, School of Life Sciences, North Maharashtra University, Jalgaon, India.

**Sudhir B. Chincholkar, PhD,** is presently Professor and Director of the School of Life Sciences at the North Maharashtra University, Jalgaon, India. He was a doctoral fellow at the USSR Academy of Sciences, Russia, and UNESCO Fellow at the Louis Pasteur University, Strasbourg, France. He has worked in various capacities, such as organizer and chairman of scientific sessions and editorial board member at the national and international level.

**Lew Christov, PhD,** Sappi Biotechnology Laboratory, Forest Products Technology Centre University of the Free State, Bloemfontain, South Africa.

**Juan Carlos Contreras-Esquivel, PhD,** has been working on polysaccharides and polysaccharidases for the last nine years. His research is focused on pectin-degrading enzymes and their use in food manufacture. He is a member of a food biochemistry team at the Universidad Autónoma de Coahuila, Mexico, researching pectinases and pectin polymers extraction, production, characterization, and application.

**Edward Crabbe, PhD,** was awarded a scholarship from the Japanese Society for Promotion of Science, and completed his doctoral studies in the Laboratory of Microbiotechnology (Ishizaki Lab), Department of Food Science and Technology, Faculty of Agriculture, the Graduate School of Kyushu University, Japan. He earned his PhD in fermentation technology in 1999. He was also a postdoctoral research fellow at Tonen Central R&D Laboratory at Saitama, Japan, 1999-2002; and a postdoctoral research associate (volunteer) at Flickinger Laboratory, Department of Biochemistry, University of Minnesota, 2001-2002.

**Ofer Danai, PhD,** Research Scientist, Maigal Kiryat Shmono, Israel.

**Carlos G. Dosoretz, PhD,** is an Associate Professor of Environmental Engineering at the Technion-Israel Institute of Technology. He has a degree in chemical engineering from the National University of Litoral, Argentina, and received his PhD in Biotechnology from Tel Aviv University. He teaches and conducts research in the area of fungal related-environmental biotechnology.

**R. S. Dubey, PhD,** is currently a research scientist in the Department of Chemical Engineering and Technology at the Institute of Technology, Banaras Hindu University, Varanasi, India. His research interests are in the areas of corrosion, microbiologically influenced corrosion, and their control.

**Guillermo Ellenrieder, PhD,** is Full Professor at the National University of Salta and Researcher of the National Research Council (CONICET), Argentina. He has published about forty articles in technical journals in the areas of chemical and enzymatic kinetics and biocatalysis applied for the utilization of bioresources.

**Ernesto Favela-Torres, PhD,** has been working on solid-state fermentations (SSF) for the past fifteen years. His research is focused on fungal physiology and metabolism for extracellular enzymes by SSF. He participates in a multidisciplinary team at Universidad Autónoma Metropolitana, Mexico, working on reactor design and microbial processes characterization for enzymes production and polluted soil bioremediation.

**Francisco J. Fernández, PhD,** Departamento de Biotecnologia, Universidad Autónoma Metropolitana-Iztapalapa, Iztapalapa, Mexico.

**Mario Fernández-Fernández, PhD,** Department of Engineering Science, Universidad de Talca, Curicó, Chile.

**Febe Francis,** Master of Technology student, Biotechnology Division, Regional Research Laboratory (CSIR), Trivandrum, India.

**Sunita Grover, PhD,** Dairy Microbiology Division, National Dairy Research Institute, Karnal, India.

**P. Gunasekaran, PhD,** Department of Microbial Technology, Centre for Advanced Studies in Functional Genomics, School of Biological Sciences, Madurai Kamaraj University, Madurai, India.

**Yitzhak Hadar, PhD,** spent most of his academic career at the Faculty of Agriculture of the Hebrew University of Jerusalem, becoming professor of soil microbiology in 1995. He is presently Dean of the Faculty of Agriculture. His research interests include environmental quality, composting, biology of edible mushrooms, and suppression of soilborne plant pathogens.

**Matt Hardin, PhD,** has worked for a number of years in a variety of food and fermentation industries. After earning his doctorate on transport phenomena in rotating drum bioreactors, he moved to the University of Auckland where his research interests included enzyme immobilisation and food processing. He is currently investigating topics in food and bioprocessing at the University of Queensland.

**Alain Houde, PhD,** earned his doctorate in microbiology from the University of Sherbrooke (1990) and worked as postdoctoral fellow at Agriculture and Agri-Food Canada's Lennoxville research station and at University of Montreal's Faculty of Veterinary Medicine. He joined the Agriculture and Agri-Food Canada's Food Research and Development Centre as a research scientist in 1995. His research is aimed at developing technologies using leading-edge techniques in microbiology, enzymology, and molecular biology to ensure sensory quality and safety of food products.

**Matina Iconomopoulou, PhD,** Food Biotechnology Group, Department of Chemistry, University of Patras, Patras, Greece.

**Adolfo M. Iribarren, PhD,** is Full Professor at University of Quilmes (Buenos Aires, Argentina), Research Member of CONICET (National Research Council of Argentina), and head of the Nucleic Acid

Chemistry Lab at Instituto de Investigaciones en Ingenieria Genetica y Biologia Molecular and National University of Quilmes.

**Ayaaki Ishizaki, PhD,** is Emeritus Professor of Kyushu University and Former Professor for the Laboratory of Microbial Technology, Department of Bioscience and Biotechnology, Graduate School, Kyushu University; President of New Century Fermentation Research, Ltd. He won the Japan Society for Bioscience and Bioengineering Prize in 1999. He has worked in the areas of fermentation technology and microbial engineering, and has published 196 original papers.

**Jefri Jaapar** is a doctoral student, Department of Chemistry, Faculty of Science, Universiti Teknologi Malaysia, Skudai, Johor, Darul Takzim, Malaysia.

**Ronald S. Jackson, PhD,** developed Canada's first wine technology course and advised the Manitoba Liquor Control Commission on sensory evaluation. His works include *Wine Tasting* (2002), *Wine Science* (2000), *Conserve Water, Drink Wine* (1997), and several technical reviews. Although retired, he devotes most of his free time to writing. He was Adjunct Professor at Brock University, St. Catharines, Ontario, and Professor and Chair, Botany Department, Brandon University, Brandon, Manitoba.

**Veeriah Jegatheesan, PhD,** is a lecturer at the School of Engineering of James Cook University. His research interests are water and wastewater treatment, network and water quality modeling for drinking water distribution systems, application of membrane technologies for wastewater reuse, and waste minimization. He has published more than sixty refereed articles in encyclopedias, journals, and conference proceedings.

**Vinod K. Joshi, PhD,** is Associate Professor in the Department of Postharvest Technology, University of Horticulture and Forestry, Nauni, Solan, India. He has twenty-four years varied experience in fruit fermentation, processing, quality control, and waste utilization; authored more than 160 publications, including seven books; and guided MSc and PhD students. He is also a wine consultant.

**Ali Kademi, PhD,** earned his doctorate in oceanology from University of Mediterranée, Marseille, France, in 1997. He then joined Agriculture and Agri-Food Canada's Food Research and Development Centre as postdoctoral fellow. His goal is the development of processes involving lipase applications.

**Haresh Keharia, PhD,** Postgraduate Department of Biosciences, Sardar Patel University, Vallabh Vidyanagar, Anand Gujarat, India.

**Yiannis Kourkoutas, PhD,** is a postdoctoral research officer in the Department of Chemistry, University of Patras, Greece. He completed his doctorate in 2002 and he has since been working in the field of food and environmental biotechnology.

**Nadia Krieger,** Departamento de Química, Universidade Federal do Paraná, Paraná, Brazil.

**Chundakkadu Krishna, PhD,** is a senior scientist at Geo-Centers, Inc. She holds a doctorate in biotechnology from India and did postdoctoral research in biochemical engineering at Delft University of Technology, The Netherlands, University of Kentucky, and Scripps Institution of Oceanography. She has received grants from the United States Department of Agriculture (USDA), United Nations Education, Scientific, and Cultural Organization (UNESCO), and the Netherlands Organization for International Cooperation in Higher Education (NUFFIC).

**Pushpa R. Kulkarni,** Food and Fermentation Technology Department, Institute of Chemical Technology, University of Mumbai, Mumbai, India.

**V. Kumar, PhD,** is Associate Professor, Department of Chemical Engineering, Thapar Institute of Technology, Patiala, India. His research interests include modeling of membrane separation processes and environmental pollution control.

**Danielle Leblanc, PhD,** earned her master's degree in veterinary microbiology from the University of Montreal in 1982. After working in the poultry science department at Iowa State University, she joined Agriculture and Agri-Food Canada in 1987. Based at the Food Research and Development Centre in St-Hyacinthe, her work as research assistant involved the enzymatic production of fruity aroma compounds and the development of molecular methods for the detection of microorganisms in foods.

6 48332 34 32 3233533644333636436336656343

**Andrzej Leonowicz, PhD,** Department of Biochemistry, Marie Curie-Sklodowska University, Lublin, Poland.

**Dan Levanon, PhD,** is Chief Scientist of the Ministry of Agriculture, Israel. His research interests are applied and agricultural microbiology, including recycling of organic wastes, bioremediation of polluted soil and water, and cultivation of edible mushrooms. His teaching experience includes courses for the BSc degree and supervision of MSc and PhD students.

**Gérard Loiseau, PhD,** CIRAD-AMIS, Agri Food Program, Montpellier, France.

**Joseph M. Lopez-Real, PhD,** Department of Agricultural Sciences, Imperial College at Wye, University of London, Wye, Ashford, Kent, United Kingdom.

**Datta Madamwar, PhD,** is Professor and Head, Postgraduate Department of Biosciences, Sardar Patel University, Vallabh Vidyanagar, India. His main research interests are in the areas of microbial energy production, industrial liquid waste nanagement, and solid-state fermentation. He has received several awards and has published more than eighty-five research papers in international journals. He is a reviewer of several international journals.

**Armando Mejía, PhD,** Departamento de Biotecnologia, Universidad Autónoma Metropolitana-Iztapalapa, Iztapalapa, Mexico.

**P. K. Mishra, PhD,** is currently Lecturer, Department of Chemical Engineering and Technology, Institute of Technology, Banaras Hindu University, Varanasi, India. He works in the areas of heat transfer, separation processes, and water pollution control.

**David A. Mitchell, PhD,** earned his degree in biotechnology from the University of Queensland in Brisbane, Australia. He has worked in solid-state fermentation since 1984, focusing on the characterization of growth kinetics and the development of mathematical models as tools for use in the scale-up of bioreactors. He is currently at the biochemistry department of Universidade Federal do Paraná, Brazil.

**Ambat Mohandas, PhD,** is Dean of the Faculty of Environmental Studies, University of Science and Technology, Cochin, India. He is an environmental biologist with research interest in pollution toxicology. His current interest includes environmental biotechnology. He has authored more than 100 publications in national and international journals and edited three books.

**Didier Montet, PhD,** is a project manager at CIRAD in Montpellier (France). He has been involved in food sciences and biotechnology research for twenty years. He is an expert on Southeast Asia for the French Embassy at Bangkok and is Associate Professor at the Asian Institute of Technology (Thailand). He has managed many international projects and has published fifty-five papers. He holds seven patents and has presented more than fifty papers in international workshops.

**Murray Moo-Young, PhD,** Distinguished Professor Emeritus, Department of Chemical Engineering, University of Waterloo, Canada. He is Editor of *Biotechnology Advances.* To date, he has produced nine patents, eleven books, and 300 papers.

**K. Madhavan Nampoothiri, PhD,** earned his doctorate in 1997 from Cochin University of Science and Technology (CUSAT), Kochi, India. He is a scientist at the Biotechnology Division, Regional Research laboratory, Council of Scientific and Industrial Research (CSIR), Trivandrum, India. He has worked in Germany as an Alexander von Humboldt fellow and in the United Kingdom as postdoctoral fellow. He has published several papers and obtained several patents. His current interests are genomes, infectious diseases, and industrial enzymes.

**Bhushan S. Naphade, PhD,** Department of Microbiology, School of Life Sciences, North Maharashtra University, Jalgaon, India.

**James Chukwuma Ogbonna, PhD,** is currently Associate Professor, Institute of Applied Biochemistry, University of Tsukuba, Japan. His research interests include development of photobioreactors and photosynthetic cell cultivation systems, renewable energy production from starch and agricultural wastes, and cell immobilization technology.

**J. S. Pai, PhD,** is Professor and Head of Food and Fermentation Technology, Institute of Chemical Technology, University Mumbai, India. His areas of teaching and research include food processing, protein technology, fermentative enzyme preparation and application, and biochemical engineering. He is a consultant to the food and fermentation industry.

**G. H. Palmer, PhD,** is Professor of Grain Science, International Centre for Brewing and Distilling, Heriot-Watt University, Edinburgh, Scotland. Professor Palmer had published extensively on the structure of cereals and the mechanism of enzymatic modification of the endosperm of barley during malting.

**Maria Papagianni, PhD,** is a fermentation biotechnologist. Her research has been in the area of microbial metabolite overproduction and food biotechnology. She is currently a lecturer in the Department of Hygiene and Technology of Food of Animal Origin, School of Veterinary Medicine, Aristotle University of Thessaloniki, Greece.

**Ricardo Pérez-Correa, PhD,** Department of Chemical and Bioprocess Engineering, Pontificia Universidad Católica de Chile, Santiago, Chile.

**Suresh D. Pillai, PhD,** is Associate Professor and Texas Agricultural Experiment Station Faculty Fellow of Food Safety and Environmental Microbiology, Texas A&M University, College Station, Texas. He also serves as Associate Director of the Institute of Food Science and Engineering at Texas A&M University. His research interest is the fate, transport, and detection of microbial pathogens in natural and man-made ecosystems.

**Flávera C. Prado** is a doctoral student, Laboratory of Biotechnological Processes, Department of Chemical Engineering, Universidade Federal do Paraná, Curitiba, Brazil.

**Poonsuk Prasertsan, PhD,** Department of Industrial Biotechnology, Prince of Songkla University, Hat Yai, Thailand.

**S. Prasertsan, PhD,** Department of Mechanical Engineering, Prince of Songkla University, Hat Yai, Thailand.

**Costas Psarianos, PhD,** Food Biotechnology Group, Department of Chemistry, University of Patras, Greece.

**B. N. Rai, PhD,** is currently Lecturer in the Department of Chemical Engineering and Technology at the Institute of Technology, Banaras Hindu University, Varanasi, India. He obtained his BE degree from the University of Mysore, and his MTech and PhD degrees from Banaras Hindu University. He works in the areas of mass transfer and water pollution control.

**Sudip Kumar Rakshit, PhD,** Associate Professor, Processing Technology Program, Asian Institute of Technology, Klong Luang, Pathumthani, Thailand.

**L. Venkateswar Rao, PhD,** Professor, Department of Microbiology, Osmania University-Hyderabad, India.

**Eldon R. Rene, PhD,** Department of Chemical Engineering, Indian Institute of Technology, Madras, Chennai, India.

**Steven C. Ricke, PhD,** is an associate professor at Texas A&M University in the Department of Poultry Science, with joint appointments in the Department of Veterinary Pathobiology, Faculty of Food Science, and Faculty of Nutrition. His research is focused on foodborne *Salmonella* spp. ecology and environmental factors that influence prevalence in the gastrointestinal systems of food animals.

**Tim Robinson** is a doctoral student, School of Biomedical Sciences, University of Ulster, Coleraine, Northern Ireland, United Kingdom.

**Jerzy Rogalski, PhD,** Department of Biochemistry, Marie Curie-Sklodowska University, Lublin, Poland.

**Hwa-Won Ryu, PhD,** is Professor at Faculty of Applied Chemical Engineering, Chonnam National University, Gwangju, South Korea. His research fields include bioconversion of renewable feedstocks to chemicals, and the bioseparation/purification process. He is Editor, *Hwahak Konghak* (Korean Journal of Chemical Engineering) and Regional President, Korean Society for Biotechnology and Bioengineering.

**Abdulhameed Sabu, PhD,** earned his doctorate in 2000 from Cochin University of Science and Technology (CUSAT), Kochi, India. He is presently Fellow Scientist at the Regional Research Laboratory, Council of Scientific and Industrial Research (CSIR), Trivandrum. He has published many research papers in reputed journals and has worked at the Technical University of Budapest (Hungary) and the University of Georgia (United States). His current research interests include the production of industrial enzymes and bioactive molecules.

**Somesh Sharma** is a doctoral student, Department of Postharvest Technology, Dr. Y. S. Parmar University of Horticulture and Forestry, Nauni, Solan, India.

**Dalel Singh, PhD,** Department of Microbiology, Choudhary Charan Singh (CCS) Haryana Agricultural University, Hisar, India.

**Poonam Nigam Singh, PhD,** is a senior lecturer at the Universtity of Ulster, Nothern Ireland. She earned a Charted Biologist title from the Institute of Biology, London, and a Postgraduate Certificate in University Teaching (PgCUT), University of Ulster, Northern Ireland. She is a biotechnology expert (Associate Advisor) for the British Council, Manchester, UK, and a board member of four international biotechnology journals. She has published 145 papers and co-authored one book.

**Rekha S. Singhal** is a lecturer with the Department of Food and Fermentation Technology, Institute of Chemical Technology, University of Mumbai. Engaged with undergraduate teaching/postgraduate and doctoral research for the past twelve years in food science and technology, she is co-author of a book and several research/review publications and book chapters.

**Carlos Ricardo Soccol, PhD,** is Head of Process Biotechnology Laboratory in the Department of Chemical Engineering, Universidade Federal do Paraná, Curitiba, Brazil. He obtained his PhD degree from the University of Technology, Compiegne, France. Industrial biotechnology has been his prime area of research and development. He has published a number of papers, supervised several master's and PhD students, and is considered a pioneer in solid-state fermentation in Brazil. He is editor of *Brazilian Archives of Biology and Technology.*

**M. Sridhar, PhD,** Department of Microbiology, University College of Science, Osmania University, Hyderabad, India.

**T. Swaminathan, PhD,** is Chemical Engineer at the Indian Institute of Technology, Madras, India. He has extensive teaching, research, and industrial experience in environmental biotechnology, membrane technology, and hazardous waste management.

**Irene K. P. Tan, PhD,** is Associate Professor, University of Malaya, where she teaches biochemistry and biotechnology. Her research in polyhydroxyalkanoates includes using palm oil as a carbon source, and isolation of indigenous bacteria and degradation of polyhydroxyalkanotes in natural environments. She was a Fulbright Scholar at Michigan State University in 2002.

**Indu Shekhar Thakur, PhD,** Department of Environmental Sciences, College of Basic Sciences and Humanities, G. B. Pant University of Agriculture and Technology, Pantnagar, Uttaranchal, India.

**Araceli Tomasini, PhD,** Departamento de Biotecnologia, Universidad Autónoma Metropolitana-Iztapalapa, Iztapalapa, Mexico.

**James M. Totten, PhD,** is Laboratory Manager for the Food Safety and Environmental Microbiology Program, Department of Poultry Science and Institute of Food Science and Engineering, Texas A&M University, College Station, Texas.

**Anil Kumar Tripathi, PhD,** School of Biotechnology, Faculty of Science, Banaras Hindu University, Varanasi, India.

**Valentina Umrania, PhD,** Mathushri Virbaima Mahila Department of Microbiology, Science and Homescience College, Rajkot, India.

**S. N. Upadhyay, PhD,** has been a member of the faculty of Banaras Hindu University, Varanasi, India, since 1967. Presently he is Professor of Chemical Engineering at the Institute of Technology, Banaras Hindu University, Varanasi, India. His research interests include catalysis, transfer processes, and pollution control.

**Luciana P. S. Vandenberghe, PhD,** Faculdade de Ciências Biológicas e da Saúde, Universidade Tuiuti do Paraná, Curitiba, Brazil.

**Juan Carlos Villar, PhD,** Departamento de Celulosas, Instituto de Investigaciones Agrarias, Carretera de la Coruña, Madrid, Spain.

**C. Visvanathan, PhD,** is Professor, School of Environment, Resources and Development, Asian Institute of Technology (Thailand). He obtained his PhD in Chemical/Environmental Engineering from the Institute National Polytechnique, Toulouse, France. His research interests include solid-liquid separation technologies for water and wastewater treatment, waste auditing, and cleaner production. He has published more than seventy papers in international journals and conference presentations.

**Oscar F. von Meien, PhD,** Departamento de Engenharia Química, Universidade Federal do Paraná, Curitiba, Paraná, Brazil.

**Kishor S. Wani** is a doctoral student, Department of Microbiology, School of Life Sciences, North Maharashtra University, Jalgaon, India.

**Gary Ward, PhD,** MIGAL-Galilee Technology Center, South Industrial Zone, Kiryat Shmona, Israel.

**Young-Jung Wee** is a doctoral student, Faculty of Chemical Engineering, Chonnam National University, Gwangiu, South Korea.

**Zwi G. Weinberg, PhD,** earned his doctorate in food science at Cornell University in 1982 and is a researcher at the Volcani Center Israel. His areas of interest are ensiling fermentation, utilization of agricultural by-products for animal feeding, and probiotic effects of lactic acid bacteria for ruminants. He conducts both laboratory and field experiments in forage preservation and utilization of by-products.

**Jong-Sun Yun, PhD,** postdoctoral fellow, Faculty of Chemical Engineering, Chonnam National University, Gwangiu, South Korea.

**Mior Ahmad Kushairi Mohd Zahari** is a doctoral student, Chemistry Department, Faculty of Science, Universiti Teknologi Malaysia, Skudai, Johor Darul Takzim, Malaysia.

**Zainul Akmar Zakaria** is a doctoral student, Chemistry Department, Faculty of Science, Universiti Teknologi Malaysia, Skudai, Johor Darul Takzim, Malaysia.

**Nadine Zakhia,** CIRAD-AMIS, Agri Food Program, Montpellier, France.

# Foreword

Biotechnology deals with living systems, including plants, animals, and microbes. It derives its strength by harnessing biological processes that sustain life. Biotechnology incorporates any technique that uses living organisms, parts of organisms, enzymes, proteins, etc., which are either naturally occurring or are derived from such living systems. Such techniques can be used to create or modify products, improve plant or animal productivity, or develop microorganisms for special use. Emerging biotechnology uses recombinant DNA, cell fusion, embryo manipulation, etc.

Biotechnology has the potential to transform people's lives through its impact on agriculture, animal husbandry, health, environmental protection, material transformation, and other areas. Thanks to our increasingly deeper understanding of the intricate biochemical interactions at cellular and molecular levels, new paradigms in health care have emerged. We have moved from "preventive" medicine (vaccines) and "curative" medicine (antibiotics) to "predictive and corrective" medicine, thanks to the unravelling of the mystery of the human genome. We can not only identify the genes that cause a disease, but also correct the defects through gene therapy. Recent breakthroughs in stem-cell research have, for the first time, provided hope that we may be able to regenerate diseased organs, thus paving the way for "regenerative" medicine.

In the agricultural sector, new biotechnology promises to find a solution to the problem of producing more from less, e.g., more food from less arable land, less water per capita, and less polluting energy sources. This could be attained by creating high-yield, disease- and drought-resistant crops.

Biofuels will provide new sources of energy. Biopesticides will provide ecologically safe pest treatments. Biofertilizers will provide safer, ecologically friendly fertilizers. In place of chemical treatments, bioremediation can now convert hazardous wastes into useful products. With the confluence of information technology and biotechnology, bioinformatics is opening exciting new opportunities of unparalleled dimensions. Indeed, the twenty-first century is truly a biofuture.

In the context of overall importance of biotechnology, the *Concise Encyclopedia of Bioresource Technology* is a useful resource, providing the state of research findings on biotechnological innovations and their potential for commercial exploitation. It has promising contributors in the fields of environmental, food, and industrial biotechnology. I hope that readers will find this encyclopedia to be informative, interesting, and useful.

*R. A. Mashelkar*
*FRS*
*Director-General, CSIR*
*New Delhi, India*

# Preface

Bioresource technology incorporates a wide spectrum of science and technology, including engineering sciences. It involves applied biological sciences for investigating the present-day subjects of biosciences, mainly for the industrial, food, and environmental sectors. Principles from such scientific disciplines as biochemistry, bioprocess technology, chemical engineering, enzyme technology, food and fermentation technology, molecular biology, microbiology, microbial technology, etc., are strongly practiced by biotechnologists, chemical engineers, resource, energy, and conservation scientists, process technologists, applied microbiologists, farm and industrial waste technologists, etc., in applying bioresource technology for industrial, food, and environmental applications. Gradual emergence of new technologies for large-scale conversions of renewable raw materials of biological origin to various industrial and energy markets has further widened the scope of bioresource technology. Thus, it was a timely decision made by The Haworth Press, Inc. to publish this encyclopedia. We have made a conscious and careful effort to select and discuss vivid topics related with the subject, including biomass, bioenergy, biowastes, production technologies, microbial growth processes, enzymatic methods, agricultural and food processing residues, municipal wastes, environmental protection, bioremediation, recycling, aerobic methods, anaerobic digestion, etc.

Forty-four chapters are covered in this encyclopedia, describing the application of bioresource technology in three sectors—environmental biotechnology, food biotechnology, and industrial biotechnology.

Part I, Environmental Biotechnology, comprises 11 chapters and 19 articles. The first chapter provides a brief overview of recent advances in biological wastewater treatment. Two related chapters are included, one on reactors for wastewater treatment (biological reactors, membrane bioreactor, rotating biological contractors, trickling filters, and waste stabilization ponds) and another on treatment of industrial effluents (distillery effluent, pulp and paper mill effluent, removal of heavy metals from wastewater, tannery effluent, and textile and dye effluent). The development of such bioprocesses as biobeneficiation, biodegradation of polycyclic aromatic hydrocarbons, biofiltration, biological control of air pollution, biomethanogenesis, bioremediation, and microbiologically influenced corrosion are discussed in other chapters in this section.

Part II, Food Biotechnology, includes 14 chapters, two of which deal with fermented products, i.e., fermented vegetables products and fermented milk products. Food products production is an important area of food biotechnology, hence several chapters cover the production of food additives, food-grade yeast, mushrooms, nutraceuticals, prebiotics, probiotics, single-cell protein, vitamins, and xanthan gum. A chapter on kefir yeast technology provides information on recent technological developments in this area. The section also includes three chapters on biopolymer application, biotransformations of citrus flavone glycosides, and molecular methods for microbial detection and characterization for food safety.

The third and final part, Industrial Biotechnology, includes 19 chapters, incorporating 22 articles. The first chapter in this section, which covers alcoholic fermentation, describes bacterial alcoholic fermentation, fruit-based alcoholic beverages, fuel ethanol from renewable biomass resources, grape-based alcoholic beverages, malted barley, Scotch whiskey, beer, and thermotolerant and osmo-tolerant yeasts for alcoholic fermentation. Three chapters dealing with the production of alkaloids, aflatoxins and other secondary metabolites, amino acids, and antibiotics follow. A chapter on the application of agro-industrial residues for bioprocesses describes specific examples of industrial residues from the cassava industry, coffee industry, palm oil industry, and seafood industry. Two related chapters discuss pretreatment of lignocellulosic substrates and recycling of agricultural by-products and residues for animal feeding. Yet another related chapter discusses solid-state fermentation for the bioconversion of biomass, providing insight about the general aspects, design, engineering, and modeling of solid-state fermentation. Several chapters describe the production of commercially important microbial metabolites and products, such as aroma compounds, biodiesel, biofertilizers, biosurfactants, pigments, polyhydroxyalkanoates, and xylitol. The process of biopulping, outlined in yet another chapter, is significant because it is environmentally friendly and offers several advantages. Enzymes and organic acids from microbial sources have important industrial applications. Several therapeutic enzymes have found new applications to treat dreaded diseases such as cancer. Articles in this section describe the production and application of important enzymes, such as inulinase, laccase, lignin peroxidase, lipase, pectinase, phytase, proteases, xylanase, and L-glutaminase, and organic acids, such as citric acid, gallic acid, and lactic acid.

Thanks to the authors of the articles included herein for their cooperation in submitting manuscripts and revising them in a timely and friendly manner. The support extended by my wife, Sushama, and children, Rahul and Neha, cannot be expressed in words. Thanks to my students and colleagues,

Sumitra, Babitha, Roopesh, Sandhya, Binod, and Sumantha for their help in preparing the encyclopedia.Thanks to Bill Palmer, Vice-President and Publications Director, and Amarjit Basra of The Haworth Press for inviting me to prepare this encyclopedia. Thanks also to Amy Rentner, Rebecca Browne, and Christine Corey of The Haworth Press for their cooperation and friendly attitudes. Finally, thanks to Peg Marr and her team at The Haworth Press for their exceptional efforts in producing this encyclopedia.

# PART I:
# ENVIRONMENTAL BIOTECHNOLOGY

# Advances in Biological Wastewater Treatment

Veeriah Jegatheesan
C. Visvanathan
R. Ben Aim

## INTRODUCTION

Population increases since the nineteenth century have been accompanied by demand for more food products and housing. Thus the production of wastewater and the subsequent deterioration of environment due to wastewater being discharged into watercourses have been increasing since the 1800s. As a result, biological wastewater treatment emerged in the 1880s in the form of trickling filters, septic tanks, and sedimentation tanks. The activated sludge process for treating wastewater was introduced in the beginning of the twentieth century. In the 1960s, an increase in nitrogen in wastewater was attributed to the rapid increase in the production of $NH_3$ fertilizers, whereas an increase in phosphorous levels was credited to the increased production of detergents.

In biological wastewater treatment, microorganisms are utilized to treat wastewater because they can uptake organic matter and nutrients, such as nitrogen and phosphorus. Thus the organic and inorganic contaminants are removed from biologically treated wastewater to a great extent. The microorganisms that treat wastewater require carbon sources for their cell synthesis (growth) and energy sources for both cell synthesis and maintenance. The principal carbon sources used in cell synthesis are either carbon dioxide or organic substances that are present in wastewater, and the source for energy production is either light or chemical compounds that are present in wastewater. Thus microorganisms are classified according to the carbon and energy sources they use for their cell synthesis and maintenance (see Table I.1).

To adsorb substrates that are present in wastewater, microbial cells first secrete extracellular enzymes called *hydrolases*. These enzymes hydrolyze substrates that are present in the form of complex molecules (cellulose and

*3*

4 CONCISE ENCYCLOPEDIA OF BIORESOURCE TECHNOLOGY

TABLE I.1. Classification of microorganisms based on the type of energy and carbon sources they use in cell synthesis and maintenance

| Energy source | Carbon source | |
| | Carbon dioxide | Organic substances |
| --- | --- | --- |
| Light | Photoautotrophs<br>Higher plants, algae, photosynthetic bacteria | Photoheterotrophs<br>Purple and green bacteria |
| Chemical | Chemoautotrophs<br>Energy derived from reduced organic compounds such as $NH_3$, $NO_2^-$, $H_2$, reduced forms of sulphur ($H_2S$, S, $S_2O_3^{2-}$) or ferrous iron | Chemoheterotrophs<br>Carbon and energy usually derived from the metabolism of a single organic carbon |

Source: Adapted from Madican et al., 2000.

other polysaccharides, proteins, etc.) in wastewater to simple molecules (sugars, amino acids, fatty acids, etc.). The simple molecules then dialyze through the cell walls. Once entered inside the cells, the simple molecules are oxidized to produce energy. The intracellular enzymes, called *desmolases* or respiratory enzymes, act as catalysts to the oxidation-reduction reactions. Substrates, such as carbohydrates, proteins, fatty acids, methanol, etc., present in wastewater thus can act as electron donors in the oxidation-reduction reactions to produce energy and provide carbon for cell synthesis. Chemoheterotrophic microorganisms utilizing these substrates require electron acceptors such as oxygen, nitrate ($NO_3^-$), sulfate ($SO_4^{2-}$), or carbon dioxide ($CO_2$) for the oxidation process. For example, if the wastewater is under aerobic conditions, specific chemoheterotrophic microorganisms will utilize the oxygen (as an electron acceptor) and organic substances (as electron donors) present in wastewater to produce energy. Similarly, under anoxic conditions, the electron acceptor is nitrate ($NO_3^-$), and under anaerobic conditions it is either sulfate or carbon dioxide, which can oxidize organic substances (electron donors) present in wastewater. In addition, more energy is produced from oxidation-reduction reactions that occur under aerobic conditions. Therefore aerobic microorganisms have more energy for cell synthesis compared to anaerobic microorganisms. Thus the production of microbial mass (or sludge) is higher in aerobic and anoxic treatment processes than in anaerobic processes. These phenomena are brought into practice in biological wastewater treatment.

## CONVENTIONAL BIOLOGICAL WASTEWATER TREATMENT

In conventional biological treatment, microorganisms (mostly bacterial cultures) are used to uptake the dissolved organic matters from wastewater. This is carried out as secondary treatment. Prior to this process, the wastewater undergoes preliminary and primary treatments. In the preliminary treatment, large and floating objects are separated from the wastewater by screens. The wastewater is then pumped to a grit chamber where grits are allowed to settle out of the wastewater. In primary treatment, suspended solids and part of the organic matter are allowed to settle in primary sedimentation tanks. Thus the wastewater that enters the secondary treatment processes mainly contains dissolved organic matter, as well as nutrients such as nitrogen and phosphorus. The nutrients are present in both organic and inorganic forms.

The concentration of biodegradable organic matter in the wastewater is measured by biological oxygen demand (BOD). Samples of wastewater are aerated and seeded with microorganisms to observe the utilization of oxygen by the microorganisms in decomposing biologically degradable organic matters. Microbial activity in the samples is allowed to occur for five days, and the five-day biological oxygen demand ($BOD_5$) is computed. For example, a sample of municipal wastewater would contain organic matter with a $BOD_5$ content of 200 mg/l.

### *Aerobic Treatment*

In conventional secondary treatment, wastewater is treated aerobically. However, the bacterial biomass decomposing the organic matter in the wastewater can either be suspended in the wastewater or attached to a supporting medium. Although aeration tanks used for the activated sludge process allows suspended growth of bacterial biomass to occur in secondary treatment, tricking filters support attached growth of bacterial biomass. In the activated sludge process, wastewater is aerated in an aeration tank to allow suspended microbial growth to occur in the tank. Microorganisms present in the aeration tank utilize organic matter in the wastewater for their growth and cell maintenance. In tricking filters, wastewater is sprayed over a bed of crushed rocks. The bed is generally 1.8 m deep, and the bacterial growth occurs on the rock surface and forms a slime layer. As wastewater flows over the slime layer, the microorganisms in the slime layer absorb organic matter and dissolved oxygen for their growth.

Activated sludge plants operating with low organic matter (food) to microorganisms ratio (F:M) and long sludge ages may experience operational problems due to filamentous organisms causing bulking sludge. Installing a selector tank at the head of a bioreactor would reduce and control both reactions. The high F:M ratio within the selector tanks promotes the growth of floc-forming microorganisms while suppressing filamentous growth. Anoxic conditions within the selector tend to buffer nitrification, promote denitrification, and recover approximately 3.3 kg $CaCO_3$ per kg $NO_3^--N$ denitrified. The high oxygen demand in the anoxic zone is met by $NO_3^-$ instead of $O_2$ and up to 2.86 kg $O_2$ per kg $NO_3^-$ reduced can be recovered. A hydraulic retention time of 5 to 25 minutes for the selector tank is recommended to operate the activated sludge process satisfactorily.

The critical elements in designing the aeration system are:

1. sizing aeration tank volume and estimating the suitable sludge age to produce effluent that meets the required standards;
2. estimating oxygen demand requirements by the microorganisms;
3. estimating the motor power required to supply the required oxygen in the mixed liquor; and
4. estimating the excess sludge production.

Although the aerobic process is favored over the anaerobic process due to its stability, reliability, and better process understanding, the anaerobic process has some clear advantages as discussed in the next section.

### Anaerobic Treatment

Anaerobic treatment processes produce less sludge (0.1 to 0.2 kg biomass or sludge per kg BOD removed) compared to aerobic treatment processes (0.5 to 1.5 kg biomass per kg BOD removed). The methane gas produced in anaerobic processes can be used as an energy source. Further, the energy required for mixing in the anaerobic processes is less than the energy required for aeration in aerobic processes. However, slower reaction rates in anaerobic processes require larger treatment plants.

Anaerobic treatment is employed for wastewaters with high BOD and for sludge produced in conventional biological wastewater treatment plants that use either aeration basins (activated sludge process) or trickling filters. In an anaerobic treatment process, the organic matter in wastewater, such as cellulose, protein, and lipids, is first hydrolyzed by fermentative bacteria and converted to acetate, saturated fatty acids, organic acids, alcohols, $H_2$, $CO_2$, $NH_4^+$, and $S^{2-}$. The fatty acids are then converted to acetate, $H_2$, and $CO_2$ by hydrogen-producing *acetogenic* bacteria. Finally, methanogenic bacteria produce methane and $CO_2$ by utilizing acetate and hydrogen. Sulfate, sulfite, and nitrate are also reduced under anaerobic conditions by certain bacteria. Sulphur-reducing bacteria (SRB) are involved in sulfur reduction, and use sulfate or sulfite as electron acceptors and organic matters such as acetate and propionate as electron donors that produce sulfides. This causes the rotten egg smell from wastewater that is kept under anaerobic conditions for long periods. Denitrification is carried out by denitrifying bacteria (DB), which reduce nitrates to nitrogen gas using the organic matter in the wastewater.

## ADVANCED WASTEWATER TREATMENT

In order to achieve better effluent quality for different purposes, advanced wastewater treatment can be employed as detailed in Table I.2. All of the treatment technologies proposed in Table I.2 are generally followed by conventional secondary treatments. Subsequent discussions are limited to biological treatment of wastewaters that are employed to remove nutrients.

TABLE I.2. Purpose and processes involved in advanced wastewater treatment schemes

| Purpose of treatment | Target pollutants | Treatment technologies |
|---|---|---|
| Additional removal of suspended matters | BOD, COD[a], TOC[b], SS[c] | Rapid sand filtration, coagulation, ultra/membrane filtration |
| Additional removal of dissolved organics | DOC[d], TDS[e], Soluble BOD/COD | Activated carbon, coagulation, biological processes, ozonation |
| Prevention of eutrophication | Nitrogen | Ammonia stripping, ion exchange, break-point chlorination, denitrification |
| | Phosphorus | Bio-P removal, coagulation, adsorption, ion exchange, crystallization |
| Reuse | Soluble inorganics | Reverse-osmosis, filtration, electrodialysis, and ion exchange |
| | Virus, bacteria | Ozonation, UV radiation, chlorination |

[a]Chemical oxygen demand
[b]Total organic carbon
[c]Suspended solids
[d]Dissolved oxygen concentration
[e]Total dissolved solids

## NUTRIENTS IN WASTEWATER

Nitrogen and phosphorus are the major nutrients in wastewater. If treated wastewater is discharged into receiving water bodies with high levels of nitrogen and phosphorus, it can cause adverse effects on the aquatic environments. Algal growth in lakes and reservoirs is one example of the excessive presence of nitrogen and phosphorus. If excessive nitrogen and phosphorus cause eutrophication in a marine environment, e.g., in reefs, then the algal growth can shade the corals from sunlight that is essential for their growth. Excessive phosphorus can also weaken the coral skeleton and makes it more susceptible to storm damage. Although algal growth depends on the availability of organic carbon, nitrogen, and phosphorus in the water, one of them becomes a critical nutrient to trigger or limit algal bloom. It is unlikely that all three nutrients become limiting simultaneously, so in any given case, only one would be critical. Usually phosphorus is the limiting nutrient in freshwater and nitrogen is the limiting nutrient in seawater. Algal synthesis can be expressed by the following chemical equation, in order to identify the limiting nutrient as illustrated in this example:

$$106\ CO_2 + 16\ NO_3^- + HPO_4^{2-} + 122\ H_2O + 18\ H^+ \xrightarrow[\text{Trace elements}]{\text{Sunlight}} C_{106}H_{263}O_{110}N_{16}P\ \text{(algae)} + 138\ O_2 \quad (I.1)$$

For example, if a population of 10,000 produces 200 liters per person per day of wastewater that contains 15 mg/l $NO_3$–N and 5 mg/l $PO_4$–P, the preceeding chemical equation can be used to find the nutrient that limits the algal growth. The amounts of nitrogen and phosphorus required to produce 3,550 kg algae are 224 kg and 31 kg, respectively. However, the community discharges 30 kg nitrogen and 10 kg phosphorus per day. Therefore, algal production is limited by nitrogen to 475 kg per day. Of the four basic elements (nitrogen, phosphorus, carbon dioxide, and sunlight) that are involved in algal bloom, only nitrogen and phosphorus can be controlled to a certain extent.

### Biological Nitrogen Removal

Organic nitrogen present in the wastewater is hydrolyzed and converted to ammonia nitrogen ($NH_4^+$–N) under aerobic conditions, and $NH_4^+$–N is oxidized to nitrite-nitrogen ($NO_2^-$–N) by *Nitrosomonas* and thereafter to nitrate-nitrogen ($NO_3^-$–N) by *Nitrobacter*. The conversion of $NH_4^+$–N to $NO_3^-$–N is called *nitrification*. Under anaerobic conditions $NO_3^-$–N is reduced to nitrogen gas by denitrifying bacteria (denitrifiers), which is called *denitrification*. Although *Nitrosomonas* and *Nitrobacter* are autotrophs, the denitrifiers *(Pseudomonas)* are heterotrophs. Therefore, in order to remove nitrogen from wastewater by an activated sludge process, it is necessary to create both anaerobic as well as aerobic zones in the treatment process. Also, the sludge retention time, $\theta_c$, required in an activated sludge process for the removal of BOD and denitrification are different than that for nitrification. For example, $\theta_c$ required for organic removal is around two to five days (in the activated sludge process) and for denitrification is around one to five days. However, $\theta_c$ for nitrification is around 10 to 20 days. An arrangement similar to that shown in Figure I.1a will provide BOD reduction as well as nitrification and denitrification. In reality this is achieved by oxidation ditches, rotating biological contactors, and sequence batch reactors (SBR), which can provide aerobic, anoxic, and anaerobic zones (see Figure I.1b-d).

### Biological Phosphorus Removal

Discharge of nitrogen and/or phosphorus stimulates algal growth. The threshold concentration of phosphorus causing eutrophication in lakes is about 0.02 mg phosphorus per liter. Therefore, in most countries the effluent discharge limit for phosphorus is set as 0.2 to 1.0 mg/l. A phosphorus balance and a carbon (or $BOD_5$) balance performed for a secondary treatment process, as shown in Figure I.2, can be used to find ways to increase phosphorus removal. From the final expression shown in Figure I.2, the following can be considered to increase the removal of phosphorus:

1. Increased BOD removal (which is not practical)
2. Increased yield coefficient, $Y$ (which is difficult to control)
3. Increased phosphorus content, $P_X$, in the sludge

To increase $P_x$, an anaerobic zone at the influent end of the aeration basin should be introduced. This would induce a metabolic function in the microorganisms to release phosphorus in the anaerobic phase and to uptake phosphorus in the aerobic phase drastically. Organic matter (or BOD) will be uptaken anaerobically (Figure I.3a). Thus, phosphorus accumulation in the sludge is stimulated and sludge with high $P_x$ (3 to 10 percent) could be produced. Although the overall performance of biological phosphorus removal is satisfactory and inexpensive, accidental increase of effluent phosphorus concentration is unavoidable. However, phosphorus removal is enhanced when biological removal is combined with chemical removal (coagulation using alum, ferric chloride, or lime) as shown in Figure I.3b.

Removal of both nitrogen and phosphorus can be achieved by combining the treatment processes discussed previously. This process is termed *biological nutrient removal* (BNR). All aerobic, anoxic, and anaerobic processes are involved in the BNR of nitrogen and phosphorus.

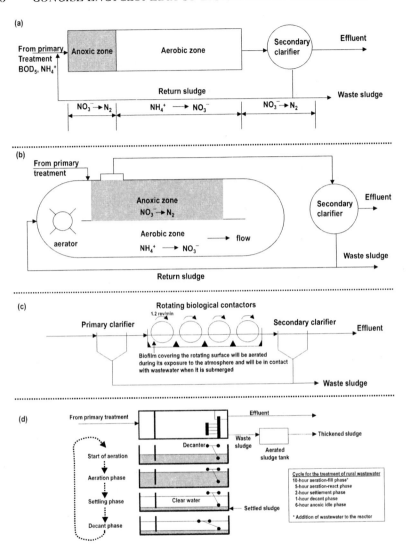

FIGURE I.1. (a) Nitrogen removal using anoxic and aerobic zones in a secondary treatment system; (b) oxidation ditch used for the removal of organic matters and nitrogen; (c) rotating biological contactors used for the removal of organic matters and nitrogen; (d) fill-and-draw method used in the sequencing batch reactor for the removal of organic matter and nitrogen. (*Source:* Adapted from Hammer, 1986.)

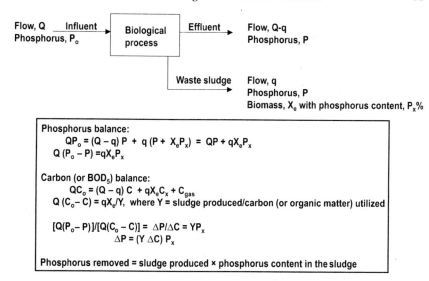

FIGURE I.2. Material balance for organic matters and phosphorus around a biological process unit

## *CONCLUSIONS*

Although application of biological wastewater treatment dates back to the late nineteenth century, advances in biological wastewater treatment are still being made due to the stringent regulations imposed by regulatory agencies on treated effluent quality. Advances in wastewater treatment encourage water reuse for both domestic and industrial purposes and contribute significantly to the efficient management of existing water resources for sustainable development. Advances made in biological wastewater treatment allow the removal of organic substances and nutrients such as nitrogen and phosphorus to a great extent, prevent eutrophication in receiving water bodies, and have increased the reuse of treated effluent significantly in most parts of the world.

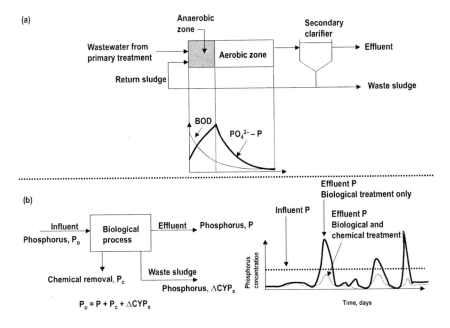

FIGURE I.3. (a) Phosphorus removal using anaerobic and aerobic zones in a secondary treatment system; (b) phosphorus removal by chemical and biological treatment

## SUGGESTED READINGS

Hammer MJ (1986). *Water and wastewater technology,* Second edition. New York: John Wiley & Sons.

Madigan MT, JM Martinko, and J Parker (2000). *Biology of microorganisms,* Ninth edition. Upper Saddle River, NJ: Prentice-Hall.

Mallevialle J, PE Odendaal, and MR Wiesner (eds.) (1996). *Water treatment membrane processes.* New York: McGraw-Hill, Inc.

Metcalf and Eddy Inc. (1991). *Wastewater engineering: Treatment, disposal and reuse.* New York: McGraw-Hill, Inc.

# Anaerobic Animal-Waste Environments: Salmonella *Species Ecology*

Steven C. Ricke

## INTRODUCTION

In addition to the chemical pollutant problems commonly identified with animal wastes are the wide variety of microorganisms originally harbored in the intestinal tracts that continue to survive in the waste materials. The microbial load originating from animal fecal material includes pathogenic bacteria, protozoa, and viruses that are capable of infecting humans. The overall focus in this review is on the study of potentially pathogenic *Salmonella* spp. in anaerobic waste streams. This is not just because of the implications regarding pathogenic *Salmonella* spp. for food safety—*Salmonella* spp. behavior may also serve as a model for understanding general bacterial pathogen persistence in animal agricultural environments. In addition, the pathological characteristics and genetics of salmonellae under these environmental conditions has largely been ignored. However, research techniques are available to assess the physiology of salmonellae in these settings and a more complete picture of *Salmonella* spp. is now feasible.

## SALMONELLA *PHYSIOLOGY IN THE ANAEROBIC WASTE ENVIRONMENT*

### Inhibitory Compounds

In general, populations of microorganisms are believed to be primarily controlled by substrate concentration and the presence of inhibitory compounds. Inhibitory compounds may range from antibacterial compounds, including antibiotics produced by indigenous soil organisms, to fermentation products produced by fermentative organisms in an anaerobic digester. Antibacterial compounds would be particularly important because animal waste-derived pathogens come in contact with anaerobic organisms in la-

*13*

goons and anaerobic digesters. Whether pathogens could become resistant to some of these compounds is possible but remains an unresolved issue. Typically, depending on how anaerobic the lagoon is, the concentration of the primary fermentation acids, acetate, propionate, and butyrate increases as the anaerobes become more established. Depending on the acidity of the effluent, exposure to these fermentation acids has the potential to limit the growth of pathogens and potentially kill them if exposure is for a long enough period of time, or other environmental stressors, such as higher temperatures, are also prevalent. In anaerobic digesters where anaerobic fermentation is more complete (as evidenced by the production of methane), inhibition of pathogens would probably also be considered more likely.

### Continuous Culture for Modeling Microbial Ecology

Microbial factors that influence competition in the environment depend on the respective organism(s) present and their ability to scavenge and grow on available nutrients. Which nutrients are consistently available versus nutrients that suddenly reach excessive amounts probably dictate when opportunistic pathogens are more likely to become prominent. A culture system that is specifically designed to examine growth physiology as a function of nutrient limitation is known as *continuous culture.* Continuous cultures are essentially flow systems in which the growth vessel containing the bacterial culture is set at a constant volume with inflow and outflow to which medium is added continuously via a mechanical pump. This results in a balanced inflow and outflow, and once such a system is in equilibrium, the bacterial cell number per unit substrate in the growth vessel is constant or at steady-state growth conditions. Most of the initial applications of continuous culture systems involved studies to understand fundamental physiological questions on single pure cultures of bacteria. However, such systems allow for the modeling of interactions among the trophic groups of bacteria and the influence of environmental factors relevant to the environment being studied. Interactions between pathogens and indigenous microbial consortia have generally been limited to interactions among intestinal bacteria and specific pathogens or cultivation of pure cultures of pathogens under anaerobic gastrointestinal incubation conditions.

### Culture Systems and Pathogen Survival

Applications more relevant to anaerobic environments have been almost exclusively focused on the development of semisolid systems that allow the flow of fluid through a reactor vessel designed to retain a solid phase. The goal of many of these studies has been to examine the efficiency of methane production as a function of the environmental restraints unique to the slow entry and turnover of solids, ambient temperatures, and high concentrations of potentially toxic fermentation intermediates. Addressing the issue of proliferation and survival of pathogens in waste streams will require combining the continuous culture methodology developed for slow-growing microbial consortia and adverse environmental conditions characteristic of waste-steam environments with a genetically constructed marker strain of the pathogen. This would allow for the ability to predict the sustainability of pathogens being emitted by confined food-animal operations, as well as the response of pathogens already present in the environment after exposure to the waste-stream effluents.

## SALMONELLA *PATHOGENICITY IN THE WASTE ENVIRONMENT*

### *Pathogenesis—General Concepts*

In the past, studies have been focused primarily on isolating and identifying *Salmonella* spp. in ecosystems. It is becoming increasingly clear that the detection of *Salmonella* spp. may only be the initial indication of a human health problem. Pathogens are distinguishable from nonpathogenic organisms because they can harm their animal or human host. This property is known as *virulence* and involves the invasion of the host by the pathogen and expression of toxicity. Only minimal direct studies have been conducted on pathogen virulence expression in animal waste streams. Most studies have focused on isolation and survival of specific pathogens or groups of pathogens. However, because pathogens may also have unusual tolerance against some environmental stresses, land application of land wastes may lead to extended survival of the pathogens.

### *Virulence Expression*

Much less is known about the relationship between virulence expression of *Salmonella* strains and its dissemination and persistence in the environment. It is known that *Salmonella* spp. have the ability to become more virulent under certain environmental conditions, such as low oxygen, high osmolarity, and slightly alkaline pH. With the knowledge gained from genetic studies, it is possible to develop methodology to investigate not only whether *Salmonella* spp. are present within anaerobic digester effluent, but also whether the genes associated with invasiveness and virulence are being expressed. Testing of effluent samples for effects on pathogen sustainability and virulence potential with in vitro assays using genetically constructed fusion strains of *Salmonella* spp. is based on previous research on understanding genetic regulation of virulence expression in salmonellae. Therefore an approach for environmental monitoring could be based on using operon fusions of these genes as indicators for quantifying environmental effects from effluent samples on virulence expression. Measured increases or decreases in the expression of these genes would be indicative of virulence potential for *Salmonella* spp. incubated under these environmental conditions. Some *Salmonella* spp. candidate genes have been identified. A *hilA* gene product possesses the ability to bind directly to a reporter gene and is also known to be vital in the invasion of epithelial cells and destruction of M cells. An *invF* gene also encodes an activator, and as with *hilA,* is required for the invasion of epithelial cells.

### Virulence and Anaerobic Waste Environments

Although anaerobic waste environments specifically have not been examined, virulence fusion strains have been used to determine the influence of the gastrointestinal conditions of chicken on invasion potential of *Salmonella* spp. The effects of short-chain fatty acids (SCFA) on the expression of *hilA* and *invF-lacZY* transcriptional fusions have been examined to determine the potential role of SCFA in the pathogenesis of *S. typhimurium.* Consequently, it is possible that SCFA may serve as an environmental signal that triggers the expression of invasion genes in the gastrointestinal tract. This would also suggest that waste-stream environments in which fermentation might occur, such as environments characteristic of deeply stacked litter, deep sediments in lagoons, or anaerobic digesters, could be conducive to enhanced virulence.

Similar scenarios could be hypothesized for these *Salmonella* species' virulence expression responses after *Salmonella* ssp. are excreted and exposed to the fluctuations of nutrients, inhibitory substances, pH, water activity, and other changes characteristic of physical and chemical conditions associated with anaerobic animal waste. Ideally, simulating environmental conditions comparable to anaerobic manure slurries with soil and water microcosms and using virulence fusion marker strains would contribute to a much more definitive picture on whether waste management systems influence the pattern of pathogenicity. In addition, the question would need to be answered on the transitory nature of virulence expression and whether the more virulent strains (compared to avirulent strains) would have survivability advantages.

## CONCLUSIONS

A long-term need exists to develop a comprehensive ecological picture of the contamination potential, growth, survival, and genetic stability of *Salmonella* spp in anaerobic animal-waste effluents. Understanding the ecology of *Salmonella* species' growth and survival in these environments will lead to explanations and possible preventative strategies for sudden blooms of nonindigenous pathogens that may occur during alterations in the dilution of inhibitory compounds present in lagoons. To address the issue of proliferation and survival of pathogens in anaerobic waste streams will require inoculating continuous culture systems that simulate slow-growing microbial consortia characteristic of these waste steam environments contaminated with *Salmonella* spp. This will allow for the ability to predict the physiological response of pathogens being emitted by confined food-animal operations, as well as the response of pathogens already present in the environment after exposure to the waste-stream effluents. A considerable amount is known about environmental signals that impact starvation and survivability, as well as the signals that control growth during and after invasion of human intestinal cells. Combining this body of knowledge with the information known regarding chemical and physical parameters of anaerobic lagoons and waste streams could lead to predictive models of components in waste disposal that have potential for controlling pathogen levels.

## SUGGESTED READINGS

Bajaj V, RL Lucas, C Hwang, and CA Lee (1996). Co-ordinate regulation of *Salmonella typhimurium* invasion genes by environmental and regulatory factors is mediated by control of *hilA* expression. *Mol. Microbiol.* 22:703-714.

Caldwell DE, GM Wolffaardt, DR Korber, and JR Lawrence (1997). Cultivation of microbial consortia and communities. In *Manual of environmental microbiology,* CJ Hurst, GR Knudsen, MJ McInerny, LD Stetzenbach, MV Walter (eds.). Washington, DC: American Society of Microbiology Press, pp. 79-90.

Lee CA (1994). Genetic approaches to understanding *Salmonella* pathogenicity. In *Molecular genetics of bacterial pathogenesis,* VL Miller, JB Kaper, DA Portnoy, RR Isberg (eds.). Washington, DC: American Society of Microbiology Press, pp. 215-234.

Mekalanos JJ (1992). Environmental signals controlling expression of virulence determinants in bacteria. *J. Bacteriol.* 174:1-7.

Pell AN (1997). Manure and microbes: Public and animal health problem? *J. Dairy Sci.* 80:2673-2681.

Pirt SJ (1975). *Principles of microbe and cell cultivation.* Oxford, UK: Blackwell Scientific Publications.

# Biobeneficiation

Valentina Umrania
A. D. Agate

## INTRODUCTION

Bioprocessing involves the use of microbial, plant, or animal cells for the production of chemical and biological compounds. It exploits a number of biological phenomena encompassing production of organic compounds, pharmaceuticals, and even precious metals. It has a higher energy efficiency and product specificity, and is more environmentally friendly. One of the bioprocessing technologies involves extraction of minerals, or bioleaching, in which microbes are used to leach out the metals from the minerals. In some natural ores, the bioprocessing technology achieves enrichment of the metal value instead of bioextracting the metal itself. This process is known as *biobeneficiation.*

To increase the efficacy of biobeneficiation, the search is on for bacterial strains that are better suited to large-scale operations, which tolerate high concentrations of metal values (increase in pulp density) and high temperatures, as reaction rates are faster at high temperature. Researchers are turning to heat-loving, thermophilic, acidophilic bacteria as agents for bioleaching and biobeneficiation. Ore-concentrate treatment with hyperthermophiles in a reactor has improved recovery rates and reduced operating costs.

## POSSIBLE MECHANISMS

For biobenefication, two modes of bacterial attack are postulated: an indirect and a direct mode.

In the indirect mode, the principle of bioleaching applies; i.e., $Fe^{+3}$ is the oxidant, whereas in the direct mode it is the $O_2$. In the indirect mode, the chief function of *Thiobacillus ferrooxidans,* the principal chemolithotrophic, bioleaching organism, is to generate ferric ion from ferrous ion in the bulk phase:

$$2Fe^{2+} + 0.5O_2 + 2H^+ \rightarrow Fe^{3+} + H_2O \qquad (I.2)$$

The ferric ion carries out the chemical oxidation of the metal sulfide (MS) in the ore and forms the divalent metal ion, where $M = Cu^{2+}$, $Zn^{2+}$, $Ni^{2+}$, etc., and elemental sulfur:

$$2Fe^{3+} + MS_2 \rightarrow M^{2+} + S_0 \qquad (I.3)$$

In addition to oxidizing $Fe^{2+}$, *T. ferrooxidans* and/or *T. thiooxidans*, which also participate in bioleaching processes, oxidize the $S_0$ formed in the chemical oxidation in reaction (I.3) to $H_2SO_4$:

$$S_0 + 1.5O_2 \rightarrow H_2O + H_2SO_4 \qquad (I.4)$$

Thus, if an ore such as gold arsenopyrite ($Au-As-FeS_2$) is exposed to bacterial action, the –As and –$FeS_2$ moiety could be oxidized by the mechanism in I.4, leaving the "Au" part unreacted. Gold is refractory by nature and is not affected by sulfuric acid formed in the process. Therefore, gold is said to be biobeneficiated.

In the direct method, low-grade ores are oxidized to their highest forms, for example, hausmanite, which contains $MnO$, $Mn_2O_3$, and $Mn_3O_4$, could be oxidized directly to pyrolusite, which contains $MnO_2$. The same holds true for those minerals, such as bauxite or excess silicate-containing minerals, in which either the excess iron present is directly reduced anaerobically by using iron-reducing bacteria to biobeneficiate bauxite ore or clay, or extra silicate is directly removed from low-grade ores using silicate degraders (biobeneficiation).

A third type of biobeneficiation mechanism postulated recently involves direct microbial attack on the metal and removes impurities. In the case of high phosphorus- (P) containing manganese ores, it was observed that the P is tightly bound (perhaps covalently) to Mn ions in the crystal lattice structure of the ore. The manganese-oxidizing bacteria, belonging to *Arthrobacter* sp. could change the Mn valence during oxidation, thereby, releasing the P moiety from the lattice. Here, the biobeneficiation indirectly attempted to get desired results (P impurity removed) without directly attacking the impurity by solubilization, etc., from the ores.

## THE PRACTICE

Some specific examples of biobeneficiation of refractory ores are given in this section.

### Gold Ores

Ore enrichment flotation is a widely adopted beneficiation technique to upgrade metal values in sulfide ores. Gold-bearing sulfides, containing pyrite, pyrrhotite, and arsenopyrite, are often floated to yield a gold-rich concentrate before leaching. Conditioning the finely ground ore with *T. ferrooxidans* prior to flotation would modify the surface properties of the sulfide minerals so as to enhance their recovery in the concentrate. Because the gold values in the refractory sulfide ores are locked up in the sulfides, microbially aided flotation can result in a gold-rich concentrate, eliminating the need for handling large tonnages of low-grade materials. The air/$CO_2$ ratio, in addition to the pulp density and temperature, plays a major role in determining the iron oxidation capability of *T. ferrooxidans*. In a recent study, results showed that with biooxidation the gold recovery from the concentrate increased from 45 percent to more than 85 percent. Similarly, the silver recovery increased from 62 to 97 percent. The study demonstrates that biobeneficiation can be used for treating refractory gold concentrates successfully.

The heterotrophic, anaerobic, sulfate-reducing organisms of the *Desulfovibrio* sp. aid in the production of flotation modifiers, such as several types of organic acids and surface active agents, that could be used as flotation reagents. By controlled bacterial conditioning, the desired mineral in an ore can be selectively enriched while the unwanted deleterious components are removed. Because many of the essential reagents are generated in situ by the organisms, microbially aided floatation offers the possibility of mineral beneficiation, even without the necessity of adding costly reagents from the outside. Ores such as molybdenum, chromite, and titanium can be upgraded (biobeneficiated) by such a process; i.e., the ore is enriched in metal value instead of the metal value being extracted out.

### Bauxite Ores

Scaling up of biobeneficiation of bauxite has been reported using a soil bacterium *Paenibacillus (Bacillus) polymyxa*. The bacterium can selectively remove calcium and iron impurities from low-grade bauxite (25 percent Al) for abrasive and refractory applications, respectively. Two types of operations were attempted in bioreactors: cascade and uncascade operation. In a cascade-leaching experiment with a pregrown culture, calcium removal was observed to occur solely by an indirect mechanism in an initial rapid phase lasting a few minutes, followed by a gradual phase comprising of a direct attack, as well as an indirect mechanism. An alternative mechanism of indirect leaching is proposed based on solubilization of accessible calcium in the culture metabolite, up to a saturation solubility limit. Some recent advances are likely to enable successful commercialization of bauxite biobeneficiation for application in refractories and ceramic industries.

## CONCLUSIONS

Although these processes have not been successfully commercialized, it is expected that the knowledge gained so far can be exploited to yield rich dividends.

## SUGGESTED READINGS

Agate AD (1996). Recent advances in microbial mining. *World J. Microbiol. Biotechnol.* 12:487-495.

Ehrlich HL (2001). Past, present, and future of biohydrometallurgy. *Hydrometallurgy* 59:127-134.

Ehrlich HL and CL Brierley (eds.) (1990). *Microbial mineral recovery.* New York: McGraw-Hill.

Karavaiko GI and SN Groudev (eds.) (1985). *Biogeotecnology of metals.* Moscow: Center for International Projects.

Rossi G (1990). *Biohydromtallurgy.* Hamburg, Germany: McGraw-Hill.

Vasan SS, J Modaka, and KA Natarajan (2001). Some recent advances in bioprocessing of bauxite. *Intl. J. Mineral Processing* 62:173-186.

# Biodegradation of Polycyclic Aromatic Hydrocarbons

Rodolfo Canet-Castello
Joseph M. Lopez-Real
Angus J. Beck

## *INTRODUCTION*

Polycyclic aromatic hydrocarbons (PAHs) are organic compounds comprising benzene rings arranged linearly, angularly, or in clusters. Naphthalene is the simplest form, with only two aromatic rings, but very recalcitrant forms comprising five or more rings also occur. Some PAHs are known or suspected to have carcinogenic and/or mutagenic effects. Their lipophilicity also implies a high risk of bioaccumulation in adipose tissue.

PAHs are released into the environment by motor emissions, volcanic activity, power and heat generation, petroleum spillage, and cigarette smoking. Thus they are ubiquitous in the environment, with soils and sediments being the major sinks. Although PAHs can be found in urban estuaries in concentrations as high as 100 mg/kg, with concomitant potential risks to the aquatic ecosystem, it can be argued that the issue of greatest concern is the large amount of land in Europe and North America, e.g., in the vicinity of manufactured gas plants, that has been contaminated by them. Environmental or human health risks aside, cleanup of such land has become a major priority for many landowners because many contaminated sites are located close to the center of cities, where land values are high and represent major capital assets. The typical size of such sites renders the use of common remediation procedures, such as soil incineration or removal, too expensive to be economically viable. Therefore, on-site bioremediation techniques are strongly encouraged by the environmental industry as an alternative, because costs derived from soil handling prior to treatment (excavation, storage) would be minimized and the pollutants ultimately removed through degradation.

The recalcitrant nature of many PAHs stems from their low water-solubility, soil-sorption kinetic constraints to their solubilization, and their resistance to microbial degradation by native soil microflora under "normal" environmental conditions. Many abiotic factors influence their degradation, such as temperature, redox conditions, pH, electron acceptors and, particularly, the overall toxicity of the medium, which may be very high in contaminated soils or sediments. All of these factors, combined with the presence, type, and number of PAH-degrading microorganisms, account for the final extent and rate of biodegradation that is possible.

Many types of PAH-degrading microorganisms exist including bacteria, fungi, and algae, which vary in their degradation effectiveness and methods depending on the aforementioned conditions. For example, many bacteria may use PAHs as their sole source of carbon and energy, whereas fungi and algae transform PAHs cometabolically to nontoxic or more readily degraded products. Furthermore, special groups of bacteria may degrade PAHs in different anaerobic conditions, playing the main role in the cleanup of materials where oxygen is so limited that aerobic decomposition is inhibited, such as in marine and lacustrine sediments. By contrast, fungi are mostly limited to soil, but the nonspecific nature of their exocellular degradation mechanisms, together with the characteristics of their typical mycelial growth, makes them the most promising organisms to be used for PAH-contaminated soil cleanup.

## *BIODEGRADATION OF PAHs BY AEROBIC BACTERIA*

Many aerobic bacteria, both Gram-positive and Gram-negative, are able to metabolize PAHs. They can be readily isolated in larger numbers from soils, natural waters, and surficial sediments where levels of these pollutants are high. Nevertheless, the highest molecular-weight PAHs that are mineralized as a sole source of carbon and energy by bacteria contain four benzene rings, such as chrysene and pyrene. One case of full liberalization of a five-ring form (benzo[$\alpha$]pyrene) by *Sphingomonas paucimobilis* has been documented, but additional sources of carbon and energy must be present (Table I.3).

The biochemical pathways and genes involved in the bacterial degradation of PAHs have been extensively investigated, and very detailed information about the simpler PAHs is already available. By contrast, knowledge of higher molecular-weight PAHs' degradation is still fragmentary and further investigation is needed. The initial steps of PAH degradation are catalyzed by multicomponent dioxygenases, which introduce two atoms of oxygen to form *cis*-hydrodiols. Ring cleavage enzymes oxidize PAHs to substrates,

TABLE I.3. Selected genera of PAH-degrading microorganisms

| Microorganism type | Genera |
|---|---|
| Aerobic bacteria | *Pseudomonas, Vibrio, Alcaligenes, Aeromonas, Bacillus, Staphylococcus* |
| Anaerobic bacteria | *Pseudomonaceae, Geobacteraceae* |
| Nonligninolytic fungi | *Cunninghamella, Aspergillus, Candida, Penicillium* |
| Ligninolytic fungi | *Phanerochaete, Bjerkandera, Pleurotus, Coriolus, Dichomitus, Phlebia, Lentinula* |
| Cyanobacteria | *Oscillatoria, Agmenellum, Anabaena, Nostoc* |
| Eucaryotic algae | *Selenastrum, Chlorella, Amphora, Navicula, Nitzschia* |

which finally enter the tricarboxylic acid cycle. Monooxygenases are also known to oxidize PAHs, however *trans*-dihydrodiols are formed instead.

Different laboratory techniques to screen and isolate PAH-degrading bacteria and benchmark their degradation potentials are available, from the simpler tests based on traditional culturing methods to the newer genetic and molecular biology analysis that was developed after the biochemical pathways of degradation were elucidated. For example, several methodologies are based on the detection of dioxygenase genes.

## BIODEGRADATION OF PAHs BY ANAEROBIC BACTERIA

Many environments exist where molecular oxygen is not readily available because its limited diffusion makes it scarce or because it is rapidly depleted by active aerobic microflora. Aerobic PAH degradation is therefore inhibited, because oxygen is not only an electron acceptor, but also it is incorporated into the aromatic ring as the first step of degradation. Although its importance has been acknowledged only very recently, and the mechanisms involved are not completely understood, anaerobic transformations may play a significant role in the removal of PAHs in oxygen-poor environments, such as deep soil, groundwater, or marine and lacustrine sediments.

When molecular oxygen is absent, the critical factor determining the metabolic diversity of microbial populations is redox potential. Accordingly, it is usual to distinguish between three categories of redox conditions leading to different pathways of PAH degradation (Figure I.4).

1. Nitrate-reducing conditions: Although evidence relating to rates and mechanisms is rather conflicting, nitrate-reducing conditions have been conclusively demonstrated in natural samples and pure cultures. Nitrate excess and a source of carbon are needed, and PAH removal

rates in denitrifying conditions seem to be similar to those of aerobic degradation when cell densities are similar.

2. Iron-reducing conditions: These are being actively investigated, but so far only naphthalene has been found to be degraded in Fe (III)-reducing conditions in some petroleum-contaminated aquifers.

3. Sulphate-reducing conditions: Degradation under these conditions was not demonstrated until the mid-1990s, but it may be one of the most important mechanisms of PAH removal from marine sediments, since sulphate reduction often serves as the predominant terminal electron-accepting process in the marine environment, given the depletion of oxygen, nitrate, and Fe (III) in marine sediments and the sulphate abundance in seawater. Although biochemical pathways for degradation are still largely unknown, carboxylation of PAHs has been shown as the initial reaction, leading to the formation of benzoate-like intermediates, which are activated by means of coenzyme A ligation and finally mineralized to $CO_2$ after ring reduction.

Although PAH degradation under methanogenic conditions is possible (since monoaromatic compounds have been found to be completely mineralized), no reports have been published to date.

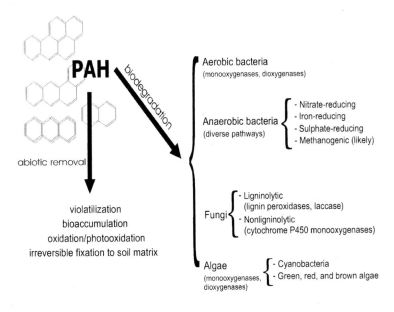

FIGURE I.4. Biodegradation of PAHs

## BIODEGRADATION OF PAHs BY FUNGI

Although bacterial degradation has been more rigorously investigated, fungi also have the capacity to degrade PAHs. Many nonligninolytic fungi are able to degrade PAHs ranging from naphthalene to benzo[α]pyrene. The white-rot fungi, which naturally degrade lignin to obtain the cellulose that is inside wood fiber, are reportedly also capable of degrading PAHs nonspecifically. Some of these fungi are originally from tropical areas and are therefore able to thrive at high temperatures, providing potential opportunities for high rates of biodegradation (Table I.3).

Lignin degradation is carried out through the action of extracellular enzymes, the best characterized of which are laccase, lignin peroxidases (LiP), and manganese peroxidases (MnP). According to their typical production patterns of extracellular ligninolytic enzymes, white-rot fungi may be divided into three main groups: (1) LiP-MnP, (2) MnP-laccase, and (3) LiP-laccase, although overlaps and exceptions occur. A fourth group may be the laccase-aryl alcohol oxidase group. Peroxidases use hydrogen peroxide to promote the one-electron oxidation of chemicals to form free radicals. Nevertheless, it seems that many compounds are not directly accessible to the heme group of peroxidases, and their direct oxidation cannot proceed. Some chemicals can, however, be oxidized to form free radicals by the peroxidases and subsequently oxidize those that cannot be oxidized directly by the enzyme. Veratryl alcohol appears to act as a peroxidase substrate, particularly when LiP is involved, although other chemicals and mechanisms are likely to occur as well.

PAH degradation by nonligninolytic fungi is carried out by another nonspecific enzyme group involving the cytochrome P-450 monooxygenases. One atom of molecular oxygen is introduced into the PAH molecule by means of cytochrome P-450, yielding an arene oxide that spontaneously isomerizes to form a phenol, which will be further modified to finally form a *trans*-dihydrodiol.

The environmental industry has become interested in fungal PAH degradation for its potential application in bioremediation. The release of enzymes to the extracellular medium allows the fungi to degrade large molecules that they would otherwise be unable to incorporate within the cell given their inability to transfer large molecules across cell walls. Furthermore, their nonspecific mode of enzyme action does not require preconditioning to individual pollutants and avoids the uptake of potentially toxic substances, improving the likelihood that the fungi will survive in contaminated environments. Furthermore, the induction of degradative enzymes is independent of the presence of pollutants, therefore degradation may continue even though degradative enzymes occur at low concentrations. Fungal growth and the subsequent production and release of enzymes may be promoted by adding cheap lignin-rich substrates such as cereal straw or corn cobs. The degradative action of fungal exoenzymes is also increased by micelle breakdown due to mechanical pressure by the elongating hyphae.

PAH-degrading fungi may be screened and benchmarked by different methodologies, most frequently the R-478 dye test. This red dye, with a chemical structure closely resembling that of the aromatic core of the lignin molecule, develops a yellow colour when attacked by ligninolytic enzymes. Potential PAH-degrading fungi may be distinguished by the appearance of yellow colonies in agar plates prepared with an N-limited basal medium and benchmarked by colorimetric methodologies when grown in a similar liquid medium.

## BIODEGRADATION OF PAHs BY ALGAE

Both prokaryotic (cyanobacteria) and eucaryotic (green, red, and brown) algae may degrade PAHs in photoautotrophic conditions. Although this happens in the surficial layer of wet soils, the major environmental significance of PAH transformation by algae lies on shallow aquatic environments, such as running waters, lakes, or coastal waters. PAH degradation by algae has not been investigated as rigorously as bacterial and fungal degradation, thus the enzymes and mechanisms involved are largely unknown. It seems, however, that degradation by cyanobacteria uses monooxygenase-catalyzed reactions more similar to those found in eucaryotic cells than those catalyzed by true bacteria, whereas some green algae uses dioxygenase-catalyzed reactions similar to those found in heterotrophic prokaryotes.

## CONCLUSIONS

Given the ubiquity of PAHs and the risks they pose to wildlife and human health, their biodegradation has many implications.

From an environmental perspective, natural disappearance is the only planetary-scale mechanism of pollutant clean up. Although photooxidation, chemical oxidation, and irreversible fixation to the soil matrix account for an important fraction of natural losses, biodegradation undoubtedly plays a significant role in the natural removal of PAHs from the environment.

For environmental engineering and related industries, PAH biodegradation has become a subject of extreme interest given the wide range of potential future applications, particularly in the field of contaminated soils.

However, it could be argued that only in situ techniques may be relevant, because when soil must be excavated before treatment, procedures based in chemical washing are most likely to be cheaper, easier and more predictable than any other biological process, whatever its efficiency may be. In fact, bacteria have been successfully used since the mid-1970s for in situ bioremediation of sites contaminated by oils, fuel, and related organic pollutants when the hydrogeological properties of the site were appropriate. However, this technique is not suitable for large areas contaminated by long-time atmospheric deposition of pollutants, a typical pattern of PAH contamination. White-rot fungi are nonetheless particularly promising for the remediation of this type of contaminated site for the reasons previously mentioned in the corresponding section of the text. Although biodegradation is currently in use for the remediation of contaminated sites, the future will bring enormous advances over the results already achieved, since there are many fields open to active investigation, including isolation and benchmarking of PAH-degrading microorganisms, use of combinations of microorganisms with complementary metabolic abilities *(consortia),* and genetic engineering based on the identification of genes involved in the biochemical pathways of degradation.

## SUGGESTED READINGS

Barr DP and SD Aust (1994). Mechanisms white rot fungi use to degrade pollutants. *Environmental Science and Technology* 28:78-87.
Canet R, JM Lopez-Real, and AJ Beck (1999). Overview of polycyclic aromatic hydrocarbon biodegradation by white-rot fungi. *Land Contamination and Reclamation* 7:191-197.
Cerniglia CE (1993). Biodegradation of polycyclic aromatic hydrocarbons. *Current Opinion in Biotechnology* 4:331-338.
Müncnerová D and J Augustin (1994). Fungal metabolism and detoxification of polycyclic aromatic hydrocarbons: A review. *Bioresource Technology* 48:97-106.

# Biofiltration

Eldon R. Rene
D. Arulneyam
T. Swaminathan

## INTRODUCTION

In general, air pollution control strategies and regulations worldwide have focused on the acute effects of air pollutants. In the past fifty years, however, advances in medical and environmental sciences have led to a better understanding of the deleterious chronic effects of air pollutants. Among these, the environmental and health effects of volatile organic compounds (VOCs) have led to increasingly stringent national and regional regulations. The low and variable contaminant concentration of VOCs in industrial emissions make traditional technologies such as absorption, incineration, catalytic combustion, and carbon adsorption costly, less effective, and wasteful in terms of energy consumption. When compared with conventional technologies, biological waste-gas treatment appears to be a cost-effective and environmentally sound approach, as it does not produce any secondary pollutants to the water, air, and soil environment. Two major processes, bioscrubbing and biofiltration are used to biologically treat air contaminants. The bioscrubbing process is primarily used for contaminants that are highly soluble in water. Contaminants are scrubbed from the waste gas in an absorption unit and then passed to a separate oxidation reactor employing a standard water treatment method to aerobically degrade the contaminant. The biofiltration process utilizes a biological microbial film fixed on a support matrix within a single process reactor, where the contaminants are both absorbed and adsorbed from the waste gas and converted to benign end products, such as carbon dioxide and water. The simplicity of the biofiltration process has resulted in its emergence as a more practical, cost-effective technology for the treatment of large volumes of air contaminated with low concentrations of biologically degradable compounds. The low operating cost is mainly due to the utilization of microbial oxidation at ambient conditions, rather than oxidation by thermal or chemical means. The main industries which apply biofiltration systems for waste-gas purification are the paint and dye industries, chemical pesticide industry, pharmaceutical industry, paper mills, refineries, sewage treatment, and solid-waste composting.

## HISTORY OF BIOFILTRATION

Although biological wastewater treatment systems have been in existence for more than a century, the advent of the biological waste-gas treatment system is of recent origin. Some of the earliest biofilter systems were constructed as open pits filled with porous soil. The contaminated gas stream was passed through the bed using a distribution system of perforated pipes at the base of the soil bed. The impetus for research on biofilters came in the 1960s. In the 1970s, propelled by stricter air quality standards, biofilters for odor and VOC control were successfully implemented in Germany and the Netherlands. During the 1980s and 1990s, biofiltration progressed rapidly in Europe and North America, as many of the VOCs were identified as toxic and hazardous and stricter regulations for their control came into force. In addition, advanced design techniques and mathematical modeling led to a transformation of biofiltration research from a black-box approach to a scientific and analytical method. Presently, biofiltration is a proven technology for VOC control, and is being adopted all over the world. Hundreds of biofilters are operating with areas between 1 and 3,000 $m^2$, treating gas volumes between 100 and 150,000 $m^3/h$. Recent research on biofilters has focused on understanding the mechanism of degradation and its pathway, mixed pollutant treatment, transient behavior, inhibition effects, and process modeling.

## PROCESS DESCRIPTION

Biofiltration utilizes a support media for microbial growth to remove odors and contaminants from air streams. A typical biofilter (Figure I.5) consists of a closed chamber containing contaminant-degrading microbes and absorbed moisture suspended in a filter medium. The solid support matrix (compost, peat moss, heather, bark, wood chips, coconut fibers, etc.) provides a high capacity for water uptake, has a long working life, and provides a low-pressure drop for the gases to pass through the media. The contaminated air is moistened by a humidifier and is pumped through a grid of perforated pipes into the filter bed. The contaminants in the air stream are absorbed and metabolized by the microbial flora. Treatment begins with the

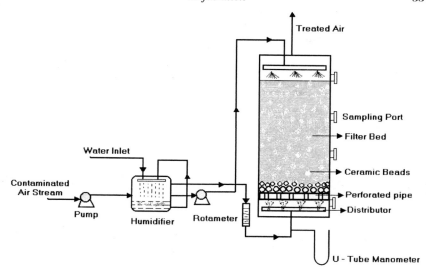

FIGURE I.5. Schematic representation of a conventional biofiltration unit

transfer of the contaminants from the air stream to the water phase. The treated air stream passes through an outlet at the top of the biofilter and into the atmosphere. Most biofilters that are in operation today can treat odors and VOCs effectively with efficiencies greater than 90 percent.

## *MECHANISM OF BIOFILTRATION*

Biofiltration is a two-phase process consisting of transfer of the compounds from the air phase to the water phase and oxidation of the absorbed compound by the microorganisms present in the filter. The dissolved contaminant is transported by diffusion and by advection in the air. When air flows around the particles, a continuous mass transfer occurs between the gas phase and the biofilm. As it passes through the filter bed, the contaminant will adsorb onto either the filter medium or the biomass itself. The rate of biodegradation of these contaminants is ultimately limited by the rate of mass transfer from the gas phase to the biofilm and by the rate of diffusion within the biomass. In general, the degradation rate for various chemicals depends on their chemical complexity. The lower the degradation rate, the longer the time required to degrade the target pollutant.

Biodegradation is influenced by a mixed microflora of degraders, competitors, and predators that are at least partially organized in a biofilm. This active biofilm supplies essential nutrients for biological activity, maintains an aqueous environment for microbial growth, acts as the air/water interface for mass transport, and receives various by-products of the reaction. A schematic of various phenomena involved within a biofilter is shown in Figure I.6.

## MICROBIAL ASPECTS OF BIOFILTRATION

Microbial activity transforms hazardous pollutants to harmless end products within a biofilter. The elimination of organic substrates by microorganisms results from the fact that these organisms use organic compounds as their sole energy (catabolism) and carbon source (anabolism). Knowledge of the species that are present, their densities, metabolic transformations, and interactions with the environment is fundamental to biofilter operation.

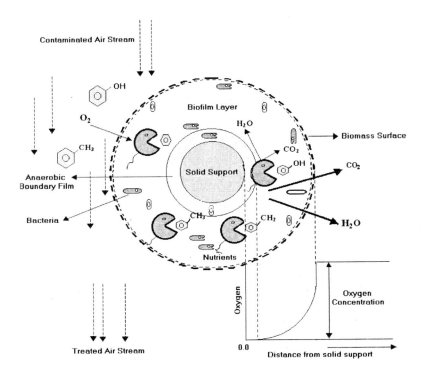

FIGURE I.6. Biofilm schematic representation

When presented with a new substrate, the organism must go through a series of biochemical changes in order to begin using the compound for food. However, the performance of a continuously operating biofilter is the ultimate result of a combined complex interaction between the microbial and physical phenomena, often described as the *macrokinetics* of the process. Some of the microbial phenomena are often represented in terms of the rate of substrate degradation, substrate inhibition, and diauxic growth. The physical phenomena include mass transport between the gas and liquid phase, mass transport to the organisms, and the average residence time of the mobile phases. The microkinetics of the degradation process are generally investigated and modeled with pure cultures of suspended microorganisms. However, in a biofilter, a heterogeneous, mixed culture of microorganisms is present rather than a monoculture. Some of the predominant microorganisms in biofilters treating specific volatile compounds are given in Table I.4.

## BIOFILTER MEDIA

The overall effectiveness of a biofilter is largely governed by the property and characteristics of the support medium. The moist filter medium provides physical and chemical conditions appropriate for the transfer of contaminants from the air to the liquid phase, and the biodegradation of the contaminants in the biofilm layer. Typical biofilter media material includes compost-based materials, plastic- or wood-product-based materials, coconut fibers, peat, and mixtures of all these. The media also serves as a nutrient source for the microbial population. In fact, some types of media lack proper nutrients and will require additional nutrients (e.g., nitrogen and

TABLE I.4. Frequently identified microorganisms in a biofilter

| Microorganism | Substrate |
|---|---|
| *Pseudomonas putida* BU2 | Butyraldehyde |
| Coryneformic bacterium AT | 2-Ethyl hexanol |
| *Pseudomonas* DI | Diethylamine |
| Bacillus TP1 | Thiophenol |
| *Alcaligenes* IN3 | Indole |
| *Pseudomonas* WR 1306 | Chlorobenzene |
| *Pseudomonas* GJ 60 | 1,2-Dichlorobenzene |
| *Methylobacterium* DM11 | Dichloromethane |
| *Mycobacterium* L1 | Vinyl chloride |
| *P. putida* and *P. fluorescens* | BTEX |

phosphorous) to sustain microbial life. All of these types of media have been successful to a great extent in degrading a wide variety of hazardous air pollutants (HAPs) in a biofilter.

Major considerations when determining the appropriate filter media include the following:

1. Ability to retain moisture to sustain biofilm layer
2. Large surface area, both for contaminant absorption and microbial growth
3. Ability to retain nutrients and supply them to microbes as required
4. Low resistance to air flow
5. Physical characteristics, such as physical stability and ease of handling

## CHARACTERISTICS OF AN "IDEAL" BIOFILTER

The following list, which may be considered an evaluation checklist, contains the most pertinent characteristics of a good biofilter. In practice, however, it may be necessary to trade one feature for another.

- *Compactness and portability:* The biofilter should occupy as little space as possible. It should also be modular to offer flexibility in design and operation. The biofilter should be easily moveable to facilitate changes in operation.
- *Inert construction materials:* All materials used in the biofilters should be noncorrosive, UV-resistant, resistant to rot or decay, and generally impervious to chemical attack. In general, marine-grade construction materials are required for reasonable working lifetimes.
- *Low operational cost:* The biofilter should have self-cleaning capacity and minimum energy requirements. The main energy requirement should lie in the operation of pumps.
- *Safety and Reliability:* Ideally, a biofilter should have no moving parts that could fail at an inopportune time. If the biofilter does have moving parts, they should be rugged and designed for a continuous operating life of several years.
- *Monitorabilty:* It should be easy to observe the operation of the biofilter to ensure that it is operating correctly.
- *Controllability:* It should be easy to change operating variables to ensure optimum performance.

## PERFORMANCE PARAMETERS

Critical biofilter performance parameters include the following.

- *Constituents and concentrations:* Analysis of chemical constituents and their concentrations are required to determine the effectiveness of biofiltration. Hydrophilic compounds in low concentrations (<1000 ppm) are treated best. Chemicals such as chlorinated compounds are degraded at low rates, which require units to be oversized.
- *Residence time:* Residence time represents the contact time between the microbes and the contaminated air stream, and is defined by the ratio of void volume to volumetric flow rate. Longer residence times produce higher efficiencies, but design constraints require minimum residence time to allow the biofilter to accommodate larger flow rates. For most biofilters, residence time ranges between 30 to 60 seconds.
- *Humidity:* The humidity of the gas stream is important for maintaining the moisture content of the biofilter media. Gas streams introduced to the biofiltration system are usually pumped through a humidifier prior to entering the biofilter.
- *pH control:* The by-products of microbial degradation are mostly organic acids. In order to maintain the pH of the biofilter media, neutral buffering material may be added.
- *Pressure drop:* Pressure drop across the biofilter should be minimized, since an increase in pressure drop requires more pumping energy and can result in air channelling through the media. Pressure drop is directly related to the moisture content in the media and the media pore size. Increased moisture and decreased pore size result in increased pressure drop. Consequently, media filter selection and watering is critical to biofilter performance and energy efficiency. For a typical biofilter, pressure drops range between 0.2 and 1.0 cm (water gauge).
- *Operation and maintenance:* The operation and maintenance of the biofiltration system would require regular inspection during its start-up/initiation. However, after acclimation, the system may operate with very little maintenance.

Typical operational parameters for a conventional biofilter are

Superficial gas velocity = 10 to 100 $m^3/m^2$ per hour
Gas contact time = 30 to 60 seconds
Biofilter height = 0.5 to 1.5 m
Biofilter area = 1 to 3000 $m^2$

Bed void volume = 50 percent
Pressure drop = 0.2 to 1.0 cm (water gauge)
Operating temperature = 15 to 40°C
Relative humidity of inlet air = >95 percent
pH of the filter media = 6.5 to 7.5
Water content = 25 to 70 percent (w/w)
Typical removal efficiencies = 60 to 100 percent (usually >90 percent)

## ADVANTAGES AND DISADVANTAGES OF BIOFILTRATION

### Advantages

- The main advantages of using biofiltration over other conventional control methods are low capital costs, low operating costs, less chemical usage, and low energy requirements.
- Biofiltration units can be designed to physically fit into any industrial setting. A biofiltration unit can be designed in any shape and size, including an open field with the piping and delivery system underground. In addition, biofilters can be designed with stacked beds to minimize space requirements, and multiple units can be run in parallel.
- Biofiltration is versatile enough to treat odors, toxic compounds, and VOCs. The treatment efficiencies are above 90 percent for low concentrations of contaminants (<1000 ppm).
- Different media, microbes, and operating conditions can be used to tailor a biofilter system for many emission points.

### Disadvantages

- Biofiltration cannot successfully treat some organic compounds, particularly those that have low adsorption or degradation rates. This is especially true for chlorinated VOCs.
- Contaminant sources with high chemical emissions would require large biofilter units or open areas to install a biofiltration system.
- Sources with emissions that fluctuate severely or produce large spikes can be detrimental to the biofilters' microbial population and overall performance.
- Acclimation periods for the microbial population may take weeks or even months, especially for VOC treatment.

## COMMERCIAL APPLICATION OF BIOFILTERS

Commercial applications to date have included the following: the chemical and petrochemical industry, oil and gas industry, synthetic resins, paints and inks, pharmaceutical industry, wastewater treatment, soil and groundwater remediation, sewage treatment, slaughter houses, gelatin and glue plants, agricultural and meat-processing industries, tobacco, cocoa, and sugar industries, and flavor and fragrance industries.

## CONCLUSIONS

Biofiltration is proving to be an attractive way of eliminating waste-gas contaminants, such as odors and VOCs. Although the biological mechanisms involved in water, gas, or soil treatment are similar, the gaseous state of the pollutant to be treated in waste gas biotreatment forces a new engineering conception, and has led to new applications in the field of environmental biotechnology. This new engineering concept introduced by biological gas treatment offers challenges for the development of novel bioreactors, new support materials, and scale up to large systems. Further, the application of genetic engineering also is a potential possibility for the development of more effective biofiltration.

## SUGGESTED READINGS

Alley ER, Jr. (ed.) (1998). *Biofiltration of gaseous compounds: Air quality handbook.* New York: McGraw-Hill.

Devinny JS, MA Deshusses, and TS Webster (1999). *Biofiltration for air pollution control.* New York: CRC Lewis.

Ottengraf SPP (1986). Exhaust gas purification. In *Biotechnology,* volume 8, HJ Rehm, G Reed (eds.). Weinheim, Germany: VCH Verlagsgesellschaft.

# Biological Control of Air Pollution

S. N. Upadhyay
V. Kumar

## INTRODUCTION

Removing water-soluble and biodegradable volatile organic compounds (VOCs), hazardous air pollutants (HAPs), and odorous organic compounds present in air emissions at low-to-moderate concentrations, through microbial processes has been a useful concept of air pollution control for decades. However, only recently has this concept been applied to large-scale practice. Three types of control devices can be used for this purpose: (1) biofilters, (2) biotrickling filters, and (3) bioscrubbers.

Biofilters and biotrickling filters, the more commonly used units for controlling VOCs, are similar to the packed-bed and trickling-filter bioreactors used for wastewater treatment. In biofilters and biotrickling filters, wet microbial films are supported on a bed of porous media (compost, peat, soil, ceramic or plastic packings) in a packed-bed bioreactor. The polluted gas is allowed to pass through this biologically active bed, where air pollutants are dissolved into the aqueous phase and microorganisms present in the wet biofilm degrade the pollutants. In biotrickling filters, liquid-phase-containing nutrients trickle downward through the porous media, whereas in biofilters they are stationary. Bioscrubbers, on the other hand, are essentially two-stage units. Absorption of organic pollutants takes place mostly in the first stage, which may be a packed bed, spray tower, or a bubble-column absorber, whereas biodegradation takes place in the second stage, which occurs in a suspended-cell type of bioreactor that is similar to the activated sludge units used for wastewater treatment.

Oxygen present in the contaminated air helps in maintaining aerobic conditions within the biofilter unit. Nitrogen, phosphorous, and other nutrients are required to sustain microbial growth. Usually an aqueous solution is sprayed onto the biofilter to supply both moisture and nutrients. Further, the contaminated air stream may have to be humidified prior to its application into the biofilter. Water-evaporation losses are counterbalanced by the humidification and aqueous nutrient spray. A typical biofilter system includes an air-distribution system, a bed of filter media, a blower, a humidifier, and a nutrient supply system.

Biofilters have been in use for odor control at wastewater treatment plants, composting plants, slaughter houses, rendering plants, and confined animal facilities since the 1950s. Biofilters and biotrickling filters have been used for controlling VOCs only since the early 1980s. Industries using biological air-pollution control techniques include adhesive plants, breweries and bakeries, chemical plants, chemical storage, domestic and industrial wastewater treatment plants, electronic units, film-coating plants, fish rendering, flavor- and fragrance-producing units, iron foundries, pet-food manufacturing units, petroleum refineries, plastic manufacturing units, printing units, pulp and paper mills, soil and ground-water remediation operations, tobacco-processing units, textile mills, and waste-oil recycling units. Compounds such as ammonia, hydrogen sulphide, methylmercaptan, dimethyl sulphides and disulphides, carbon disulphide, ethenol, methenol, butanol, formaldehyde, phenol, acetaldehyde, acetone, methyl ethyl ketone, methyl isobutyl ketone, ethyl acetate, gasoline and jet-fuel vapors, benzene, toluene, xylenes, and styrene have been successfully removed. A properly designed and well-maintained system may have a removal efficiency as high as 95 percent.

Low operating cost, absence of residuals and by-products, and extremely low $CO_2$ and $NO_x$ emissions compared to thermal processes are the major advantages of biological air-pollution control processes. Due to complete mineralization of pollutants, compounds produced in the system include $CO_2$, $H_2O$, and inorganic ions such as $Cl^-$, $SO_4^-$, and $NO_3^-$, unlike other air-pollution control systems, which produce spent adsorbents and chemical sludge. Biological air-pollution control processes operate at ambient pressure and temperature, thus requiring little power. In addition, low-pressure drops across the biofilter bed (~10 cm of $H_2O$/meter of packed-bed depth) requires less power for the blower. Some pumping is required for humidification, water addition, and dosing of nutrients and buffer. Filter media may require periodic replacement.

The major disadvantages of biological control systems are their moderate to high capital costs and relatively high area requirements. Further, only biologically assimilable gaseous pollutants can be controlled by this technique.

## *PROCESS DESCRIPTION*

The gaseous pollutants present in the emission must be biodegradable under aerobic conditions. Heterotrophic microorganisms use volatile organic compounds as carbon and energy sources, and $H_2S$ and $NH_3$ are used as electron donors by chemolithotrophic metabolism. Molecules having amine, methoxy, sulfonate, and nitro groups, highly halogenated molecules, meta position substituted benzene, ether linkages, and branched carbon chains act like organic refractories and require long residence times to biodegrade.

For biological treatment, it is essential that VOCs get dissolved into the aqueous phase. The extent of dissolution is expressed in terms of Henry's law (H), the ratio of the gas and liquid phase concentrations ($C_G/C_L$). Pollutants with large Henry's law constants (e.g., hexane, H = 74 at m/l per mole) are difficult to degrade and require longer residence times than those with small Henry's law constant (e.g., ethanol, H = $2.6 \times 10^{-4}$ at m/l per mole). The recommended VOC loading rates for biological control systems are less than 100–150 $g/m^3$ per h. At high VOC loading rates, excessive microbial growth results in clogging of the filter, causing high-pressure drops and uneven gas distribution. Some constituents of VOCs may be toxic and inhibitory to microbial growth and biodegradation.

Common microorganisms in biofilters are mesophils with an optimum growth temperature of 25 to 35°C. In cold climates, inlet gases may need to be heated and reactors insulated for stable operation throughout the year. On the other hand very hot gases need to be cooled prior to treatment. Thermophilic species (50 to 65°C) have been tried in some cases. In some situations, complete mineralization of biodegradable organics may not occur. However, the biocontrol may be able to reduce odor or toxicity. Inorganic acids (HCl, $H_2SO_4$) or organic acids may also form and reduce the pH to as low as 1. Use of buffers on the packing media or in the liquid phase can help in maintaining a relatively neutral pH.

An acclimation period of several days to weeks may be required for the microbes to reach maximum biodegradation efficiency. The acclimation period can be shortened by using acclimated active sludge from an operating activated-sludge treatment plant. Reacclimation may be required when the plant had been nonoperational for several days and no air flow was maintained through the unit. Under frequent shut-down and transient operating conditions, the microbial population adapts to the conditions and reacclimation periods are short. Shock loadings and toxic compounds should be avoided.

During biodegradation of mixed organic compounds, more readily biodegradable compounds are removed prior to less biodegradable ones. Thus a deeper bed is required to facilitate degradation of more biodegradable compounds near the inlet and less biodegradable ones deeper in the bed. Prediction of performance for mixture of compounds, however, is difficult and pilot tests may be required. Gaseous emissions loaded with particulate matter and grease (e.g., those from wood products and bakeries) clog the biofilters and lead to excessive pressure drops. A pretreatment unit comprising wet collectors or an electrostatic precipitator is used before the biological unit.

In a biotrickling filter a recirculating nutrient/buffer solution is continuously or intermittently trickled down over the porous medium. A portion of the recirculating solution is discarded continuously or intermittently and automated control of pH/nutrient concentration is possible. Biotrickling filters are used at higher inlet-loading rates [100–150 $g/(m^3/h)$] and/or where continuous pH control is required.

### Filter Media

A good filter media should have a high pore volume ($\geq$80 percent), near-neutral pH (7 to 8), appropriate particle-size distribution ($d_{60} > 40$mm) and high organic-matter content ($\geq$55 percent). Compost, soil, or peat, mixed with a bulking agent, are commonly used as the porous packing media in biofilters. Nutrients and pH buffers are added to improve the performance. Such a medium serves both as a support and as source of nutrients for the microorganisms. Biotrickling filters use porous ceramic pellets, granular activated carbon, plastic or fibrous packing, or polyurethane foam porous support media. The nature of filter media has substantial influence on the cost of construction and operation of a biofilter. The pressure drop across the bed and its compaction during operation, as well as excessive microbial growth, lead to an increase in power consumption.

### Media for Biofilters

Compost-filled biofilters are used to treat low-mass loadings of VOCs and odorous compounds [<40–50 $g/(m^3/h)$], and for processes in which pH control is not important. Compost beds have a high surface area for microbial growth attachment and adsorption of pollutants, low pressure drop, high nutrient composition, high microbial diversity, good water-retaining capacity, and low capital and running costs that have proved extremely effective.

Properties of different types of compost, however, vary widely and affect biofilter performance. Municipal solid waste, industrial sludge, garden wastes, animal manures, and food and agricultural residues can be used to produce compost. Compost stability is a key parameter affecting long-term performance of the biofilter. Degradation of bioavailable carbon in unstable compost may result in decrease in bed volume and cause compaction. Further, heat released during biooxidation of compost makes it dry, causing subsequent acidification and proliferation of fungi. A stable compost is characterized by oxygen uptake rates of 200 mg $O_2$/kg total solids per ha or below.

Peat has an extremely large surface area, allows relatively free flow of air, holds moisture well and provides an excellent support for the growth of microbial population. In particular, sphagnum peat supports a microbial population with a high fraction of fungal species that are highly effective in breaking down certain air pollutants. It is, however, a hydrophobic and acidic material that has a low nutrient content and low indigenous microbial population. Moisture control in pit beds is difficult and requires supplemental nutrients and buffering.

Soil is a cheap media that has a high indigenous microbial population. It is more structurally stable than compost or peat and permits use of deeper beds. Its hydrophilic nature permits ease of moisture control. Low degradative capacity and low air permeability requires larger beds than compost-based units. It is suitable for large land areas.

## Bulking Agents

A coarse granular material is commonly added to the biofilter media to prevent compaction, promote drainage, reduce pressure drops, and improve permeability. A large fraction of coarse material increases the permeability but reduces the surface area for microbial growth and attachment and adsorption of pollutants. Further, bulking agents have lower nutrient contents than compost material. Wood chips and wood bark (2 to 6 cm in size), polystyrene beads, pearlite, vermiculite, and shredded tires have also been used as bulking agents. The fraction of bulking agent could be as low as 20 percent or as high as 80 percent, the average being 50 to 60 percent.

## Media for Biotrickling Filters

Pall rings, polyurethane foam cubes, fibrous packing materials, ceramic balls, granular activated carbon, porous lava rocks, and structured plastic or ceramic media are commonly used as packing media in biotrickling filters. High specific surface area (7200 $m^2/m^3$), high bed voidage for minimizing pressure drops and eliminating clogging, chemical resistance, light weight, and cost help determine the selection of packing media for a given application.

## Nutrients

Microorganisms need several nutrients ($N_2$, P, S, K, Ca, Mg, Fe, etc.) and micronutrients (Cu, Se, Zn, etc.) for their growth. In biofilters, the nutrient requirements are either met by the compost media or by adding a nutrient solution to the media. In biotrickling filters, a nutrient solution is continuously or intermittently trickled over the porous media bed. Most of the nitrogen requirement in a biofilter is met by the biosolids present in compost, which have an N content of 20 to 30 g/kg total solids. Adding ammonia to the inlet gas, or adding slow-release nutrient granules or $NO_3^-$ solution to the media improves the VOCs' elimination capacity.

## pH Control

Slaked lime [$Ca(OH)_2$], lime (CaO), limestone ($CaCO_3$), crushed oyster shell ($CaCO_3$), dolomite [$CaMg(CO_3)_2$], marl (soil + $CaCO_3$), and slags ($CaSiO_3$) can be used to neutralize the acidic substances formed in the media. Chemical composition and particle size of these additives control the buffering capacity. About 10 percent by weight of crushed oyster shells are mixed with compost media as pH buffer. A large quantity of buffering agent is needed for systems having high acidic product formation. In biotrickling filters pH is maintained near 7 by injecting a controlled amount of caustic solution using a feedback control system.

## Humidification, Irrigation, and Leachate Collection

Manual or automatic devices for spraying water over the bed and humidification of influent gas streams are used to keep the system moist. Open biofilter units are also irregularly irrigated by precipitation. The humidification device is placed upstream of the biofilter, preferably after the blower. The system should be capable of maintaining over 95 percent relative humidity (RH) at the inlet of the bed. Simultaneous removal of particulate matter and/or heating or cooling of the influent stream is also possible. Humidification is accomplished by using steam injection systems, spray chambers, venturi scrubbers, and packed-bed towers.

Loss of water from the bed occurs due to (1) evaporation to an unsaturated influent gas stream, (2) biooxidation caused by bed heating, (3) metabolic water requirements, and (4) heat exchange with the environment. Irrigation systems are used to sprinkle water uniformly over the bed to compensate for this loss. An over-the-bed sprinkler system, soaker hoses, and pressure compensated soaker hoses are used for this purpose. Care should be taken to avoid clogging or freezing of sprinkler heads.

The quantity of liquid fed into and maintained within the filter bed affects the performance of the unit. Too high of an inflow of liquid into the bed will lead to flooding and anoxic or anaerobic microbial growths. If the liquid inflow is insufficient, the dissolution of pollutants will be low and treatment will be ineffective. The leachate, which trickles down and out of the media bed, is collected in the tapered bottom of the unit and pumped to the sewerage system for treatment with wastewater.

### Distribution and Flow of Gas

Uniform distribution of the influent polluted gas during its flow through the biofilter or biotrickling filter is essential for better performance of the unit. Short circuiting or channeling may lead to reduced removal efficiency. A smoke test is used to test channeling in the full scale unit.

A network of perforated PVC pipes (or pipes made of any other chemically resistant material) buried in a layer of gravel at the base of the filter is often used as the gas distributor. Specially fabricated, perforated concrete blocks can also be arranged to distribute gas. These arrangements permit movement of heavy equipment. In fully enclosed column biofilters, the inlet gas stream can be distributed in a properly designed plenum chamber located either at the top or bottom of the unit.

Biofilters can be operated either in down-flow or up-flow mode. In down-flow mode, any moisture added at the inlet is carried down the depth of filter, however, acidic and toxic products produced near the inlet are also transported downward and affect filter performance. In up-flow mode, undesirable substances produced near the inlet or particulates can be more easily removed from the system. The addition of moisture, however, becomes difficult. At high flow rates, any water added at the top of a filter bed that is operating in up-flow mode becomes trapped, causing flooding and uneven gas distribution. This results in the development of anaerobic zones in the bed.

To avoid such problems, biofilters are usually operated in dual mode. During moisture addition, the system is operated in down-flow mode to aid in the distribution of moisture, whereas during regular operation, it is operated in up-flow mode. This periodic switching of flow also helps achieve a more uniform distribution of microorganism growth throughout the bed.

Biotrickling filters are usually operated with both gas and liquid flowing downward to avoid stripping VOCs from the recirculating liquid into the outlet gases.

## PROCESS MODELING AND DESIGN

The primary aim of process modeling is to understand the effects of various process parameters, such as media surface area, biofilm thickness, and biodegradation kinetic constants on the removal of pollutants. All models assume equilibrium at the gas-biofilm interface, transport of pollutants through the biofilm by diffusion, and a simple biodegradation reaction kinetics. These models, however have not been used for design purposes.

The design and operation of biofilters and biotrickling filters are based on five parameters: gas residence time, gas flux, liquid hold-up, pollutant mass loading rate, and degradation capacity. The nature and quantity of nutrients to be supplied, temperature control, pH control, and excess liquid withdrawal are some other design parameters, though of lesser significance. The gas residence time, $t_g$, is the ratio of the bed volume to the volumetric gas flow rate $(V_b/Q)$. The effective residence time, $t_e$, is much shorter and is equal to the product of bed porosity, $\in$ and $t_g$. The gas residence time for biological systems varies from a few seconds to several minutes depending upon the biodegradability and solubility of the pollutant. The gas residence time has a direct bearing on the cost of the system. The gas flux (Q/A) has a significant effect on the pressure drop across the unit. It has been established that a filter-bed depth of about one meter is optimum. Successful biofilter systems have filter areas ranging from 10 to 2,000 $m^2$ and contaminated gas flow rates from 1,000 to 150,000 $m^3$ per hr. The corresponding surface loading rates are up to 300 $m^3$ hr per $m^2$, and removal rates are 10 to 100 $g/m^3$ per hr. However, the optimal value of these parameters for any given application depends upon the filter media, nature and concentration of contaminant, pH, and temperature.

## OPERATION AND MAINTENANCE

During operation and maintenance, one has to consider the acclimation period, response to transients, moisture monitoring and control, biomass accumulation and control, off-gas and filter-bed temperatures, media replacement, and bed pH.

### Acclimation

An acclimation period following start-up is required to reach optimum pollutant removal capacity. This period generally ranges from days to weeks depending upon the system used and pollutants being treated. Low loading rates or a precontrol unit may be necessary during this period. During the acclimation period, appropriate pollutant-degradation enzymes are induced within the microbial population, the microorganisms grow, and a biofilm is established on the media surface. The acclimation period can be shortened by inoculating the filter with organisms already acclimated to and actively degrading the pollutants present in the gas stream. Cultures isolated from already running biofilters, biotrickling filters, or even activated-sludge plants can be used for inoculation purposes. Inoculation is almost necessary for biotrickling filters in which the filter media is devoid of microorganisms. Inoculation is easily accomplished in these systems by recirculating the microbial suspension through the packing medium. Biofilters do not require inoculation because the packing media itself contains enough indigenous microorganisms that can easily adapt to the organic pollutants. However, inoculation shortens the acclimation period considerably, and for some calcitrant organic pollutants, inoculation with specific microorganisms may be required.

### Operation Under Transient Conditions

Most operating biofilters are subjected to varying feed conditions such as process shutdowns, start-up, and surges in influent pollutant concentrations. During shutdown or low inlet pollutant concentrations, microbial growth starves and undergoes endogenous decay, resulting in decreased pollutant-degrading activity. The longer the period of nonoperation, the longer the duration of acclimation after restart to restore full activity. If the shutdown and transients are too frequent, microorganisms adapt to the situation and restart acclimation periods are shorter. Continuation of air flow through the filter during shutdowns helps maintain aerobic conditions and reduce the destruction of aerobic microorganism film. Unstable or transient feed conditions during start-up are the most detrimental because they can resist the formation of microbial growth and result in excessively long acclimation periods.

A sudden increase in influent pollutant concentration is also detrimental to biofilter performance, leading to pollutant breakthrough, toxic inhibition, or even death of the microorganisms in the biofilter. For moderate and continuous surges in concentration, the microbial population adopts itself to the higher concentrations. An intermediate acclimation period is, however, required for gaining full degradation capacity.

### Monitoring and Control of Moisture

Improper moisture control often leads to failure of the biofilter. Biotrickling filters are less prone to drying because a liquid phase is continuously or semicontinuously trickled over the packing media. Media moisture content plays a critical role in affecting biodegradation, microbial ecology, pH, mass transfer rates, and compost physical structure. Optimum moisture content in compost ranges from 41 to 63 percent.

Insufficient moisture enhances drying-up of the liquid film surrounding the biofilm, resulting in a loss of biological activity. Too much moisture, on the other hand, affects the transport of $O_2$, VOCs, and waste products in and out of the biofilm. Oxygen deficiency results in the development of anaerobic zones, leading to acidification and odor formation.

Excessive drying may result in the development of hydrophobic zones and growth of hydrophobic fungi, which makes wetting difficult. After significant drying, the biofilter media needs to be replaced. Several gravimetric, electrical, and optical methods have been developed to measure moisture content.

## Accumulation and Control of Biomass

The biomass yield is a strong function of microbial community present, the contaminants being degraded, as well as nutrient and oxygen supply available to the microorganisms. The greater the mass loading rate and average biomass yield in a biofilter, the greater the potential to accumulate excess biomass within the packing material, which can lead to clogging problems. Aerobic biodegradation of organic compounds results in a higher biomass yield than anaerobic biodegradation or biodegradation of inorganic pollutants such as $H_2S$ or $NH_3$.

Adequate nutrient supplies and VOC loadings higher than 30 to 50 g VOC m$^3$/ha may accumulate excess biomass within the packing media. Due to higher inlet concentration, this accumulation occurs near the biofilter inlet. Biomass buildup also occurs on plates used to support the media within the bioreactor. Biomass accumulation reduces effective porosity, residence time, and specific surface area of the packing media. This results in an increase in $\Delta P$ and decrease in pollutant removal efficiency. Biomass accumulation in biotrickling filters is observed for moderate to high VOC loadings. Biofilters are normally less prone to biomass overgrowth.

Biomass accumulation can be controlled by limiting the supply of one or more key nutrients, such as nitrogen and/or potassium, physical removal of the biomass and/or mixing of the packing material, and intermittent operation of the filter unit. Regulation of the nutrient supply helps in controlling the microbial growth, but also reduces the removal efficiency if nutrients become limiting. By monitoring nutrient consumption, it is possible to identify the nutrients that limit growth. Nutrients also get recycled within the biofilm, and this process must be considered in maintaining a nutrient balance. Regulating the nitrogen supply limits the biomass growth effectively, but has a detrimental effect on degradation of pollutants. Potassium is more effective in controlling biomass accumulation and has only a moderate effect on the degradation capacity.

Periodic washing with water or an aqueous solution (e.g., 0.1 M NaOH) helps in removing excess biomass from biotrickling filters. Backwashing with water is another frequently used technique. This, however, will require backup air pollution control systems. The restart periods, however, become longer after washings with chemical solutions.

Physical removal of biomass in conjunction with nutrient regulation is used to control biomass and distribute it evenly for uniform biodegradation of contaminants throughout the bed. This is more conveniently achieved by switching periodically the nutrient feed from top to bottom and vice versa. This strategy also prevents bed clogging.

### *Media Replacement*

Biofilter media are usually replaced every two to five years with fresh media. Two different approaches are followed. According to one procedure, media are replaced every two years, and according to the second procedure, a decrease in treatment capacity, an increase in pressure drop, decrease in media pH, or signs of significant compaction are used as guidelines for media replacement. Reasons for changes in media performance include utilization, volatilization and/or leaching of nutrients, acidification, increase in media hydrophobicity, biomass accumulation, degradation of media and compaction, improper moisture control, high temperature, and high VOC loading rates.

## CONCLUSIONS

Biological systems such as biofilters, biotrickling filters, and bioscrubbers offer effective and low-cost solutions to controlling air pollution caused by low-to-moderate concentrations of reduced sulphur compounds, certain VOCs, and many other biodegradable organic vapors from industries and service facilities. The polluted air stream is compressed and passed through a humidifier and biofilter bed. Humidification helps in keeping the bed moist. Activated carbon, compost, peat, sawdust, soil, sand, etc., are used as filter media. Nutrients are sprayed periodically on to the bed to let the microorganisms grow, as the VOCs rarely provide enough food or nutrients for microbial growth. The microorganisms adsorb and eat the VOCs as the gas passes through the bed. The major operating parameters include humidity and temperature of off-gas, filter temperature, back pressure, filter moisture content, pH, etc.

## SUGGESTED READINGS

Davis WT (ed.) (2000). *Air Pollution Engineering Manual,* Second Edition. John Wiley and Sons, Inc., New York: Air and Waste Management Association, pp. 55-65.

Devinny JS, MA Deshussess, and TS Webster (1999). *Biofiltration for Air Pollution Control.* Boca Raton, LA: Lewis Publishers.

Epstein, E (1997). *Compost Science and Technology.* Lancaster, PA: Technomic.

Eweis JB, SJ Ergas, DPY Chang, and ED Schroeder (1998). *Bioremediation Principles.* New York: McGraw-Hill, Inc.

Heinsohn RJ and RL Kabel (1999). *Sources and Control of Air Pollution.* Engelwood Cliffs, NJ: Prentice-Hall, Inc.

# Biomethanogenesis

Dalel Singh
Poonam Nigam Singh

## INTRODUCTION

Methanogenesis, most commonly used anaerobic digestion process in organic waste disposal, results in the formation of biogas containing methane and carbon dioxide. Biogas (or methane), being insoluble, can be readily removed from treatment systems or digesters and used as a source of energy. In all agricultural situations, the disposal of residues could be a profiting exercise in which the recovered biogas is utilized as a cheaper source of energy, and optimization of process for the disposal of residues is achieved for the maximization of methane yields.

Methane production has been used for many years to stabilize municipal sewage sludge for disposal. The process involves two kinds of bacteria: acidogenic and methanogenic. Complex organic compounds are first converted to soluble products that have a lower molecular weight. These hydrolysis products are primarily carboxylic acids produced in the water slurry by the acidogenic bacteria present in the digester, which are then converted by methanogenic bacteria to biogas. Depending on its methane content, biogas may have heating values from about 19.6 to 29.4 MJ/cubic meters (500-750 Btu/SCF). Residual solids generally have good manure value and can be used for agricultural purposes. The conventional high-rate digestion process is conducted under nonsterile conditions in large tanks at near atmospheric pressure and at about 30 to 35°C (mesophilic range) or above 55°C in thermophillic range. The usual residence time in digesters could be 10 to 20 days, and the pH is maintained in the range of 6.8 to 7.2.

### Historical Developments

A large number of Euryarchaeota produce methane as an integral part of their energy metabolism. Such microorganisms are known as *methanogens* and this process of methane formation is called *methanogenesis*. Methane was first discovered as a type of "combustible air" by Italian physicist Alessandro Volta (1745-1827). Volta collected gas from marsh sediments and showed that it could burn in flames. Methanogenesis is the terminal step in the biodegradation of organic matter in many natural anoxic habitats, such as swamps.

The habitats of methanogens include anoxic sediments (marshes, swamps, lake sediments, moist landfills, and paddy fields) and animal digestive tracts (the large intestines of monogastric animals, such as humans, dogs, and swine; rumen of ruminant animals, such as cattle, sheep, elk, camel, and deer; cecum of cecal animals, such as rabbits and horses; and hindgut of cellulolytic insects, termites). Other habitats include geothermal sources of hydrogen and carbon dioxide, hydrothermal vents, and artificial biodegradation facilities such as sewage sludge digestors.

### Methane

Methanogenesis is the biological production of methane from the reduction of carbon dioxide with hydrogen or from methylated compounds. A variety of unique coenzymes are involved in methanogenesis, and the process is strictly anaerobic. During the process, energy conservation involves both sodium ion and proton gradients. Biogas can be upgraded to pure methane or synthetic natural gas (SNG) by scrubbing the carbon dioxide or by other processes. The overall thermal efficiency of the anaerobic digestion of biomass to methane is dependent on the process design and on the type of raw material used as feed in the digester. The feed can generally be gasified at overall thermal efficiencies of about 30 to 60 percent without the pretreatment of the feed or the addition of recycled ungasified solids to increase biodegradability. Methane yields are generally up to 0.30 $m^3$/kg of volatile solids added to the digesters.

## BIOMETHANATION PLANTS AND DIGESTORS

A typical biological gasification unit or biomethanation plant may have many subunits for different steps. These subunits include hydrolysis units with an optional pretreatment stage, anaerobic digesters, gas clean-up and dehydration units, and liquid effluent treatment units. Advanced designs presently being used include two-phase, plug-flow, packed-bed, and fluidized-bed digestors.

Anaerobic installations for waste treatment are called *digestors.* The primary process in methanogenesis is the digestion of organic material to soluble and gaseous products. In many waste treatment systems, the main objective has not been the production of methane as an energy source, but the stabilization of sludge so that it can be safely disposed of in the environment. In such systems, little attention has been paid to optimizing the methanogenesis process. Various treatment plants collect biogas generated in digestors, which is then used to fuel the plants. In these anaerobic digestors, contrary to aerobic processes, some significant advantages exist. Energy expenditure for aeration is not required, which saves considerably on operating costs. In such digestors, organic wastes and residues are converted more than 90 percent to methane and carbon dioxide. Bacterial biomass formation is very low under anaerobic conditions; consequently, the cost of sludge disposal is lower. In addition, odor problems are decreased since the digestion process is carried out in closed digestors and the methane is collected. Therefore, the advantage of these digestors is that the produced gas can be easily removed from the top of the system and stored for its utilization as an energy source. However, solid wastes and residues are the suitable starting materials for anaerobic digestions. The more diluted liquid wastes are primarily treated in aerobic activated-sludge processes.

Because of the low microbial biomass formed in such fermentation processes and low energy yield, the rate of the digestion process is slow. The average residence time in the digestor may exceed 20 days. Immobilization of microorganisms in a fixed-bed reactor can be used to increase the concentration of cells. Such fixed-bed reactors are very useful in treating solutions with very high organic loads in shorter periods. Some research has been carried out using porous sintered glass as carrier material for fixed-bed reactors. Using such a reactor with a capacity of 1000 litres, a considerable reduction in the biological oxygen demand (BOD) from 6.4 to 1.3 $kg/m^3$ could be achieved in just 4.8 hours.

In a different installation for the treatment of high-concentration wastes obtained from a fermentation plant, the digestion process was carried out in two stages. The first digestor was used for acid production and the second reactor was used for biomethanogenesis. The size of both reactors was 380 $m^3$, and sand was used as the carrier. In a two-stage system such as this, waste volumes of 150-200 $m^3$ per hour could be treated within 1 to 1.5 hours, and the digestion of wastes could be achieved up to 30 kg chemical oxygen demand (COD) per $m^3$ per day.

## SUBSTRATES FOR BIOGAS PRODUCTION

### Substrates for Anaerobic Digestion

The most commonly used substrates for anaerobic digestion are agricultural residues, food and agro-industrial wastes, cattle dung, poultry and piggery wastes, sewage, and sludge. The types of wastes may include crop wastes and residues, vegetables and tubers, sugar, starch, and confectionery; grains, legumes, oilseeds, wastes from distilleries, wineries, and breweries; plantation products, milk and dairy wastes, meat, poultry, fish wastes, marine products, and eggs. Many other sources of biomass exist that have a load of organic matter suitable for digestion. Studies have been done to produce biogas from the biomass of the water hyacinth, which grows in excessive amount in canals and streams in tropical countries. In theory, 800 $m^3$ of biogas can be produced under optimal conditions from the digestion of about two tons dry mass per day.

### Substrates for Methanogenesis

Methanogenic bacteria constitute a unique group of organisms that are the final and key link in the breakdown of organic matter in the anaerobic food chain. These bacteria are able to utilize only a restricted group of substrates for the synthesis of methane, including acetate, methanol, formate, hydrogen, and carbon dioxide. In waste disposal systems, about 75 percent of the methane is synthesized from acetate, and most of the rest from hydrogen and carbon dioxide. Although the starting materials of the anaerobic decomposition process are complex polymeric materials, such as cellulose, starch, fats, and proteins, none of these can be utilized by methanogenic bacteria. Therefore, other anaerobic fermentative organisms are required for the initial breakdown of polysaccharide and polymer compounds for the production of intermediate substrates, which can then be utilized by methanogenic bacteria.

### Effect of Substrates

The rate of methanogenesis is affected by the nature of the substrate used in digesters as well as the temperature of digestion. With mixed sludge, up to 600 litres of biogas per kg dry substrate can be produced. This biogas consists of about 60 to 70 percent methane and 25 to 30 percent carbon dioxide with the rest being hydrogen and nitrogen. Tropical countries have a wide variety of agro-industrial residues from agriculture and food industries, which are the most useful substrates for anaerobic digestion. Developing countries present the most promising areas for the development of biogas production, particularly because energy is in short supply and waste disposal is generally difficult to be carried out by those processes that are in operation in developed countries. Therefore, the efficiency of the process in developing countries is not as important as the energy produced.

Among the intermediary compounds produced in the digestion process, acetate is the main precursor, since two moles of methane are produced from acetate and one mole from carbon dioxide and hydrogen. Acetate is produced from the degradation of lipids and many fatty acids, including propionic, butyric, valeric, and long-chain fatty acids. These substrates undergo the following chemical reactions during methanogenesis:

Acetic acid
$$CH_3COOH \Rightarrow CH_4 \text{ (methane)} + CO_2 \qquad (I.5)$$
Propionic acid
$$4CH_3CH_2COOH + 2H_2O \Rightarrow 7CH_4 + 5\,CO_2 \qquad (I.6)$$
Butyric acid
$$2CH_3CH_2CH_2COOH + 2H_2O \Rightarrow 5CH_4 + 3CO_2 \qquad (I.7)$$
Ethanol
$$2CH_3CH_2OH \Rightarrow 3CH_4 + CO_2 \qquad (I.8)$$
Acetone
$$CH_3COCH_3 + H_2O \Rightarrow 2CH_4 + CO_2 \qquad (I.9)$$

Virtually any organic compound can be converted to methane and carbon dioxide in cooperative reactions involving methanogens and other anaerobic bacteria. At least ten substrates have been shown to be converted to methane by pure cultures of methanogens. These substrates do not include common compounds such as glucose and organic or fatty acids (other than acetate). Three groups of compounds are included in the list of ten methanogenic substrates.

The first group includes $CO_2$-type compounds: carbon dioxide (with electrons derived from hydrogen, certain alcohols, or pyruvate), formate, and carbon monoxide. Carbon dioxide is reduced to methane using hydrogen as an electron donor:

$$CO_2 + 4H_2 \Rightarrow CH_4 + 2H_2O \quad \Delta G^{0\prime} = -131 \text{ kJ} \qquad (I.10)$$

The second group of compounds includes methyl substrates such as methanol, methylamine, dimethylamine, trimethylamine, methylmercaptan, and dimethylsulfide. Using methanol as a model, the formation of methane can occur in either of two ways. First, methanol can be reduced using an external electron donor such as hydrogen:

$$CH_3OH + H_2 \Rightarrow CH_4 + H_2O \quad \Delta G^{0\prime} = -113 \text{ kJ} \qquad (I.11)$$

In the absence of hydrogen, some methanol can be oxidized to carbon dioxide in order to generate some electrons needed to reduce other molecules of methanol to methane:

$$4CH_3OH \Rightarrow 3CH_4 + CO_2 + 2H_2O \quad \Delta G^{0\prime} = -319 \text{ kJ} \qquad (I.12)$$

The third group includes acetotrophic substrates such as acetates. The final methanogenic process is the cleavage of acetate to carbon dioxide and methane. This process is known as the *acetotrophic reaction:*

$$CH_3COO + H_2O \Rightarrow CH_4 + HCO_3 \quad \Delta G^{0\prime} = -31 \text{ kJ} \qquad (I.13)$$

Very few methanogens are acetotrophic, but experimental measurements of methane formation in methanogenic habitats, e.g., sewage sludge, have revealed that about two-thirds of the methane is actually formed from acetate and one-third from hydrogen and carbon dioxide. Although lacking in terms of known diversity, acetotrophic methanogens are obviously very ecologically significant organisms in nature.

## *MICROBIOLOGY OF BIOMETHANATION*

The biological production of methane is carried out by a group of strictly anaerobic archaea called *methanogens.* Research on the biochemistry and bioenergetics of methanogenesis has revealed that biological production of methane occurs by a group of microorganisms through a series of reactions, which involve novel coenzymes and amazing complexity. Three groups of microorganisms participate in the anaerobic process.

### *First Group of Microorganisms*

A large number of bacteria are involved in the breakdown of the original organic polymeric constituent of the substrates, such as starch, carbohydrates, fats, and protein. These organisms hydrolyze the substrates into organic acids, such as propionic, butyric, acetic, lactic, and valeric acid, alcohol, hydrogen, and carbon dioxide. Any lignocellulosic material in feed-starting material is metabolized very slowly, because one of the constituents of lignocellulosics, lignin, is not broken down anaerobically. The group of bacteria involved in this initial breakdown of organic matter includes obligate anaerobes, such as clostridia, and facultative anaerobes, such as streptococci and enteric bacteria. Their total number and types differ according to the physiochemical nature of feedstock used in the digestors. About 400 strains of cellulolytic bacteria have been detected in cattle-waste-fed digesters. All cellulolytic strains that have been isolated so far as cellulase producers possess varying (high or low) capabilities of enzyme production.

Anaerobic microorganisms that produce cellulolytic enzymes include *Ruminococcus flavefaciens, R. albus, R. callidus, Clostridium cellobioparum, C. glycolicum, C. polysaccharolyticum, Bacteroides succinogenes, Eubacterium cellulosolven,* and *B. buccae.* Anaerobic microorganisms that produce xylanase enzymes include *C. botulinum, C. absonum, C. roseum, C. hastiformis, C. lituseburense, C. barkeri, C. titani, Butyrivibrio fibriosolvens, Fusobacterium nucleatum, F. russei,* and *Eubacterium alactolyticum.* The main protein hydrolyzers in the biogas digestors include *Peptococcus, Bifidobacterium,* and several sporolactobacilli.

### Second Group of Microorganisms

The second group includes bacteria that convert longer-chain fatty acids, such as propionic acid and butyric acid, and alcohols to acetic acid, hydrogen, and carbon dioxide. This conversion is endergonic at pH 7 and can occur only when coupled with exergonic reactions. Such reactions occur in mixed cultures. For example, ethanol is converted to acetic acid and hydrogen by an acetic acid bacterium, whereas a second reaction is accomplished by a methane bacterium utilizing hydrogen in the following reaction:

$$CH_3CH_2OH + H_2O \Rightarrow CH_3COO^- + H^+ + 2H_2 \qquad (I.14)$$
$$4H_2 + CO_2 \Rightarrow CH_4 + 2H_2O \qquad (I.15)$$

### Third Group of Microorganisms

The third group of bacteria are the strict anaerobic methanogens. Since methanogenesis is an ubiquitous process occurring in an anaerobic environment, methanogens involved in this process are very specific to their requirements of a carbon source. Only a limited range of substrates are utilized by these bacteria. Most methanogens utilize hydrogen as an energy source, and use carbon dioxide as a carbon source and electron acceptor. A few species from such morphologically diverse groups as cocci, sarcinae, and spirillae, also metabolize formic acid, methanol, or methylamine. The most important organic substrate of methanogenic bacteria is acetic acid. Acetic acid is fermented in a reaction that is weakly favorable energetically:

$$CH_3COO^- + H^+ \Rightarrow CH_4 + CO_2 \; \Delta G^{0'} = -37 \text{ kJ} \qquad (I.16)$$

Due to this characteristic, anaerobic methanogenic bacteria grow very slowly and are the most critical organisms in the mixed culture of the anaerobic digestor. Their morphology also differs considerably, which include sarcina rods, spheres, and spirals. Some of the important methanogens are *Methanobacterium ruminantium, Methanothermoautotrophicum, Methanospirillum hungatii, Methanogenium cariaci, Methanotrix sohngenii, Methanomicrobium mobile, Methanobrevibacterium smithii, Methylosinus trichosporium, Methylobacter capsulatus, Methylomonas albus, Methanosarcina barkeri, Methanococcus vannieli,* and *Methanobacterium formicicum.* Methanogenic bacteria are tentatively identified by fluorescence microscopy. These organisms possess some special coenzymes, such as $F_{420}$ and $F_{350}$, and are common in abundance in mesophilic digestors. Contrary to these organisms, two bacteria are predominantly found in thermophillic digestors operated at 60°C and above. These include *Clostridium thermocellum,* which are Gram-positive sporogenous rods, and *Thermoanaerobium* sp., which are Gram-positive asporogenous rods.

## BIOCHEMISTRY OF METHANE SYNTHESIS

### Reduction of Carbon Dioxide to Methane

The reduction of carbon dioxide to methane is generally hydrogen dependent, but electrons required for carbon dioxide reduction can be supplied by formate, carbon monoxide, and even certain organic compounds, such as alcohols. For example, 2-propanol can be oxidized to acetone, yielding electrons for methanogenesis in certain species of microorganisms. In general, the production of methane from carbon dioxide is driven by molecular hydrogen. The reduction of carbon dioxide occurs in the following steps:

- Carbon dioxide is activated by a methanofuran-containing enzyme and subsequently reduced to the formyl level.
- The formyl group is transferred to an enzyme-containing methanopterin from a methanofuran-containing enzyme. The formyl group is then dehydrated and reduced to methylene and methyl levels in two individual steps.

- Methanopterin transfers the methyl group to an enzyme containing coenzyme M (CoM).
- The methyl reductase system reduces methyl-CoM to methane with the involvement of $F_{430}$ and coenzyme B (CoB).
- Coenzyme $F_{430}$ removes the methyl group from methyl-CoM, forming a $Ni^{+2}$–$CH_3$ complex.
- The $Ni^{+2}$–$CH_3$ complex is reduced by electrons from CoB, which generates methane and a disulphide complex of CoM and CoB (CoM-S–S-CoB).
- The disulphide complex is reduced with hydrogen to generate free CoM and CoB. This reaction allows for energy conservation in the process of methanogenesis.

### Methanogenesis from Methyl Compounds and Acetate

In addition to hydrogen and carbon dioxide, methane can be produced from a variety of methylated compounds. Methyl compounds are catabolized by donating methyl groups to a corrinoid protein to form methyl-corrinoid. Corrinoids contain a porphyrinlike corrin ring with a central cobalt atom, and these act as parent structures of compounds such as vitamin $B_{12}$. The methyl group is donated by the methyl-corrinoid complex to CoM to produce methyl-CoM, from which methane is produced. If a reducing power such as hydrogen is not available to drive the terminal step, some of the methanol must be oxidized to carbon dioxide to yield electrons. This process occurs by reversing the steps in methanogenesis. If acetate is being used as the substrate for methanogenesis, it is first activated to acetyl-CoA, which can interact with carbon monoxide dehydrogenase of the acetyl-CoA pathway. Subsequently, methyl-corrinoid is produced with the transfer of the methyl group of acetate to the corrinoid enzyme. From there the methyl group then goes through the CoM-mediated terminal step of methanogenesis.

### Coenzymes Involved in Methanogenesis

Two classes of coenzymes are involved in the process of methanogenesis. The first class carries the $C_1$ unit from the initial substrate, carbon dioxide, to the final product, methane. The second class functions in redox reactions to supply the electrons that are required for the reduction of carbon dioxide to methane.

Methanofuran is the coenzyme involved in the first step of methanogenesis. Methanofuran contains the five-membered furan ring and an amino nitrogen atom that binds carbon dioxide. Another coenzyme is methanopterin, a methanogenic coenzyme that resembles the vitamin folic acid. Methanopterin acts as the $C_1$ carrier in the intermediate steps of reducing carbon dioxide to methane. Coenzyme M is a small molecule that is involved in the terminal step of methanogenesis. CoM plays its role in the conversion of a methyl group to methane. Another compound involved in methanogenesis is $F_{430}$, a nickel-containing tetrapyrrole coenzyme. $F_{430}$ is not a $C_1$ carrier, but is involved in the terminal step of methanogenesis as part of the methyl reductase enzyme complex.

### Redox Coenzymes

Two coenzymes, coenzyme B or 7-mercaptoheptanoyl-threonine phosphate, and $F_{420}$ are electron donors in methanogenesis. The structure of CoB is rather simple, and this coenzyme resembles the vitamin pantothenic acid. Coenzyme $F_{420}$ is a flavin derivative, and its structure resembles the common flavin coenzyme flavin mononucleotide (FMN). During methanogenesis, $F_{420}$ acts as an electron donor in several steps of carbon dioxide reduction. $F_{420}$ absorbs light at 420 nm in its oxidized form showing blue-green fluorescence. This phenomenon is used as a useful tool for microscopic identification of an organism as a methanogen.

## CONCLUSIONS

Biogas generation from locally available agricultural residues and animal dung is one of the answers to energy promotion strategies in most rural areas of developing countries. This technology offers several advantages, such as providing clean fuel for rural areas, promoting a safe and clean environment by the recycling of waste materials, and producing nutrient-rich organic manure. Biomethanogenesis or biogas technology has important implications in the area of energy, agriculture, farming, and pollution control for a cleaner environment, hence there is a need for vigorous efforts to promote its usefulness.

## SUGGESTED READINGS

Grayson M (ed.) (1984). *Recycling, fuel and resource recovery: Economic and environmental factors* (Encyclopedia Reprint Series). East Sussex, UK: Wiley Interscience Publication.
Madigan MT, JM Martinko, and J Parker (2000). *Biology of microorganisms*, Ninth edition. London: Prentice Hall International (UK) Ltd.

# Bioremediation

Wan Azlina Ahmad
Zainul Akmar Zakaria

## INTRODUCTION

Bioremediation is defined as the use of living organisms to reduce or eliminate environmental hazards resulting from accumulations of toxic chemicals and other hazardous wastes. The key element in any bioremediation process is the aerobic or anaerobic heterotrophs whose activity is affected by a number of physicochemical environmental parameters, namely, energy sources (electron donors), electron acceptors, nutrients, pH, temperature, moisture, and inhibitory substrates or metabolites. Heterotrophs are organisms that require organic or a complex source of carbon as substrates for metabolism. The substrates serve as an electron donor resulting in microbial growth. However, the application of cometabolism is required when the substrate cannot serve as a source of carbon and energy by nature of the molecular structure. A good example of such substrates are xenobiotics, a persistent contaminant in nature.

Aerobic processes are characterized by metabolic activities involving oxygen as a reactant. Dioxygenases and monooxygenases are two of the primary enzymes employed by aerobic organisms during the transformation and mineralization of xenobiotics. Anaerobic microbes take advantage of a range of electron acceptors, which, depending on their availability and the prevailing redox conditions, include nitrate, iron, manganese, sulphate and $CO_2$.

A chemical may or may not be classified as a hazard depending on other factors besides its chemical structure (U.S. Environmental Protection Agency). *Solid waste* is any material that is discarded or disposed. Solid waste does not need to be solid; it may be semisolid, liquid, or a contained gaseous material. Based on the guide provided by the 1976 Resource Conservation and Recovery Act (RCRA), United States, a solid waste is a hazardous waste if it is listed or exhibits one of the following characteristics: ignitability, corrosivity, reactivity, and toxicity. It is also considered hazardous even if it was a mixture between a listed hazardous waste and a nonhazardous solid waste, or it is derived from storage, treatment, or disposal of a hazardous waste.

## BIOREMEDIATION METHODS

Bioremediation methods fall into three broad categories: (1) land farming, (2) bioreactors, and (3) in situ treatment.

### Land Farming

Land farming is usually conducted on the surface (upper soil zone) or in a biotreatment cell in an open environment. The process consists of controlled degradation of contaminated materials in an above ground system or with in situ treatment near the soil's surface. Land-farming activities cultivate and enhance microbial degradation of hazardous compounds in place. Among hazardous compounds treatable using this method are pesticides, fuels, and polynuclear aromatic hydrocarbons. In composting, methods employed include in-ground trenches, rotating drums, circular tanks, open bins, silos, windrows, and open piles. As opposed to the treatment of sewage sludge compounds, which utilizes aerobic organisms, an anaerobic process is more preferred in treating hazardous waste compounds. Many composting systems utilize a bulking agent to increase porosity of the media to be treated and decrease moisture levels. Modern composting systems are usually divided into three process configurations: the windrow system, static-pile system, and the in-vessel system. The windrow system is the simplest to operate and least costly, but requires greater space and produces volatile emissions. The in-vessel systems provides excellent captures of emissions, but has low flexibility whereas the static-pile system can be considered an intermediary between the in-vessel and windrow systems.

### Bioreactors

Bioreactors consist of two basic physical systems: suspended growth and fixed film. Suspended growth bioreactors can be designed as batch, plug-flow, or a complete-mix system. Fixed-film bioreactors are designed as fixed-beds, fluidized beds, or rotating media. In suspended-growth reactors, the microorganisms are suspended as microbial aggregates in the liquid. This suspension is called biomass, activated sludge, mixed liquor suspended solid (MLSS), or mixed liquor volatile suspended solids (MLVSS). For these systems, the biomass must be removed, usually by settling, where a portion will be recycled back to the bioreactor. For fixed-film reactors, the biomass growth occurs on or within a solid medium that acts as a support. However, maintaining an effective biomass level is difficult when dealing with hazardous chemicals. First, these chemicals are typically found at low concentrations and may have little energy for supporting biomass growth. Second, most hazardous chemicals provide a low growth rate plus a decrease in influent chemical concentration due to the life of the project.

## *In Situ Treatment*

Another type of bioremediation, in situ remediation, utilizes the growth of indigenous, contaminant-degrading microorganisms that are present at the contaminated site. These organisms are capable of some degradation of contaminants. Unfortunately, their decontaminating action proceeds at too low a level and too slow a rate to effectively decontaminate the area. In addition, the organisms may only be able to chemically change one contaminant in a mixed collection of pollutants, or make only a few chemical changes in a chemically complex contaminating molecule. The growth of the naturally occurring microorganisms must be enhanced by the addition of oxygen and nutrients.

A major problem with in situ treatment using indigenous microorganisms is that the conditions of the site cannot be controlled, as with those of the bioreactor. This lack of control of such conditions as temperature, pH, and nutrient levels leads to a much longer decontamination time for the site. It is also much harder to predict what the outcome of the treatment will be, how long the decontamination will take, how the contaminants will be changed, and how much will be changed.

## *Other Methods*

Other methods practiced in bioremediation are as follows:

- *Bioventing:* Treatment of contaminated soil by drawing oxygen through the soil to stimulate microbial activity
- *Biofilter:* Use of microbial stripping columns to treat air emissions
- *Bioaugmentation:* Addition of bacterial cultures to a contaminated medium, especially in the in situ and ex situ systems
- *Biostimulation:* Stimulation of indigenous microbial populations in soil or groundwater by providing necessary nutrients

## APPLICATIONS OF BIOREMEDIATION

### Methane Degradation

Two novel methanotrophs, which actively degrade methane under environmental conditions, have been identified using isotope-labeled DNA. Molecular approaches that target the 16S rRNA gene (16S rDNA) and gene-encoding enzymes involved in key metabolic steps, e.g., methane monooxygenase, have been applied to the analysis of methanotrophs in rice-field soil, lake sediments, and forest soil. Methanotrophs are considered to be important for reducing the emission of methane, a greenhouse gas, from soil and sediment. In addition, methanotrophs cometabolize tricholoroethylene (TCE); therefore, TCE bioremediation often employs methane injection as a means to stimulate the TCE-degrading activity of indigenous methanotrophs.

### Marine Petroleum Hydrocarbon Degradation

Spilled-oil bioremediation experiments conducted at a sandy beach found that phylotypes affiliated with the α subclass of Proteobacteria appeared in the DGGE (denaturing gradient gel electrophoresis) fingerprints obtained for oiled plots, but not in those of unoiled plots. Another oil-spill experiment at a beach in the Norwegian Arctic showed that 16S rDNA types affiliated with the γ Proteobacteria, especially those belonging to the *Pseudomonas* and *Cycloclasticus* groups, were abundant in fertilized oil sands. These studies have indicated that some groups of bacteria commonly occurred in oil-marine environments, although other populations change under different environmental conditions.

### Anaerobic Petroleum Hydrocarbon Degradation

Because petroleum hydrocarbons are persistent under anaerobic conditions, their contamination of groundwater is a serious environmental problem. The microbial diversity in a hydrocarbon- and chlorinated-solvent-contaminated aquifer undergoing intrinsic bioremediation was assessed by cloning and sequencing bacterial and archaeal 16S rDNA fragments. This study detected phylotypes that were closely related to *Syntrophus* spp. and *Methanosaeta* spp., suggesting their syntrophic association. A toluene-degrading methanogenic consortium was characterized by rRNA approaches. The consortium comprised two archaeal species related to the genera *Methanosaeta* and *Methanospirillum*, and two bacterial species, one related to the genus *Desulfotomaculum* and the other not related to any previously described genus. Fluorescence in situ hybridization (FISH) with group-specific rRNA probes was used to analyze a denitrifying microbial community degrading alkylbenzenes and n-alkanes. Microbial communities associated with anaerobic benzene degradation under Fe (III)-reducing conditions in a petroleum-contaminated subsurface aquifer were also analyzed by DGGE analysis, and it has been suggested that Fe (III)-reducing *Geobacter* spp. play an important role in the anaerobic oxidation of benzene. The available electron acceptors are the principal determinants for the types of microorganisms that occur in anaerobic environments, and the microbial populations mentioned previously are considered important for petroleum hydrocarbon degradation in subsurface environments under respective conditions.

### Polycyclic Aromatic Hydrocarbon Degradation

Polycyclic aromatic hydrocarbons (PAHs) are compounds of intense public concern owing to their persistence in the environment and potentially deleterious effects on human health. A soil-derived microbial consortium capable of rapidly mineralizing benzo[$\alpha$]pyrene was analyzed by DGGE profiling of PCR-amplified 16S rDNA fragments. The analysis detected 16S rDNA sequence types that represented organisms closely related to known high-molecular-weight PAH-degrading bacteria (e.g., *Burkholderia, Sphingomonas,* and *Mycobacterium*), although the degradation mechanisms have yet to be resolved. In soil environments, the reduced bioavailability of PAHs due to sorption to natural organic matter is an important factor controlling their biodegradation. It has also been shown that the application of surfactants to soil enrichments that degrade phenanthrene and hexadecane altered the microbial populations responsible for the degradation. These results seem to suggest that nature harbors diverse microbial populations capable of pollutant degradation, from which a few are selected according to bioremediation strategies.

### Metal Bioremediation

Contamination of the environment by heavy metals has received a lot of attention lately due to its deleterious effects to animals and humans. Common sources of metal-contaminated waste include mining, electroplating, electronics, and nuclear industries. Conventional techniques for heavy metal removal from wastewaters including precipitation and ion exchange are limited only to metal concentrations greater than 100 mg/L. Hence biological processes are recommended to deal with the low metal concentrations in order to meet the discharge limits set by relevant authorities. Biological processes can either solubilize metals, thereby increasing their bioavailability and potential toxicity, or immobilize them and reduce their bioavailability. Metal mobilization can be carried out by a range of microorganisms, and processes include autotrophic and heterotrophic leaching, chelation by microbial metabolites and siderophores, and methylation, which can result in volatilization. Similarly, many organisms can contribute to immobilization by sorption to cell components or exopolymers, transport and intracellular sequestration, or precipitation as insoluble organic and inorganic compounds, e.g., oxalates, sulfides, or phosphates. Among the microorganisms reported to be present in metal-comtaminated environments are α-Proteobacteria, Actinobacteria, and sulfate-reducing bacteria (SRB), of which *Desulfovibrio* is a good example. Recently a genetically engineered strain of *Ralstonia eutropha* was found to decrease the toxic effects of Cd on the growth of tobacco plants.

## FEATURES OF BIOREMEDIATION

### Advantages of Bioremediation

Bioremediation is a natural process whereby indigenous microorganisms act on the contaminants present to release harmless products, namely $CO_2$, $H_2O$, and fatty acids. This process can be carried out in situ, i.e., where the problem is located. This eliminates the need to transport large quantities of contaminated waste off site and the potential threats to human health and the environment that can arise during such transportation. Bioremediation is less expensive than other technologies that are often used to clean up hazardous waste. For example, a bioremediation process only cost half as much compared with building an incinerator to treat the waste.

### Limitations of Bioremediation

Lack of expertise exists in the area of bioremediation, as it is a relatively new field. In order for the bioremediation program to be successful, a multidisciplinary approach incorporating fields such as microbiology, chemistry, engineering, geology, soil science, etc., needs to be addressed. Unlike other industries, bioremediation does not result in the production of high value-added products. Thus, venture capital has been slow to invest in the technology, and as a consequence, commercial activity in research and development has lagged far behind other industrial sectors. Some chemicals, e.g., PCBs, pesticides, coal tars, heavy metals, chlorinated solvents, and radionuclides, are not degraded so readily. Hence, more intensive research is needed with the limited funds available. In some cases, microbial metabolism of contaminants may produce toxic metabolites. Bioremediation is a scientifically intensive procedure that must be tailored to site-specific conditions, meaning that one has to do treatability studies on a small scale before the actual cleanup of the sites.

## BIOREMEDIATION—SUCCESS STORIES

One of the most famous cases of bioremediation was the cleanup of the Exxon Valdez oil spill in Alaska in 1989. Cleanup of the spill, which contaminated some 350 miles of shoreline, was accelerated through a federally supported biotechnology demonstration project. In the bioremediation project, nitrogen and phosphorous-rich nutrients were applied to shorelines to stimulate the growth of naturally occurring, oil-degrading microorganisms. Lab studies and visual observation confirmed that added nutrients enhanced the extent and rate of oil degradation. Oil samples showed changes in hydrocarbon composition, indicating that extensive biodegradation had occurred. Another case involved the use of sulfate-reducing bacteria (SRB) in 2003 to treat contaminated groundwater at the Budelco zinc-smelting works in the Netherlands. The pilot plant comprised a 9 $m^3$ stainless-steel sludge-blanket reactor using SRB and was developed by Shell Research Ltd. and Budelco B.V. This plant successfully removed toxic metals, primarily Zn and sulfate, from contaminated groundwater at the longstanding smelter site by precipitation as metal sulfides.

## CONCLUSIONS

Bioremediation as a site-specific technology has long been addressed as a potential solution to treat contaminated areas. However, among the more important issues are the application of bioremediation as a site-specific technology, monitoring and process control and also measuring effectiveness. However, additional research at the laboratory and a pilot-scale study has to be carried out before translating the results into a meaningful larger-scale treatment technology. A site-specific approach tends to require guidelines or expert systems for interfacing site characteristics with treatability information derived from tests using samples taken directly from the site concerned. Monitoring and control of chemical processes are important in bioremediation because they would indicate the sustainability of the process as a whole. Current applied techniques are expensive, which necessitates the development of other monitoring tools. One of the alternatives is biotechnology, an area in which techniques such as the nucleic acid probe, immunological assays, microbial diversity measures, gene expression, and stress promoter activation promise a high potential of application. Measuring effectiveness is the last and most difficult aspect in bioremediation work because it involves controls and assumptions in judging the success of the work.

## SUGGESTED READINGS

Bender JA and PC Phillips (1999). Compositions of constructed microbial mats. U.S. Patent 6008028.

Cookson JT, Jr. (1995). *Bioremediation engineering: Design and application.* New York: McGraw-Hill Inc.

Falthman EP, DE Jerger, and JH Exner (eds.) (1994). *Bioremediation: Field experience.* Boca Raton, FL: CRC Press, Inc.

Watanabe K (2001). Microorganisms relevant to bioremediation. *Current Opinion in Biotechnology* 12:237-241.

White C, JA Sayer, and GM Gadd (1997). Microbial solubilization and immobilization of toxic metals: Key biogeochemical processes for treatment of contamination. *FEMS Microbiology Reviews* 20:503-516.

# Methods for the Biological Treatment of Wastewater

## Biological Reactors

P. K. Mishra
B. N. Rai
S. N. Upadhyay

### PRINCIPLES OF BIOLOGICAL TREATMENT

Biological treatment of wastewater has developed into a highly efficient technology based on sound engineering and scientific principles. Biological treatment processes can be of two broad types: aerobic and anaerobic. The aerobic processes use oxygen as an electron acceptor. The general schematic reaction of the process is as follows:

$$COHNS + O_2 + cell + nutrient \rightarrow CO_2 + NH_3 + C_5H_7NO_2 + \cdots \quad (I.17)$$

(pollutant)                                        (new cell)

The cells die in the endogenous phase according to this scheme:

$$C_5H_7NO_2 + 5 O_2 \rightarrow 5 CO_2 + 2 H_2O + NH_3 + energy \quad (I.18)$$

Under anaerobic conditions, the complex organic compounds are first hydrolyzed to acids, which are then converted to methane:

Acid-forming bacteria
$$4 C_3H_7O_2 NS + 8 H_2O \rightarrow 4 CH_3COOH + 4 CO_2 + 4 NH_3 + 4 H_2S + 8 H \quad (I.19)$$

Methane-forming bacteria
$$4 CH_3COOH + 8 H \rightarrow 5 CH_4 + 3 CO_2 + 2H_2O \quad (I.20)$$

Acid-forming bacteria grow much faster (doubling time = a few hours) than methane-producing bacteria (doubling time = a few days). Acid-forming bacteria cause odor problems and also inhibit the growth of methane-producing species. Thus, it is necessary to maintain conditions for promoting the growth of methane producers.

Organic nitrogen (protein, urea) present in domestic wastewater is easily biodegraded and hydrolyzed to ammonia. A part of this ammonia is used for cell synthesis, and the remainder undergoes biooxidation. During biooxidation, ammonia is oxidized first to nitrite and then to nitrate by *Nitrosomonas* and *Nitrobacter*, respectively. *Nitrosomonas* are obligately aerobic lithoautitrophic bacteria, whereas *Nitrobacter* are chemoautotrophic. Both, however, use carbon dioxide as a carbon source. The schematic conversion equations are as follows:

$$\textit{Nitrosomonas}$$
$$NH^+_4 + 1.5\ O_2 \rightarrow NO^-_2 + 2H^+ + H_2O \qquad (I.21)$$

$$\textit{Nitrobacter}$$
$$NO^-_2 + 0.5\ O_2 \rightarrow NO^-_3 \qquad (I.22)$$

Nitrifying bacteria are mesophilic and grow very slowly (doubling time = 1 to 2 days). They generally proliferate in biological wastewater treatment units that have long hydraulic retention times (e.g., aerated lagoons, stabilization ponds, and oxidation ditches) or when the biological oxygen demand (BOD) in the wastewater is low (e.g., at the bottom of a low-rate trickling filter). The nitrification process is sensitive to disturbance. Several inorganic and organic substances (e.g., metals, phenols) act as inhibitors. A high concentration of ammonia and nitrous acid can also be inhibitory. The optimal pH range is 7.5 to 8.6. Temperature has a significant effect on the growth of nitrifying bacteria. The dissolved oxygen (DO) levels above 1 mg/l are essential for effective nitrification. Below this level, oxygen becomes limiting and nitrification slows down. Nitrate formed during the nitrification step is reduced to nitrogen by nitrate, reducing facultative anaerobic (denitrifying) bacteria in the presence of a carbonaceous energy source (e.g., $CH_3OH$).

Denitrifying bacteria

$$NO^-_3 + CH_3OH \rightarrow 0.5\ N_2 + 0.83\ CO_2 + 1.17\ H_2O + OH^- \qquad (I.23)$$

Phosphorus occurs in wastewater as orthophosphate ($PO_4^{-3}$), polyphosphate ($P_2O_7$) and organic phosphorus. The last two forms account for 70 percent of phosphorus in the influent wastewater. Microorganisms utilize phosphorus for cell synthesis and energy transport and also store it for subsequent use. About 10 to 30 percent of the influent phosphorus is removed during secondary biological treatment.

*Acinetobacter* are the primary microorganisms responsible for the removal of phosphorus. In presence of volatile fatty acids (VFAs), these organisms release stored phosphorus under anaerobic conditions. Under appropriate anaerobic-aerobic conditions, more phosphorus than needed for cell synthesis, energy transport, and storage may be taken up by the microorganisms. Anoxic conditions lead to the release of phosphorus from cells. The sludge containing excess phosphorus is either wasted or removed and treated separately under anoxic conditions to release the excess phosphorus. The symbiosis between aerobic and anaerobic organisms help in phosphorus removal. Thus biological phosphorus removal requires both anaerobic and aerobic reactors or zones within the same reactor.

Biological treatment processes necessitate a high microbial growth rate and sustainability to have a high cell density. A satisfactory growth rate requires that the concentration of all substrates be reasonably high (above 10 mg/l) and all necessary macro- and micronutrients are present. The microbial growth rates are also dependent upon environmental conditions, such as mixing and hydraulic regime, dissolved oxygen concentration (for aerobic processes), pH, availability of nutrients (N, P, trace elements, etc.), temperature, and BOD level.

For sustaining the growth of microorganisms, the BOD level should be above 10 mg/l. For domestic wastewaters it ranges from 200 to 500 mg/l, whereas for industrial wastewaters it could be up to 50,000 mg/l.

Nutrient requirements for the conventional activated-sludge process are higher than those for the extended aeration process due to more recycling and less sludge withdrawal. In facultative aerated lagoons and oxidation ponds, no sludge is withdrawn and some nitrogen and phosphorus is released back through the anaerobic decomposition of settled sludge in the bottom layers. Some nitrogen loss through denitrification may, however, occur in these units.

Domestic wastewater has all the necessary nutrients needed for bacterial growth, but some industrial wastewaters require the addition of nutrients. For an activated-sludge unit, the optimal BOD:N:P should be 100:5:1.

Mixing and hydraulic regimes control the availability of the substrate and other substances to the cells. The more intense the mixing, the faster the growth of microorganisms. Aerobic reactions take place at higher rates when dissolved oxygen concentration is the highest under the prevailing environmental conditions. The optimum pH range for most anaerobic reactions is 6 to 8. Only some anaerobic biological reactions occur beyond this range. In general, microorganisms grow optimally between 25 to 35°C. The microbial growth rate nearly doubles for every 10°C rise in temperature.

## *REACTION KINETICS*

The interrelationship between the rate of energy or substrate utilization and energy supply determines the rates at which microorganisms can grow, metabolize, and multiply. These rates are controlled by the enzymes that catalyze various metabolic pathways. The rate of an enzymatically catalyzed reaction can be expressed by Michaelis-Menten kinetics:

$$V = \frac{V_m [S]}{K_m + [S]} \qquad (I.24)$$

where $K_m$ is the Michaelis-Menten constant, numerically equal to the substrate concentration at which $V = V_m/2$, $[S]$ is the substrate concentration, $V$ is the rate of enzymatically catalyzed reaction, and $V_m$ is the maximum possible rate of reaction.

According to the Monod model for biological reactions occurring in the presence of microorganisms, the source of enzymes, $V_m$ is no longer a constant but a function of microbial cell concentration and can be replaced by

$$V_m = \mu_m [X_a], \qquad (I.25)$$

where $\mu_m$ is the maximum specific growth rate and $[X_a]$ is the concentration of active (or viable) cells. Thus, the Monod model gives

$$\frac{d[X_a]}{dt} \cdot \frac{1}{[X_a]} = \frac{\mu_m [S]}{K_s + [S]}, \qquad (I.26)$$

where $K_s$ is the substrate saturation constant and is equal to the substrate concentration at which $\mu = \mu_m/2$. Thus, the specific growth rate is expressed as follows:

$$\mu = \frac{\mu_m [S]}{K_s + [S]} \qquad (I.27)$$

The rate of substrate consumption and the rate of cell formation are related through

$$\frac{d[X_a]}{dt} = -Y\frac{d[S]}{dt},$$ (I.28)

where $Y$ is the yield coefficient and is the mass of microorganisms formed per unit mass of substrate consumed. The rate of removal of substrate expressed as BOD, COD, TOC, etc., can be represented as follows:

$$-r = -\frac{1}{Y}\left[\frac{\mu_m[X_a][S]}{K_s + [S]}\right]$$ (I.29)

The biodegradation kinetics are affected by the relative values of $K_s$ and $[S]$ when $[S] > K_s$:

$$-r = \frac{\mu_{max}}{Y}[X_a]$$ (I.30)

Here the biodegradation is independent of substrate concentration and depends only on the mass of microbial solids present in the bioreactor. When $[S] < K_s$

$$-r = \frac{\mu_{max}}{Y}[S][X_a]$$ (I.31)

$$= K[S][X_a],$$ (I.32)

and when $[X_a]$ is constant,

$$-r = K'[S]$$ (I.33)

Here $K'$ is the first order rate constant. Equation (I.33) is useful in determining the BOD level of a wastewater in laboratory conditions and is also widely used for designing waste stabilization ponds.

The Monod model was developed using experimental data obtained with a single species culture and single organic compound as the substrate. In wastewater treatment units, a mixed population of microbial species persists and metabolize scores of organic compounds. Thus, the Monod model is of limited applicability. However, because of its simplicity, it is widely used for designing practically all wastewater treatment units.

The microbial population must adjust itself to the organic compounds, particularly organic refractories, if present in the influent. The rate constants calculated using data generated with nonacclimated organisms would be unable to provide proper substrate removal rate. For example, phenols are toxic to most microbes, however, acclimated species can easily degrade it.

Some organic pollutants can be toxic or inhibitory beyond certain concentration levels. This causes metabolic processes to decline, leading to a reduction in growth rates and hence the biodegradation rate. The Monod model fails to describe such situations and needs to be modified. Halden's model takes into account various inhibitory situations. For mixed microbial populations, the effect of inhibition can be predicted successfully by operating a bench or a pilot-scale bioreactor.

Primary substrate acts as electron donor which on oxidation provides energy and electrons for all synthesis and growth. It can be a pure compound such as glucose or a mixture of compounds collectively expressed as BOD, chemical oxygen demand (COD) or total organic carbon (TOC).

There is a minimum primary substrate concentration below which cells have a negative growth rate under steady-state concentrations. Removal of primary substrate to levels below 1 mg/L (expressed as $BOD_{lim}$) would be impossible to achieve. However, it is possible to remove organic compounds below $[S_{min}]$ levels of target compounds when the target compound is not the primary substrate, but the secondary substrate. The secondary substrate is removed by secondary utilization, which is controlled by the intrinsic kinetics of the secondary substrate and the amount of biomass. The amount of biomass generated, however, is determined by the primary substrate utilization.

## BIOREACTORS FOR WASTEWATER TREATMENT

Aerobic and anaerobic bioreactors are of two types: suspended microbial growth bioreactors and supported growth (or fixed film) bioreactors. Figure I.7 shows various common bioreactor configurations under each category.

### Suspended Microbial Growth Bioreactors

In these bioreactors, microorganisms are kept in suspension through agitation and/or mixing in order to have the best possible contact with the substrate. Microorganisms grow as suspended cells or cell flocs. Suspended microbial growth bioreactors can be operated under three different modes: the batch, the chemostat, and the recycle bioreactor (or activated sludge).

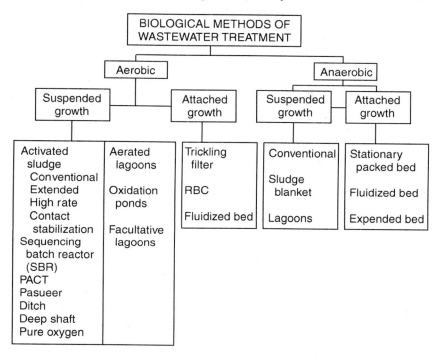

FIGURE I.7. Biological methods of wastewater treatment

Batch reactors are the oldest type of bioreactors. Sequencing batch reactors (SBR) are the commonly used batch bioreactors. The wastewater is treated in four steps:

1. contact with microorganisms
2. biological reaction
3. settling of the sludge
4. draining of the clarified treated liquid

All four operations can be performed either in the same unit turn by turn or by using four different units. The wastewater is added to the first bioreactor having some microbial sludge. The contents of the bioreactor are agitated and oxygen (or air) is sparged in to it so that microorganisms can grow and metabolize the organic pollutants in the wastewater. After some time (depending on the type of microorganism used), mixing and aeration are stopped and the suspended microbial mass is allowed to settle. The clarified supernatant liquid is then removed, leaving the settled sludge behind. Excess sludge is removed leaving some residual in the bioreactor to act as seed for initiating the operation with the next batch. The sludge may also be given some treatment to stabilize it. Sequencing batch reactors are preferred by industries. The major advantage of these units is that the effluent can be analyzed before its discharge. Continuous biological treatment units do not provide this advantage where samples can be withdrawn only from the treated effluent.

High rate aerobic and anaerobic digesters and stabilizers, aerated lagoons, and other type of ponds and lagoons fall under the category of chemostats. The *chemostat* is a simple flow-through device in which the microbial growth rate ($\mu$) is controlled solely by the dilution rate or residence time. The *dilution rate* is defined as the ratio of the volumetric flow rate and volume of the bioreactor. The *residence time* is the reciprocal of the dilution rate (D) and is equal to the rate of cell growth. The effluent from such a bioreactor contains microbial cells and residual substrate. The microbial cells must be removed to realize treatment goals.

The activated-sludge process is the most widely used, continuous suspended-growth biological treatment process. Normally it refers to an aerobic biological treatment unit, however, in more general terms it can refer to any process having an integration of sludge removal, sludge recycle, sludge wastage, and biomass accumulation. A biomass separator follows the main biological treatment unit and is used for removing biomass from the effluent. The biomass from the separator is recycled back to the biological reactor to maintain a particular level of microbial concentration with respect to substrate concentration. This is characterized in terms of food to microorganisms (F:M) ratio. The (F:M) ratio is maintained by controlling the sludge-wasting and recycling rates. Recycling helps maintain a higher microbial concentration in the bioreactor in comparison to batch or chemostat bioreactors. This results in lower cell growth compared to the dilution rate, and thus a bioreactor of relatively smaller size is required. These bioreactors, however, require much elaborate process control and monitoring for optimizing the sludge recycle and wastage rates, sludge accumulation rates, and easily settleable solids.

### Attached Microbiological Growth Bioreactors

Attached microbial growth bioreactors are characterized by a microbial growth attached to a solid support (or media), and rely on the metabolic activity of active microorganisms in the growth layer that have contact with a downward-moving film of wastewater. As the wastewater flows over the microbial growth, organic pollutants and other nutrients diffuse into it, and are used as food by the microbial cells. In aerobic processes, oxygen from the air also diffuses into the microbial layer. The microbial species grow and increase the thickness of microbial layer.

In due time, the microbial layer becomes so thick that oxygen is consumed much before it can diffuse up to the surface of the support media. An anaerobic (or anoxic) zone thus develops on the inner side of the microbial growth layer. This anaerobic or anoxic layer consumes the organic pollutants diffusing up to this layer, as well as aerobic cells growing in the outer aerobic zone. This process reduces the quantity of waste sludge that must be handled and disposed of. Some excess microbial growth continues sloughing off from the media surface and a clarifier is usually included in attached growth bioreactor systems to remove such biomass.

Attachment of the microbial growth on a solid medium provides a much higher cell density than realized in suspended microbial growth bioreactors. This permits the use of a smaller bioreactor compared to suspended growth systems as well as very low specific growth rates. Attached microbial growth bioreactors are useful when the influent wastewater has a very high substrate concentration, requiring a high cell density for efficient biodegradation. These are also useful for anaerobic processes in which cell growth rates are slower and more difficult to maintain. Due to attached growth, enough microorganisms remain in the system and it is less susceptible to flow fluctuations.

Three general types of attached microbial growth bioreactors are in common use today: the plug-flow bioreactor, the well-mixed bioreactor, and the fluidized-bed bioreactor. Plug-flow bioreactors allow the wastewater to flow over and/or through the media. Microorganisms grow on the support media and metabolize pollutants. The media could be made of a variety of materials, e.g., rocks, plastic, wood slabs, etc. Trickling filters, biological towers, the biological activated filter (BAF), and multistage rotating biological contactors (RBC) are common examples of this type of bioreactor.

A well-mixed bioreactor can be designed by recycling the effluent around a fixed-bed bioreactor or by using a single-stage RBC. The fluidized-bed bioreactor utilizes a media that can support microbial growth and can also be expanded, fluidized, and suspended by the upward flow of wastewater through the bioreactor. Activated carbon, coal, ion-exchange beads, metal-oxide particles, sand, etc., have been used as support media. Recycling of the effluent may be required to maintain a fluidized state. Fluidization helps in mixing the media, provided the particle size is uniform and flow distribution is even.

### Anaerobic Treatment

Anaerobic treatment is recommended for high-BOD wastewaters. These units take less space than aerobic units and are generally more energy efficient. It is usually used as a pretreatment unit to reduce BOD from 600 or more to 200 to 300 mg/l. Anaerobic organisms are highly sensitive to certain chemicals, pH, and temperatures, than aerobic organisms. Thus a laboratory treatability study is generally carried out to determine whether the wastewater is amenable to anaerobic degradation. The wastewaters from chemical and plastic units are not suitable for anaerobic degradation.

### Facultative Treatment

A trickling filter is the traditional facultative treatment device. Two main forms of these units are the packed tower and the rotating biological contactor (RBC). These units are suitable for roughing purposes to reduce BOD from 600 to 1000 mg/l to 50 to 70 mg/l. When used with recycling, these units are capable of producing treated effluent similar to that produced by the activated-sludge process. Installations treating industrial effluent often use packed towers and RBCs for roughing purposes. When operated under anoxic conditions, they can also be used for removing nitrogen and phosphorous from aerobically treated wastewater. Nitrate is reduced to nitrogen gas, which is released into the atmosphere. The phosphorous forms a part of the sludge and must be handled in the sludge disposal system.

Facultative lagoons are used as tertiary treatment devices or as polishing ponds at the end of the treatment train.

## CONCLUSIONS

Wastewater treatment in one of the most widely used biotechnological processes. Wastewater treatment methods vary widely, but all have a microbiological basis to break down the organic pollutants in wastewater and convert them into harmless products that can be safely discharged onto land or into rivers or seas. In biological treatment, microorganisms are efficiently used in aerobic or anaerobic bioreactors to stabilize biodegradable organic pollutants. Aerobic processes convert organic matter into $CO_2$, $H_2O$, and new cells, whereas anaerobic processes convert organic matter primarily into methane and more cells. Nitrogen and phosphorous-bearing compounds also can be mineralized and removed. The cells of microorganisms can either be in suspension or as an attached layer. The reactors could be a simple system, such as an oxidation pond, or a complex and mechanized unit, such as an activated-sludge plant. The Monod model is effectively used to model the behavior of these bioreactors.

## SUGGESTED READINGS

Benefield LD and CW Randall (1980). *Biological process design for wastewater treatment.* Englewood Cliffs, NJ: Prentice-Hall.

Eckenfelder WW, Jr. (1989). *Industrial water pollution control.* New York: McGraw-Hill Book Co.

Gardy CPL, Jr. and HC Lim (1980). *Biological wastewater treatment: Theory and applications.* New York: Marcell Dekker.

Metcalf & Eddy, Inc. (1991). *Wastewater engineering: Treatment, disposal, and re-use* (revised by G Tchobanglous and FL Burton). New York: McGraw-Hill, Inc.

Sundstorm DW and HE Klei (1979). *Wastewater treatment.* Englewood Cliffs, NJ: Prentice-Hall, Inc.

# Membrane Bioreactor

C. Visvanathan
R. Ben Aim

## *INTRODUCTION*

A *membrane* is a material that forms a thin wall capable of selectively resisting the transfer of different constituents of a fluid and thus effecting a separation of the constituents. Thus, membranes should be produced with a material of reasonable mechanical strength that can maintain a high throughput of a desired permeate with a high degree of selectivity. The optimal physical structure of the membrane is based on a thin layer of material with a narrow range of pore size and a high surface porosity. This concept is extended to include the separation of dissolved solutes in liquid streams and the separation of gas mixtures for membrane filtration.

Membranes can be classified by

1. the driving force used for the separation of impurities, such as pressure, temperature, concentration gradient, partial pressure, electrical potential;
2. the structure and chemical composition;
3. the mechanism of separation; and
4. the construction geometry of the membrane.

Microfiltration (MF) and ultrafiltration (UF) are low-pressure-driven processes in which feed water is driven through a microporous synthetic membrane and divided into permeate, which passes through the membrane, and retain or reject the nonpermeating species. In wastewater treatment applications, these membrane processes are more effective in the removal of particles and microorganisms. Reverse osmosis (RO) is a high-pressure-driven process designed to remove salts and low molecular weight organic and inorganic pollutants. Nanofiltration (NF) operates at a pressure range in between RO and UF, targeting the removal of divalent ion impurities. Figure I.8 illustrates the size range of various impurities and the application range of the membrane processes.

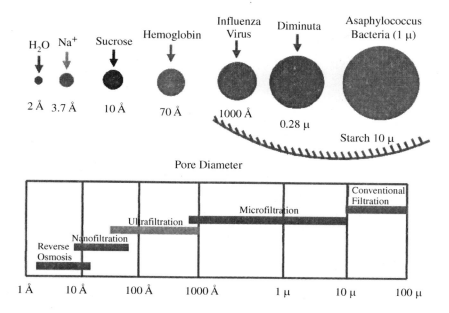

FIGURE I.8. Size and application ranges of membrane processes

## *MEMBRANE BIOREACTOR SYSTEMS*

Membrane bioreactor (MBR) systems essentially consist of a combination of membrane and biological reactor systems. These systems are emerging technologies, currently developed for a variety of advanced wastewater treatment processes. In general, MBR applications for wastewater treatment can be classified into four groups, namely, extractive membrane bioreactors, bubbleless aeration membrane bioreactors, membrane recycle bioreactors, and membrane-separation bioreactors

### *Extractive Membrane Bioreactors*

Extractive membrane bioreactors (EMBR) enhance the performance capabilities of biological treatment of wastewater by exploiting the membrane's ability to achieve a high degree of separation while allowing transport of components from one phase to another. This separation aids in maintaining optimal conditions within the bioreactor for the biological degradation of wastewater pollutants. For example, degradable toxic organic pollutants from a wastewater could be transferred through a nonporous membrane to a growth biomedium for subsequent degradation. In this case the mass transfer of toxic compounds across the membrane takes place due to the presence of a concentration gradient, while the biomedium functions as a sink.

The extractive membrane bioreactor can be operated in two modes, as illustrated in Figure I.9:

- Mode 1: the membrane is immersed in the biomedium tank. Here the toxic wastewater is circulated through the membranes, and due to the concentration gradient, the toxic compounds are selectively transported to the surrounding biomedium. Specialized microbial cultures could be cultivated in the bioreactor, which could be easily optimized for the degradation of the pollutants.
- Mode 2: the membrane forms an external circuit with the biomedium tank. The wastewater containing toxic organic pollutants is circulated on the shell side of the membrane modules. While the biomedium liquid is pumped through the membrane lumens. Due to the presence of a concentration gradient, the toxic pollutant is transferred to the medium. Within the medium, the toxic pollutant is continuously degraded by specialized microorganisms operating in optimum conditions, such as pH, temperatures, dissolved oxygen, and nutrient concentration. The organic, extracted wastewater is removed on the other end of the membrane shell.

In both the systems, because the bioreactor is unaffected by the toxic wastewater within the membranes, the conditions within the bioreactor can be optimized to ensure efficient degradation of the toxic compounds. This technology has been successfully demonstrated for the treatment of priority pollutants, such as chloroethanes, chlorobenzenes, chloroanilines, and toluene.

### *Bubbleless Aeration Membrane Bioreactors*

In a conventional aerobic wastewater treatment unit, such as an activated-sludge unit, the process efficiency is controlled by the availability of air. Due to an inefficient mode of air supply, 80 to 90 percent of the oxygen diffused as air in an activated sludge process is vented to the atmosphere.

Oxygenation with pure oxygen, as opposed to air as an aeration medium, would lead to an increase in the overall mass transfer and biodegradation rate. However, since conventional aeration devices have high power require-

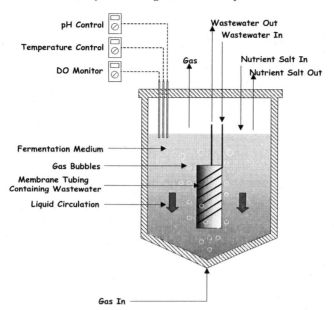

EMBR  System with Internal  Membrane Module (Mode 1)

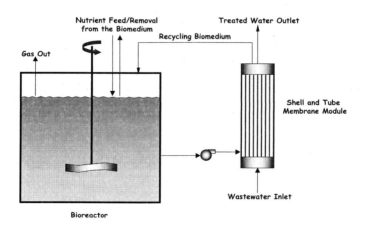

EMBR  System with External  Membrane Module (Mode 2)

FIGURE I.9. Extractive bioreactor membrane modes

ments due to the high rate of mixing, these devices cannot be used with biofilm processes. Biofilm processes are advantageous because they enable retention of high concentrations of active bacteria. The membrane aeration bioreactor (MABR) process uses gas-permeable membranes to directly supply high purity oxygen without bubble formation to a biofilm. Here the bubble-free aeration is achieved by placing a synthetic polymer membrane between a gas phase and a liquid phase. This membrane is used to transfer large quantities of air/oxygen into the wastewater. Because the gas is practically diffused through the membrane, a very high air transfer rate is attained. The membranes are generally configured in either a plate-and-frame or hollow-fiber module. However, current research has focused on the hollow fiber arrangement with gas on the lumen side and wastewater on the shell side. The hollow-fiber modules are preferred because the membrane provides a high surface area for oxygen transfer while occupying a small volume within the reactor. Here the membrane also acts as a support medium for the bioflim formation, which reduces the potential for bubble formation and air transfer rate.

### Membrane Recycle Bioreactors

The membrane recycle bioreactor consists of a reaction vessel operated as a stirred tank reactor and an externally attached membrane module. The substrate (feed wastewater) and biocatalyst are added to the reaction vessel in predetermined concentrations. Thereafter the mixture is continuously pumped through the external membrane circuit. The smaller molecular compounds, the end products of the biodegradation reaction, are permeated through the membrane, wherease the large molecular-sized biocatalysts are rejected and recycled back into the reaction tank.

Traditionally, batch processes are used in biotechnological applications. Due to this, the efficiency is lower than continuous processes, with a batch-to-batch variation in products. In batch processes, the microbial population would have to be separated out at the end of the run because the microbial species are attached to the membrane via adsorption, entrapment, microencapsulation, etc. However, membrane recycle reactors are continuous processes that are being adopted for biotechnology applications. The advantages of adopting a continuous process are lower operating costs, since the enzymes are more effectively utilized and the product more uniform and consistent. Inhibitory end products are continuously removed from the system, which results in a reduced likelihood of biocatalyst poisoning. A disadvantage of the membrane recycle process is the loss of activity (between 10 to 90 percent) due to enzyme substrate orientation and diffusional resistances.

However, research efforts of late have been directed toward the effective adsorption of biocatalysts onto the membrane surface, thereby maximizing the degradation potential of the recycle membrane reactor.

In industrial applications, recycle membrane bioreactors are utilized essentially in two basic configurations: tubular and beaker. In the beaker type system, the feed wastewater and the biocatalyst are placed in a beaker, which serves as the reaction vessel. A u-shaped bundle of fibers immersed into the beaker and product is continuously filtered through the membranes. Tubular configurations are preferred in large-scale industrial applications where the biocatalysts can be loaded or trapped either in the shell side (annular space between the membrane fibers and the housing) or the tube side of a tubular membrane module. If the biocatalyst is trapped inside the membrane tube, the feed substrate is pumped through the shell side. The pumping rate has to be controlled to maintain a residence time within the membrane tubes for total biodegradation. This type of bioreactor has been tested on industrial scale for bioremediation activities, for the removal of aromatic pollutants and pesticides.

### *Membrane Separation Bioreactors*

The activated-sludge process is the most widely used aerobic wastewater treatment system to treat both municipal and industrial wastewater. Its operational reliability is one of the major reasons for the success of this technology. However, the quality of the final effluent from this treatment system is highly dependent on the hydrodynamic conditions in the sedimentation tank and the settling characteristics of the sludge. Consequently, large-volume sedimentation tanks offering several hours of residence time are required to obtain adequate solid/liquid separation. At the same time, close control of the biological treatment unit is necessary to avoid conditions, which could lead to poor settling ability and/or bulking of sludge.

Application of membrane separation (micro or ultra filtration) techniques for biosolid separation in a conventional activated-sludge process can overcome the disadvantages of the sedimentation and biological treatment steps. The membrane offers a complete barrier to suspended solids and yields higher quality effluent. Although the concept of an activated-sludge process coupled with ultrafiltration was commercialized by Dorr-Oliver in the late 1960s, the application started to attract serious attention over the last ten years.

The biomass separation bioreactor is a combination of a suspended growth reactor for biodegradation of wastes and membrane filtration. In this system, the solid-liquid membrane separation bioreactor employ filtration modules as effective barriers. The membrane unit can be configured either external to or immersed in the bioreactor.

Figure I.10 schematically represents the various stages of development of this MBR system for biological wastewater treatment. The conventional approach to attain reusable quality water from an activated-sludge process is by applying tertiary treatment techniques, such as multimedia filtration and carbon adsorption, on biologically treated secondary effluents. As a first step, these tertiary treatment methods were replaced with membrane (ultra/micro) filtration, which ensures almost bacterial- and viral-free effluent in addition to colloids and solid removal without modifying existing treatment facilities. This type of coupling of membrane technology provides good quality effluent.

Later, in view of utilizing membrane technology more effectively, the secondary sedimentation tanks were replaced with cross-flow membrane filtration. Here membranes are placed in an external circuit, where the biomass is circulated at a higher velocity on the membrane surface. The higher energy cost to maintain the cross-flow velocity led to the development of

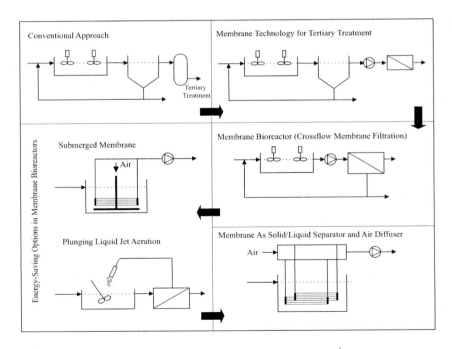

FIGURE I.10. Developments in membrane separation bioreactors

submerging externally skinned membranes in the reactor itself and withdrawing the treated water through the membranes. As a further attempt at energy saving in membrane-coupled bioreactors, the possibility of using jet aeration in the bioreactor was introduced. The main feature of this bioreactor is that the membrane module is incorporated into the liquid circulation line for the formation of the liquid jet, thereby accomplishing both operations of aeration and membrane separation using only one pump. After passing through a gas layer, the liquid jet plunges into a liquid bath, entraining considerable amounts of air. Recently, the invention of the air back washing technique for membrane de-clogging led to the novel approach of using the membrane itself as a clarifier as well as an air diffuser.

The major advantages of the membrane separation bioreactors are as follows:

- Because suspended solids are totally eliminated through membrane separation, the settling ability of the sludge, which is a problem in conventional activated sludge, has absolutely no effect on the quality of the treated effluent. Consequently, the system is easy to operate and maintain.
- Sludge retention time (SRT) is independent of hydraulic retention time (HRT). Therefore a very long SRT can be maintained, resulting in complete retention of slowly growing microorganisms, such as nitrifying bacteria, in the system.
- The overall activity level can be raised, since it is possible to maintain high concentrations in bioreactors while keeping the microorganisms dispersed as long as desired. As a result, reactor volume will be reduced. In addition, the system requires neither sedimentation nor any posttreatment equipment to achieve reusable quality water, so the space-saving potential is enormous.
- Treatment efficiency is also improved by preventing leakage of undecomposed polymer substances. If these polymer substances are biodegradable, there will be no endless accumulation of substances within the treatment process. On the other hand, dissolved organic substances with low molecular weights that cannot be eliminated by membrane separation alone can be taken up, broken down, and gasified by microorganisms or converted into polymers as constituents of bacterial cells, thereby raising the quality of treated water.
- Removal of bacteria and viruses can be expected, so the disinfection process is ecologically sound.
- Compared to conventional activated-sludge processes, maintaining a low F/M (food/microorganisms) ratio will produce less excess sludge to be handled and treated.

- The fluctuations on volumetric loading have no effect on the system. Hence a high sludge capacity can be maintained.
- Because all process equipment can be tightly closed, no odor dispersion will occur.

Table I.5 presents the overall performance of immersed MBR systems in terms of influent and effluent concentrations. Considering the guidelines and criteria for reclaimed water use for various purposes in Japan, the effluent of MBR comply with every aspect of the reported values. In this pilot-scale unit, it was also noted that the reactor performance was not affected at various operating conditions. This indicates that the improvement in membrane flux can result in undisturbed water quality even at a hydraulic retention time of three hours, thus reducing the size of the treatment unit. The effectiveness of the process was proven, since both effluent turbidity and pathogen removal were detected below drinking water standards. If necessary, a small dosage of chlorine could be added to maintain a residual chlorine concentration in the distribution system of the main water supply.

TABLE I.5. Comparison of reclaimed water quality of the MBR with reuse guidelines

| | Concentration | | Criteria/guidelines | | |
| | | | Toilet flush | Landscape | Environmental |
| Parameters | Influent | Effluent | water | irrigation | water |
| --- | --- | --- | --- | --- | --- |
| Total coliform (count/mL) | $>10^7$ | ND | $\leq 10$ | ND | ND |
| Fecal coliform (count/mL) | $>10^5$ | ND | – | – | – |
| Chlorine residual combined (mg/L) | – | – | TA | $\leq 0.4$ | – |
| Appearance | NP | NU | NU | NU | NU |
| Turbidity (NTU) | $>1000$ | $<0.3$ | – | – | $\leq 10$ |
| Biological oxygen demand (BOD) (mg/L) | 295-375 | $<4$ | – | – | $\leq 10$ |
| Odor | NP | NU | NU | NU | NU |
| pH | 7.6-8.5 | 7.3-8.4 | 5.8-8.6 | 5.8-8.6 | 5.8-8.6 |
| Chemical oxygen demand (COD) (mg/L) | 530-625 | $<25$ | – | – | – |
| Total Kjeldahl nitrogen (TKN) (mg/L) | 26-165 | $<3$ | – | – | – |
| Total nitrogen (TN) (mg/L) | 26-165 | $<6$ | – | – | – |
| Total phosphate (TP) (mg/L) | 2.2-9.0 | 0.2-4 | – | – | – |
| Color (Hazen color unit) | $>5000$ | $<30$ | – | – | – |

Source: Criteria/guidelines adapted from Japan Sewage Work Association, 1993.
NP = not pleasant; NU = not unpleasant; ND = not detected; TA = trace amount

## CONCLUSIONS

This review of membrane bioreactors for the application of wastewater treatment has shown that this emerging technology has developed a niche in the wastewater treatment sector. Whereas research efforts of late have been directed toward application of membrane separation bioreactors to various wastewaters, the next step in their development would be to develop a membrane bioreactor process that is both robust and efficient for various wastewater applications.

## SUGGESTED READINGS

Asano T, M Maeda, and M Takaki (1996). Wastewater reclamation and reuse in Japan: Overview and implementation examples. *Water Science Technology* 34 (11):219-226.

Belfort G (1989). Membranes and bioreactors: A technical challenge in biotechnology. *Biotechnology and Bioengineering* 33:1047-1066.

Gunder B (2001). *The membrane coupled activated sludge process in municipal wastewater treatment.* Lancaster, PA: Technomic Publishing Co.

Japan Sewage Works Association (JSWA) (1993). *Sewerage in Japan—Its status and plans.* Tokyo, Japan: JSWA.

Stephenson T, S Judd, B Jefferson, and K Brindle (2000). *Membrane bioreactors for wastewater treatment.* London: IWA Publishing.

Visvanathan C, R Ben Aim, and K Parameshwaran (2000). Membrane separation bioreactors for wastewater treatment. *Environmental Science and Technology* 30(1):1-48.

# Rotating Biological Contactors

S. N. Upadhyay
P. K. Mishra
B. N. Rai

## INTRODUCTION

Rotating biological contactors (RBCs) or "biodiscs" are attached microbial growth bioreactors consisting of an assembly of equally spaced (2 to 3 cm apart) molded polyvinyl chloride or polystyrene foam discs (up to about 4 m in diameter) mounted on a metallic shaft. The disc-shaft assembly is mounted inside a semicylindrical vessel (basin) containing the wastewater to be treated. Only a portion (about 30 to 40 percent) of the disc surface is immersed in the wastewater. The disc assembly is rotated at a slow speed (1 to 6 rpm). As the discs rotate, microbes grow and attach themselves to the surface and a thick layer of microbial growth is soon established. During the course of rotation a portion of discs alternately comes out of wastewater pool and gets exposed to the air above the disc assembly, which supplies the oxygen needed for microbial assimilation of organic pollutants present in the wastewater. The duration of contact between the microbial growth attached to the disc surface and wastewater is determined by the depth of submergence and speed of rotation. The former determines the duration and the latter the actual time. The depth of immersion is both a design and an operating parameter, whereas speed of rotation is only a design parameter. Although the depth of immersion can be varied by adjusting the overflow weirs, the speed of rotation is prefixed by the manufacturer. The excess microbial growth is sloughed off by the shearing action and is kept in suspension by the mixing caused by the rotation of discs. The flow of treated wastewater out of the unit eventually carries the sloughed microbial biomass into a classifier, where it is separated. RBC basins are usually made of concrete or steel. Steel is preferred for smaller plants. For small installations, RBC drive shafts are oriented parallel to the direction of the flow with disc assemblies separated by baffles. In larger installations, shafts are mounted perpendicular to the flow, with several stages operating in series. In order to avoid excessive loading on the initial units, a step-feed or a tapered-feed system may be used. Two or more parallel flow trains are installed to isolate units for turndown or repair and maintenance.

The RBC system can be a single-stage or a multistage unit. In the single-stage unit, one or more disc assemblies rotate in a single basin, whereas in the multi-stage unit, more than one basin, each containing one or more disc assemblies, operate in series. Better performance has been reported when three or four stages of disc assemblies are used to promote plug flow condition. The final effluent from the unit(s) flows into a secondary clarifier for the removal of suspended solids. Recycling of flow is not essential. Unlike single-stage units, the more easily biodegradable substances are assimilated in the first stage of multistage units, and so on through the final stage. As a result, different microbial populations persist in each stage. Accordingly, the reaction kinetics also progressively change. This characteristic feature of RBC units is used in proliferating *Nitrosomonas* organisms in the final stage to carry out nitrification. Staging also eliminates short-circuiting and dampens shock loadings. If required, the effluent from the nitrification unit is fed into an anoxic RBC unit, where discs are completely submerged in wastewater and covered to operate in anoxic mode. By controlling the hydraulic residence time through recycle, anaerobic conditions and resultant odor nuisance in the denitrification unit can be avoided. A higher recycle rate will prevent anoxic respiration from reaching the completion stage.

The major advantages offered by RBC systems include large surface areas and short contact periods (<1 h), capabilities to handle a wide range of flows (3 to 400 million l/d), no requirement for recycling, good settling characteristics of sloughed microbial biomass, and low operating costs. Lower energy requirements, ease of maintenance, and a modular nature are the major advantages of RBC units over activated-sludge or trickling filter units, making RBCs attractive for several industrial wastewaters. Further, because the microbial growth is exposed to air 50 percent of the time, these units can treat concentrated wastewaters without becoming anaerobic. A properly designed RBC unit is generally quite reliable because of the large amount of microbial biomass present, and can withstand hydraulic and organic shock loads more effectively. The land requirement is quite small (<0.1 $m^2$/person per d) if no sludge disposal is on site. Head loss is quite low, making RBC units suitable for flat terrain. The unit may be covered, if desired, and forced ventilation should be provided to take care of possible malodor.

Two serious problems are (1) physical failure of the shaft or drive assembly that runs the assembly and rotates the shaft, and (2) odor nuisance usually encountered in RBC installations, which can be prevented by appropriate design and proper operation. Past experience of the designer and manufacturer with operating units helps in selecting proper material for the shaft and an appropriate drive system to avoid such failure problems.

Odor problems usually occur due to excessive microbial slime growth on the discs, resulting in the bridging of air gap between adjacent discs. This prevents air (or oxygen) from entering into the interior space and results in anoxic or anaerobic conditions, causing formation of $H_2S$, volatile organic acids, and other malodorous compounds. Due to volatile acids, the pH becomes acidic and reduces the solubility of $H_2S$, which escapes to the atmosphere as a gas, causing odor problems. This can be prevented by preventing the slime layer from bridging the gap between the discs. One way of achieving this is by bubbling air below the disc assembly. The bubbles travel up through the space between the discs and maintain the aerobic condition in addition to disrupting the growing microbial layer. In an alternative method, a small amount of $H_2O_2$ is added to kill the odor-causing anaerobic microbes.

## PROCESS MODELING

The attached microbial growth model under reaction controlling state can be readily adopted to RBCs. Assuming a well-mixed liquid phase in contact with the disc surface, absence of mass transfer limitations, and applicability of the Monod model, a material balance on the substrate gives

$$QS_i - QS_e - \frac{\mu_m X_b S_e}{K_s + S_e Y} V_b = 0, \qquad (1.34)$$

where, $K_S$ is the substrate constant, $Q$ is the steady-state flow rate, $S_i$ and $S_e$ are the biological oxygen demand (BOD) levels in inlet and exit wastewater flows, respectively, $\mu_m$ is the maximum specific cell growth rate, $V_b$ is the volume of active biomass on the disc surface, $X_b$ is the concentration of active biomass, and $Y$ is the yield factor. Here,

$$V_b = aV \delta, \qquad (1.35)$$

where $a$ is the biofilm surface area per unit volume of liquid, $\delta$ is the thickness of active biomass film, and $V$ is the liquid volume in the basin. Thus,

$$Q(S_i - S_e) - \left[ \frac{\mu_m X_b S_e}{(K_s + S_e)Y} \right](aV\delta) = 0. \qquad (1.36)$$

Substituting $P = \mu_m \delta X_b / Y$, Equation (I.36) gives

$$\frac{S_e}{S_i} = \frac{1}{1 + \dfrac{Pa\theta}{K_s + S_e}}, \qquad (I.37)$$

where, $\theta$ is the liquid residence time, $(V/Q)$.

For liquid velocities below 0.8 m/s, the external diffusion is the rate limiting reaction, and the overall rate will be controlled by the transfer of substrate to the liquid-biofilm interface. The mass balance across a microbial-liquid film element gives

$$QS_i - QS_e - K_l a\left( S_e - S_f \right)V = 0. \qquad (I.38)$$

Here, $a$ is the specific surface area, $K_l$ is the mass transfer coefficient, and $S_f$ is the substrate concentration at the interface. Due to fast reaction, the substrate concentration $S_f$ at the interface would be zero. Hence, from Equation (I.38) comes

$$\frac{S_e}{S_i} = \frac{1}{1 + K_l a\theta} \quad \text{and} \qquad (I.39)$$

for an RBC unit having $N$ stages with the same liquid residence time

$$\frac{S_e}{S_i} = \left( \frac{1}{1 + K_l a\theta} \right)^N. \qquad (I.40)$$

Attempts have been made to further improve the previous models by considering substrate removal by microbial suspension in a liquid pool. However, the removal by the microbial growth attached to the surface is much greater than that by the suspended biomass. Due to the complex nature of the process and difficulty in establishing values of kinetic parameters, the design of RBC units is still largely based on empirical approaches and past experience.

## PROCESS DESIGN

The design parameters required for the selection of an off-the-shelf RBC unit are

1. organic loading rate (kg BOD per 1000 m$^2$ disc surface per day);
2. hydraulic loading rate (m$^3$/day);

3. number of stages;
4. number of shafts per stage;
5. diameter of discs (m);
6. number of discs per shaft;
7. depth of submergence of each rotating disc assembly (m);
8. rate of rotation of each shaft (rps); and
9. hydraulic retention time for each stage (day).

A wide range of loading rates and liquid residence times are encountered in practice. Thus, knowledge about the degree of success and problems of operating units helps in deciding the required organic and hydraulic loading rates. The designer's own judgment and manufacturer's recommendations should be taken into account in deciding about these parameters. Efficiency of removal in various successive stages, past experience with operating units, and other relevant parameters are used to determine the required number of stages. It should be kept in mind that the first stage, which removes the most easily degradable organics, needs the most oxygen. The following stages are characterized by successively lower reaction rates: hydraulic retention time, depths of submergence, and speed of rotation. Each stage's reaction rate should be appropriate to have maximum efficiency.

Usually one or more proprietary systems are selected, the design procedures laid down by the manufacturers are carefully examined, and required wastewater characteristics are established. A full-scale wastewater characterization may be in order for existing wastewater generating systems, but an appropriate estimate will have to be carried out for new industrial units. Staging of the RBC units, loading criteria, and settling tank requirements also need to be considered.

The RBC units cannot be designed following the approach used for activated-sludge systems because neither the active biomass nor the sludge age can be determined. For this reason, the amount of soluble BOD removal per unit surface area for each stage is taken as a design parameter. The design of RBCs is comparatively simple and straightforward compared to activated-sludge units. Most industrial wastewaters have soluble BODs of 150 mg/l or more and two-stage units are needed. The first stage should have enough surface area to reduce soluble BOD to 50 mg/l or less for mechanically driven units and 70 mg/l or less for air-driven units at the corresponding surface loading rates. For a high strength wastewater, the rate of oxygen input to the first stage or influent end of the disc section is not sufficient enough to metabolize the large amount of substrate diffusing into the microbial film. The BOD removal rate is maximum and the process follows a zero order kinetics. At some intermediate point in the basin or in the next stage, the BOD is reduced to a point that more than enough oxygen is available for metabolization and the process shows a first or second order behavior. The BOD level at which zero order behavior is exhibited and maximum substrate removal is obtained varies with the type of wastewater drive and method. For mechanically driven units, it generally starts at 50 mg/l soluble BOD and for air-driven units at 70 mg/l. The corresponding surface loading rates are 12.206 kg/1000 m² (2.5 lb/1000 ft²) and 14.65 kg/1000 m² (3.0 lb/1000 ft²), respectively. The second stage is designed to reduce the BOD (50 or 70 mg/l) to the desired effluent value. The required number of stages for a soluble BOD level of <10 mg/l is three to four, for 10-15 mg/l it is two or three, and for 15-25 mg/l it is one or two. Above this level a single-stage unit is used. Manufacturers usually provide process design curves for helping in arriving at such decisions.

The RBC systems have a much higher microbial cell density than trickling filters and thus require less surface area for cell support. The thickness of microbial growth on the disc surface can be controlled more efficiently and is usually kept at around 2 to 4 mm. The biomass concentration attached to the disc surface is as high as 50,000 mg/l, and on being sloughed off from the surface provides a suspended microbial cell concentration of 10,000 to 20,000 mg/l. At such a high microbial cell concentration, the degree of BOD removal is very high even with a relatively short retention time. This high biomass also permits RBC units to withstand hydraulic and organic shocks more effectively.

The shear force achieved in RBC units is larger than that in trickling filters. Typically the Reynolds number of water mass moving past the disc surface varies from around 8,000 at the outer perimeter of the disc to around 5,000 at the inner edge of the microbial growth on the surface. This exerts more shearing force than in trickling filters, and, in turn, results in reduced mass transfer resistance for oxygen and substrate and increased BOD removal rates. On the average, BOD removal rates in RBC units are two to three times greater than in standard trickling filters.

The disc media selected for assembling the RBC unit should have a sufficiently large surface area. The media could be packed up to 8 to 9 m long on a single shaft and can have up to 9000-10,000 m² of surface area. High density media, having 50 percent more surface area than conventional media, are also available, but are unsuitable for high strength wastewater because microbial overgrowth leads to clogging. However, they are useful for low strength wastewater and for nitrification.

*Disc Drive*

The disc assembly is rotated either by a geared electric motor belt or chain drive or by air buoyancy. In air-driven units, discs are provided with buckets on the outer rim to trap air bubbles rising into them from the air bubblers. The buoyancy of the air causes the buckets to move up and the discs to rotate. This is similar to the rotation of a water wheel in reverse, in which the buckets are under water and receive air. The air bubbles also help in aeration in addition to that taking place through the unsubmerged disc surface exposed to the atmosphere. Air-driven units have several advantages over gear-chain/belt-driven units. They are simpler in design and easy to maintain, provide increased BOD removal due to higher DO concentrations, have thinner microbial growth due to increased shearing, lead to increased shearing due to rising bubbles, and provide increased operating flexibility through variation of speed by varying air input rates. Air-driven systems are, however, less efficient than the mechanically driven units when it comes to power consumption. Power requirements increase exponentially with decreasing hydraulic loading. For a given BOD removal and/or nitrification efficiency, RBC units need less power than required for other comparable processes.

## NITRIFICATION AND DENITRIFICATION

Nitrification requires additional stages/units. The first two stages/units are similar to those described previously and provide the surface area required for reducing the BOD to a level capable of promoting growth of nitrifying bacteria. The surface area required for nitrification depends upon the ammonia-N concentration. For wastewaters with high total Kjeldahl nitrogen (TKN) content, hydrolysis of soluble TKN to ammonia-N is an important design factor. For wastewaters with TKN < 100 mg/l, it is expected that half of the TKN should get hydrolyzed to ammonia. This value should be added to the influent TKN for design purposes. For wastewaters with high TKN (>100 mg/l), it would be appropriate to generate data through pilot units. Because the retention time is so short, organic-N does not have enough time to degrade to ammonia and passes through the unit. A part of organic-N, however, is adsorbed on the biomass, flocculates, and is removed in the final clarifier. The biodegradable ammonia-N is converted to nitrate, which depends on the ammonia-N concentration in the effluent and not on TKN. This occurs when the TKN:$NH_3$-N ratio is not more than 2 percent. For ratios higher than this, other design considerations are observed.

In general, biodegradable ammonia-N appears only when the soluble BOD value drops down to less than 15 mg/l. Under this condition, the ammonia removal rate is directly proportional to ammonia concentration, and up to 5 mg/l ammonia-N is possible. However, hydraulic loading is important and staging is required. For obtaining effluents with ammonia-N concentration above 5 mg/l, the ammonia-N mass loading is the important design criteria and staging is of no use. It has been established that the optimum basin volume is 0.18 l/m$^2$ of media. Increasing the volume beyond this amount will not increase removal rates. However, decreasing the basin volume below this value will decrease removal rates.

The RBCs can also be used for denitrification. This is accomplished by completely submerging the disc assembly in wastewater and adding an organic substance as the carbon source. The microbial growths on the disc surface and in suspension utilize the nitrates formed by nitrification as an oxygen source and reduce them to nitrogen. Denitrifying bacteria grow on the discs in anoxic or reduced oxygen conditions. No sludge circulation is required. Staged systems give better treatment. Surface loading of denitrifying units varies with influent and effluent nitrate-N concentrations.

The organic carbon source required for denitrification should be cheap and readily available. Methanol is generally added for this purpose. Stoichiometrically, 2.5 mg/l of methanol per mg/l of nitrate-N reduced is required. In practice, however, this amount is around 3 mg/l per mg/l of nitrate-N removed, because the facultative organisms, which grow in the system due to some oxygen entering the denitrification unit with nitrified influent, consume some of the methanol. The anoxic unit can precede the aerobic unit, thus reducing or eliminating the requirement of a carbon source. Here the biodegradable organics in the influent themselves become the carbon source. Recycling the effluent from the aerobic unit to the anoxic unit increases the process efficiency. Pilot tests have indicated that at a recirculation rate of 200 percent, 70 to 80 percent nitrogen removal is possible, resulting in an effluent with 5 to 10 mg/l of total nitrogen. For mixed or purely industrial wastewaters, a pilot test is required. Most sludge is produced up to the nitrification stage only. No sludge is produced during denitrification. An estimate of sludge production can be made using an appropriate design graph provided by manufacturers. The sludge separator (secondary clarifier) is similar in design and operation to that used for activated-sludge systems.

## EFFECT OF TEMPERATURE

Between 13 to 32°C, there is no effect of temperature on the performance of RBC units. Above 32°C, the decrease in oxygen solubility causes a decrease in performance. Further, the microbial population also shifts from more efficient mesophilic to less efficient thermophilic organisms. RBC units operating in cold climates should be enclosed to prevent heat loss and freezing and to avoid the negative impact of low temperatures on the microbial growth rate. In hot climates, covers are recommended to avoid photosynthesis, resultant algal growth, and UV-mediated degradation of disc media.

BOD removal, nitrification, and denitrification all are temperature-dependent processes, and thus a temperature correction may be required. To compensate for temperature effects, the surface area required for RBC may need to be modified. Manufacturers provide surface area correction factor graphs for this purpose.

## CONCLUSIONS

Rotating biological contactors (RBC) are attached microbial growth bioreactors. They are modular in nature and are specially suited for small communities, army units, camping sites, picnic places, etc. An RBC consists of large plastic discs mounted on a horizontal shaft. The disc assembly rotates slowly with approximately 40 percent submergence. A 1 to 4 mm thick layer of biomass grows on the media. As the discs rotate, they carry a film of wastewater through the air, resulting in oxygen and nutrient transfer into the biofilm. Additional removal occurs as the contactor rotates through the liquid in the tank. Shearing forces cause excess biomass to be stripped from the surface of the media in a manner similar to the trickling filter. This biomass is removed in a clarifier. The attached biomass is shaggy with small filaments, resulting in a high surface area for organic removal to occur. The primary variables affecting performance are rotational speed, disc submergence, wastewater retention time, staging, and temperature. Increasing the rotational speed increases contact, aeration, and mixing, and would therefore improve efficiency. However, increasing rotational speed rapidly increases power consumption, thus an economic evaluation should be made between increased power consumption and increased aeration.

## SUGGESTED READINGS:

Arceivala SJ (1998). *Wastewater treatment for pollution control*. New Delhi: Tata McGraw-Hill Pub. Co.

Benefield LD and CW Randall (1980). *Biological process design for wastewater treatment*. Englewood Cliffs, NJ: Prentice-Hall.

Eckenfelder WW, Jr. (1989). *Industrial water pollution control*. New York: McGraw-Hill Book Co.

Stephenson RL and JB Blackburn Jr. (1997). *The industrial wastewater systems— Handbook*. Boca Raton, LA: Lewis Publishers.

Sundstorm DW and HE Klei (1979). *Wastewater treatment*. Englewood Cliffs, NJ: Prentice-Hall.

# Trickling Filters

B. N. Rai
P. K. Mishra
S. N. Upadhyay

## INTRODUCTION

Trickling filters are attached microbiological growth packed-bed bio-reactors. They are made of steel or concrete tanks that are round, square, rectangular, etc., with perforated bottom, and are filled with a packing media. Wastewater, fed into the filter at the top of the packed media by a distributor device, trickles down the media's surface. Air flows up from the bottom, through the media, and supplies the oxygen. Although air blowers can be used to maintain an upward flow of air, natural circulation of the air is maintained due to metabolic heat generated in the unit. Some trickling filters employ horizontal flow, referred to as *cross-flow.*

Up to the 1950s, the packing media used in trickling filters was made of stone pieces of 2.54 to 10.16 cm in size. Stone, coal, or slag is still used, but packing media made of polymeric materials are becoming popular. Trickling filters employing stone pieces as packing media are normally 1 to 3 meter in depth, whereas those using plastic packings are normally 2 to 14 meters deep.

The wastewater distribution device mounted over the top of the media can be either stationary or movable. A grid of stationary nozzles, supplied with the wastewater by pumps, is common with trickling filters that use plastic media. Rotary distributors are normally used with both stone media and plastic media. The rotary distributor is fed from the center of the circular filter. The wastewater coming out from one side of the distributor arm provides the reactive force to rotate the distributor, thus providing an uniform distribution of wastewater over the top of the filter bed media.

The contact time between the trickling wastewater and the microbiological film can last from a few minutes to about an hour. The organic pollutants present in the wastewater are transferred to the microbiological film, where biodegradation and synthesis of new cells occur and the end products are carried out with the trickling wastewater stream. Cell synthesis leads to an increase in the microbiological film thickness, which eventually sloughs off and is carried out of the filter by the effluent wastewater stream.

Depending upon hydraulic and organic loading rates, trickling filters can be classified into low-rate and high-rate filters. When these are used for pretreatment prior to treatment in an aeration unit, they are referred to as *roughing filters*. Low-rate trickling filters are best used for treating wastewater from small communities or single residential units, where simple and stable operations are required. Packing materials used in these units are usually rock, gravel, slag, etc., and bed depth is of the order of 2 to 3 meters. An inflow system is a simple piping system or dosing siphon. These units are specially suited for poor communities located on high-altitude, hilly terrain and where energy conservation is required.

High-rate trickling filters are more commonly used for treating domestic sewage from large communities. They involve more mechanization due to pretreatment and postfiltration settling, continuous sludge withdrawal, recirculation pumping, etc. Excess sludge also needs further treatment. Figure I.11(a) shows a secondary treatment unit incorporating a trickling filter, and I.11(b) shows the schematic configuration of the trickling filter unit. Both stone and plastic packing media can be used. In the case of stone media, filter depth is generally limited to 3 m to support ventilation. Plastic media have more void spaces and deeper beds; up to 12 m deep can be used. This reduces land requirements and makes these units attractive for industrial wastewaters. Removal efficiency depends upon BOD load, recirculation rates, media, etc., and is typically in the range 65 to 85 percent.

## RECIRCULATION

It is essential to regulate the operation of a trickling filter for controlling the thickness of the microbial growth layer. If the microbial growth is too thin, the number of microorganisms will be too few to cause effective treatment. The flow rate of wastewater down the filter will be too fast to reduce contact time, hence lowering the degree of treatment. If the microbial growth is too thick, the reduced free space in the media impedes wastewater and airflow rates. For efficient operation of the trickling filter unit, a proper balance between organic and hydraulic loading rates is required. This is realized by recycling a part of the treated effluent from the unit.

Figure I.12 shows recirculation patterns in single- and two-stage trickling filters. By regulating the recycle rate, it is possible to regulate both hydraulic and organic loading rates, as well as microbial growth thickness. The recirculation ratio, R (ratio of the fresh influent wastewater flow to recycle flow), is usually in the range of 0.5 to 6.0, with 1.0 being more common. For domestic wastewaters, R greater than 2 is uneconomical.

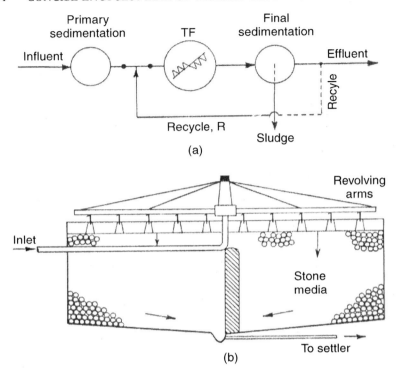

FIGURE I.11. Secondary treatment unit incorporating a trickling filter

The odor nuisance mentioned earlier is minimal during normal operation of the trickling filter. The outer aerobic growth is capable of oxidizing malodorous compounds forming in the inner anoxic/anaerobic microbial layer. However, when the organic loading rate is too high with respect to the hydraulic loading rate, the microbial growth becomes too thick, and the air flow rate becomes too low to meet the oxygen requirement of the aerobic oxidation in the outer aerobic layer, causing an odor problem. This problem can be overcome by increasing the recycle rate and causing hydraulic shearing of the microbial growth to reduce its thickness.

## PROCESS MICROBIOLOGY

Microbial fauna in the packing media growth includes aerobic, anaerobic, and facultative bacteria, fungi, algae, and protozoa. Higher species,

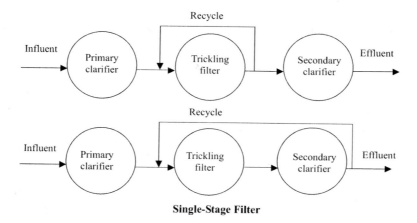

**Single-Stage Filter**

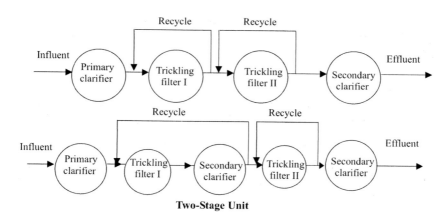

**Two-Stage Unit**

FIGURE I.12. Various recirculation patterns in trickling filters

such as worms, insect larva, and snails are also present. The individual population of the biological community varies throughout the depth of the filter due to changes in organic loading, influent wastewater composition, pH, temperature, air availability, etc. The predominant microorganisms, however, are facultative bacteria. *Achromobacter, Flavobacterium, Pseudomonas,* and *Alcaligenes* are the common bacterial species found in the growth. Filamentous species such as *Sphaerotilus natans* and *Beggiota* are present in the slime layer, where growth conditions are adverse. *Nitrosomonas* and *Nitrobacter* are present in the lower reaches of the unit.

Fungal species such as *Fusarium, Mucor, Penicillium, Geotrichum, Sporotrichum,* and various yeasts are also present. These can poliferate at low pH or with certain industrial wastewaters and may clog the filter and restrict the ventilation.

In the upper layers of the media, where sunlight is available, algal species such as *Phormidium, Chlorella,* and *Ulothrix* predominate. They add oxygen to the wastewater percolating down the unit, and thus take part in the treatment indirectly. However, they can cause the filters to clog and may lead to odor nuisance.

Ciliate protozoan species, including *Verticella, Opercularia,* and *Epistylis* predominate in trickling filters and help in controlling the bacterial population. Insects, snails, and worms feed on the biological films and keep the bacterial population in a state of rapid growth. High-rate trickling filters normally do not have these animal forms. Snails, if present in the nitrifying filters, consume most of the growth of the nitrifying bacteria.

## PROCESS MODELING AND DESIGN

Hydraulic and organic loading rates and the degree of treatment are some of the important factors that must be considered for predicting the performance of trickling filters. Theoretical mass balance approach-based models and empirical models based on field data are used for this purpose.

### Theoretical Models

Mathematical modeling for trickling filter performance can be done using two different approaches: (1) reaction controlling and (2) mass transfer controlling.

#### Reaction Controlling

Let us consider a trickling filter unit as sketched in Figure I.13. For a differential element of filter bed of thickness $dz$, mass balance on the substrate gives

$$QS - Q(S - ds) - \frac{\mu_{max}X_b\delta aS}{Y(K_s + S)}Adz = 0. \qquad (I.41)$$

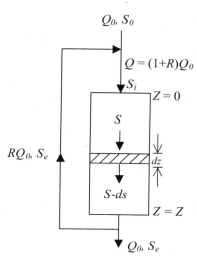

FIGURE I.13. Schematic diagram of a trickling filter with a differential bed element

Here $a$ is area of packing per unit volume of the filter, $\mu_{max}$, $Y$, and $K_s$ are the kinetic constants, $X_b$ is the concentration of active biomass, $\delta$ is the thickness of the active biomass layer, and $A$ is the area of cross section of the filter unit. The active biomass film thickness depends upon BOD and hydraulic loadings. A higher BOD loading will give rise to a thinner aerobic zone due to oxygen depletion, and a higher flow rate will result in a thicker aerobic zone. Formation of an anaerobic zone will cause $CH_4$ and $H_2S$ to release resulting in odor problems. A hydraulic loading of 15 to 150 l/m$^2$ per min (0.4 to 4.0 gal/min per ft$^2$) is generally used. The presence of larvae indicates good working conditions. From Equation (I.41) comes

$$Qds - \frac{\mu_{max} X_b \delta aS}{Y(K_s + S)} A dz = 0. \tag{I.42}$$

For $S_0 > 500$ mg/l, $\delta$ is constant and integration of Equation (I.42) after separating the variables gives

$$K_s ln \frac{S_i}{S_e} + (S_i - S_e) = \frac{A\mu_{max} a\delta X_b Z}{QY} \tag{I.43}$$

or

$$ln \frac{S_e}{S_i} = \frac{S_i - S_e}{K_S} - \frac{PaAZ}{QK_S},$$ (I.44)

where

$$P = \frac{\mu_{max} \delta X_b}{Y}.$$ (I.45)

For $S_o < 500$ mg/l, $\delta = \delta_o$ and from Equation (I.42) we get

$$Qds - \frac{\mu_{max} X_b \delta_o S^2 aAdZ}{Y(K_s + S)} = 0.$$ (I.46)

Integration after separation of variables gives

$$ln \frac{S_e}{S_i} = K_S \left( \frac{1}{S_e} - \frac{1}{S_i} \right) - \frac{paAZ\hat{e}}{Q_o}.$$ (I.47)

*Mass Transfer Controlling*

It is assumed that diffusion into the microbial growth layer controls the rate of reaction and no concentration gradient exists across the liquid film. Mass balance on the BOD across the differential element of the unit gives

$$QS_o - Q(S - dS) + k_l aA(S - S_f)dZ = 0.$$ (I.48)

Here $S_f$ is the BOD value at the film surface. This gives

$$Qds = -k_l aA(S - S_f)dZ.$$ (I.49)

Under mass transfer limitation $S_f = 0$, hence integration after separation of variables gives

$$ln \frac{S_e}{S_i} = -\frac{k_l aZ}{\left( \dfrac{Q}{A} \right)}.$$ (I.50)

For turbulent flow,

$$k_l \alpha \left( \frac{Q}{A} \right) = k_o \left( \frac{Q}{A} \right)^m,$$ (I.51)

where $m$ varies from 0.5 to 0.7

$$ln \frac{S_e}{S_i} = -\frac{k_o aZ}{\left(\dfrac{Q}{A}\right)^n}, \qquad (I.52)$$

where $n$ varies from 0.3 to 0.5 or

$$\frac{S_e}{S_i} = e^{-\left[k_o aZ/(Q_o/A)^n\right]}. \qquad (I.53)$$

Due to oversimplification and inherent limitations, these approaches are not that popular in practice.

### *Empirical Approaches*

Several empirical approaches can also be used for designing a trickling filter system. For domestic wastewaters, past experience with an operating unit is used for designing a new unit. However, for industrial wastewaters, laboratory studies followed by studies with pilot-scale units are recommended. Several manufacturers have mobile pilot-scale trickling filter units, which are operated on sites for a few months to generate the data needed for designing larger units.

### *NRC Equation*

Data collected from a large number of trickling filter units at military installations were analyzed during the 1940s to develop an empirical method. This approach is suitable for domestic wastewater as well as for wastewater from some food processing units. The BOD removal efficiency is given by

$$E_1 = \frac{100}{1 + 0.44\sqrt{\dfrac{W}{VF}}} \qquad (I.54)$$

where $E_1$ is percent BOD removal efficiency, $W$ is organic loading rate (kg/day), $V$ is volume of filter media (m$^3$), and $F$ is the recirculation factor. The recirculation factor, $F$, is given by

$$F = \frac{1 + R}{\left[1 + \left(\dfrac{R}{10}\right)\right]^2}, \qquad (I.55)$$

where $R$ is recirculation ratio ($=Q_r/Q$), $Q$ is influent flow rate (liquid flow rate per min [LPM]), and $Q_r$ is recycle flow rate (LPM). For the second stage Equation (I.52) will become

$$E_2 = \frac{100}{1 + \dfrac{0.44}{(1-E)}\left(\dfrac{W'}{VF}\right)}, \tag{I.56}$$

where W' is the organic loading rate applied to the second stage. These relations are applicable to single- and multi-stage rock filter units with varying recirculation rates.

Wastewater characterization is done to determine organic loading. For new industrial installations, the organic loading is determined using the information from an existing plant, having similar wastewater characteristics. The National Research Council (NRC) equation yields reasonably good estimates for domestic wastewater having a temperature near 20°C. At other temperatures, the estimated efficiencies will be significantly different for a given organic loading rate.

*Eckenfelder's Approach*

Eckenfelder developed an empirical design approach by analyzing data from laboratory and full-scale trickling filters having various types of plastic packing media, and treating various industrial wastewaters. The proposed equation is

$$\frac{S_e}{S_i} = \exp\left[-Ka^{m'}Z(Q_a)^{-n'}\right], \tag{I.57}$$

where $Z$ is the depth of the trickling filter, $K$ is a reaction rate constant, $m'$ and $n'$ are empirical constants, $Q_a$ is surface loading rate ($= Q/A$). The parameter $K$ is specific for a given depth of trickling filter. It would be appropriate to add here that Equation (I.57) is essentially similar to Equation (I.53). The local rate of removal decreases with the increasing depth; consequently the localized value of $K$ decreases with increasing depth. Deeper filter units have better BOD removal. This results in a higher $K$ value. The rate of increase in the value of $K$ declines with increasing depth. This declining rate of increase in overall reaction rate can not be predicted without laboratory and pilot-scale data. Thus, the $K$ values calculated using the data for a particular depth obtained with a working unit are applicable only for that filter. Empirical constants $m$ and $n$ are specific for the operating conditions, temperature, depth, wastewater, and filter media used for generating the data. Published data available in the literature can, at best, serve as guidelines, but are not useful for designing a new system or retrofitting an existing system, unless all the physical and operating conditions are the same.

### Trickling Filters As Roughing Units

Quite often trickling filters are used to reduce or "knock down" the BOD of industrial wastewaters prior to main biological treatment. The robust nature, better relative resiliency, and requirement of little operator's attention make trickling filters a cost-effective method for reducing BOD prior to additional biological treatment.

Trickling filters are operated at high hydraulic loading rates to avoid creating anaerobic conditions and odors. Usually, high recycle rates are used for this purpose. Roughing filters have also been used to absorb "shock" loads resulting out of occasional spills, daily washings, and accidents. In this situation trickling filters protect the main treatment unit.

Roughing filters remove the most easily biodegradable organics, thus their effect on the reaction kinetics of the main unit must be considered. At high hydraulic loading rates and the higher microbiological growth rates, sloughing of biomass is relatively high and this also needs to be considered in the design of the main unit. Roughing filters pirmarily use plastic media, and typical operating depths are 12 to 14 m.

### CONCLUSIONS

Trickling filters are attached microbial growth bioreactors, in which the microorganisms grow on a solid support (or media). The media could be made of a variety of materials, e.g., rock, plastic, wood slab, etc. As the wastewater flows over the microbial growth-covered bed of media, organic pollutants and other nutrients diffuse into it and are used as food for the microorganisms. Oxygen from the air also diffuses into the microbial growth. This aerobic processes reduces the quantity of pollutants in the wastewater. Attachment of the microbial growth on a solid medium provides a much higher cell density than realized in suspended-growth bioreactors. This permits the use of a smaller bioreactor compared to suspended growth, as well as provides very low specific growth rates. Trickling filters are useful when the influent BOD load is high and the system needs a high cell density for efficient biodegradation. Due to attached growth, enough microorganisms remain in the system and it is less susceptible to flow fluctuations.

## SUGGESTED READINGS

Benefield LD and CW Randall (1980). *Biological process design for wastewater treatment.* Englewood Cliffs, NJ: Prentice-Hall.

Grady CPL, Jr. and HC Lim (1980). *Biological wastewater treatment: Theory and applications.* New York: Marcel Dekker.

Metcalf and Eddy, Inc. (1991). *Wastewater engineering: Treatment, disposal and reuse,* Third edition. New York: McGraw-Hill Inc.

Saren E (1980). *Plastic packed trickling filters.* Ann Arbor, MI: Ann Arbor Science Publications.

# Waste Stabilization Ponds

P. K. Mishra
B. N. Rai
S. N. Upadhyay

## INTRODUCTION

Waste stabilization ponds are shallow earthen basins used for wastewater treatment through natural aerobic and anaerobic processes. The term *oxidation pond* is synonymous with waste stabilization ponds. Their low construction and operating costs offer significant advantages over other biological wastewater treatment techniques and make them specifically suited for small communities and tropical countries. Waste stabilization ponds are also used extensively for the treatment of industrial and mixed wastewaters. For some industrial wastewaters, it may be necessary to supplement nitrogen and phophorous sources from outside. These elements are used in oil refineries, slaughterhouses, dairies, poultry plants, rendering plants, etc.

## CLASSIFICATION OF POND SYSTEMS

Waste stabilization ponds are classified according to the nature of microbial activity taking place within them, such as aerobic, anaerobic, or facultative (aerobic-anaerobic). Sometimes the type of influent (untreated, screened, or settled wastewater or activated-sludge effluent), the pond overflow condition (non-existent, intermittent, continuous), and the method of oxygenation (photosynthetic, atmospheric, surface reaeration, or mechanical aeration) are also used as the basis for classification. Table I.6 lists types of waste stabilization ponds and their applications.

### Aerobic Ponds

Aerobic waste stabilization ponds are large, shallow earthen basins that are used for the treatment of wastewaters by natural algal-bacterial symbiosis. They are useful primarily for the treatment of soluble organics and effluents from wastewater treatment plants. In these ponds, algae and bacte-

TABLE I.6. Types and applications of waste stabilization ponds

| Type of Pond System | Common Name | Identifying Characteristics | Application |
|---|---|---|---|
| Aerobic | Low-rate pond | Designed to maintain aerobic conditions throughout the liquid depth | Treatment of soluble organic wastes and secondary effluents |
| | High-rate pond | Designed to optimize the production of algae cell tissue and achieve high yields of harvestable protein | Nutrient removal, treatment of soluble organic wastes, conversion of wastes |
| | Maturation or tertiary pond | Similar to low-rate ponds but very lightly loaded | Used for polishing effluent from conventional secondary treatment processes, such as trickling filters or activated sludge |
| Aerobic-anaerobic (oxygen source supplemental aeration) | Facultative pond with aeration | Deeper than high-rate pond Aeration and photosynthesis provide oxygen for aerobic stabilization in upper layers. Lower layers are facultative. The bottom layer of solids undergoes anaerobic digestion. | Treatment of screened untreated or primary settled wastewater or industrial wastes |
| Aerobic-anaerobic (oxygen source algae) | Facultative pond | As above, except without supplemental aeration Photosynthesis and surface reaeration provide oxygen for upper layers. | Treatment of screened untreated primary settled wastewater or industrial wastes |
| Anaerobic | Anaerobic lagoon Anaerobic pretreatment pond | Anaerobic conditions prevail throughout, usually followed by aerobic or facultative pond. | Treatment of municipal wastewater and industrial wastes |
| Anaerobic followed by aerobic-anaerobic | Advanced Integrated Wastewater Pond System (AIWPS) | Combination of pond types described above Aerobic–anaerobic ponds may be followed by an aerobic pond. Recirculation frequently used from aerobic to anaerobic ponds. | Complete treatment of municipal wastewater and industrial wastes with high bacterial removal |

ria are in suspension and aerobic conditions prevail throughout the basin. For their energy needs, aeorbic waste stabilization ponds depend primarily on solar insolation. Climatic conditions and geographical locations govern availability of solar insolation.

Aerobic waste stabilization ponds are of two basic types. In the first type, the production of algae is maximized, hence the ponds are shallow with depth varying from 0.15 to 0.45 m. In the second type, photosynthetic oxygen production is maximized. These ponds are about 1.5 m in depth. In both pond types, oxygen enters the wastewater through atmospheric aeration. In order to improve performance, periodic mixing of pond contents using pumps or surface aerators is also carried out. The pond cross-section could be circular, rectangular, or square. The bottom of the pond should be level and impervious. Inlet to and outlet from the pond should be appropriately located to avoid a short circuit.

In addition to algal species, other biological communities present in waste stabilization ponds are similar to those persisting in activated-sludge systems. Dissolved oxygen in the wastewater and atmospheric aeration are used by the bacteria in the aerobic biodegradation of organic pollutants. The carbon dioxide and nutrients (phosphate and sulphate) produced through this process are used by the algae. Higher species—rotifers and protozoa, that are present in the pond help in the polishing of the treated wastewater. In aerobic ponds, the upper aerobic layer predominates.

Organic loading, degree of mixing in the pond, pH, nutrients, sunlight, and temperature are important factors, that control the presence of algal, bacterial, and animal species. Solar irradiance and temperature have a profound effect on the pond's performance, particularly in cold climates. Depending upon location, the hydraulic detention time may vary from 20 to 50 days.

The soluble BOD removal efficiency is up to 95 percent. The presence of algae and bacteria in the treated effluent may exert a higher BOD load than the original wastewater. Thus algal species must be carefully removed before discharging the treated effluent into a receiving water body.

A number of factors affecting pond performance make it difficult to analyze this system mathematically, however, some efforts have been made. The system's design is still based on empirical approaches and data obtained from pilot plants and full size operating units. Organic loading rates and hydraulic retention times are used as design parameters. Large units are designed as ideal, well-mixed bioreactors using two or three bioreactors operating in a series. In another approach, a first order rate expression using a nonideal flow situation is used. A graphical design method has also been developed.

### Facultative Ponds

Facultative ponds are the most common pond systems. In these treatment ponds, aerobic, anaerobic, and facultative bacteria stabilize organic wastes.

Facultative ponds have been used for the treatment of domestic wastewaters and a wide variety of industrial wastewaters for decades. The wastewater, which has received only preliminary treatment from septic tanks and anaerobic treatment ponds, can be successfully handled in faculative ponds.

Facultative ponds have three zones: (1) an upper aerobic surface zone, where algal-bacterial symbiosis helps in biodegradation, (2) a partly aerobic and partly anaerobic zone in the middle, where biodegradation of organic waste is carried out by facultative bacteria, and (3) an anaerobic bottom zone, where organic sludge is digested by anaerobic bacteria.

Conventional facultative ponds are earthen basins that are 1 to 3 m deep. The effective liquid depth may vary from about 0.9 to 2.0 m. Hydraulic detention time varies from 20 days (in warm climate) to 180 days (in cold climate). Screened or comminuted wastewater or effluent from the primary settling tank is filled into this basin. Larger solids settle at the bottom of the basin as a sludge layer and are digested anaerobically. This results in the production of soluble organics and gases, such as $CO_2$, $H_2S$, and $CH_4$, which are either oxidized by the aerobic bacteria or released into the atmosphere. Using the oxygen produced by the algae growing abundantly near the surface of the pond, colloidal and soluble organic pollutants are biologically degraded by aerobic and facultative bacteria. Carbon dioxide produced during biodegradation serves as a carbon source for the algae.

Photosynthetic activity of algal species and surface reaeration supplies oxygen to the upper layer. Under certain situations, surface aerators are also used, and algae has no role to play. Such systems can handle higher BOD loadings. However, the BOD load must not exceed the amount of oxygen that can be supplied by the aerators without disturbing the bottom and middle zones.

The microbial species in the upper aerobic zone are similar to those in an aerobic pond. The middle and bottom zones have facultative and anaerobic organisms. Respiration also occurs in the presence of sunlight, however, the net reaction is the production of oxygen. The simplified photosynthetic and respiration reactions are as follows:

Photosynthesis
$$CO_2 + 2H_2O = (CH_2O) + O_2 + H_2O \tag{I.58}$$
$$\text{(new algal cell)}$$

Respiration
$$CH_2O + O_2 = CO_2 + H_2O \tag{I.59}$$

Use of carbon dioxide by algae in photosynthesis results in high pH, especially in wastewaters with low alkalinity. Under several conditions, algae in facultative ponds use carbon from bicarbonate ions for cell growth, causing high diurnal variation in the pH. As the pH increases, the alkaline components change, and carbonate and hydroxide alkalinity tend to predominate. In wastewaters with high $Ca^{2+}$ concentration, calcium carbonate will precipitate when the product of $CO_3^{--}$ and $Ca^{++}$ concentrations exceeds the solubility limit. This precipitation helps in keeping the pH constant.

Facultative ponds are capable of handling small flows (equivalent to 5,000 or fewer persons per day), concentrations of effluent, and flow fluctuations, and have long retention times. The surface loading may vary from 16 to 80 kg BOD/d/ha. The treatment system may have a single facultative pond or several ponds in parallel or series.

Despite the great deal of work on facultative ponds and development of equations for their design, no universal design equation exists. Windy conditions mix the wastewater mass and resuspend the settled solids, making the use of a design equation difficult. Thus, facultative ponds are usually designed on the basis of loading factors developed from field experience.

Design methodology for facultative ponds is, in fact, similar to that of aerobic ponds. The dispersion factor for these ponds varies from 0.3 to 1.0 to permit settling of solids. Sludge accumulation controls oxygen requirements and overall performance of the faculative ponds. During the winter, some of the influent organic pollution remains in the settled sludge. During spring and summer, this pollution degrades anaerobically, producing acids and gases that put a heavy demand on dissolved oxygen. Under such situations, surface aerators, capable of providing oxygen to satisfy 175 to 225 percent of incoming organic pollution, should be used. Accumulated sludge reduces the performance of facultative ponds and more solids remain in a suspended state.

Heat and wind affect the degree of mixing in the pond. Mixing helps in minimizing hydraulic short-circuiting, and formation of stagnant regions, and in ensuring reasonably uniform distribution of BOD, $O_2$, and algae. Wind-induced mixing depends upon the extent (fetch) to which air is in unobstructed contact with water. This is usually 100 m for effective wind-induced mixing.

If the temperature is >15°C, the sludge building in the bottom is controlled through anaerobic activity. The sludge layer's thickness is usually ≤ 250 mm. Desludging is required once or twice every 10 to 15 years. For temperatures >22°C, the evolution of methane gas is sufficiently rapid. Rising gas bubbles take up sludge particles, which form a mat on the surface that will have to be removed to allow light penetration.

If the depth is <1 m, vegetation grows and the pond becomes a breeding ground for mosquitoes and midges. For depths >1.5 m, oxypause is too close to the surface and the pond becomes predominantly anaerobic. In arid climates, the depth is increased to 2 m and the surface area is reduced to minimize evaporation losses. At higher altitudes, deeper ponds help in storing the thermal energy of incoming wastewater.

A hot climate is ideal for pond operation. For design purposes, the mean temperature of the coldest month is used as the design temperature.

*Recirculation*

Recirculation of pond effluent improves the performance of ponds operating in series. The recirculation rates vary from 0.5 to 2.0 times the fresh wastewater flow rate of influent. Occasionally internal recirculation is also used. If three facultative ponds are used in series, the normal mode of operation involves recirculation of effluents from the second or third pond to the first pond. The same methodology is followed if the first facultative pond is replaced by an anaerobic pond.

Waste stabilization ponds may be used in parallel or series mode to achieve special objectives. Series operation is performed for high levels of BOD or coliform removal. The algal concentration and the resultant order and turbidity in the influent from facultative ponds operated in series are lower than those operated in parallel. Multiple-pond systems, operating in parallel or series, also provide either complete treatment or retention with water evaporating into the air or percolating under the ground. Parallel units permit better distribution of settled solids. Smaller ponds permit better circulation and less wave action. The cost of additional equipment for both configurations is low.

## Maturation Ponds

Maturation ponds are low-rate aerobic stabilization ponds that permit the polishing of secondary effluent and seasonal nitrification. The residual microbial species are endogenously respired, and ammonia is converted to nitrate using oxygen supplied from surface reaeration and algal photosynthesis. Fecal bacteria and viruses are killed by the inhospitable environment. The cyst and ova of intestinal parasites settle to the bottom and die off. However, the BOD removal is small. A detention period of 18 to 20 days has been found to be the minimum period required to provide for complete endogenous respiration of the residual biological solids. Greater than 99.99 percent destruction of coliforms is possible with proper design. In order to maintain aerobic conditions, the applied loadings should be quite low. If properly designed, aerobic conditions can be maintained up to 3 m. For design convenience, the depth is normally kept the same (1 to 1.5 m) as in facultative ponds.

## Anaerobic Ponds

Anaerobic wastewater treatment ponds are used for the treatment of high BOD wastewaters that also contain a high concentration of solids and are usually completely devoid of oxygen. These ponds are much deeper earthen basins than aerobic or facultative ponds. The typical depth is 2 to 4 m. The solids present in the wastewater settle to the bottom and are digested anaerobically. The clarified wastewater is transported to the next unit, usually a facultative pond, for further treatment. A temperature greater than 15°C and pH greater than 6 is essential for effective operation.

Anaerobic activity persists throughout the depth of the basin, except for the upper shallow surface zone. A combination of precipitation and anaerobic biodegradation of organic wastes to $CO_2$, $CH_4$, other gaseous end products, organic acids, and new cells removes BOD. The average BOD conversion efficiency is about 70 percent, and under optimum conditions it could be as high as 85 percent. Usually anaerobic ponds are used in combination with facultative ponds to provide complete treatment.

## Advanced Integrated Wastewater Pond System (AIWPS)

AIWPS consists of a series of four ponds designed to perform one or more of the best basic wastewater treatment processes.

### Facultative Pond (FP)

The first AIWPS unit is a facultative pond with an aerobic surface and an extremely anoxic pit for sedimentation and fermentation. Anaerobic microbes in the pit are protected by surrounding walls from the intrusion of cold surface water containing dissolved oxygen. Raw sewage is introduced directly into the pits, where sedimentation and methane fermentation occur. Overflow velocity in the pits is maintained at such a low level that suspended solids removal approaches 100 percent and BOD removal approaches 70 percent. A low overflow velocity of 1 to 2 m/d results in the settling of helminth ova and parasitic cysts, which are thus permanently removed from the effluent. Chlorinated hydrocarbons are converted into forms that may be biodegradable in an anaerobic environment. Due to the large pit volume and reducing environment, settled solids ferment to a point where only an ashlike material remains. Hardly any sludge removal is needed.

*High Rate Pond (HRP)*

The second pond of the AIWPS series is a paddle wheel-mixed shallow raceway called a high rate pond. Microalgae grow profusely, releasing oxygen from the water by photosynthesis. Bacteria utilize this oxygen to oxidize most of the soluble and biodegradable BOD remaining in the effluent from the facultative pond.

Because algae produced during paddle wheel mixing are highly settleable, the remaining water after algae removal by sedimentation has a BOD that is generally less than 20 mg/l. The recirculation of algae-bearing water from a high rate pond to a facultative pond provides an oxygen-rich cap on the facultative pond. This oxygen quickly oxidizes reduced gases emerging from the fermentation pit, thus reducing the odor. It also reduces the presence of mosquito larvae. The algae, which is recycled to the facultative pond, absorbs the heavy metals in the incoming effluent pond and settles there. Thus HRPs provide the benefit of high BOD removal, low consumption of energy, and further absorption of metals.

*Algae Settling Pond (ASP)*

The third pond in AIWPS series is an algae settling pond. Algae, which settle, tend to hibernate and thus do not immediately decompose or produce nuisance. Two settling ponds can be used in tandem. One or the other can be drained or dried every three or four years to remove concentrated algal sludge. This dried algal sludge is rich in nitrogen, phosphorous, and potassium, and hence is an excellent fertilizer for fast-growing plants. No evidence has been found of infectious organisms, but to be on the safe side, this sludge should be used on ornamental plants and crops that are not eaten raw.

The waters emerging from ASPs are sufficiently low in BOD and suspended solids (SS) to be used for irrigation. They are, however, likely to contain a most probable number (MPN) *(E. coli)*>1000 per 100 ml, and hence may require additional storage prior to use.

*Maturation Pond (MP)*

The primary function of a maturation pond is to store the reclaimed effluent and improve further its quality by the continued die-off of bacterial pathogens by time and exposure to UV radiation.

The AIWPS combines the simplicity and reliability of ponds while managing their disadvantages. Table I.7 compares AIWPS with other techniques of wastewater treatment. The AIWPS provides special advantage for

TABLE I.7. Comparison of waste stabilization ponds (WSPs) and advanced integrated wastewater pond systems (AIWPSs)

| WSP | AIWPS |
|---|---|
| The basic mechanism of BOD removal in WSP and AIWPS is essentially the same; however, AIWPS is more efficient. | |
| Pathogen removal varies from 4-log units to nearly 100 percent, generally 4-logs. | Pathogen removal is superior. |
| Nitrogen removal is 80 percent and phosphorous removal is 45 percent. | Nitrogen removal is nearly 100 percent and phosphorous removal is 63 to 65 percent. |
| Energy is required for sewage pumping and 50 percent recirculation. | Energy is required for sewage pumping and 25 percent recirculation. |
| Around 50 percent recirculation of the treated effluent fermentation pond is required at the inlet end for removing odor. This requires higher energy and piping costs. | Around 25 percent recirculation of the wastewater from the HRP is required for this purpose. This requires lower energy and piping costs. |
| Desludging is required every year. | Desludging has never been done, even after running plants for 30 years. |
| The hydraulic detention time is 12 days. | The hydraulic detention time is higher. |
| Needs about 1.5 ha of land per MLD. | Needs about 1.0 ha of land per MLD. |
| Odor problems occur due to $H_2S$ production in the first unit, i.e., the anaerobic pond. | No such problem. |
| Heavy metals such as Cd, Cu, Zn, Ni, Pb, Cr, and Fe are removed only to some extent. | These metals are removed up to 50 to 92 percent. |
| The anaerobic pond is exposed to the atmosphere and may not have effective anaerobic conditions. It would become facultative once 50 percent of water from the maturation pond is recirculated and mixed in influent. | There is no such problem because the fermentation pits are deep under water and are protected by baffled plastic walls. |
| Algae removal is carried out by filtering through rock filters where the trapped algae decays to produce humus. | Algae is harvested in ASPs and dried under sand filters. It is used as cattle feed or fish feed. |

developing countries such as India. The AIWPS is not only nuisance- and pollution-free, but also cost-effective. Transmission of helminth ova, breeding of mosquitoes, and subsequent diseases are major problems in India. The AIWPS mitigates these problems to some extent. As a system of wastewater treatment, AIWPS deserves special consideration.

## CONCLUSIONS

Waste stabilization ponds or oxidation ponds are shallow earthen basins in which wastewater is treated through natural aerobic and/or anaerobic processes. Due to their low cost of construction and operation, these ponds are especially suited for treating domestic wastewater from small communities and in tropical climates. They are also used for treating wastewater from oil refineries, dairies, poultry plants, slaughterhouses, etc. If properly designed and synthesized, advanced versions (AIWPS) are capable of providing the most efficient and economical treatment with a very high grade of treated effluent.

## SUGGESTED READINGS

Arcevala SJ (1998). *Wastewater treatment for pollution control.* New Delhi: Tata McGraw-Hill Pub. Co. Ltd.

Benefield LD and CW Randall (1980). *Biological process design for wastewater treatment.* Englewood Cliffs, NJ: Prentice-Hall.

Metcalf and Eddy, Inc. (1991). *Wastewater engineering: Treatment, disposal, and reuse* (revised by G Tchobainglous and FL Burton). New York: McGraw-Hill, Inc.

# Microbiologically Influenced Corrosion

R. S. Dubey
S. N. Upadhyay

## INTRODUCTION

Microbiologically influenced corrosion (MIC) is the deterioration of metals by corrosion processes that occur directly or indirectly as a result of metabolic activity of microorganisms. Alternatively, MIC may also be defined as the degradation or deterioration of structures due to the activity of various organisms that either produce aggressive metabolites to render the environment corrosive or are able to participate directly in the electrochemical reactions occurring on the metal surface. The presence of microbial growths or deposits on a metal surface encourages the formation of differential aeration or concentration cells between the deposits and the surrounding environment that stimulate the corrosion process.

In an aqueous environment, biofouling by algae, barnacles, mussels, microbial slime, mosses or seaweeds provides potential microhabitats that may allow proliferation of other bacterial species whose metabolic activity results in localized corrosion beneath the biofilms. Pits observed on the metal surface often contain a soft black product with a strong smell of sulfide. This type of corrosion is caused by sulfate-reducing bacteria (SRB). Another significant microbial corrosion problem is associated with buried metals. In freshwater transmission pipelines, the first indication of the problem may be excessive tuberculation on the inner side of the pipe.

Biofouling and MIC can affect nearly all materials. Microbial corrosion is a significant cause of corrosion of underground structures, especially pipelines. According to one estimate, nearly 50 percent of all metal corrosion worldwide is caused by MIC. Sulfate-reducing bacteria are associated with the corrosion of 70 percent of all the seriously corroded water mains. Some industries affected by microbial corrosion are listed in Table I.8. In the petroleum industry, well casings, pumps, oil tanks, refinery equipment, and gas storage tanks may be seriously corroded as a result of SRB. The cor-

TABLE I.8. Microbial corrosion in some industrial activities

| Industry | Problem areas |
|---|---|
| Chemical processing units | Stainless steel tanks, pipelines, and flanged joints, particularly in welded areas after hydrotesting with natural river or well waters |
| Nuclear power plants | Carbon and stainless steel piping and tanks; copper, nickel, and stainless steel; brass, aluminium, bronze cooling water pipes and tubes, especially during construction, hydrotest, and outage periods |
| Onshore and offshore oil and gas installations | Mothballed and waterflood systems; oil and gas handling systems, particularly in environments soured by sulfate-reducing bacteria (SRB)-produced sulfides |
| Underground pipelines | Water-saturated clay-type soils at near neutral pH with decaying organic matter and a source of SRB |
| Water treatment plants | Heat exchangers and pipelines |
| Sewage collection and treatment | Concrete and reinforced concrete structures |
| Highway maintenance | Culvert piping |
| Aircraft | Aluminium integeral wing tanks and fuel storage tanks |
| Metal working units | Increased wear from breakdown of cutting fluids and machining oil |

*Source:* Based on Dexter, 1987, p. 118.

rosion of aircraft fuel tanks and lower-wing skin panels is a serious problem for aircraft operators and related industries. Microbes can invade any fuel tank because air, water, or the fuel itself can carry spores. Such spores can grow rapidly inside a tank if the temperature is appropriate and water is present.

Some environmental conditions help in predicting the involvement of microorganisms in the corrosion process. These are

1. proper environment—suitable pH values ranging between 4 to 9 (some sulphur oxidizers tolerate a lower pH), temperature generally below 50 to 60°C, approximately redox conditions, and an appropriate nutrient for the activity of the microorganisms;
2. morphology and chemistry of corrosion products; and
3. changes in the environment due to microbial activity, e.g., marked changes in pH in either an acidic or alkaline medium.

## BIOFOULING

Biofouling and MIC are mediated by microorganisms attached to a metal surface that is embedded in a gelatinous organic matrix, commonly called the biofilm. The formation of biofilm at the metal/solution interface is initiated with the adsorption of biologically produced organic materials on the metal surface, exposure to some suitable medium, and a supply of microorganisms. The microorganisms can attach to the surface, with growth occurring through the assimilation of nutrients. This growth increases the thickness of the biofilm. Eventually, some of the biofilm is sheared away and reintroduced to the solution to repeat the process of biofilm development.

Typical examples of the microflora identified for biofouling include the filamentous algae chlorophyta and bacteria (*Pseudomonas aeruginosa*, species of *Flavobacterium, Gallionella,* and *Sphaerotilus*). Fungal genera often identified include *Trichoderma, Monilia, Aspergillus,* and *Penicillium*. Almost any type of microorganism that adheres to the metal surface plays a critical role in the corrosion process. The mechanism of the corrosion is simply the formation of differential aeration cells due to the uptake of oxygen by the microbial colony, with the oxygen concentration under such a mass becoming depleted. The poorly aerated surface becomes the anode of the cell, whereas the better aerated regions, away from the deposits, provide the balancing cathodic reactions.

Several parameters govern the adhesion of microorganisms, including suspended substances and, ultimately, the accumulation of biofilms on the surface. Generally, a clean, virgin surface first makes contact with nonsterile water or other liquid having soluble and suspended substances. Microbial cells are transported to that surface before biofilm development can begin. The microbial cells are transported through the resistant, viscous sublayer present near the surface of the substratum by a simple diffusion process. The mass transport of microbial cells and nutrients with suspended organic and inorganic materials in a liquid system occurs through diffusion, as systematically described by Ficks' first law. As the main portion of the biofilm, sessile microorganisms can also influence perturbation in the flow system if microbes are moving faster than the liquid between the regions of the wall. An initial force directs the microbes towards the wall region. Thermal gradients may also contribute to the transport of the microbial cells to or away from the surface. However, molecular diffusion seems to depend more on thermal effects than on the movement of microbial cells. Some chemical species present in the environment influence the transport and attachment to the surface. Sublethal concentrations of the variety of microbial toxicants are also responsible and indirectly play a key role in the development of biofilm on the surface.

Efforts have been made to explain microbial adhesion and its stability in terms of the Derjaguin-Landau-Verwey-Overbeek (DLVO) theory. According to this concept, when a microbe approaches the surface a net force of interaction occurs at the living/nonliving interface. This is due to van der Waals forces of attraction and forces of electrostatic double layer, which have a repulsive effect and directly relate to the nature and size of the microbe and exopolysaccharides (EPS). The nature of biofilm is influenced by the presence of copious amounts of EPSs, and is dependent on the microbial species present beneath the biofilm. EPSs have been shown to influence the physical properties of the biofilm, including diffusivity, thermal conductivity, and rheological properties.

## MICROORGANISMS ASSOCIATED WITH CORROSION

Microorganisms associated with microbial corrosion may be classified into three categories:

1. Aerobic and anaerobic bacteria
2. Algae
3. Fungi

Aerobic bacteria serve one or more functions:

1. Formation of slime
2. Oxidation of sulfide
3. Oxidation of iron
4. Generation of acidic by-products that cause corrosion

Filamentous fungi, algae, protozoa, and diatoms also produce slime. Slime, comprised mostly of extracellular polymers, enhances the growth environment and adherence to the surface. Hydrated biofouling slimes shield the surface, create differential aeration cells, and eventually provide a sheltered environment for anaerobic bacteria to exist and cause corrosion.

### Aerobic and Anaerobic Bacteria

Several aerobic and anaerobic bacteria play active roles in MIC. In the presence of sulfate/sulfide, oxidizers may produce slime that provide a localized anaerobic environment and support SRB.

## Sulfur-Oxidizing Bacteria

*Thiobacillus* spp. are autotrophic aerobic bacteria commonly occurring in soil. They thrive well within 10 to 40°C and at pH 1.5 to 8. Two main species involved in microbial corrosion are *T. thioparus* and *T. thiooxidans*. *T. thiooxidans* are responsible for the degradation of iron, steel, copper alloys, concrete and building stones. The chemical reactions by which these organisms oxidize sulfur and sulfides to produce sulfuric acid responsible for the deterioration are as follows:

$$2H_2S + 2O_2 \rightarrow H_2S_2O_3 + H_2O \qquad (I.60)$$

$$5\,Na_2S_2O_3 + 4O_2 + 4H_2O \rightarrow 5\,Na_2SO_4 + H_2SO_4 + 4S \qquad (I.61)$$

$$4S + 6O_2 + 4H_2O \rightarrow 4H_2SO_4 \qquad (I.62)$$

The sulfuric acid formed by these reactions causes corrosion of metals. Despite its toxicity, copper can also be affected by certain bacteria (e.g., *T. thiooxidans*) that have a tolerance for $Cu^{2+}$. It has been reported that *T. thiooxidans* can tolerate copper concentrations up to 2 percent.

## Sulfate-Reducing Bacteria

*Desulfovibrio* spp. (pH = 4 to 8, temp. = 10 to 40°C), *Desulfotomaculum* spp., and *Desulfomonas* spp. (pH = 6 to 8, temp. = 10 to 40°C) are common sulfate-reducing anaerobic bacteria. *Desulfovibrio sapovorans, Desulfobulbus propionicus, Desulfotomaculum acetooxidans, Desulfomonas acetooxidans, Desulfobacter postgatiae, Desulfosarcins variabiei,* and *Desulfuronema magnum* are newly identified sulfate-reducing bacteria. Iron, steel, and stainless steels are corroded by all sulfate-reducing bacteria. *Desulfovibrio* spp. also attack aluminium, copper alloys, and zinc. These bacteria reduce sulfate to sulfide and $H_2S$ according to the following schematic reactions:

$$SO_4^{2-} + 4H_2 \rightarrow S^{2-} + 4H_2O \qquad (I.63)$$

$$S^{2-} + 2H^+ \rightarrow H_2S \qquad (I.64)$$

The molecular hydrogen used as a reducer in the previous reaction may be the hydrogen that evolved during the corrosion reaction or hydrogen derived from cellulose, sugars, or other organic products present in the soil. Anaerobic sulfate-reducing bacteria present in saturated soils and deaerated cooling waters support relatively high corrosion rates. SRB are the most notorious and harmful of the microorganisms known to enhance corrosion. They are strict anaerobes, although many can survive for long periods as spores under aerated conditions and become activated under favorable conditions. They thrive well in a wide range of environments and may appear as mesophilic, thermophilic, or halophilic strains. The presence of sulfide ions markedly influence both cathodic and anodic reactions occurring on metal surfaces. Sulfide tends to retard cathodic reactions particularly hydrogen evolution, and accelerates anodic dissolution.

### *Iron-Oxidizing Bacteria*

Prominent iron-oxidizing species are *Thiobacillus ferrooxidans* (pH = 1 to 7, temp. = 10 to 40°C), *Gallionella* (pH = 7 to 10, temp.= 20 to 40°C) and *Sphaerotilus* (pH = 7 to 10, temp.= 20 to 40°C). Iron-oxidizing bacteria are aerobic chemolithotrophs and attack iron, steel, and stainless steel by oxidizing soluble $Fe^{2+}$ to less soluble $Fe^{3+}$. *Gallionella* and *Sphaerotilus* also oxidize manganous to manganic and promote tubercule formation. Aerobic *Pseudomonas* sp. (pH = 4 to 9, temp. =20 to 40°C) also oxidize $Fe^{2+}$ to $Fe^{3+}$ and attack iron, steel, and stainless steels. The lower $Fe^{2+}$ activity increases the rate of anodic reaction and iron oxidizers convert significant amount of $Fe^{2+}$ to $Fe^{3+}$ at anode sites leading to the formation of tubercules.

### *Algae, Diatoms, and Fungi*

Algae are a heterogeneous group of chlorophyll-containing plants found in marine water and freshwater. Algae and diatoms are generally found in cooling water systems. Similar to fungi, algae and diatoms adhere to metal surfaces, forming differential aeration and concentration cells and thereby accelerating the corrosion process. Fungi associated with metallic corrosion are filamentous or yeastlike. Branched filaments form a tangled mass generally referred to as *mycelium,* which require oxygen for growth. Energy required for their growth is obtained by aerobic oxidation or anaerobic fermentation of an organic substrate. In general, metabolites such as citric acid and tartaric acid are formed by fungi, and are corrosive in nature. *Cladosporium resinae* (pH = 3 to 7, temp. = 10 to 45°C), cause the corrosion of fuel tanks made of aluminium alloy by degrading hydrocarbons in the fuel and producing acids that dissolve in the contaminating water and attack the fuel body.

## MECHANISM OF MICROBIAL CORROSION

When a metal is immersed in water, damp soil, or other aqueous environment, the initial reaction is the dissolution of the metal as metallic cations, which release an excess of electrons:

$$Fe \rightarrow Fe^{2+} + 2e^- \qquad (I.65)$$

The electrons produced are consumed at a cathodic site, balancing the reaction, which in near neutral solution is usually the reduction of oxygen to hydroxyl ions:

$$O_2 + 2H_2O + 4e^- \rightarrow 40H^- \qquad (I.66)$$

In the absence of oxygen, the usual cathodic reaction for corrosion processes is the reduction of hydrogen as follows:

$$2H^+ + 2e^- \rightarrow H_2 \qquad (I.67)$$

The role of microorganisms is to participate directly or indirectly or in one or both of the previous electrochemical reactions on the metal surface, thereby initiating or exacerbating the reactions responsible for MIC on the basis of metabolism or organisms through the following processes:

1. Absorption of nutrients (oxygen) by microbial growth adhering to the metal surface
2. Liberation of corrosive metabolites or end products of fermentative growth
3. Production of sulphuric acid
4. Interference in the cathodic process under oxygen-free conditions by obligate anaerobes

## CONTROL AND MONITORING OF MICROBIAL CORROSION

Prevention of MIC requires surface cleaning and treatment with biocides to control the bacterial population. Biocide treatment without surface cleaning may not be effective, because chemicals may not reach the inner depths of the microbial film. The choice of biocide depends upon the nature of the microorganisms and surrounding environment.

Cathodic protection can prevent or arrest MIC. It may, however, persist at low cathodic currents at points remote from the anodes or under already established deposits. Cathodic protection systems should be carefully designed with added current capacity to new or freshly cleaned surfaces, especially when biological activity is known or suspected.

### Use of Biocides

Biocides have the ability to kill the organisms or inhibit their growth and reproductive cycles. Biocides perform their functions in various ways. Some biocides alter the permeability of the microbe cell walls, thus interfering with their vital life processes. Others damage the cell by interfering with the normal flow of nutrients and discharge of waste.

Biocides can be classified broadly into two groups: oxidizing biocides and nonoxidizing biocides. In general, oxidizing biocides are used only in freshwater systems because their activities are rapidly changed during the reactions. The nonoxidizing biocides cover a wide variety of chemical compounds that can be used in various environments. Chlorination of freshwater and seawater is effective, and chlorine is less persistent than other biocide systems. Chlorine also has the advantage of easy application as a gas or as salts of hypochlorous acid. Chlorine is the most prevalent industrial oxidizing biocide. It rapidly hydrolyzes in water to form HClO and HCl. At pH 7.5, equal concentrations of HClO and hypochlorous ions (ClO$^-$) exist. Above this pH, ClO$^-$ predominates, with essentially total ionization at pH 9.5. Therefore, chlorine becomes less effective in more alkaline environments. In general, the pH range of 6.5 to 7.5 is considered practical when chlorine is used as a biocide. Lower pH will accelerate corrosion. Continuous treatment levels of 0.1 to 0.2 mg/L are common, but intermittent treatment requires higher levels, typically 0.5 to 1.0 mg/L. Chlorine is both an excellent algaecide and bactericide. However, *Desulfovibrio* can develop a strong resistance, requiring an increase in chlorine concentration or a change to an alternate biocide. Other sources of chlorine are salts of HClO, such as sodium hypochlorite (NaClO) and calcium hypochlorite [Ca(ClO)$_2$]. These salts function in much the same way as chlorine gas.

Another oxidizing biocide is chlorine dioxide (ClO$_2$). This gas does not form HClO in water, but exists solely as ClO$_2$ in solution. It is used more extensively in the pulp and paper industry for bleaching than as a biocide. However, ClO$_2$ is extensively used in cooling waters contaminated with NH$_3$ or phenols due to the low demand for reaction with species such as *Desulfovibrio*. Brominated compounds that form hypobromous acid (HBrO) are very effective over a broader pH range than HClO. At pH 7.5, 50 percent of the HClO is present, but over 90 percent of the HBrO is present. Increasing the pH to 8.7 reduces the HClO concentration to 10 percent, but 50 percent of the HBrO remains. Nonoxidizing biocides can be more effective than oxidizing biocides because of the overall control of algae, bacteria, and fungi. Nonoxidizing biocides also have greater persistence, with many of them being pH independent. 2,2-dibromo-3-nitrolopropianamide (DBNPA) is an organobromine broad spectrum nonoxidizing toxicant. This molecule is an extremely potent bactericide and is only slightly effective as an algaecide. It has little fungicidal activity. The toxicity of DBNPA decreases with an increase in alkaline pH.

Organosulfur compounds include a wide variety of different biocides, of which methylene bisthiocyanate (MBT) is the most common. Their mode of activity is through the inhibition of cell growth by preventing the transfer of energy of life-sustaining chemical reactions from occurring within the cell. MBT is effective in controlling algae, fungi, and bacteria, most notably *Desulfovibrio*. A shortcoming of MBT is its pH range. Therefore, it is not recommended for use in cooling water systems having a pH above 8. Under broader alkaline conditions, sulfur-based biocides, such as bis-trichloro-methylsulfone and tetrahydro-3,5-dimethyl-2H-1,3,3-thiodiazine-2-thione are more appropriate. The former is active in the pH range of 6.5 to 8 and the latter in more alkaline cooling water systems. Isothiazolinone can be used over a broad pH range with no decrease in activity. Some $N_2O_2$ and $N_2S_2$ donor Schiff bases are also found to be effective in controlling the MIC of the metals. Their inhibition efficiency increases with increasing polymethylene chain length. Quaternary ammonium salts are generally most effective against algae and bacteria in the alkaline pH range.

### Use of Microorganisms

As discussed previously, microorganisms influence the corrosion of metals in many ways. The genus *Pseudomonas* is reported to enhance corrosion because of its production of biofilm. Bacterial exopolymers may have metal-ion-binding properties that can affect the metal surface. *Pseudomonas* strain S9 and *Serratia marcescens* have been reported to enhance the corrosion of iron and nickel in comparison to sterile conditions. However, many investigations have shown that the effect of *Pseudomonas* S9 and *S. marcescens* on metals can be dominated by protective factors under certain conditions. The bacterial film may prevent diffusion of corrosive species such as oxygen ($O_2$) to the metal surface, thereby reducing the corrosion rate. Under laboratory conditions, the corrosion rate may be reduced if the metal is immersed in a bacterial suspension. The mechanism of the protective action of microorganisms is not yet fully understood.

### Microbial Corrosion Monitoring by Biosensor

All common electrochemical techniques, e.g., direct current (DC) corrosion measurement, alternating current (AC) impedance, and cyclic voltammetry, can be used for the investigation of MIC, but they are not suitable for online measurements of the metabolic activities of microorganisms. Recently, several biosensors have been developed for online corrosion monitoring in various environments. A biosensor is a type of probe in which a biological component, such as an enzyme, antibody, or nucleic acid, interacts with an analyte, which is then detected by an electronic component and translated into a measurable signal. Enzyme-based biosensors are highly specific for the substrate of interest and are more expensive and unstable. Microbial biosensors are composed of immobilized microorganisms attached to the electrochemical device and are more suitable for the online monitoring of biochemical processes. The microorganism-based biosensors have been developed on the basis of assimilation of compounds by microbes, change in respiration activities, or the production of electroactive metabolites during redox reactions. The detection and confirmation of microbial corrosion is not straightforward because the microbial environment and its effect on metallic corrosion processes are very complex. For analyzing the exact role of factors that influence metallic biodeterioration, online detection techniques are required to obtain quick results about redox reactions occurring at the metal/environment interface. Electrochemical- and other corrosion-monitoring techniques provide useful and quick responses when combined with biosensor technology. The applications of microbial biosensors also have an edge over enzyme-based biosensors due to their low cost and relatively wider specificity for monitoring MIC.

## CONCLUSIONS

Microorganisms play an important role in the corrosion process. Microbial corrosion, for any system, must be treated as an interdisciplinary pursuit. A precise value for biocorrosion is yet to be well established, since corrosion due to chemically corrosive species cannot be separated from microbial corrosion. Laboratory screening and field monitoring are necessary to have success in controlling microbial corrosion. A wide range of products are available for controlling MIC in various environments. Biosensor-based techniques are most suitable for online monitoring of biocorrosion.

## SUGGESTED READINGS

Borenstein SW (1994). *Microbiologically influenced corrosion handbook.* Cambridge, UK: Woodhead Publishing Ltd.

Dexter SC (1987). *Metal handbook,* Volume 13, *Corrosion,* Ninth edition. ASM International.

Dubey RS and SN Upadhyay (2001). Microbial corrosion monitoring by an amperometric microbial sensor developed using whole cell of *Pseudomonas* sp. *Biosensors and Bioelectronics,* 16: 995-1000.

Fontana MG (1987). *Corrosion engineering.* New York: McGraw-Hill Book Co.

Jones DA (1996). *Principles and prevention of corrosion,* Second edition. New Jersey: Prentice-Hall, pp. 372-384.

Videla HA (1996). *Manual of biocorrosion.* New York: Lewis Publisher.

# Treatment of Industrial Effluents

## Distillery Effluent

Poonam Nigam Singh
Tim Robinson
Dalel Singh

### INTRODUCTION

Distilleries for ethanol production are among the biggest water polluters in the world, with 28 to 36 billion liters of effluent produced for every 2.4 billion liters of alcohol per year. Ethanol is produced as a result of the fermentation of sugars, starch, or cellulose. Sugarcane or beet can be fermented to produce rum and grain starch for whiskey or brandy. Although mainly used for alcoholic beverages, ethanol has been produced as a potentially renewable biofuel substitute for petroleum. This has been widely implemented by Brazil.

After the distillation stage, which yields ethanol, a residual liquid waste remains. This effluent, also known as "slops," "stillage," "vinnase," or "dunder," poses disposal problems for distilling industries due to its high volume and poor nutrient content. In a typical distillation process, 10 to 15 liters of effluent is produced per liter of ethanol recovered. Distillery effluent is acidic and dark brown in color, rich in nitrogen and phosphorous, and contains fermentable sugars. Many treatment technologies employed by distilling industries are expensive and their effectiveness is limited, falling short of the national and international standards set for distillery effluents. With government policies on pollution control becoming more and more stringent, distilling industries have been forced to look at more effective treatment technologies, which would not only be beneficial to the environment, but also reduce capitol costs and avoid government penalty fines for ineffective treatments.

## PROBLEMS ASSOCIATED
## WITH DISTILLERY EFFLUENT

The problems associated with disposing of distillery effluent wastewaters are particularly evident in developing countries such as Brazil and India, which produce enormous volumes of ethanol and effluent. In such countries ethanol is produced principally using sugarcane molasses, a by-product of the sugar industry. A substantial quantity of sugar is still present in molasses (~40 percent), but in a form that cannot be recovered or recrystalized by the sugar industry. Bacteria and yeasts are the only microorganisms capable of producing fermentation products from this acidic liquid.

After fermentation of the molasses, a thick acidic effluent remains, which has a high biological oxygen demand (BOD) and chemical oxygen demand (COD). The high BOD and COD indicate the effluent's high pollution potential and its bioremediation resistance. Table I.9 shows the characteristics of a typical distillery effluent. This organically rich effluent must be treated before being discharged into natural water bodies in order to prevent damage to the natural aquatic flora and fauna. Such damage may include eutrophication or photosynthesis inhibition due to the effluent's dark coloration. Untreated effluent released into the natural environment has an effect on the pH and color of the water, while also depleting the available oxygen for natural organisms.

TABLE I.9. Typical composition of untreated distillery effluent

| Parameter | Value |
| --- | --- |
| BOD (ppm) | 50,000-70,000 |
| COD (ppm) | 100,000-120,000 |
| Color | Red/brown |
| pH | 4-5 |
| Specific gravity | ~1 |
| Nitrogen | ~1 percent |
| Phosphates | ~0.03 percent |
| Potash | 0.8-1.0 percent |
| Sulfates | ~0.04 percent |
| Chlorides | ~0.06 percent |
| Total suspended solids | 11-13 percent |
| Ash content | 3-4 percent |

# TREATMENT TECHNOLOGIES

A number of technologies have been explored for reducing the pollution load of distillery effluent. The level of technology used and its effectiveness is dependent on the distillery and ultimately by national and international legislation. The advantages and disadvantages of various effluent treatment technologies can be seen in Table I.10.

## Physiochemical Treatments

The use of physiochemical treatments on distillery effluents has been limited due to their complex and specific nature coupled with high capital costs. The distillery effluent can be treated through evaporation in order to recover the solid organic components. The solids can then be incinerated, yielding energy that is available for recovery. Incineration can also be used to obtain potash or potassium salts that can be used as fertilizer. Considering the economic viability of evaporation and incineration for fertilizer components, it should be kept in mind that handling and transport costs are reduced. However, the amount of energy input required to achieve this ultimate product must also be taken into account.

TABLE I.10. Advantages and disadvantages of various methods used for the treatment of distillery effluent

| Effluent treatment | Advantages | Disadvantages |
|---|---|---|
| Lagooning | Cheap and effective | Foul odor<br>Requires large spaces<br>Effluent held for weeks<br>Requires dilution before discharge<br>Possible groundwater pollution |
| Dilution | Simple<br>No need for holding tanks | Requires large volumes of freshwater |
| Fixed bed | Little biomass production<br>Low energy requirements | Toxicity and pH problems |
| Sludge blanket | Effective for low-strength effluents | Large volume of sludge produced |
| Fluidized bed | High methane production | Foaming and flotation due to gas production |
| Evaporation | Sediment used as fertilizer | Requires large surface area<br>Foul odor<br>Possible groundwater pollution |

The simplest and easiest method of dealing with concentrated effluents is by diluting them with large volumes of freshwater, which would reduce the strength of the salts present as well as the pH and BOD. However, this method is limited by the availability of freshwater, and may therefore not be a plausible option for developing countries in tropical locations. Approximately 150 to 200 liters of freshwater would be required per liter of effluent to produce a satisfactory quality fit for discharge. An advantage of this method is that the effluent does not need to be held in large holding tanks for treatment.

Sedimentation in large tanks is another alternative, but it also has been generally unsatisfactory as settling leads to the production of odorous gases through the formation of anaerobic degradation conditions, which are unacceptable to the environment. Flocculation of the effluent through centrifugation allowed sludge to be recovered for animal feed, but is unpractical for large volumes. Reverse osmosis and electroflocculation have also been attempted with little effectiveness in a large-scale setting.

### Biological Treatments

A typical COD/BOD ratio of 1.8 to 1.9 indicates the suitability of effluents for biological treatment. Moreover, a BOD:N:P ratio of 100:2.4:0.3 suggests that anaerobic treatment methods will be more effective than aerobic methods for reducing the polluting potential of the distillery effluent.

### Lagooning

Distillery effluent treatment by lagooning requires large open or closed holding tanks of 2 to 6 meters in depth with residence time for weeks or months. Decomposition of the organic matter in closed lagoons is exclusively an anaerobic process, but in open lagoons, some aerobic reactions occur on and near the surface. Gaseous decomposition products may be formed as a result of these reactions, and foul-smelling odors are released into the atmosphere. This problem can be remedied by using closed lagoons.

A major limiting factor of lagoons is the requirement of large space in order to treat large volumes of effluent. To help prevent groundwater pollution, lagoons need to be adequately lined, which may in turn add to the cost. Even after lagooning, many distillery effluents are required to be diluted before discharge.

## Anaerobic Biomethanation

This method is similar to lagooning in many respects, in which the effluent is held in large closed tanks. Biomethanation decomposes the organic material anaerobically under controlled conditions. The period of holding is lower for this technology in comparison to lagooning. Methane and carbon dioxide (biogas) are produced as products of the process, which can be utilized by the distillery for fuel. Around 1.5 cubic meters of biogas is produced per kg of organic load. This process allows faster degradation of pollutants with a high percentage reduction in BOD (~85 percent) and COD (~70 percent). The remaining BOD (~15 percent) is difficult to degrade biologically and the effluent is either subjected to a secondary process or diluted before being discharged. Biomethanation can be carried out in either a one- or two-step system:

- *Single-step process:* This is the simplest and cheapest method for biomethanation. The distillery effluent can be fed continuously into a single tank and degraded before being discharged. Biogas is retrieved from the same tank and careful monitoring is required in order to prevent any decline in the rate of the biomethanation process. Typically, a period of 15 days is required for an 80-85 percent reduction in BOD.
- *Two-step process:* This involves separating the production of raw materials for methanogenesis from the organic matter, known as *acidification,* from the actual phase of methanogenesis. This is seen as being advantageous because the degradation of the organic material is more efficient and, therefore, faster than the methanogenesis stage. A disadvantage of the two-step process is cost. Twice as many holding tanks would be required, as well as more space, maintenance, and monitoring. A reduction of ~85 percent in BOD can be achieved in the two-step process.

## Fixed-Bed Reactor

In this system, the microorganisms responsible for the decomposition process are attached to an inert support. The distillery effluent is passed over the bed and excess sludge and treated wastewater is removed simultaneously. An advantage of fixed-bed anaerobic reactors is that biomass production is small, with sludge production less than that from an aerobic system. The electricity requirements for such a system are also less than that required for a similar aerobic process. A two-step reactor may also be employed for a higher degree of COD reduction.

*Sludge Blanket*

In this system, distillery effluent is pumped into the bottom of the reactor via a series of pipes. This allows an even distribution at the bottom of the reactor. Large quantities of sludge tend to accumulate at the bottom of the reactor, forming a highly concentrated deposit. A disadvantage of this system is the buildup of sludge causing variations in sludge concentration in the reactor.

*Moving Bed*

In this system, micororganisms are attached to an inert support that is moved through the effluent. Excess sludge and treated distillery effluent leave the reactor together, with ~70 percent COD being removed. A multiple phase system also exists for increased BOD and COD removals.

## BIOREMEDIATION OF DISTILLERY EFFLUENT

As a secondary treatment procedure, the treated effluent is often diluted before discharge in order to reduce its pollution potential. It can be used for irrigation purposes, although gradual darkening of soil occurs over time. Research in recent years has examined the possibility of combining anaerobic digestion and bioremediation to reduce the COD content as well as decolorizing the effluent. The recalcitrant nature of the effluent is mainly due to the presence of melanoidins. The chemical composition of a typical raw and digested distillery effluent can be seen in Table I.11.

Fungi were initially tested for their ability to reduce the pollution capacity of distillery effluent by effectively removing melanoidins. *Aspergillus* spp. were shown to be capable of decolorizing effluents by removing melanoidins by adsorption to their mycelia. The melanoidin-adsorbed fungi could be isolated from the treated wastewater, dried, and incinerated for power generation.

Bacterial strains have also been used for effective decolorization and degradation purposes. These strains use the nitrogen present in the effluent to grow and simultaneously degrade the melanoidins. The *Lactobacillus* genus has been found to be efficient in this regard, with as much as 30 percent decolorization occurring. A disadvantage of such a process is the requirement of an external source of carbon for the growing cultures, thereby increasing running costs.

TABLE I.11. Comparison of the characteristics of undigested and digested distillery effluent in a typical sample

| Parameter | Undigested effluent | Digested effluent |
|---|---|---|
| pH | 4.4 | 7.5 |
| Density | 1.1 | 1.0 |
| Electrical conductivity | 16.3 | 14.0 |
| Total solids (g/l) | 110.7 | 29.6 |
| Volatile solids (g/l) | 84.5 | 14.2 |
| Total carbon (g/l) | 48.0 | 8.3 |
| Total nitrogen (g/l) | 3.4 | 1.7 |
| Total phosphorus (g/l) | 0.1 | 0.1 |
| Total sugar (g/l) | 25.0 | 12.5 |
| Crude protein (mg/l) | 21.2 | 10.6 |
| COD (mg/l) | 128,000 | 20,600 |

## *RECYCLING TREATED DISTILLERY EFFLUENT*

By-products formed as a result of effluent treatment can be utilized by the distilling industry to help reduce the cost of the actual process. Energy from the treatment process in the form of biogas, which is high in methane content (60 to 70 percent), can be recovered and used for many purposes in the distilling plant, such as for gas-powered appliances. Treated wastewater (with or without dilution), depending on its level of pollutants, may be used directly for irrigation. This is especially beneficial if the distillery uses sugar molasses from a nearby or joint sugar-processing plant. A recycling system that could be adopted by ethanol-producing industries can be seen in Figure I.14. The system allows the high pollutant level of the distillery effluent to be treated effectively while also facilitating the retrieval of energy and useful by-products.

## *CONCLUSIONS*

It can be seen that a wide range of suitable technologies exists for the effective treatment of distillery effluent—spanning from the simple to the more high tech. Anaerobic degradation of this acidic, high BOD, nitrogen/phosphorous-rich waste appears to be the best current treatment. Although many of the treatments effectively reduced the BOD content, it should be emphasized that these processes are still only applicable in a multistage process ultimately involving dilution.

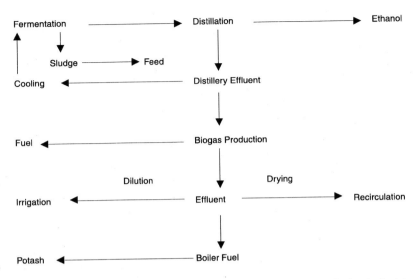

FIGURE I.14. Potential recycling system for distillery effluent-producing industries

Although the initial costs of adopting an ethanol-producing plant for the recycling of by-products is high, this can be achieved by government incentives. Long-term energy savings and valuable by-product recovery means that overhead costs will eventually be reduced.

## SUGGESTED READINGS

Kaul, SN, T Nandy, and RK Trivedy (1997). *Pollution control in distilleries.* Karad, India: Enviro Media.

Singh D, V Kumar, P Nigam, IM Banat, and R Marchant (1998). Microbial decolorisation and bioremediation of anaerobically digested molasses distillery effluent spentwash from methane-producing effluent treatment plants. In *Advances in Biotechnology,* A Pandey (ed.). New Delhi, India: Educational Publishers and Distributors.

Singh D and P Nigam (1996). Treatment and disposal of distillery effluents in India. In *Environmental biotechnology: Principles and applications,* M Moo (ed.). London: Kluwer Academic.

# Pulp and Paper Mill Effluent

Indu Shekhar Thakur

## *INTRODUCTION*

Pulp and paper are manufactured from wood, nonwood fibers, and recycled fibers. The primary raw material in paper manufacture is cellulose fiber, which constitutes 50 percent of wood. The pulp and paper industry is huge and technically diverse, using a wide variety of manufacturing processes on a range of fiber types from tropical hard woods to straw. Worldwide pulp production from wood is $10^6$ metric tons per day, which is also responsible for the discharge of a considerable volume of effluent (200 m$^3$/ metric tons). The product is screened and the chemicals are washed out and recovered. The resulting pulp is frequently bleached to increase the brightness of the finished paper product. The pulp is dried and sent to a paper mill onsite or sold as bales for papermaking elsewhere. Paper manufactured for diversified purposes includes printing paper used in catalogs, books, and magazines; writing paper used for photocopying, computer printing, and other office purposes; kraft paper used for products such as grocery bags and envelopes; paperboard used to make boxboard and container board; and newsprint used to print daily and weekly newspapers, inserts, flyers, and directories.

The paper industry is a notorious polluter of the environment. The wastewater (effluent) from the mill process contains many potentially hazardous chemicals. The most important problem the pulp and paper industries are facing today is disposal of tremendous volumes of wastewater. The effluents are heavily loaded with chlorinated lignosulfonics, resin acid, phenols, and aliphatic and aromatic hydrocarbons, which can have a profound impact on the environment. Numerous physicochemical methods have been used for the treatment of bleach-plant effluents. Although biotechnological methods have the potential to reduce the problems associated with physicochemical methods, major organochlorinated and color-containing compounds are not degraded in the effluent.

## PROCEDURE OF PULPING

The objective of pulping is to separate wood into discrete fibers. The process can be mechanical, thermal, chemical, or a combination of all three. In mechanical pulping, the wood is broken down into fibers (or pulp) by mechanical action. The quality of pulp is low. In chemical pulping, sulfate (kraft) and sulfite are used. This pulping process separates the lignin and wood resin from the cellulose fiber pulp, which is then washed and bleached. Oxygen delignification is the step just before the pulp enters the bleach plant. Its purpose is to reduce the amount of lignin that passes through to the bleach plant and thus lower the bleaching chemical consumption, increase pulp brightness, and reduce waste loading to the wastewater treatment facility. The commonly used kraft process debarks the logs, chips them, and heats the chips in a strong broth of chemicals to separate the fibers from the binding agents in the wood (lignin), producing high-quality fibers. The fibers are then matted together and combined with papermaking chemicals to make a variety of paper products. This process is carried out using a variety of different processes.

## BLEACHING

Chemicals are used to bleach pulps to make the paper white. The bleaching process includes hydrogen peroxide brightening, chlorine bleaching, TCF (totally chlorine free) bleaching, and ECF (elemental chlorine free) bleaching. Bleaching alters the chemical structure of lignin, lightening its color but leaving its presence in the pulp. The most widely used bleach is chlorine. Ozone bleaching offers the ability to produce totally chlorine-free pulp. To ensure the lowest evaluated cost of supplying a mill with ozone, a total mill impact study must be conducted that considers the overall oxygen and ozone requirements and fiber-line constraints. Oxygen alkali extraction (EO) is a stage in a pulp bleach plant in which oxygen is used together with alkali to lower consumption of other, more expensive bleaching chemicals.

## CHARACTERISTICS OF EFFLUENT

The manufacturing steps produce substantial amounts of liquid and other wastes. The effluents of paper-manufacturing industries contain stray wood chips, bits of work, cellular fibers, dissolved lignin, and a wide variety of chemical compounds. Bleaching liquors contain free chlorine and sulphur dioxide. The wastes also contain highly poisonous compounds, such as methyl mercaptans, pentachlorophenol, and sodium pentachlorophenate. They also contain readily settleable solids such as dust, grit, and sand. The major part of this effluent is contributed by pulp washing and bleaching operations. The effluents are strong and dark brown in color, alkaline with a high pH, and possess an appreciable biological oxygen demand (BOD), high chemical oxygen demand (COD), and suspended solids. COD discharge can range from 25 to 125 kg/ton of pulp. The combined effluent from chlorinating and hypochlorite treatments contains chlorine compounds. Recovery plant effluent is a combination of three individual effluents, e.g., effluents from the surface condenser, barometric condenser, and floor washes.

## PROBLEMS RELATED
## TO THE PULP AND PAPER INDUSTRY

The main wastes generated in large, integrated paper mills are as follows.

### Solid Wastes

The major contributors of solid wastes in pulp- and paper-mill effluent are bamboos, wood dust, line sludge, coal ash, fly ash, and other rejects. Of these, lime sludge and ash are generated to the extent of 1,250 to 1,500 kg and 400 to 500 kg per MT respectively of paper produced. Under high-temperature combustion, organic compounds containing carbon, hydrogen, and often chlorine are oxidized. Other substances potentially incinerated include sulfur, arsenic, and metals such as chromium, mercury, and lead. Both the toxic emissions produced during the burning process (sometimes from accidents) and toxic ash left over after combustion are often more hazardous than the original materials. These emissions consist of products of incomplete combustion, escaping heavy metals, and new combinations of materials as a result of the burning process.

### Liquid Wastes

Enormous amounts of wastewater (i.e., effluent) laden with organic matters are generated in pulp and paper mills. They are wood reaction, spent cooking, bleaching chemicals, chlorine compounds (dissolved substances), fibers, and organic compounds (suspended solids). Organochlorine compounds have been a matter of great concern in the pulp and paper industry for the last two decades. These compounds are produced mainly by the reactions between residual lignin present in the wood fiber and chlorine used for bleaching. The fraction of AOX (absorbable organic halogen) that is extractable by a nonpolar organic solvent is referred to as EOX (extractable organically bound halogen), accounts for about 1 to 3 percent of the total organically bound chlorine. This fraction contains relatively lipophilic (i.e., fat-soluble) neutral organic compounds, primarily of low molecular weight. Resin acids, including chlorinated dehydroabietic acid (DhA) are commonly found in pulp and paper mills, as well as in the effluent (230 m$^3$ to 500 m$^3$ water for one ton of paper). Chlorobleaching (using $Cl_2$, $ClO_2$, or other chlorine compounds) of wood pulp causes the formation of chlorinated dioxins and furans, which were found to be produced when certain compounds present in the materials used to manufacture wood pulp reacted with chlorine. Dioxins and furans are persistent and tend to accumulate in sediments and human and animal tissues. In addition, effluent also contains major trace clement such as Hg, Pb, and Cr, depending upon the manufacturing process. The effluents are generally very alkaline and have high chemical and biological $O_2$ demands. Thus, the effluents discharged to the water system make the water unfit for use and cause health hazards.

### Gaseous Emissions

Air pollution from pulp mills is not well studied. Mills usually do not monitor their emissions, such as particulate matter, carbon dioxide, sulfur dioxide, hydrogen sulfide, volatile organic compounds, chlorine, chloroform, and chlorine dioxide. The general gaseous wastes are digester relief gases, digester blow tank and water hood vent gases, chemical recovery furnace emissions, smelt dissolving tank gases, and power/steam boiler emissions. Emissions from pulp and paper mills using the sulfate method of pulping contain malodorous gases, such as mercaptans and hydrogen sulfide. Therefore, odor problems exist in all mills. An increase in temperature of the chlorination resulted in an increase in pollution loadings in chlorination and extraction effluent. An increase in the end pH and temperature of chlorination and chlorine charge increases the formation of chloroform, potential mutagens, and mutagens in the chloroform liquor.

## ENVIRONMENTAL IMPACT
## OF THE PULP AND PAPER MILL

Pulp mills are voracious water users. Their consumption of freshwater can seriously harm habitats near mills, reduce water levels necessary for fish, and alter water temperature. The conventional chlorine bleaching of kraft pulp has been estimated to produce approximately 100 to 300 g of chlorinated phenolic compounds per ton of pulp. Because of extensive chlorination, water bodies receiving such effluents contain different chemical compounds in their sediments. About 300 different chemical compounds have been identified in pulp and paper mill effluents, but these represent only 10 to 40 percent of the total chlorinated organic compounds present. The toxicity of chlorinated compounds increases with increasing numbers of chlorine atoms on the organic compounds. Chlorinated neutral compounds with low molecular masses are major contributors to mutagenicity. This fraction includes chlorocatechols, chloroguaicols, chlorinated vanillins, and syringaldehyde. The toxic and environmentally persistent dioxinlike compounds and coplanar polychlorinated biphenyl (PCBs) arise as trace pollutants in the manufacture of chlorinated organic compounds, chlorinated waste incineration, wood and coal burning, metal recycling, and wood pulp and paper bleaching. Chlorate is yet another pollutant that has recently aroused environmental concern. Pulp mill and bleach plant effluents are highly colored due to polymeric lignin degradation products, and contain chlorinated aromatics.

Chlorinated aromatic compounds are present throughout the ecosystem, in the air, water, and soil, and in the food that humans and animals eat. The effluent, even upon dilution by receiving waters can cause adverse effects on the reproduction and behavior of aquatic organisms. Effluents from pulp mills using bleaching were identified as a priority for assessment of their human health and environmental effects. The impact of pulp mill effluent on human health has not been completely established, but a significant body of knowledge has been gathered on two related classes of compounds of the effluent: phenols, and dioxins and furans. Mill effluent causes reproductive impairment in zooplankton, invertebrates, and shellfish. It also causes genetic damage and immune system reactions in fish. Air discharges from pulp mills contain hormone-disrupting and carcinogenic chemicals, such as chlorinated phenols, polycyclic aromatic hydrocarbons, and volatile organic compounds. Rainbow trout exposed to effluent exhibit signs of distress during the first hours of exposure.

## EFFLUENT TREATMENT IN THE PULP AND PAPER MILL

### Treatment of Air Pollutants

Boilers, furnaces, incinerators, and electrical generating units are common sources of contaminants. Particulates are a major air pollutant from many industries, and improved removal can reduce the impact of the industry. Electrostatic precipitators, thermal precipitators, and bioscrubbers are used for removal of air pollutants from pulp and paper mills. Wet scrubbers are applied to provide more effective removal of very fine particles (0.1 to 2.0 μm radius) from an exhaust gas stream. The research is focused on ways to improve drop size and distribution in a venturi scrubber to optimize particle removal. Postcyclones, which use the energy in an exhaust stream, leaving a cyclone to further remove fine particles, may provide a cost-effective means of improving particle removal. The research involves both laboratory tests and computer modeling of air and particulate movement through the cyclones.

### Wastewater Treatments

Wastewater treatment is divided into pretreatments, primary treatments, secondary treatments, and tertiary treatment.

#### Pretreatment

In a treatment system, the process efficiency of successive stages is interrelated, and hence any upset created in the beginning may affect overall performance of the system. In addition to removing lignin and chlorine compounds, other biotechnological approaches are adopted to remove major toxicants. Pretreatment with fungi, such as *Phanerochaete chrysosporium, Coriolus versicolor, Phellinus pini, Pleurotus eryngii,* and *Lentinus edodes* have significantly reduced pollution. Pretreatment of pulp with xylanase and ligninase enzymes from bacteria and fungi has also been adopted. A commercial preparation from Lignozyme GmbH, Germany has been purified and applied for treatment.

#### Primary Treatment

Primary treatment plants are designed principally to remove suspended matter from wastewater. The large and heavy objects present in the wastewater can obstruct pipelines and pumps, interfere with flow-metering units, or cause other mechanical problems. Screening is used to protect pump values, pipelines, and other appliances from damage by rags and large objects. The screening element may consist of parallel bars. The screen could be distinguished as medium screening with spacing. The wastewater having high suspended solids are allowed to pass through a gravity settling tank. Based on the characteristics of the suspended solids, their concentration and flow, settling may occur in the tank. This is also known as a *clarifier.* Suspended matter with a specific gravity greater than water settles to the bottom of the settling basin and is removed as sludge, whereas particles lighter than water rise to the surface and are skimmed off. In a circular primary settling basin, the influent enters a circular baffled compartment at the center of the tank and flows outward to overflow over a well extending around the basin's periphery. A baffle near the well retains floating scum in the tank. A rotating device moves it to a point where it is withdrawn for treatment and disposal. Sludge settling to the bottom is moved to the center of the tank by flows, suspended from a rotating structure, and pumped to other units for treatment and disposal.

*Secondary Treatment*

The liquid effluents contain thousands of organic and inorganic substances, in soluble and insoluble forms. Controlled populations of aerobic and anaerobic microorganisms degrade complex chemicals into simpler and less harmful compounds and elements. The solid materials in the waste stream are separated out and removed as sludge, which must then receive proper handling and disposal as solid waste. The contaminants in the waste can be divided into two main groups: chlorinated organics and traditionally regulated parameters (e.g., BOD, TSS, toxicity). Chlorinated organics can be further subdivided into two groups: those that are measured as part of AOX and those that are not.

Biological treatment is known to be effective in reducing BOD and simultaneously the toxicity of kraft-mill effluents. It involves lower capital investment and shows better performance for sludge settling, odor control, and removal of colors and refractory organics (nonbiodegradable CODS). Most biological wastewater treatment plants in the pulp and paper industry have traditionally operated within the mesophilic temperature range of 20 to 30°C. However, the feasibility of treating pulp- and paper-mill effluent at higher temperatures (e.g., 40 to 45°C) has been demonstrated. Complete or partial biodegradation of resin acids (a major source of acute toxicity) and chlorophenolic compounds could be achieved. Trichlorophenol, pentachlorophenol, and polychlorinated dibenzo-*p*-dioxins (PCDDs) and dibenzofurans are recalcitrant compounds that are highly toxic. Anaerobic biological treatment can also efficiently destroy chlorophenolic compounds, mutagenecity, and acute toxicity.

As mentioned previously, white-rot fungi produce extracellular enzymes, which can degrade high molecular mass chlorolignins effectively. The culture conditions favoring lignin degradation are similar to fungal decolorization. The addition of carbon and nitrogen improves decolorizing efficiency of the fungus and also results in reduction of the BOD and COD of the effluent. A white-rot fungus, *Tinctoporia borbonica,* has been reported to decolorize kraft waste liquor to a light yellow color. About 90 percent color reduction was achieved after four days of cultivation.

Some enzymes also seem to have the potential to remove color and AOX from pulp- and paper-mill effluents. Lignin peroxidase, manganese peroxidase, and laccase are most important among them.

*Activated-Sludge Process.* The process consists of an aeration tank, solid liquid separator, and recycling sludge pumps. Activated sludge is comprised of 95 percent bacteria and 5 percent of higher microorganisms. The bacteria in activated sludge decompose resin acids, carbohydrate sugars, and complex organic molecules, and reduce BOD. Two types of sludge form depending on how the bacteria form communities: flocs or conglomerates that sink to the bottom, forming a dense sludge and a clear effluent, and filamentous bacteria that develop with fungi. The most dominant type of bacterium is the filamentous *Haliscomenobacter hydrossis,* whose presence is an indicator of low oxygen content. Another less common type of bacterium is the *Thiothrix* spp., a sulfur-based genus. The bacteria are prey to larger microorganisms, including amoeba *(Sarcodina),* free-swimming ciliates *(Ciliata),* stalked ciliates *(Vorticella),* and *Suctoria.*

Immobilized cells can be used for the biodegradation of phenols and chlorinated phenols in a series of batch reactors, including the dechlorination of chlorophenol (CP) compounds using an upflow anaerobic sludge blanket reactor.

*Tertiary Treatment*

Tertiary treatments include precipitation with lime, alum, and metal ions and synthetic polymeric coagulants, adsorption on activated carbon, natural clays and polymeric adsorbents, membrane techniques, rapid filtration on soil, UV irradiation, and oxidation using oxygen, sulfur dioxide, hydrogen peroxide, and sodium hypochlorite. Photodegradation efficiencies of polynuclear aromatic hydrocarbons, chlorinated phenols, and polychlorinated dibenzo-*p*-dioxins are investigated. Aluminum oxide, ferric oxide, and polyelectrolyte assist coagulation of waste in the effluents, which are then sand filtered. Activated carbons saturated with a wide range of organic compounds can be dealt with using this technique. White liquor oxidation (WLO) is a technology that is primarily used in conjunction with oxygen delignification and oxygen alkali extraction. Lime kiln enrichment (LKE) is an economical alternative for increasing lime kiln capacity and/or reducing total reduced sulfur (TRS) emissions from this recovery process. Supplemental oxygen is introduced into the kiln burner to promote more efficient combustion. Black liquor oxidation (BLO) is used in the chemical recovery process to lower TRS emissions (which contribute to the characteristic kraft-mill odor) to levels in compliance with government regulations. The THR (total heat recovery) process is a patented, energy-efficient black liquor-oxidation technology that recovers nearly all of the heat of oxidation to reduce evaporator steam requirements.

## CONCLUSIONS

Pulp and paper mills are using enormous amounts of plant material and depleting our natural resources quite rapidly. The residual lignin molecule combines with chlorine and other chemicals, transformed into highly toxic recalcitrant chlorinated lignosulphonics, resin acid, phenols, aliphatic and aromatic hydrocarbons, dibenzo-*p*-dioxin, and dibenzofuran. Other major pollutants containing coloring materials are not degradable. Biotechnological approaches related to bacteria, fungi, and algae, and more expensive tertiary methods have been adopted recently. However, we still do not have a proper explanation about the degradation of various chemical compounds in the paper mill effluent for controlling pollution.

## SUGGESTED READINGS

Bajpai P and PK Bajpai (1997). Reduction of organochlorine compounds in bleach plant effluent. In *Advances in biochemical engineering biotechnology,* J Scheper (ed.), Vol. 57. Berlin: Springer-Verlag, pp. 213-260.

Leuenberger, C, W Giger, R Coney, JW Graydon, and E Molnar-Kubica (1985). Persistent chemicals in pulp and paper mill effluents: Occurrence and behaviour in an activated sludge treatment plant. *Water Technology* 19:885-894.

Mohn, WW (1995). Bacteria obtained from a sequencing bioreactor that are capable of growth on dehydroabietic acid. *Applied Environmental Microbiology* 61: 2145-2150.

Valenzuela, J, U Burman, R Cespedes, L Padilla, and B Gonzaloz (1997). Degradation of chlorophenols by *Alcaligenes eutrophus* JMP 134 (pJP4) in bleached Kraft mill effluent. *Applied Environmental Microbiology* 63:227-232.

# Removal of Heavy Metals from Wastewater

Wan Azlina Ahmad
Jefri Jaapar
Mior Ahmad Khushairi Mohd Zahari

## INTRODUCTION

Human demands for water may be classified into six groups: domestic use, industrial consumption, agricultural production, recreation, transport, and fisheries. The total amount of water on earth is huge, $1.4 \times 10^9$ km$^3$, but only a fraction of this, represented by $2.9 \times 10^6$ km$^3$ of freshwater, could be utilized for the purposes mentioned previously. This is further restricted by the availability of freshwater and its degree of pollution. Nearly 99 percent of the stock of freshwater is held in glaciers. The remaining freshwater is held in lakes, rivers, the atmosphere, soil, and underground. However, most of these remaining freshwater sources are intensively contaminated and polluted by various wastes produced as a result of human activity.

The disposal of wastewaters became a necessity as soon as humans began to live in organized communities. The development of industries and the installation of water closets led to the development of drainage systems for the removal of offensive wastes from sewage. The original goal of sewage disposal was the removal of waterborne wastes from domestic and industrial communities without causing any danger to health. Disposal does not necessarily include treatment. The principle aim of sewage treatment is to remove as much of the solids content as is practicable and economical, and then to oxidize (and subsequently remove) the colloidal and dissolved solids. When discharged, the effluent should not pollute the stream, be a danger to public health, or cause a local nuisance.

Chemical as well as biological processes have been used to remove heavy metals from wastewaters.

## CHEMICAL REMOVAL PROCESSES

Various techniques have been developed to remove heavy metals from wastewater. Conventional techniques, e.g., solvent extraction, electrolysis, evaporation, cementation, flotation, and stripping, are limited to processing small volumes of water at high concentrations of metal ions. Many technologies are used today to treat large volumes of diluted metal ion-containing solution, i.e., reverse osmosis, membrane filtration, ion exchange, and adsorption. However, these processes are very expensive and require a high level of expertise to operate and maintain the process.

### Adsorption and Ion Exchange

These are the most widely used techniques in wastewater treatment process. Activated carbon, silica sand, coal, and alumina are usually used as an adsorbent. The effectiveness of an adsorbent depends on the adsorptive properties of its surface. Adsorption takes place when a solid surface is contacted with a solution and tends to accumulate a surface layer of solute molecules created by the unbalanced surface forces. Activated carbon has been reported to remove heavy metals such as Cd(II), Zn(II), Hg (I), Pb(II), Ni(II), Cu(II), Pb(II), Cr(III) and Mn(II). However, from the different types of activated carbon found commercially, very few are selective for heavy metals, and they are also very costly.

Ion exchange is a reversible chemical reaction in which an ion from solution is exchanged for a similarly charged ion attached to an immobile solid particle. Most of the resins used are synthetic, made by polymerization of organic compounds in a porous three-dimensional structure. For the purpose of heavy metal removal, a polystyrene matrix-type resin with a chelating functional group is widely used.

The disadvantage of using the heavy-metal-selective chelating resins is their high cost. Ion exchange is not practical to handle multiple waste streams due to the high selectivity of resin.

### Reverse Osmosis (RO) and Membrane Filtration

Reports on the use of reverse osmosis and membrane filtration techniques for heavy metal removal from wastewater are scanty. Both of these techniques are very selective on certain metal ions based on the type of membranes used. Their capability normally does not meet trends toward zero metal limits. Frequent membrane cleaning also creates a new stream in an operational plant. The use of sulfonated polysulfone RO membrane has been reported to remove only Zn(II) and Cu(II) from the waste water. Studies have shown that polyvinylidene membrane with polyethyleneimine and polyvinylalcohol (PVA) as a polymeric macroligands are efficient for removal of heavy metal.

Low-quality feed water fed into the membrane unit may damage the unit. The damage is usually caused by ammonia, chlorine, iron and manganese. A pretreatment step consisting of dechlorination, lime softening or ultra violet radiation is required before the feed water passes through the membrane unit.

## BIOLOGICAL REMOVAL PROCESSES

### Mechanisms

The biological removal of heavy metals from wastewater encompasses two basic mechanisms: biosorption and bioaccumulation.

### Biosorption

The term *biosorption* is used to describe the accumulation of metal ions from the solution by material of biological origin, particularly microorganisms and plant products. A variety of uptake mechanisms are involved, including adsorption and ion exchange. In developing a biosorption process, the first step involves biomass contact with the metal-contaminated wastewater, whereas the second step involves separating the metal-loaded biosorbent from the metal-depleted effluent. This is normally achieved by immobilizing the biomass in the form of beads, which are used in either a packed-bed or fluidized-bed reactor.

Most metal ion-sequestering processes using microbial or plant biomass involve either a batch or column configuration. Batch systems involve the mixing of free or immobilized cells with the metal ion solution to be pumped through a column packed with cells. A suitable eluant is then used to separate the metals from the biosorbent, and the metals can be recovered electroanalytically.

### Bioaccumulation

The active mode of metal accumulation by living cells is usually referred to as *bioaccumulation*. This process is metabolically dependent and can be significantly affected by the metallic ions. The use of living systems certainly has application in a selected metal recovery system. However, the toxicity and complexity of many wastes may limit the use of living systems. The mechanisms by which bacteria actively accumulate metals include precipitation, intracellular accumulation, and oxidation or reduction.

Precipitation of metal results when living bacteria produce and excrete substances that chemically react with metals present in solution to produce an insoluble metal compound. An example of metal precipitation is the production of hydrogen sulfide by sulfate-reducing bacteria. The $H_2S$ reacts with metals to form insoluble metal sulfide compounds. The active intracellular accumulation of metals by bacteria is a two-stage process. Metals are first bound passively to the cell surface by physicochemical processes. Next, the metals are accumulated inside the cell, usually by an energy-dependent transport system. Metal-binding proteins, such as metallothionein, have been shown to accumulate metals intracellularly.

Oxidation and reduction results in a change in the valence state of a metal. Though oxidation and reduction generally require the functions of living micororganisms, some metal ion reduction can occur passively by chemically reactive sites on the cell walls of micororganisms. Extracellular complexing of metals occurs when bacteria produce or excrete metal-binding substances. Examples of these substances are siderophores, an ion specific ligand, and emulsin, an emulsifying agent.

## Fixed Film Systems (Attached Growth Systems)

Fixed film systems grow micororganisms on substrates, such as rocks, sand, or plastic. The wastewater is spread over the substrate, allowing it to flow past the film of micororganisms fixed to the substrate. As organic matter and nutrients are absorbed from the wastewater, the film of microorganisms grows and thickens. Trickling filters, sand filters, and rotating biological contactors are examples of film systems.

### Rotating Biological Contactors (RBC)

The rotating biological contactor (RBC) represents a viable means for the secondary treatment of both municipal and industrial wastewaters by exploiting the advantages of both fixed film and suspended growth systems. Although RBCs entail high initial capital costs, their low costs of operation and maintenance, as well as their simple process control, increase their economic viability. Metals are removed by biosorption onto the microbial film, and the metal-loaded biomass may either be periodically removed for controlled disposal or suitably treated to recover sorbed metals, such that the biofilm may be reused in multiple cycles.

## Suspended Film Systems

Suspended film systems stir and suspend micororganisms in wastewater. As the micororganisms absorb organic matter and nutrients from the wastewater, they grow in size and number. After the micororganisms have been suspended in the wastewater for several hours, they are settled out as sludge. Some of the sludge is pumped back into the incoming wastewater to provide "seed" micororganisms. The remainder is wasted and sent on to a sludge treatment process. Activated-sludge, extended aeration, oxidation ditch, and sequential batch reactor systems are all examples of suspended film systems.

## Activated Sludge Process (ASP)

Activated sludge can be defined as a mixture of micororganisms, which contact and digest biodegradable materials from wastewater. The process consists of the wastewater source (inflow), aerobic biological treatment (aeration), and the secondary clarification or sedimentation.

In the aerobic biological treatment processes, micororganisms degrade the organics present into free energy $CO_2$ and $H_2O$ or cellular material. Nitrogen and phosphorous are also removed by the micororganisms. This process generates surplus sludge, which must be removed from the reactor. The valuable bacteria in the form of sludge flocs are returned to the aeration unit. The outflow consists of the treated wastewater without the sludge.

## Emerging Technology—Wetlands

Wetlands are commonly known as biological filters, providing protection for water resources, such as lakes, estuaries, and ground water. Although wetlands have always served this purpose, research and development of wetland treatment technology is a relatively recent phenomenon. Wetlands have proven to be well suited for treating municipal wastewater (sewage), agricultural wastewater and runoff, and industrial wastewater. A number of physical, chemical, and biological processes operate currently in constructed and natural wetlands to provide contaminant removal. With the advent of large industries, the need to dispose of increasing amounts of waste has become a major concern. Failing to deal with these wastes in the past led to contaminated surface and subsurface waters. A constructed wetland is one method used to help purify wastewaters.

Biological removal is perhaps the most important pathway for contaminant removal in wetlands. Probably the most widely recognized biological process for contaminant removal in wetlands is plant uptake. Contaminants that are also essential plant nutrients, e.g., nitrate, ammonium, and phosphate, are readily taken up by wetland plants. However, many wetland plant species are also capable of uptake and even significant accumulation of certain toxic metals such as cadmium and lead.

Constructed wetlands are based on, but different from, natural wetlands. A plot of land is chosen near the wastewater that is to be purified. A shallow pond is built, and plants found in natural wetlands, such as cattails, reeds, and rushes are set out. The wastewater is then routed through the wetland. Microbial utilization and plant uptake of nutrients results in cleaner water leaving the constructed wetland. In practice, a constructed wetland was used to treat metals and acid mine drainage near Idaho Springs, Colorado. The principle components of the wetlands include organic soils, microbial fauna, algae, and vascular plants. The precipitated and adsorbed metals in the form of hydroxides and sulfides settle in quiescent ponds or are filtered out as water percolates through the soil or the plant substrate. This process can be adapted to treat neutral and basic tailing solutions.

## CONCLUSIONS

The goal of wastewater treatment systems is to produce clean and safe water for consumption and other purposes. This can be achieved by a combination of existing conventional processes, namely ion exchange and adsorption with the biological processes. The biological treatment process is gaining wider acceptance mainly due to its relatively low cost. However, more research needs to be carried out in this area to fully utilize the potential of micororganisms in the removal of heavy metals from wastewaters.

### SUGGESTED READINGS

de Oliveira E and MJS Yabe (2003). Heavy metal removal in industrial effluents by sequential adsorbent treatment. *Advances in Environmental Research* 7:263-272.

Gupta G and N Torres (1997). Use of fly in reducing toxicity of and heavy metals in wastewater effluent. *Journal of Hazardous Materials* 57:243-248.

Stevenson DG (1997). *Water treatment unit processes.* London: Imperial College Press.

Tebbutt THY (1990). *Basic water and wastewater treatment.* London: Butterworth and Co.

# Tannery Effluent

Indu Shekhar Thakur

## INTRODUCTION

The basic scientific methods applied for leather production go back about a century. Modern leather production is a complex industrial process that involves chemical transformation and stabilization of protein components. The process involves tanning, which is the chemical process of converting the semisoluble protein collagen present in the corium of animal skins and hides into tough, flexible, and highly durable leather. In tanning, the hide substance is treated with chemicals that cross-link to the collagen molecules to form stable materials, i.e., leather. The tanned leathers are then dyed and finished.

The tannery industries are considered polluters due to the inherent manufacturing processes, as well as the type of technology employed in the manufacture of hides and skin into leather. The several processes employed during manufacture are causes of solid and liquid waste and air pollution. Tannery waste from various processes contains different chemicals and materials that are toxic to flora, fauna, and human health. Various methods have been developed for the removal of major contaminants from the waste.

## LEATHER INDUSTRY—WORLD SCENARIO

The world trade in leather goods has increased almost tenfold since the 1980s. The economies of developed and developing countries are dependent upon leather goods production. Since the 1960s, the leather marketing of developing countries has doubled, whereas developed countries' economic share reduced by half in this same period. The tanning industry is scattered unevenly in various countries, and exists in the large, medium, and small cottage section.

## TANNING PROCESSES

The tanning process involves cleaning and washing off dirt, blood, flesh, etc., from rawhides and skins before preserving them with salt until they are transported to the tannery. The salts are removed by soaking, liming, deliming, and fleshing. Hides are delivered to the tannery, where they are soaked in water and detergent to wash away dirt and salt. They are then treated with various chemicals, including sodium hydroxide and calcium hydroxide. Tanning of hides leads to stabilization, retanning, and dyeing to impart special properties into the hides, increases penetration of tanning solution for replenishment of oils and color, and finally finishing of hides to specifications and preparing them for sale. Two types of tanning processes are mainly followed: chrome tanning and vegetable tanning. As a consequence, two types of effluents are discharged.

### Chrome Tanning

Leather production involves chrome tanning, which is the chemical process of converting collagen, the semisoluble protein present in the corium of animal skins and hides. In this process, hides are placed in a salt-and-acid solution, and then chromium sulfate is added. After completion of chrome tannage, the leather is washed with running water. The treated skin surface is cleaned by adding a small quantity of acid. The tanned leather is removed from a drum, wrung, and twisted storngly. The leather is then split to the desired thickness. This results in two layers of leather: the grain and the split. The grain layer is the larger and more valuable layer. The split is trimmed and further processed in the same manner as the grain leather.

### Vegetable Tanning Process

The complex wastewater from the chrome tanning industry is ranked among the most polluting of all industrial wastewater. This complexity is evident in the presence of excess concentrations of suspended and dissolved forms of organic solids, inorganic impurities, and the numerous chemicals and additives used in converting animal skin to leather. As an alternative, the vegetable tanning process is used. In this process, the hides are separated after liming. The hides that are to be vegetable tanned are cut into sections for bellies, shoulder, and bends to ensure the most efficient use of the expensive vegetable tanning materials. Vegetable tanning is done without the use of chromium.

## EXISTING POLLUTION PROBLEMS

A great difference exists in respect to the pollution load between effluent generated from vegetable tanning and effluent derived from chrome tanning. The effluent from chrome tanning generally contains much higher concentrations of total dissolved salts, suspended solids, chloride, etc., as compared to vegetable tanning. Untreated wastewater is typically turbid, colored, and foul smelling. Significant volumes of solid waste, chromium discharge, volatile organic compounds, sulfide waste, and suspended solids, including hair and trimmings, are major source of pollution. In addition, dyes and leather-lubricating oils used in the tanning process are also found in the effluent. Air quality is also a frequent concern due to the release of solvents. The concentration levels of organic materials and ammonia-nitrogen in tannery effluents are also high. During tannery processing, 30 to 40 liters of effluent per kg of skin or hide is discharged, however, in the case of finishing, the quantity can reach up to 50 liters per kg. Industrial discharge sludge contains elevated levels of arsenic, cadmium, chromium, lead, pentachlorophenol (PLP), chlorobenzene, and trichloroethylene. Organochlorine compounds, used mainly for the preservation of leather, have been a matter of great concern because they are highly toxic and recalcitrant.

## IMPACTS OF TANNERY EFFLUENT

The tanning industry discharges different types of waste, primarily in the form of liquid effluent containing organic matters, chromium, sulfide ammonium, and other salts, which affect the quality of the environment.

### On Soil Health

Tannery effluents have undesirable effects on soil properties. The total porosity and hydraulic conductivity of soil decrease as a result of the addition of effluent, whereas the bulk density of soil increases. This may be attributed to the twin effect of direct accumulation of large quantities of organic and inorganic materials, as well as the interaction of Na which causes the deflocculation. Soil treated with tannery effluent was found to be rich in Mg, Mn, Fe, Na, and K. The pollution of soil by arsenic contained in tannery waste has also been reported.

### On Crops

Effluents emanating from the chrome tanning process contain much higher concentration of chromium, which may affect the metabolic processes of plants. Excess quantities of sulfide present in tannery effluent may induce the deficiency of cationic micronutrients, e.g., Zn, Cu, Fe, and Mn. Among the growth processes, seed germination and early seedling growth have been considered critical for raising a successful agricultural crop. The retardation of germination and overall seedling growth of a crop can be attributed to high salinity and other ingredients of effluent, such as sodium chloride, pentachlorophenol, and chromium.

### On Water Bodies

Tannery is one of the major industries responsible for high magnitude water pollution problems. The effluents reach the river, and from there, seep into the earth. The wells and bore wells in the area thus tap the contaminated water. The potential environmental impact of tanning is significant. High levels of chromium are frequently found in effluent. Serious deterioration in the quality of groundwater occurs as a result of the effluents discharged from the tanneries.

### On Human Health

The contamination of water with toxic chemicals from runoff waste, sewage, and industrial wastes and its effect on the environment has generated considerable interest. Pentachlorophenol present in tannery effluent is highly toxics. Pentachlorophenol and its biotransformation products manifest adverse toxic effects. Pentachlorophenol may cause irritation of the skin, conjunctiva, and upper respiratory tract and impairs oxidative phosphorylation pathways and membrane properties, hemolytic anemia, and aplastic anemia. Only two of the several oxidation states of chromium, Cr(III) and Cr(VI), are present in the tannery effluent. Chromium (III) is poorly absorbed, regardless of the route of exposure, whereas chromium (VI) is more readily absorbed. Humans and animals localize chromium in the lung, liver, kidney, spleen, adrenals, plasma, bone marrow, and red blood cells. No evidence suggests that chromium is biotransformed, but Cr(VI) does undergo enzymatic reduction, resulting in the formation of reactive intermediates and Cr(III). The respiratory and dermal toxicity of chromium are well documented. Among the general population, contact dermatitis has been associated with the use of bleaches and detergents. Compounds of both Cr(VI) and Cr(III) have induced developmental effects in experimental animals, including neural tube defects, malformations, cancer, and fetal deaths.

## POLLUTION PREVENTION OPPORTUNITIES

### Primary Treatment of the Effluent

In all processes dealing with solid and liquids, it is very important to define the optimum conditions to carry out solid-liquid separation, including type of flocculants, the type of filter used, and all the other operational variables. The suspended solids' requirements make the primary treatment system essential. The mixing of the acid and alkaline wastes at a controlled pH will result in a coagulation of the suspended solids. The removal of the coagulated materials by primary treatment will result in a decrease of suspended solids by about 80 percent and BOD by 50 to 70 percent. This approach has been successfully used in many tanneries. A Bauxsol blend has been successfully used to treat acidic chromium-rich tannery wastes. The application of modest quantities of Bauxsol raised the pH of the effluent from 3.6 to 8.5 and reduced the total chromium concentration.

### Chemical Treatment of the Effluent

Sulfides are deadly toxic materials and must be destroyed chemically. The normal treatment system in the tanning industry is to collect the sulfide-containing wastes and oxidize the sulfides with air using a manganese sulfate catalyst. The lime solution, free of sulfide, can be used to neutralize the acid wastes to adjust the pH to an acceptable range. Various chemical techniques are used to remove PCP from effluent, such as coagulation and precipitation. A chemical method for oxidative degradation of PCP in soil under unsaturated conditions and neutral pH was developed. Reagents used were heme ($Fe^{++}$), a catalyst, and hydrogen peroxide, an oxidant. The heme and peroxide (Fenton reagent) can degrade PCP efficiently in a short period of time, either in liquid or unsaturated soil systems.

Chrome tanning wastes contain valuable chrome tanning materials. Recycling chrome tanning solutions have technical benefits for the tanner. The effect of solution pH, adsorbent and solute concentration on the extent of $Cr^{+6}$ removal has been reported. Reduction precipitation and adsorption processes have been studied for the removal $Cr^{+6}$ from synthetic wastewater. The treatment of soil contaminated with spent solvents, such as trichloroethylene (TCE), has been emphasized in the past ten years. The treatment can be achieved by a comparison of the removal efficiencies attained through emerging in situ technologies and more traditional ex situ treatment.

## Biological Treatment Methods of the Effluent

The anaerobic and aerobic treatment methods applied for reducing the pollution load have proven successful to some extent, but removal of chlorinated phenols and related major toxicants from tannery effluent has not been successful so far.

### Fungal degradation

Despite the toxicity of the effluent, the microbial flora of tannery liquid wastes are relatively rich, with the *Aspergillus niger* group predominant. Sixteen fungal species belonging to six genera and two yeasts belonging to one genus were isolated. Extracellular enzymes and cell mass from pre-grown *Phanerochaete chrysosporium* cultures were used for the degradation of PCP. The lignin-degrading fungi *P. chrysosporium, P. sordida, Trametes hirsuta,* and *Ceriporiopsis subvermispora* were evaluated for their ability to decrease the concentration of PCP and to cause dry weight loss in PCP-treated wood. Twelve species of white-rot fungi were able to absorb and remove PCP formation. *P. chrysosporium, T. versicolor,* and four *Ganoderma* spp. removed up to 50 percent of PCP within 24 h, though *Inonotus rickii* achieved a 96 percent overall reduction.

### Bacterial Degradation

A variety of bacteria, including *Arthrobacteria, Flavobacterium, Pseudomonas* spp., and *Sphingomonas,* have been isolated and applied for the degradation of pentachlorophenol. A *Pseudomonas* strain capable of degrading pentachlorophenol isolated from tannery effluent was able to utilize the PCP at a concentration of 1500 mg/l. Reduction of toxic hexavalent chromium to trivalent chromium by *Enterobacter cloacae, Bacillus simplex, B. subtilis, Pseudomonas mendocina, P. putida,* and *Pseudomonas* sp. has been carried out in industrial effluent. Trichloroethylene can be degraded to $CO_2$ through a series of reductive dehalogenations via dichloroethylene and vinyl chloride. The obligate anaerobes *Methanosarcina* dechlorinate TCE to yield tricarboxylic acid cycle intermediates. Chlorobenzene is degraded via deoxygenation to from chlorocatechols, which is degraded further following ortho cleavage pathways. *Pseudomonas putida,* a chlorobenzene-utilizing recombinant strain, was isolated from the mixed culture of toluene-grown *Pseudomonas putida* and benzoate-grown *Pseudomonas alcaligenes.*

*Degradation by Mixed Culture or Consortium*

Mixed cultures or consortia might overcome some of the problems of degradation monocultures face in the environment, such as nutrient limitation and unutilizable or toxic substrates. Consortia may be based on the exchange of specific nutrients, removal of growth-inhibitory products and cometabolism. The association of microorganisms to completely mineralize toxic compounds by sequential metabolism is generally referred to as *microbial communities, consortia, syntrophic association,* or *synergistic association.* A PCP-degrading mixed culture contained three predominant strains, identified as *Flavobacterium gleum, Agrobacterium radiobacter,* and *Pseudomonas* sp. Reactors operated under aerobic/methanogenic and anaerobic/denitrifying conditions were inoculated with bacterial consortia obtained from anaerobic granular sludge, long-term PCP-contaminated soil.

### Bioreactors: Place of Action of Microbes

Experiments were conducted by operating a laboratory-scale, completely mixed, continuous flow, activated-sludge system to treat settled chrome tannery wastewater and to develop biokinetic parameters for the same. BOD and COD removal ranges from 84 to 96 percent under steady-state operations, indicating that settled chrome tannery effluent can be treated by a controlled activated-sludge system. After the removal of phenolics and elimination of color-causing compounds, the wastewater is tested for nitrification both at batch scale and in a continuously fed, completely mixed, activated-sludge system. The activated carbon prepared by carbonisation of groundnut husk with sulphuric acid followed by thermal activation showed 80 percent removal of chromium (VI) at optimum pH 2.0.

The immobilization of microbial cells on solid supports is an important biotechnological approach introduced only recently in bioremediation studies. Various bioreactors have been designed for the application of microbial consortium for the treatment of tannery effluent. UASB reactors were used to treat tannery wastewater containing high sulfate concentration. Bench-scale, continuous flow, activated-sludge reactors were used to study the removal of PCP mixed with municipal wastewater.

*Flavobacterium* cells were immobilized on polyurethane and studied for the degradation of PCP in a semicontinuous batch reactor. The ability of *Arthrobacter* cells to degrade PCP in a mineral salt medium was evaluated for immobilized, nonimmobilized, and coimmobilized cells. The immobilized cells were encapsulated in alginate. A microbial consortium able to degrade PCP in contaminated soil was used in a fed batch bioreactor. The microorganisms in the biofilm employ natural biological processes to efficiently degrade complex chemical process and can remediate high volume of waste more cheaply than other available clean-up procedures.

## Advanced Methods

Membrane technology, freeze concentration, solar evaporation, and various methods of steam-assisted evaporation have been evaluated for practicality and economic feasibility for the treatment of tannery effluent. Ultrafiltration reverse osmosis (UFRO) may be used for treatment of the combined pretreated final tannery effluent. Microfiltration reverse osmosis (MFRO) could be used for treatment of the soak-paddle effluent and UFRO could be used for treatment of the dye-house effluent, liming effluent, and deliming effluent. Chromium, iron, sulphate, fats, and oils were removed with UF treatment of the effluent. Freeze concentration was found to be impractical at present as a method of concentrating chrome liquors. Traditional clean-up methods for removal of PCP from the effluent included use of activated charcoal and carbonized pine bark. The decomposition of PCP by sonication has been investigated. Solar evaporation, although attractive from an energy perspective, is not viable for several months of the year when rainfall exceeds evaporation. The solar evaporating pond would have to be significantly cheaper than a steam evaporator.

## In Situ Bioremediation

It has long been recognized that microorganisms have distinct and unique roles in the detoxification of polluted soil environments. In recent years, this process has been termed *bioremediation* or *bioreclammation*. Application of the principles of microbial ecology will improve methodology. The enhancement of microbial degradation as a means of bringing about the in situ clean-up of contaminated soils has spurred much research. The rhizosphere, in particular, is an area of increased microbial activity that may enhance transformation and degradation of pollutants. The most common methods to stimulate degradation rates include supplying inorganic nutrients and oxygen. However, the addition of degradative microbial inocula or enzymes as well as the use of plants should also be considered.

## Phytoremediation by Aquatic Weed

*Phytoremediation* is the use of green plant-based systems to remediate contaminated soils, sediments, and water. Some aquatic macrophytes, such as *Hydriila verticillata, Bacopa monnieri,* and *Nymphaea alba* have been found to be effective in reducing the chromium concentration in the effluent under monoculture. The adsorption of chromium (VI) by *Cladophora crispate, Zoogloea ramigera, Chlorella vulgaris,* and *Sphagnum* sp. has been reported. *Eichornia crassipes* has been used to degrade PCP. The potential to accumulate chromium by *Scirpus lacustris, Phragmites karka,* and *Bacopa monnieri* was assessed by subjecting these species to different chromium concentrations under laboratory conditions.

## CONCLUSIONS

In leather processing, large quantities of chemicals, such as sodium chloride, chromium sulfate, calcium salts, ammonium salts, acids, alkali, fat liquor and organic dyes sludge, arsenic, cadmium, chromium, lead, pentachlorophenol, chlorobenzene, and trichloroethylene are applied. Physical, chemical, and biological treatment methods together with biological reactors are designed to contain the toxic compounds present in tannery effluent. Despite considerable speculation and research on the potential for biotechnology to improve the treatment of hazardous wastes, little progress has been made to date in developing commercially available treatment methods and recovery of products and processes.

## SUGGESTED READINGS

Park CH, M Keyhan, B Wielinga, C Fendore, and A Matin (2000). Purification to homogeneity and characterization of a novel *Pseudomonas putida* chromate reductase. *Applied Environmetal Microbiology* 66:1788-1795.

Pellerin C and MS Booker (2000). Reflection on hexavalent chromium. *Environmental Health Perspective* 108:403-406.

Rose, PD, BA Mart, KM Dunn, RA Rowswell, P Britz, DD Mara, and HW Pearson (1996). High rate of algal oxidation ponding for the treatment of tannery effluent. *Water Science Technology* 33:219-227.

Shukla S, R Sharma, and IS Thakur (2001). Enrichment and characterization of pentachlorophenol degrading microbial community for the treatment of tannery effluent. *Pollution Research* 20:353-363.

Thakur IS, P Verma, and KC Upadhyay (2001). Involvement of plasmid in degradation of pentachlorophenol by *Pseudomonas* sp. from a chemostat. *Biochemical Biophysical Research Communication* 286:109-113.

# Textile and Dye Effluent

Haresh Keharia
Datta Madamwar

## *INTRODUCTION*

Textile plants, particularly those involved in finishing processes, are major water consumers and sources of considerable pollution. Wastewaters from the textile industry consist of a variety of pollutants, such as dyes, detergents, insecticides, fungicides, grease and oils, sulfide compounds, solvents, heavy metals, and inorganic salts and fibers. In general, the chemical oxygen demand (COD)/biological oxygen demand (BOD) ratio of textile industry effluent ranges from 3 to 4, meaning that effluent is moderately biodegradable. The main recalcitrant component of textile industry wastewaters is dye. Textile dyes are classified as azo, diazo, cationic, basic, anthraquinone-based, or metal complex dyes based on the nature of their chemical structure. Further, depending on their application, dyes are classified as reactive, disperse, vat, mordant, etc. The presence of even a small fraction, of dyes in water is highly visible due to the color, and affects the aesthetic merit of streams and other water resources. The presence of dyes also interferes with the penetration of light in water bodies and may affect the aquatic biota. Further, some of the dyes and/or their degradation products have proven to be toxic, mutagenic, and/or carcinogenic in nature. Thus, removal of dyes from effluent has been given a top priority. These dyes are highly resistant to microbial degradation under the aerobic conditions normally found in wastewater treatment plants. This is because dyestuffs are designed to resist chemical fading and light-induced oxidative fading. Other factors involved in reducing the biodegradation of dyes include properties such as high water solubility, high molecular weight, and fused aromatic ring structures, which inhibit permeation through biological cell membranes.

In principle, decolorization may be achieved using one or a combination of the following methods: adsorption, filtration, precipitation, chemical degradation, photodegradation, and biodegradation. However, the color and chemical composition of textile effluents are usually subject to both daily and seasonal variations dictated by production routines and fashion cycles, which complicates the design of treatment processes for handling textile and dyestuff industrial wastewater.

Several industrial-scale decolorization systems are now on the market. The majority of color removal techniques work either by concentrating the color into a sludge, or by the partial to complete breakdown of the colored molecule. This section gives an account of available treatment technologies and prospective technologies being developed.

## PHYSICOCHEMICAL PROCESSES

Numerous physical and chemical techniques based on coagulation, flocculation, precipitation, membrane filtration, ion-exchange, electrochemical destruction, photochemical degradation, ozonation, and adsorption are available for the removal of color from textile wastewaters. Coagulation-flocculation, commonly employed as primary treatment for most textile effluents, yields mediocre results. Sulfur and disperse dyes are efficiently removed by coagulation-flocculation, whereas acid, direct, mordant, and reactive dyes result in poor quality floc that does not settle well, and cationic dyes do not coagulate at all.

The majority of disperse and vat dyes can be easily removed by microfiltration membranes, however, the filtration efficiency of these membranes for other classes of dyes is almost nil. Ultrafiltration can be employed for complete color removal of all classes of dye, but care is needed to avoid membrane clogging, which appears to occur rapidly. Ozone has an oxidizing effect preferentially for the double bonds of the dye molecules. As a result, color removal is fairly rapid using ozone, depending upon the class of dye. Reasonable ozone dosages (50 mg/l) usually allow very efficient color removal as well as COD removal for acid, mordant, cationic, direct, reactive, and sulfur dyes. Disperse and vat dyes are generally difficult to remove, even at high ozone dosages, thus ozone does not seem to be an efficient solution for treatment of these dyes.

Electrochemical technology provides an environmentally sound method of reducing color and removing BOD, COD, total suspended solids, and heavy metal pollution from textile wastes. Surface complexation, electrostatic attraction, chemical modification, and precipitation have been described as the four primary mechanisms by which color is electrochemically removed, although cost is the main constraint.

Higher decolorization efficiency (greater than 90 percent) can be achieved using activated carbon for cationic, mordant, and acid dyes, whereas for direct, sulfur, disperse, and reactive dyes, efficiency is about 40 percent, which can be improved using massive dosages of activated carbon. For vat dyes, color removal using activated carbon is poor (less than 20 percent).

Photocatalytic oxidative degradation processes based on the generation of OH radicals from $H_2O_2$ in the presence of Fe ions and light have attracted considerable attention since the 1990s. The hydroxyl radicals attack the unsaturated dye module, resulting in the destruction of the chromophore and decolorization. The most likely side reaction in this process is dimerization of dye molecules, which will also aid in decolorization. The Fenton oxidation process not only possesses the advantages of both oxidation and coagulation processes, but can also increase the amount of oxygen in water. This method is efficient and effective to all dye wastewaters, but the use of the Fenton reagent alone to treat whole dye wastewater would increase treatment costs.

Though some of the physicochemical processes have been shown to be effective, their application is limited due to the excess usage of chemicals, sludge generation with subsequent disposal problems, and high installation as well as operating costs and sensitivity to a variable wastewater input.

## BIOLOGICAL TREATMENT PROCESSES

Despite the existence of a variety of chemical and physical treatment processes, bioremediation of textile effluent is still seen as an attractive solution due to its reputation as a low-cost, environmentally friendly, and publicly acceptable treatment technology. Biological treatment for decolorization of textile effluents may be either aerobic, anaerobic, or a combination of both, depending on the type of microorganisms being employed. Various biotechnological processes for treatment of textile effluents are discussed.

### Aerobic Treatment Processes

The majority of the fungi belonging to the white-rot group have the ability to degrade a wide variety of dyes. The dye-decolorizing activity of these fungi has been correlated to their ability to produce ligninolytic enzymes, such as laccase, lignin peroxidase, manganese peroxidase, and manganese-independent peroxidases, which exhibit broad substrate specificity. One of the most studied white-rot fungi is *Phanerochaete chrysosporium,* which has been shown to degrade a large spectrum of azo dyes with decolorization efficiencies exceeding 90 percent in most cases. The dye-decolorizing activity of *P. chrysosporium* is stimulated by the presence of veratryl alcohol, which seems to play role in the decolorization process. Dyes having hydroxyl, amino, acetamido, or nitro functional groups substituted in their aromatic rings are more susceptible to degradation by *P. chrysosporium.* Other white rot fungi, such as *Trametes versicolor, Pleurotus ostreatus, Bjerkandera adusta,* and *Pycnoporus cinnabarinus,* have also been shown to efficiently degrade industrially relevant complex azo dyes. The majority of white rot fungi described require nitrogen-limiting conditions and long time periods to decolorize dyes, which limits their application to the laboratory level. Decolorization of chemical industry effluent containing a diazo-linked chromophore was demonstrated using white rot fungi. All strains tested were shown to cause 70 to 80 percent decolorization of effluent (40 percent v/v) in nitrogen-limited medium. Different reactor configurations have been tested for the application of white rot fungi in treatment of dye-bearing wastewaters. Among various configurations, a fed batch-fluidized bed bioreactor was found to be most efficient, and showed 97 percent color removal at a dye (orange II) loading rate of 1000 mg/l per day. The reasearch also justified the suitability of a fluidized bed bioreactor employing mycelial beads of *T. versicolor* for decolorization of sulfonated azo dyes. The reactor performance was found to be highly stable when operated continuously, with more than 95 percent dye removal efficiency at dye loading rates of 100 mg/l per day for 30 days.

A recent study has demonstrated the use of immobilized laccase for decolorization and detoxification of textile dyes. The toxicity of dyes was reduced by 80 percent. When decolorized with immobilized laccase, the textile effluents could be successfully reused for dyeing. Thus a closed-loop technology with reuse of enzymatically treated dyeing effluent to reduce water consumption was demonstrated.

Streptomyces also produce extracellular peroxidases and have the ability to degrade various xenobiotic compounds, including dyestuffs. Further, mechanisms of azo dye degradation by ligninolytic peroxidases of *Phanerochaete chrysosporium* and extracellular peroxidases of *Streptomyces chromofuscus* are found to be similar. The azo dyes are converted to cation radicals enzymatically, which then exhibit increased susceptibility to nucleophilic attack by $H_2O$ or $H_2O_2$ as a result of which dye molecule is cleaved.

A bacterium belonging to *Kurthia* sp. was reported to decolorize dyes belonging to the triphenylmethane group. It was also shown to decolorize textile and dyestuff effluent with a maximum decolorization efficiency of 58 percent and COD reduction of 56 percent within 90 hours of incubation. The Gram-negative *Shewanella* spp. isolated from industrial effluent stream was shown to degrade a range of reactive dyestuffs, including the commercially important dye Remazol Black B. A new process involving *Corynebacterium* and *Mycobacterium* sp. for degradation of dyes belonging to the triphenylmethane group has obtained a German patent. A *Mycobacterium* sp. was precultured in 1 percent methanol as a sole carbon source for three days. Harvested cells were resuspended in tap water and were used for decolorization of malachite green (20 mg/ml). The resting cells caused 53 percent reduction of the initial dye within 2 h of incubation. A process based on a combination of activated-sludge treatment followed by chemical coagulation may be effective in the treatment of dye wastewater. A polyurethane fluidized bed biofilm activated-sludge process resulted in 75 percent $COD_{Mn}$ removal in the loading range of 0.16 to 0.32 kg $COD_{Mn}$/kg VSS per day. In a subsequent coagulation process using alum, 92 percent of total $COD_{Mn}$ removal was observed with a final effluent $COD_{Mn}$ of 65 mg/l.

A fixed film bioreactor was used to demonstrate the treatment of dyestuff wastewater containing phenol and methyl violet at the site of a dye factory near Pune, India. The brick pieces were used as a supporting media in a concrete tank 9.5 m length × 7.3 m breadth × 1.5 m height. The mixed culture of *Pseudomonas alcaligenes* and *Pseudomonas mendocina* cultured in dyestuff wastewater was spread on the brick media. The wastewater was showered through the bed at a loading rate of 1.44 $m^3/m^2$ of brick bed area per day, carrying phenol and COD loading rates of 0.9 kg phenol/$m^2$ per day and 5.67 kg COD/$m^2$ per day, respectively. The reactor performance was found to be highly stable with phenol, methyl violet, and COD reduction of 97.5 percent, 63 percent and 54.4 percent, respectively.

A lab-scale rotating drum biofilm reactor was evaluated for decolorization of three azo dyes—acid orange 8, acid orange 10, and acid red 14. Dye removal efficiency varied from 20 to 90 percent under different conditions of operation, with higher removal rates observed at either high bulk-phase dissolved oxygen and low COD-removal flux, or at low dissolved oxygen and high COD flux, as determined with a statistical model.

A novel technology known as *bioflotation* has proven to be successful in the treatment of effluents from dyeing and finishing processes. To date, about 35 plants are operating in Italy and Spain, where the technology has produced impressive results. Bioflotation leads to the transformation of tensioactive compounds present in wastewaters into activated foam that acts as a supporting structure with a high surface area for bacterial activity. The efficiency of bioflotation is based on the breathing capability of the bacterial pool working within this activated foam, which transforms organic waste into carbon dioxide and water at a faster rate than conventional systems. The efficiency of COD removal varies from 50 to 62 percent using only one phase, but rises to between 90 and 94 percent using two phases in series. Due to its simplicity of use and low sludge production, the bioflotation process is ideal for treating wastewaters from dyeing and finishing operations.

## Anaerobic Treatment Processes

Biodegradability studies on various dyes have shown that anaerobic processes could be used to decolorize dye-containing wastewaters and improve wastewater biodegradability for subsequent aerobic treatment. The advantages of anaerobic biological processes are their simplicity and low running cost.

A fed-batch bioprocess using *Pseudomonas luteola* was shown to effectively decolorize reactive red 22. Since the dye decolorization by this culture was inhibited by oxygen, the culture was aerated during the growth phase only. Gentle agitation was then applied. The continuous feeding of dye (200 mg/h) to a 2L initial culture volume and a yeast extract to dye ratio (Y/D) of 1.25 were found to be optimum conditions for dye decolorization, with a specific decolorization rate of 113.7 g/cell per hour. The Y/D ratio was found to be a critical parameter for dye decolorization, and a Y/D ratio higher than 0.5 was recommended because lower ratios would result in an insufficient yeast extract supply and decreased dye decolorization efficiency.

An upflow aerobic sludge blanket (UASB) reactor consisting of a PVC column (100 cm in height and 140 cm in diameter) seeded with municipal wastewater treatment plant sludge and fed with a synthetic medium containing glucose and sucrose as a carbon source, showed an average color removal efficiency of 80 and 90 percent for acid dyes (CI acid red 42 and CI acid red 73) and 81 percent for CI direct red 80. The reactor performance was adversely affected when an anthraquinone-based disperse dye was fed to the reactor, leading to accumulation of dye in the reactor above inhibitory concentration, and finally causing reactor failure.

A pilot, scale, two-stage, upflow anaerobic sludge blanket bioreactor, consisting of an acidification tank and a UASB reactor with a hydraulic retention time of about 12 hours for each phase, effectively decolorized three different reactive dyebath effluents with color- and COD-removal efficiencies of 56 percent and 90 percent, respectively, using tapioca (500 mg/l) as a co-substrate. Color removal was observed during the acidification and methanogenic phases, suggesting the role of both acid producing as well as strictly anaerobic methanogenic bacteria for color reduction. Experiments have demonstrated the decolorization of a reactive dyestuff industrial effluent using an anaerobic upflow fixed film reactor, with bone char seeded with cattle dung slurry as a support material. Upon biofilm development, microorganisms were acclimatized to dyestuff effluent by gradually decreasing the hydraulic retention time and increasing the organic loading rate. Average color removal efficiency and COD reduction were found to be 70 and 50 percent, respectively, at an organic loading rate of 1,960 mg/l per day.

Anionic dyes have a strong affinity for cellulosic or lignocellulosic ion exchangers, which makes subsequent regeneration of the adsorbent bed difficult. The adsorbed dye can be reduced using chemical reductants, which would add to the cost. The cheaper alternative would be regeneration of the dye-adsorbed resin using anaerobic bacteria for dye reduction. Such a process using a combination of dye adsorption on cellulosic anion-exchange resin and anaerobic dye reduction was demonstrated for effective removal of anionic dyes from wastewater. Cells of *Burkholderia cepacia* ($1.4 \times 10^{10}$ cfu/ml) were filled in a dialysis tubing and suspended in a large column (2.5 × 30 cm internal diameter) containing a glucose-mineral medium along with 1 mM of sodium anthraquinone-2-sulfonate (AQS), which was connected to a small column (0.8 × 6 cm) loaded with a 3-(N-Morpholino)-propanesulfonic acid (MOPS) buffer-washed quaternary ammonium cellulose (100 mg dry weight). The resin was then loaded with 10 μmol of Remazol Red $F_3B$. After about 12 hours of incubation, the medium from the large column was then pumped through the dye-loaded resin, which resulted in 80 percent dye reduction within 50 minutes, demonstrating the continuous use of the resin bed for dye adsorption with periodic brief interruptions for a regeneration cycle involving the passing of microbially reduced AQS. The AQS served as an electron shuttle between the bacterium and dye, thus overcoming the constraints of having microorganisms compatible with variety of dyes typically present in textile wastewaters.

Under anaerobic conditions, bacteria mediate decolorization of azo dyes by causing reductive cleavage of azo linkage. The process of azo bond reduction is catalyzed by a variety of soluble cytoplasmic enzymes with low substrate specifities, known as *azoreductases*. These azoreductases facilitate the transfer of electrons via soluble flavins or other redox mediators to the azo dye, which is then reduced. The role of cytoplasmic azoreductases in dye reduction in vivo is uncertain because transport of polymeric dye molecules or highly charged sulfonated azo dyes across the cytoplasmic membrane is unlikely. Reduced flavins that are products of cytoplasmic flavin reductases may function as intermediates in azo dye degradation. It is also possible that reduced inorganic compounds, such as $Fe^{2+}$, $H_2S$, etc., which are formed extracellularly as end products of certain strictly anaerobic bacterial metabolisms, may cause azo dye reduction.

### Anaerobic/Aerobic Treatment Processes

Although the anaerobic reduction of azo dyes is relatively easy to achieve, complete mineralization of dye molecules is difficult and generally results in an accumulation of aromatic amines. With the exception of a few aromatic amines, most are generally recalcitrant to anaerobic degradation and pose a threat to human and animal health, as their toxic, mutagenic, and/or carcinogenic nature is well documented. Aerobic bacteria mineralize these aromatic amines easily. Thus aerobic treatment after anaerobic dye reduction would be preferable for complete mineralization of dyestuffs in textile wastewaters.

Technologies based on a combination of reductive and oxidative processes for complete mineralization of azo dyes have been proposed. One such technology, which uses cocultivation of oxygen-tolerant, anaerobic granular sludge with aromatic amine-degrading, aerobic enrichment cultures, demonstrated mineralization of azo dyes, mordant yellow 10, and 4-phenylazophenol in the presence of ethanol as a cosubstrate.

A sequencing batch reactor, namely the "anaerobic-aerobic" tandem system was used to demonstrate decolorization of synthetic dye wastewater containing reactive turquoise blue (RTB). The anaerobic and aerobic phases were performed separately in two reactors. A retention time of 20 hours was allowed for each phase, followed by 2 hours each of settling after anaerobic phase and feeding for the aerobic phase, and a settling period of 4 hours after the aerobic phase. The overall RTB removal efficiency was observed to be 80.8 percent with a mean dye removal efficiency of 50.4 percent and 30.4 percent for the anaerobic phase and aerobic phase, respectively.

Treatability of simulated textile effluent was demonstrated using anaerobic and aerobic treatment processes. Seventy-eight percent of true color removal occurred during the anaerobic phase using a UASB reactor at an initial dye concentration of 1500 ppm, whereas no decolorization occurred during the subsequent aerobic stage. An average COD removal of 35 percent and a BOD removal of 71 percent occurred during the anaerobic stage alone whereas an overall COD removal of 57 percent and a BOD removal of 86 percent occurred after the combined anaerobic-aerobic treatment.

A biodegradability analysis of wastewater streams produced by individual production steps showed that the $BOD_5$/COD ratio for different streams was found to vary from 0.01 to 0.612. It was further demonstrated that the biodegradability of streams having a $BOD_5$/COD of less than 0.4 can be increased by Fenton's oxidation pretreatment and activated carbon. The resulting effluent could then be effectively treated with a fixed film bioreactor, acclimatized with dyestuff effluent. Thus, a process involving chemical oxidation, activated carbon adsorption, and fixed bed biofilm process with optional Fenton oxidation as a posttreatment system seems to be a practical approach for treatment of dyestuff wastewater having high salinity, color, and nonbiodegradable organic compounds.

The removal of azo dyes in sludges has been evaluated using three vinyl sulfone-based reactive dyes: Remazol Black B, Remazol Red RB, and Remazol Golden Yellow 3RA. Under aerobic conditions, unhydrolyzed Remazol Black B can be removed efficiently, whereas hydrolyzed dye, which often results during alkaline conditions prevailing in the dye bath, is hard to degrade. Dye removal increased with an increase in the biomass, whereas a high dye to biomass ratio inhibited color removal. Hydrolyzed dyes were found to be reduced readily under anaerobic conditions, which was apparent from the color change from purple to greenish yellow to yellow within 24 hours. Toxicity characteristic leaching procedure (TCLP) extracts showed the presence of trace amounts of dyes, suggesting degradation of dyes in sludge and safe disposal of sludge in landfills.

## *CONCLUSIONS*

No general or economically feasible method currently exists for the decolorization of wastewaters. The diverse chemical nature of dyestuffs makes it difficult to design a common treatment scheme for handling all dyestuff industry wastewaters. Major emphasis by researchers has been given on decolorization studies rather than biodegradation pathway elucidation. Intensive research needs to be carried out to understand the biodegradation pathway. Although the role of lignin peroxidase, laccase, and manganese peroxidase produced by white-rot fungi has been described for color removal, the involvement of other enzymes and microbial metabolites, such as redox mediators/siderophores, cannot be ruled out and needs thorough investigation. Genetic modification of the enzymatic systems of different microorganisms responsible for decolorization and degradation may be studied to make the system more efficient. A complete, comprehensive regime must be found to overcome problems of residual color and BOD/COD for complete mineralization of effluent.

## SUGGESTED READINGS

Banat IM, P Nigam, D Singh, and R Marchant (1996). Microbial decolorization of textile-dye-containing effluents: A review. *Bioresource Technology* 58:217-227.

McMullan G, C Meehan, A Conneely, N Kirby, T Robinson, P Nigam, IM Banat, R Marchant, and WF Smyth (2001). Microbial decolorisation and degradation of textile dyes. *Applied Microbiology and Biotechnology* 56:81-87.

Stolz A (2001). Basic and applied aspects in the microbial degradation of azo dyes. *Applied Microbiology and Biotechnology* 56:69-80.

# PART II:
# FOOD BIOTECHNOLOGY

# Biopolymer Applications

Sudip Kumar Rakshit

## INTRODUCTION

Carbohydrates, fats and oils, proteins, and the information-coded poly-deoxyribonucleic acids and polyribonucleic acids (DNA and RNA) are biological polymers (biopolymers) that have important roles in cellular function. A number of other biopolymers can be extracted from nature, however, in this section the application and use of some of the most abundantly available natural polysaccharide bioresources, such as starch, cellulose, chitin, and chitosan will be discussed.

## STARCH

Starch and flour, presumably from barley or emmer (a primitive variety of wheat), have been utilized from antiquity for the production of beer and bread. From these first applications, the use of starch has grown both in quantity and quality in a large number of applications. Starch is the second largest compound produced by plants in nature after cellulose. Both starch and cellulose are polymers of glucose. Starch has a number of distinct advantages over cellulose. The most important of these is that it can be consumed by human beings and has greater susceptibility to partial and total hydrolysis, leading to its application in a number of useful products and its easy modification to compounds of value in a variety of industries. The differences in the properties of the two carbohydrates are due to the nature of the glycosidic bonds between the monomers. Cellulose has β-1-4 linkages, which make it very difficult to digest or hydrolyze, whereas starch has an α-1-4 bond, which are relatively easily broken down. Technological advances in the use of immobilized enzyme isomerases have lead to the cheap conversion of the hydrolytic product glucose to high fructose syrups used in large quantities in food and beverage industries.

Starch is made up of two types of polymers. The amylose fraction with molecular weights varying from several thousand to half a million are straight chain polymers, which are water insoluble and typically constitute 20 percent of starch. The larger bulk of starch is amylopectin, which is chiefly distinguished from amylose by a considerable amount of 1-6 branching from the linear molecule. Amylopectin molecules are much larger than amylose, with molecular weights varying from one to two million. Amylopectin is soluble in water and forms gels by absorbing water. Another important difference between amylose and amylopectin is in their iodine binding capacity.

Various types of starch occur in higher plants as cereals (wheat, corn, rice, barley, sorghum, rye, millet, oats), tubers and roots (potato, tapioca or cassava, arrow root, yam), fruits (banana, plantain), stem, pith, and seeds. The starch available from various sources vary in the size and shape of the granule, composition of amylose and amylopectin, and other functional properties, such as pasting temperature and swelling power (Table II.1). A major portion of starch is consumed without modification in the food industries in the form of baked products, etc. The products of starch obtained by modification are used mainly in the production of hydrolytic products and sweeteners, food applications, paper and textile applications, fermentation products, etc.

Through complete hydrolysis using acids and/or enzymes, starch can be split quantitatively to glucose. Glucose syrups are hydrolysates of starch in which the reactions are stopped at intermediate levels, leaving a mixture of glucose, maltose, and a mixture of higher sugars. These sugars are commercially available at various dextrose equivalent (DE) levels, defined as the total reducing sugars expressed as dextrose (anhydrous glucose) as a percentage of the total initial dry substance. At present, hydrolyzed syrups of diffferent DE values, such as 25 to 37, 58, and 100, are produced by the combination of amylases such as alpha amylase, beta amylase, glucoamylase, isoamylase, and pullanase. Some of the products of starch hydrolysis are further modified to obtain useful products in the food, industrial, and cosmetic industries (Figure II.1). Maltitol obtained from the hydrogenation of high maltose syrup can be used as a bulk sweetener without any cooling sensation or aftertaste in the mouth. Lycasin and mannitol are obtained by hydrogenation of glucose and fructose respectively. Fat replacers derived from starch-based compounds are also now available. As with many other polysaccharides, they are marketed as bulking agents, but some have been reported to have unfavorable effects, such as laxative and gas production in the larger intestines.

The use of modified starch as a food additive is not based on its nutritional value, but on its functional properties. Modified starches confer to the

TABLE II.1. Variation in properties of starch types

| Starch properties | Potato | Maize | Sweet potato | Tapioca |
|---|---|---|---|---|
| Composition of raw materials (%) | | | | |
| Starch | 17 | 60 | 23 | 26 |
| Moisture | 78 | 16 | 68 | 66 |
| Protein ash N x 6.25 | 2 | 9 | 1.5 | 1 |
| Lipids | 0.1 | 4 | 0.3 | 0.3 |
| Fiber | 1 | 2 | – | 1 |
| Starch on dry substance | 77 | 71 | 72 | 77 |
| Starch granule properties | | | | |
| Type | Tuber | Cereal | Root | Root |
| Size, diameter ($\mu$) | 5-100 | 2-30 | 5.25 | 4-35 |
| Size, diameter (average $\mu$) | 28 | 10 | 15 | 16 |
| Size, diameter; weight average ($\mu$) | 40 | 15 | – | 25 |
| Shape | Oval, spherical | Round, polygonal | Polygonal | Oval, truncated |
| Gelatinization of native starches | | | | |
| Pasting temperature (°C) | 60-65 | 75-80 | 65-70 | 60-65 |
| Peak viscosity range (BU) | 1000-5000 | 300-1000 | – | 500-1900 |
| Peak viscosity average (5%)(BU) | 3000 | 600 | – | 1000 |
| Properties of pastes of native starch | | | | |
| Paste viscosity | Very high | Medium-low | High | High |
| Paste texture | Long | Short | Long | Long |
| Paste clarity | Clear | Opaque | Translucent | Very clear |
| Rate of retrogradation | Medium | High | Medium | Low |
| Chemical composition of granule | | | | |
| Lipid (%) | 0.1 | 0.8 | – | 0.1 |
| Protein (%) | 0.1 | 0.35 | – | 0.10 |
| Phosphorus (%) | 0.08 | 0.02 | – | 0.01 |
| Amylose (%) | 21 | 28 | – | 17 |
| DP[a] (amylose) | 4000 | 1000 | – | 4000 |
| Amylopectin (%) | 79 | 72 | – | 83 |
| DP[a] ($\times 10^6$) (amylopectin) | 2 | 2 | – | 2 |

[a]Degree of polymerization = average number of glucose residues per molecule.

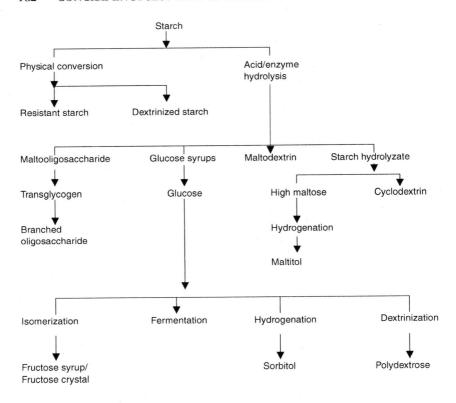

FIGURE II.1. Products of physical conversion and acid/enzyme hydrolysis of starch

food such properties as better mouth feel, thickening or gelling characteristics, and stability. Potato and cassava products yield clear pastes and a bland flavor, whereas the small amounts of proteins and lipids present in corn and wheat impart undesirable flavors to the food products. Properties such as pasting temperature, solids-viscosity relationships, gelatinization, and cooking characteristics, resistance of starch pastes to mechanical break down, mechanical shear, retrogradation tendencies, ionic characteristics, etc., have been modified. Starches are also obtained from physical modifications, such as the production of pregelatinized starches obtained by simultaneous cooking and drying. Pregelatinized starches are applied in instant puddings, pie fillings, dry gravy, etc. Also obtained by physical modification, resistant starch can play a role as a dietary fiber with an additional health benefit of being of low caloric value. Dextrinized starch's slow dispersion in cold water and rapid dispersion in hot water makes it suitable for use in infant food.

Chemical modifications are also used to produce a large number of products. Oxidation leads to low viscosity starches and soft gels with no retrogradation that can be used in salad dressings and mayonnaise or as starch batters in fish, meat, and breaded products. Cross-linked starch with improved properties, such as increased resistance to swelling and gelatinization and high viscosity, are used in bakery custard, cream pie fillings, and toppings, soup powders, salad dressings, etc. Stabilized starches obtained by etherification or esterification to products such as starch acetate and mono starch phosphate are other forms of modified starch used in the food industry.

The paper industry is the single largest consumer of modified starch. The bond strength of starch to fibers of pulp used in papermaking is greater than the fiber-fiber bonds. Sizing of paper gives mechanical strength to the paper and retards the rate of penetration of water into the finished sheet. All stages of paper production make use of physically or chemically modified starches. Cationic starches have a number of advantages over unmodified starches, including their ability to be retained more fully and consistently.

Carbohydrates serve as raw materials for fermentation to many valuable chemicals and pharmaceuticals. Very few microorganisms can directly convert starch to other useful products, though many can produce enzymes for the hydrolysis of starch to glucose, which can then be consumed. Some reports have indicated the simultaneous saccharification and fermentation of starch by lactic acid bacteria producing their own amylolytic enzyme. Aside from ethanol, the major fermentation product obtained from starch is citric acid. Other commercial products using this substrate include organic acids, such as acetic, itaconic, gluconic, 2-ketogluconic, and ascorbic acids, enzymes, penicillin antibiotics, and a host of other products.

## *CELLULOSE*

Energy is the backbone of modern societies. A number of initiatives are taking place to increase the use of other forms of energy and reduce dependence on oil. A potential renewable source of energy that biotechnologists have been trying to harness is the stored chemical energy produced by photosynthetic conversion of incident light. Lignocellulosic agricultural residues form a major part of the biomass available for this purpose. These residues are made up of cellulose, hemicellulose, and lignin. *Cellulose,* a homopolymer of 7,000 to 10,000 anhydroglucose units linked by β 1-4 linkages, is nature's most abundant polymer. *Hemicellulose* is a heteropolymer containing several sugar units. *Lignin* is a complex polymer of phenyl-propanoid units joined largely by benzylic, phenolic, and carbon-carbon linkages. Cellulose, hemicellulose, and lignin can then be used as substrates for the production of gaseous and liquid fuels and other products (Figure II.2).

Bioconversion of these ligno-cellulosic residues consists of an initial pretreatment process to separate these components. Cellulose, which is the major component of these residues, can be broken down to glucose by hydrolysis. Hydrolysis of 1 kg of cellulose yields 1.1 kg of glucose. This is the building block and substrate for further conversion to a number of useful chemicals. Hydrolysis of cellulose to glucose can be done by acid as well as by enzymatic processes. The crystalline nature of cellulose makes it resistant to hydrolysis, and is perhaps the reason for cellulose's abundance in nature. The temperature and pressure conditions for acid hydrolysis are so high that they cause decomposition of the resulting sugars to the extent of 33 percent of the initial cellulose content. This also results in large impurities, unwanted byproducts, and reversion compounds. On the other hand, the cellulase enzyme acts at moderate conditions, is specific in its activity, and produces glucose syrup of fairly pure and constant composition. The cost of the enzyme had been found to be 40 percent of the overall cost of the process. This major hurdle could be overcome with the utilization of higher yielding strains and recombinant organisms capable of producing the enzyme in the extracellular broth. Another method, developed in the 1990s, is the conversion of cellulosic biomass to synthesis gas (consisting primarily of carbon monoxide, carbon dioxide, and hydrogen) via a high-temperature gasification process. Anaerobic bacteria are then used to convert the synthesis gas into ethanol. Synthesis gas fermentation technology has been developed that can be used to produce ethanol at high yields and rates.

## CHITIN AND CHITOSAN

Chitin is a 1,4-linked 2-acetamido-2-deoxy-$\beta$-D-glucan and chitosan is *N*-deacetylated derivative of chitin. These polymers are the main structural components of the cuticles of crustaceans, insects, and mollusks and the cell wall of microorganisms. They are thus a major component of the wastes generated by the seafood industry. Because these compounds have been found to have a number of desirable characteristics, they have come under considerable research scrutiny leading to a number of applications.

Chitin is commercially produced from shrimp and crab shells by chemical methods. The shells are deproteinized (with an aqueous solution of 3 to 5 percent sodium hydroxide), demineralized (treatment with 3 to 5 percent

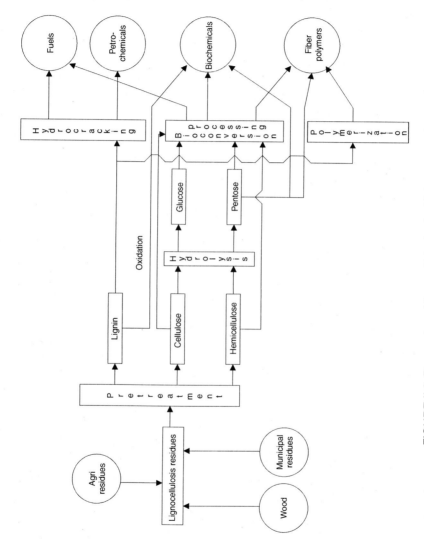

FIGURE II.2. Processing of lignocellulosics for high-value products

185

hydrochloric acid), and the chitin obtained is deacetylated (with 50 percent sodium hydroxide solution at 90 to 120°C for 4 to 5 h) to get chitosan. Attempts are being made to replace this highly polluting process with an enzymatic process. The useful characteristics of the naturally occurring amino polysaccharide chitin and chitosan are that they are biodegradable, biocompatible with organs, tissues, and cells of animals and plants, able to undergo physical transformation into a number of forms (fine powders, flakes, beads, membranes, sponges, cottons, gels, etc.) and have a number of good, functional characteristics, such as metal chelating, affinity binding, and polyelectrolyte-forming capacity.

Chitosan is used as flocculating agent in wastewater treatment and sugar manufacture, as an additive in processed and functional foods and feeds, as a seed coating and fertilizer in agricultural materials, as an antibacterial agent in textiles, fabrics, and foods, as a cosmetic ingredient for hair and skin care, as a biomedical component, as a source of oligosaccharides, such as D-glucoseamine, as a membrane material, as a paint, dye, thickener, chromatographic, and media ingredient, etc. By far the most popular use of chitosan is as a lipid absorber or slimming agent. Chitosan's mode of action is apparently to attach itself to the fat in the stomach before it is metabolized. The complex becomes a large mass, which the body cannot absorb. The Japanese market has a number of pharmaceutical and biomedical products that benefit from chitin, including bandages, sutures, dressings, sustained drug delivery systems, etc. The characteristics of both chitin and especially chitosan depend on molecular weight, degree of deacetylations, and inherent viscoelastic nature. These properties have led to a number of applications for these polymers.

## *OTHER IMPORTANT POLYMERS*

A number of other biopolymers are being used in a variety of industries. These include the derivatives of starch and cellulose, alginates, pectin, xanthan, dextran, gum arabic, gaur gum, carrageenan, locust bean gum, agar, etc. Although some are obtained from plant and seaweed sources, some are exopolysaccharides produced by microbial means. The biopolymers are used as emulsifiers, stabilizers, binders, gelling agents, coagulants, lubricants, film formers, thickeners, suspending agents, etc. Xanthan gum, for example, besides having a number of food applications, is also used in industry as a flowable pesticide, for cleaning, polishing, and as a abrasive, metal working ceramic, foundry coating, drilling fluid, and in enhanced tertiary oil recovery (polymer flooding).

## *CONCLUSIONS*

Biomaterial science is an expanding area with applications in biology, medicine, biochips, sensors, etc. Advances in genetic engineering and nanotechnology will eventually lead to the production of polysaccharides with novel superior properties, and open up new areas, applications, and demand. However, the use of the naturally occurring biopolymers is bound to increase.

## SUGGESTED READINGS

Chahal PS and DS Chahal (1998). Ligno-cellulosic wastes: Biological conversion. In *Bioconversion of waste material to industrial products,* Second edition. AM Martin (ed.). London: Blackie Academic and Professional,

Hirano S (1996). Chitin biotechnological applications. In *Biotechnological Annual Review,* Volume 2. M Raafat El-Gewely (ed.). Elsevier Press.

Mathur NK and KN Chander (1990). Chitin and chitosan: Versatile polysaccharide from marine animals. *Journal of Chemical Education* 67(11):938-942.

Whistler R, JM Bemiller, and EF Paschall (eds.) (1984). *Starch: Chemistry and technology.* New York: Academic Press.

Wurzburg OB (ed.) (1986). *Modified starches: Properties and uses.* Boca Raton, FL: CRC Press.

# Biotransformations of Citrus Flavanone Glycosides

Guillermo Ellenrieder

## *INTRODUCTION*

Flavanone glycosides are abundant constituents of citrus leaves and fruits. On a dry basis, they account for up to about 5 and 30 percent of ripe and small unripe fruit weight, respectively. In fruits they are mainly in the peel, section membranes, and other solid parts. The most common citrus flavanone glycosides are hesperidin, which is found in oranges, lemons, and other citrus; naringin in grapefruits and sour oranges; and neohesperidin in sour oranges.

Flavanones are included in a larger group of substances broadly distributed in the vegetable kingdom named *flavonoids,* which have a common basic structure of two aromatic rings linked by three carbon atoms, generally forming a third central ring. The structures of the flavanones found as glycosides in citrus are shown in Figure II.3. Like all glycosides, their molecules have two parts: a sugar moiety and an "aglycone." In most citric flavanone glycosides, the carbohydrate portion is a disaccharide made up of an *L*-rhamnose (6 deoxymannose) unit and a D-glucose unit. Both monosaccharides can be linked in two different forms: through an $\alpha(1\text{-}2)$ or an $\alpha(1\text{-}6)$ glycosidic bond from rhamnose to glucose. In the first case the resultant disaccharide is called *neohesperidose,* in the second it is called *rutinose* (Figure II.3). Rutinose or neohesperidose are linked to the aglycones by a $\beta$-glycosidic bond from the glucose carbon 1 to the position 7 of the flavonoid.

Several methods were developed for laboratory and industrial extraction and purification of these compounds from citrus wastes or by-products. These processes are generally based on the increase of solubility of the flavanone glycosides in basic solutions, at high temperatures, or on the use of nonaqueous solvents. Their retention in adsorbent resins was also used in recovery processes. Due to their properties and biological activity, these substances and some of their derivatives have important applications in

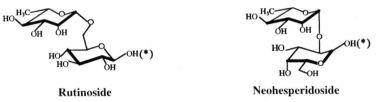

**Flavanone aglycones**

**Hesperetin**

**Naringenin**

**Eriodictyol**

**Isosakuranetin**

(*) Binding site to aglycone sugar moiety (CY)

**Sugar moieties (diglycoside groups)**

**Rutinoside**

6-*O*-α-1-rhamnosyl-β-D-glucoside

**Neohesperidoside**

2-*O*-α-1-rhamnosyl-β-D-glucoside

(*) Binding site to aglycone (C1)

**Main citrus flavanone glycosides**

| | |
|---|---|
| **Hesperidin:** | hesperetin-7-β-rutinoside |
| **Neohesperidin:** | hesperetin-7-β-neohesperidoside |
| **Narirrutin:** | naringenin-7-β-rutinoside |
| **Naringin:** | naringenin-7-β-neohesperidoside |
| **Eriocitrin:** | eriodictyol-7-β-rutinoside |
| **Neoerocitrin:** | eriodictyol-7-β-neohesperidoside |
| **Neoponcirin:** | isosakuranetin-7-β-rutinoside |
| **Poncirin:** | isosakuranetin-7-β-neohesperidoside |

FIGURE II.3. Structure of main flavanone glycosides

pharmaceutical and food industries. Drugs containing citrus flavonoids are marketed for treatments of chronic venous insufficiency, easy bruising, hemorrhoids, and nosebleeds. The reduction of cholesterol levels, control of inflammations, prevention of diabetic complications, reduction of allergic reactions, and cancer prevention are other effects also attributed to these compounds. In the food industry, naringin can be used as a flavoring substance to provide bitterness to foods, such as marmalades and tonic water or grapefruit-flavored beverages. In order to produce other valuable derivatives or to make possible the utilization of some citrus flavanone glycoside-containing bioresources, it is often necessary to transform these substances chemically or enzymatically. The following transformations are frequently carried out on citrus flavanone glycosides:

1. Enzymatic hydrolysis of flavanone glycosides to improve citrus product quality
2. Hydrolysis to produce rhamnose, flavanone glucosides, and flavanones
3. Hydrogenation in basic medium to produce dihydrochalcone sweeteners
4. Enzymatic glycosylation and esterification to synthesize new derivatives

## ENZYMATIC HYDROLYSIS OF FLAVANONE GLYCOSIDES

### Bitter Taste Reduction of Grapefruit Juices by Enzymatic Hydrolysis

The flavanone glycoside naringin and, to a lesser extent, limonin (a tetracyclic triterpenoid substance) give grapefruit juice its characteristic bitter taste. The taste threshold of naringin in water solutions is about 20 ppm. Its concentration in juices is sometimes far above this value, reducing their acceptability. In the fruit juice, the naringin concentration is low, but during juice extraction it is transferred from peel and membranes to the liquid. The level of naringin in juices depends, consequently, on the extraction process. Methods for debittering grapefruit juices are based mainly on adsorption of naringin on resins or other solids, or on its enzymatic hydrolysis. The adsorptive debittering is more economical than the enzymatic method, and for this reason is the method predominantly used. However, it can present some disadvantages, by affecting color, flavor, etc. Furthermore, the healthful effects claimed for flavonoids and other related substances would be lost if they are removed.

The enzymatic hydrolysis of naringin takes place in two steps (Figure II.4). An enzyme called α-*rhamnosidase* acts first, liberating rhamnose and "prunin," or naringenin glucoside. After that, the enzyme β-glucosidase hydrolyses prunin to glucose and the flavanone naringenin. The first step is more important because it causes a considerable reduction of the bitter taste. Prunin is essentially less bitter than naringin. Both enzymes are constituents of the enzymatic complex called *naringinase,* which is industrially produced and commercialized by several companies. Microscopic fungi, mainly *Aspergillus niger* or *Penicillium decumbens,* produce the industrial naringinase complexes. Other microorganisms can also produce these enzymes, but considering that this utilization is for the food industry, their GRAS (generally recognized as safe) character is an essential requirement. Naringinase is produced by submerged and solid fermentation cultures.

The first attempts at debittering were carried out by simply adding an enzyme solution to the juices. However, this practice is not economical because the catalyst cannot be separated from the treated juice and reused. To overcome this situation, naringinase was used immobilized on solid supports and membranes. Different supports, such as DEAE-Sephadex, chitin, glycophase-coated porous glass, dextran, alginate gels, or entrapment in hollow fibers, were tested for juice debittering. Hydrolysis of naringin present in grapefruit juice using free or immobilized enzymes shows several problems—the catalyst is inhibited by several components of the juice, solids in suspension cause the fouling of the column reactors, and some characteristics of the juice can be altered. Good results were claimed for the use of naringinase entrapped in cellulose triacetate fibers, which hydrolyzes naringin and removes limonin by adsorption. In spite of its high specificity in the reduction of naringin concentration, the enzymatic debittering of grapefruit juices has not found great application due to the high cost of the enzymes. However, a new method using enzymes to debitter is currently assuming importance: the use of so-called "bioactive packaging." The enzymes are bound on films to the package material, acting slowly on the undesirable substrate, in this case naringin, improving the taste quality of the juice. Films of cellulose triacetate were also tested to hydrolyze naringin and remove limonin simultaneously.

### Prevention of Formation of Hesperidin Crystals in Citrus Products

Hesperidin is a flavanone glycoside of very low water solubility. However, together with other insoluble substances such as oil, pectins, and proteins, it can be present in the "cloud" of some citrus juices. Citrus juices are

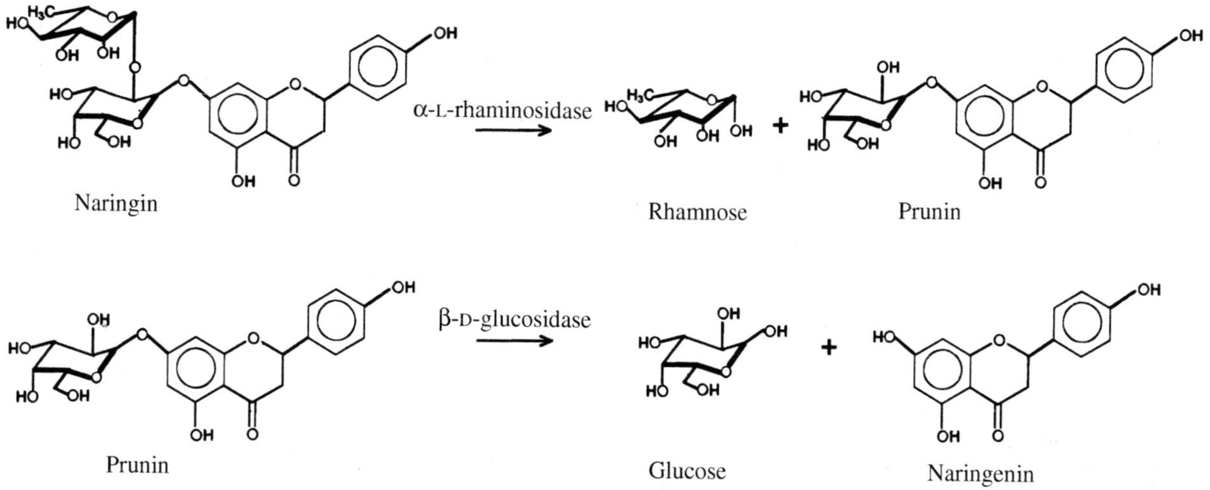

FIGURE II.4. Enzymatic hydrolysis of naringin

preferred turbid, and hesperidin has a desirable effect in the production of artificial juices from pulp or peel because it contributes to the stability of the cloud. However, in some cases solid crystals of hesperidin in the form of flakes can be formed, affecting the quality of the product. This problem is frequent in juices and "pulp wash" concentrates and on the equipment employed in the process of concentration. The enzymatic hydrolysis of hesperidin is used to prevent this problem in some syrups and other products. Hesperidin is enzymatically hydrolyzed by a mechanism similar to that of naringin, but due to its very low solubility, the process slows down. *Hesperidinases* are enzyme complexes containing α-rhamnosidase with a special ability to hydrolyze hesperidin.

## HYDROLYSIS OF THE CITRUS FLAVANONE GLYCOSIDES

Most of the hydrolysis products of the citrus flavanone glycosides are valuable substances with actual and potential applications. Rhamnose is the starting material in the synthesis of one of the most intense sweet aroma chemicals, 2,5-dimethyl-4-hydroxyfuran-3-one, a natural aroma compound of some fruits and an ingredient of commercial flavors. Prunin (naringenin β–glucoside) and hesperetin glucoside (coming from the hydrolysis of hesperidin), were proposed as sweetening substances for diabetics, and flavanone aglycones show anticancer and other biological properties.

Acids or enzymes can hydrolyze flavanone glycosides. Acid hydrolysis takes place at more rigorous conditions than enzymatic hydrolysis, requiring high temperatures. The acid process is more economical than the enzymatic one, but it can produce corrosion, undesirable by-products, and contamination problems. The glycoside molecule can be hydrolyzed at two sites: at the glycosidic bond between rhamnose and glucose or at the bond between glucose and aglycone. Five different products can result: a disaccharide, two monosaccharides, a flavanone glucoside, and an aglycone. All these products can be simultaneously formed by acid hydrolysis. Reaction conditions are known, however, that favor the predominant hydrolysis of only one of the bonds.

The commercial enzyme complexes that hydrolyze the glycosides have the two necessary enzymes for hydrolyzing both bonds. However, α-rhamnosidase can be obtained free from β-glucosidase, allowing the formation of only two products: rhamnose and the corresponding flavanone glucoside. The enzymatic hydrolysis of the different flavanone glycosides shows some distinctive aspects that depend on substrate properties, such as solubility and type of sugar moiety (rutinose or neohesperidose).

The hydrolysis of naringin for the manufacture of its products has one advantage when compared with that of hesperidin: naringin has higher water solubility and consequently a faster reaction rate. However, the solubility of naringin is not as high at the optimum temperature of the enzymes (generally 40° to 60°C). In order to obtain appreciable concentrations of products, e.g., rhamnose, it would be necessary to hydrolyze concentrated suspensions of naringin, which has some operational complications. These problems can be solved by hydrolyzing supersaturated naringin solutions. The solubility of this flavonoid increases sharply at temperatures above 70°C, it is dissolved at 80° to 90°C, and after cooling the solution to the reaction temperature, a supersaturated solution is obtained, which is stable for several hours. During this stability period the enzymatic reaction can be carried out in homogeneous solution at an acceptable rate with good yields.

Another problem for the production of rhamnose by naringin hydrolysis is the presence of the enzyme β-glucosidase, which hydrolyzes prunin to glucose and naringenin. Glucose must then be separated from rhamnose after the hydrolysis, and this additional step increases the cost. A method for the separation of glucose from rhamnose was proposed, which makes use of the inability of yeasts to ferment rhamnose. The yeast eliminates the glucose, leaving only rhamnose in the solution. However, it is preferable to use the enzyme α-rhamnosidase free from β-glucosidase for hydrolyzing naringin. The β-glucosidase can easily be eliminated from some complexes by high pH treatments. Under these conditions, the two enzymes differ appreciably in stability depending on their microbial origin. The enzyme from *Aspergillus terreus,* for example, can be freed from β-glucosidase activity by incubation for 2 hours at pH 11 at room temperature without appreciable loss of α-rhamnosidase activity. Using this treated enzyme, only rhamnose and prunin are produced by naringin hydrolysis.

Another problem observed in the manufacture of enzymatic hydrolysis products of naringin is the inhibition of the enzyme by the products. Both rhamnose and prunin can inhibit the reaction. This problem is enhanced when the products are obtained at a high concentration. The incidence of product inhibition on the yield of products depends on the enzyme origin, so the *Aspergillus niger* enzyme is less inhibited than that of *Aspergillus terreus.* This difference suggested that a less inhibited enzyme could be found by screening enzyme-producing microorganisms. Such microorganisms were indeed found: strains of *Trichoderma longibrachiatum* and *Fusarium sambucinum* produced α-rhamnosidases that are not inhibited by the products. These fungi are not GRAS. However, in addition to the use of processes that avoid the possible presence of mycotoxins, the possibility of the transference of the enzyme gene to other GRAS microorganisms exists.

Hesperidin is a flavanone that is more abundant and economical than naringin. It can also be hydrolyzed by acid or enzymes to rhamnose and hesperetin glucoside. However, the enzymatic hydrolysis is slow due to its low solubility. A screening of microorganisms may also locate appropriate enzymes in this case. The hydrolysis of the insoluble substrate or the appropriate type of rhamnose-glucose bond could be possible if an active rhamnosidase stable in basic solutions is found, because the solubility of hesperidin increases under these conditions. *Fusarium sambucinum* α-rhamnosidase, which maintains activity in basic solutions, hydrolyzes hesperidin six times faster at pH 10 than at pH 5.5, the optimum for soluble substrates hydrolysis.

## HYDROGENATION IN BASIC MEDIUM TO PRODUCE DIHYDROCHALCONE SWEETENERS

Naringin or neohesperidin can easily be transformed into the corresponding dihydrochalcones. Contrasting with the bitter taste of the flavanone neohesperidosides, the dihydrochalcones are intensely sweet substances that have been accepted as sweeteners by food regulatory organizations. The transformation can be carried out easily—the central nonaromatic ring of the flavanone is opened in basic media, conducive to the formation of chalcones. Under these conditions a catalytic hydrogenation produces the dihydrochalcones (Figure II.5). Neohesperidin dihydrochalcone is sweeter than naringin dihydrochalcone, and they are 1,500 and 100 times sweeter than sucrose, respectively. Some differences observed between their taste inten-

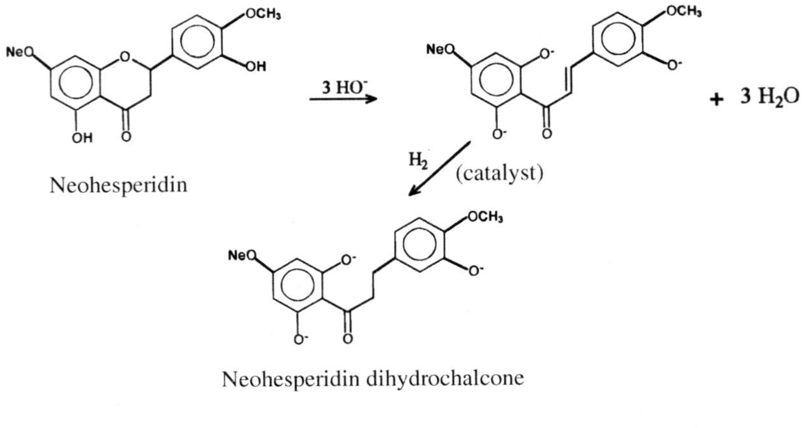

FIGURE II.5. Hydrogenation of neohesperidin in basic medium

sity profiles and that of sucrose can be corrected by the addition of other sweeteners. In additon to sweetness, neohesperidin dihydrochalcone has the characteristic of enhancing some tastes. On the other hand it masks some bitter and salty components. Sour oranges are the principal and cheaper source of neohesperidin. It can also be produced chemically from naringin, but the process is more complicated and expensive.

## ENZYMATIC GLYCOSYLATION AND ESTERIFICATION TO SYNTHESIZE NEW DERIVATIVES

Recently, a new type of biotransformation has been applied to the flavanone glycosides, which makes possible the synthesis of many new compounds with interesting properties: enzymatic glycosylations and esterifications. The enzymes catalyzing the synthesis of glycosides in nature are *glycosyl transferases,* but in vitro the glycosidases can also be used for synthesizing glycosides and oligosaccharides. Glycosyl transferases are very specific and efficient for catalyzing this type of reaction, but their stability is not always good, and they require expensive cofactors to act. Although their yields are not optimum and their specificity toward the glycosyl acceptor is not good, glycosidases are also attractive glycosylating enzymes because they are stable, economical, and easily available. The reaction catalyzed in vivo by the glycosidases is the hydrolysis of glycosides and oligosaccharides. However, they can catalyze in vitro the glycosylation of molecules having alcoholic groups in two ways: reverse hydrolysis and transglycosylation. In reverse hydrolysis, the thermodynamic conditions of the systems are changed in such a way that the spontaneous reaction is reversed. To achieve this objective, high concentrations of acceptors can be used, or the water activity can be decreased by adding a nonaqueous solvent. In transglycosylation, the enzyme transfers the glycosyl group of the donor molecule to the acceptor instead of to a water molecule to produce hydrolysis. The synthesized glycoside is, however, hydrolyzed in a process that is slower than the transglycosylation. Consequently, the yield goes through a maximum and then decreases again. The reaction is said to be "kinetically controlled," and the optimum reaction time must be properly controlled.

Hesperidin was first glycosylated by cyclodextrin glucanotransferase, an enzyme that catalyzes the cyclodextrin synthesis starting from starch. Cyclodextrin glucanotransferase also transfers glucosyl residues from starch to acceptor molecules. Hesperidin glycosides synthesized in this way have the new glucosyl residues incorporated into the sugar moiety of hesperidin. Some interesting applications were proposed for these new compounds, such as the protection of natural pigments in solution from ultraviolet radiation and prevention of hesperidin crystal formation in syrups. Glycosylation highly increases water solubility of hesperidin, allowing the preparation of concentrated glycoside solutions that properly absorb radiation and avoiding its damaging effects on natural pigments. In syrups, the presence of concentrated hesperidin glycosides prevents the formation of hesperidin crystals through their incorporation into the nascent crystals, interfering with their growth.

Naringin, neohesperidin, and neohesperidin dihydrochalcone were glycosylated by *Bacillus stearothermophilus* maltogenic amylase. Glycosylation takes place at the primary hydroxyl group (C6) of the glucosyl portion of the naringin (Figure II.6). The most significant effect of this transformation is the solubility increase of the flavonoids. Glycosylated naringin is 250 times more soluble in water and ten times less bitter than naringin. Neohesperidin dihydrochalcone solubility increases 700 times by glycosylation, whereas its sweetness decreases only seven times. These changes can find interesting applications in the food industry.

The diversity of compounds capable of being synthesized starting from citrus flavanone glycosides can also be expanded by enzymatic esterification. Many of the abundant flavonoid glycosides in natural sources are often acylated, so the synthesis of these substances can be of importance due to their possible biological properties. As with glycosylation, enzymatic esterification can be carried out by reverse hydrolysis catalyzed by lipases, generally in nonaqueous solvents. Naringin was enzymatically acylated in this way using commercial *Mucor miehei* and *Candida antarctica* lipase in nonaqueous solvents. Esterification takes place at the primary hydroxyl group of the glucosyl portion of the naringin. Other secondary sugar hydroxyl groups are esterified only with low yield.

Oligosaccharides or *p*-nitrophenylglycosides are generally used as glycosyl donors in glycoside synthesis catalyzed by glycosidases. Naringin was tested as a rhamnosyl donor for the synthesis of alkyl-α-L-rhamnosides catalyzed by α-L-rhamnosidases, because it is more economical and easily available than the glycosylating agent rhamnose. For this purpose the flavonoid was incubated in a supersaturated solution in the presence of the

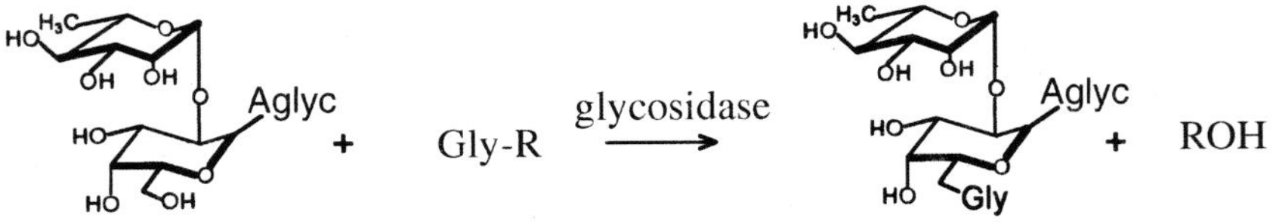

FIGURE II.6. Enzymatic glycosylation of neohesperidosides

enzyme and the appropriate water-soluble alcohol. The results were similar to those obtained by reverse hydrolysis. The rhamnosyl group can be transferred from naringin to the acceptor alcohol either by direct transglycosylation or in two steps by naringin hydrolysis followed by the reverse hydrolysis reaction between the generated rhamnose and the alcohol. The products can be separated from the rest of the flavanone glycoside and their derivatives after the reaction using anion-exchanger chromatography at pH 10. Under these conditions, the flavonoid has ionized phenolic hydroxyl groups that are retained by the anion exchanger.

## SUGGESTED READINGS

Bär A, AF Borrego, O Benavente, J Castillo, and JA del Río (1990). Neohesperidin dihydrochalcone: Properties and applications. *Lebensmittel Wissenschaft und Technologie* 23:371-376.

Braddock RJ (1999). *Handbook of citrus by-products and processing technology.* New York: John Wiley and Sons, Inc.

Cho JC, SS Yoo, TK Cheong, MJ Kim, Y Kim, and KH Park (2000). Transglycosylation of neohesperidin dihydrochalcone by *Bacillus stearothermophilus* maltogenic amylase. *Journal of Agricultural and Food Chemistry* 48:152-154.

Gao C, P Mayon, DA MacManus, and EN Vulfson (2001). Novel enzymatic approach to the synthesis of flavonoid glycosydes and their esters. *Biotechnology and Bioengineering* 71:235-243.

Puri M and UC Banerjee (2000). Production, purification, and characterization of the debittering enzyme naringinase. *Biotechnology Advances* 18:207-217.

Terada Y, T Kometani, T Nishimura, H Takii, and S Okada (1995). Prevention of hesperidin crystal formation in canned mandarin orange syrup and clarified orange juice by hesperidin glycosides. *Food Science Technology International* 1:29-33.

# Fermented Milk Products

V. K. Batish
Sunita Grover

## INTRODUCTION

Although the exact period of origin for fermented milk products is unknown, their use as dietary adjuncts dates back thousands of years. Ever since humans first learned the art of fermentation, they have exploited it with the objective of preserving milk for future use. In Euripe, Asia, and Africa, sour milk was known for its better keeping quality, stability, digestibility, and other beneficial health effects as compared to fresh milk. On the Indian subcontinent, the conservation of milk by souring with the previous day's sour milk has been a common practice ever since the Aryans invaded the land in 1500 to 1000 B.C. Today, the practice of preserving milk by fermentation has become a facile household technology and fermented milks have become an integral part of the human diet. In India, *dahi* (an indigenous fermented milk) figures invariably as a regular component of the Indian menu. The Indian medical treatise *Sushrita Samhita* (c. 600 B.C.) describes *dahi* as a food promoting appetite and strength. The use of fermented milks in human diet was also advocated by Élie Metchnikoff, who ascribed the longevity of Bulgarians to the ingestion of milk prepared with the help of *Lactobacillus bulgaricus*. It was postulated that this organism possessed the ability to combat disease-causing germs in the intestine. This exciting revelation eventually paved the way for exploring the therapeutic and biopreservative attributes of food-grade lactic acid bacteria for the preparation of fermented milks. In the process, the dairy industry, particularly in the Western world, got a boost with the introduction of a variety of fermented milk products, such as yogurt, acidophilus milk, kefir, kumiss, and cheese, in the market. The list of such fermented milks has expanded enormously during the past few decades as a result of better understanding of the fermentation characteristics of lactic acid bacteria, namely lactococci, lactobacilli, leuconostocs, pediococci, etc., which serve as starter cultures in the preparation of fermented milks. The major role of starter cultures is to ferment milk sugar (lactose) into lactic acid and flavor components, along with some antagonistics, which inhibit undesirable microorganisms in the fermented product, thereby, enhancing not only the shelf life, but also the safety of such foods. The story of fermented milks, which began with the traditional methods of preparation by various ethnic groups, blossomed into a full-fledged industry with the introduction of state-of-the-art technology for large-scale production of these specialized dairy foods in the world market.

Although only 2 to 3 percent of the total world dairy products market is in the form of fermented milks currently, their production has shown a marked increase during the last several years. The Western world, particularly Europe, continues to dominate the production of fermented milks and contributes a lion's share to the world market. A large variety of such products are now commercially available for consumption by a wide section of the human population, depending upon individual taste. Largely due to increasing consumer awareness regarding their beneficial effects in human nutrition and health, fermented milk products are now in great demand all over the world. Although a variety of fermented milk products of Western and indigenous and ethnic origin are known and commercially available, the most notable ones consumed extensively all over the world will be briefly described here.

### *YOGURT*

Yogurt is a fermented milk that originated in Eastern Europe and Asia, but is now consumed throughout the world as a popular dessert. Basic yogurt, known as "set" or "firm" yogurt, has expanded into many new products, including stirred yogurt, drinking yogurt (with various additives), frozen yogurt, and protein- and lactose-enriched yogurt products. Yogurt is made from cow's milk, sheep's milk, goat's milk, or even soya milk using the standard starter cultures, namely *Streptococcus thermophilus* and *Lactobacillus delbrueckii* ssp. *bulgaricus* in a ratio of 1:1 to 2:3 grown at temperatures in the range of 40 to 45°C. Symbiotic interaction between two microorganisms results in yogurt having a dominant acetaldehyde flavor. Lactobacilli also show lipolytic activity liberating fatty acids and contributing to flavor development. Combinations of these typical acidification bacteria with *Bifidobacterium bifidum* have resulted in products such as Bioghurt and Biogarde, which are characterized by good digestibility, low acidification performance, and longer taste stability.

The nutritional and therapeutic value of yogurt has long been known. The bonus is that protein, calcium, and phosphorus are more easily absorbed from yogurt than from milk because they are partially digested during the fermentation process. Because lactose is already converted to lactic acid during its manufacture, yogurt is more easily digested by the people with lactose intolerance. Yogurt has also been shown to have an antagonistic effect against a number of pathogenic and spoilage organisms both in vivo and in vitro. The yogurt bacteria make valuable vitamins, which in turn stimulate the growth of beneficial intestinal bacteria, discouraging and destroying harmful ones. Yogurt can restore the digestive tract to normal condition in antibiotics-associated diarrheal cases. Scientific research has documented many nutritional and healthful attributes in the live, active cultures used in the preparation of yogurts, such as antiallergenic effects to milk protein, an increase in calcium bioavailability, enhancement of bioavailability of other nutrients, conversion of lactose to lactic acid, and the presence of active cultures in the digestive tract. Additional evidence suggests that yogurt cultures are important in growth stimulations and longevity, immunostimulant activity, anticholesterolemic activity, and also have an anticancer effect.

## DAHI OR DADHI

Dahi, or dadhi, is an Indian fermented milk product that is obtained by lactic fermentation of cow or buffalo milk or mixed milk through the action of single or mixed strains of lactic acid bacteria or by lactic acid fermentation accompanied by alcoholic fermentation by yeasts. It is similar to yogurt and differs in having less acidity. The starters used in the manufacture of dahi constitute a complex and heterogeneous flora, such as *Lactococcus lactis* ssp. *lactis*, *L. lactis* ssp. *cremoris, Streptococcus thermophilus* and *Lactobacillus delbrueckii* ssp. *bulgaricus,* and lactose-fermenting yeasts. The National Dairy Culture Collection at the National Dairy Research Institute (NDRI), Karnal, India, recommends the use of LF-40 (a mixed culture) for the manufacture of superior quality dahi.

Dahi is an extremely popular fermented food on the Indian subcontinent, which includes India, Pakistan, Bangladesh, Nepal, Sri Lanka, etc. In the Indian system of medicine (Ayurveda), the use of dahi has been strongly advocated for curing ailments such as dyspepsis, dysentery, and other gastrointestinal disorders. The product is also believed to improve appetite, vitality, and increase digestibility. Some of the beneficial effects of dahi are attributed to the antibacterial components formed during fermentation and the low pH that prevents the growth of putrefactive and other undesirable organisms, including potential pathogens. As the metabolic activity of dahi starts, appreciable changes in mineral and vitamin contents occur, depending on the type of organism involved. Other fermented milk products derived from dahi include srikhand (semisolid mass obtained after drainage of water from dahi and mixing with sugar) and lassi (a liquid nourishing drink from dahi), which are consumed by a large population.

## LEBEN AND OTHER RELATED PRODUCTS

Leben is another fermented milk, which originated in the Middle East countries. It is a concentrated yogurtlike or kefirlike product. The related fermented milks are known under different names, e.g., labneh or lebneh from Lebanon or other Arabian countries; tan from Armenia; torba and tubem from Turkey; gioddu from Italy; and matzun from Russia.

### Taette

Taette is a moderately ropy and sour milk product of slightly flowing consistency that contains not more than 0.3 to 0.5 percent of alcohol. This product is extensively used in the Scandinavian countries and in Finland. In the Scandinavian countries, a bulk of taette is produced mainly in homes by fermenting fresh milk. It is mildly acidic in flavor and markedly viscous. The microflora of taette is composed of *Streptococcus lactis* var. *hollandicus* and some yeasts.

### Skyr

Skyr is a traditional Icelandic milk product that is rich in protein and low in fat. Skyr is sometimes mixed with cream and fruit. It also has potential as an ingredient for raw milk products because of its unique texture and high nutritional quality. Skyr whey is used as a drink as well as a medium for cooking and food preservation. The preservation potentials of skyr whey are considerable, as the foods preserved in such way can last for months in a cool place without loss of quality.

### Bulgarian Sour Milk and Buttermilk

Bulgarian milk, a product belonging to the yogurt family, originated from the Traki'e tradition, i.e., from the tradition of sheep breeders. Bulgarian milk is an extremely sour product prepared from boiled goat's milk or cow's milk inoculated with a portion of previously fermented milk. The commercial production of Bulgarian milk uses *Lactobacillus delbrueckii* ssp. *bulgaricus* as a single culture or mixed with *S. thermophilus*. Milk soured with *Lactobacillus delbrueckii* ssp. *bulgaricus* is marketed as Bulgarian Buttermilk in Bulgaria. It is more viscous and has a higher acidity than cultured buttermilk.

### Acidophilus Milk

Acidophilus milk is a highly acidic product made by the fermentation of milk with *Lactobacillus acidophilus*. The therapeutic and health-promoting potentials of acidophilus milk have been known since ancient times. It is also claimed that *L. acidophilus* can establish in the intestine of adults and can help combat various gastrointestinal disorders, such as constipation and diarrhea. This has beneficial effects in patients suffering from constipation, irritable colitis, and colonic ulcerative colitis, and can also reduce serum cholesterol level. The use of acidophilus milk as a therapeutic agent is attributed to its ability to combat the autointoxications caused by accumulation in the body of toxic substances elaborated by the growth of certain toxigenic bacteria. Constant use of this product is recommended for controlling several other intestinal disorders.

### Cultured Buttermilk and Sour Cream

Cultured buttermilk is the fluid remaining after ripened cream or sour cream is churned into butter. It is prepared by souring true buttermilk or skim milk with a butter starter culture that produces a desirable flavor and aroma. As with other fermented products, cultured buttermilk is also very popular in Scandinavian and other European countries. A similar product, known by the name *chach,* is equally popular on the Indian subcontinent. The starter cultures used for the preparation of cultured butter milk are generally of mixed types consisting of *Lactobacillus lactis* ssp. *lactis, L. lactis* ssp. *diacetylactis, L. lactis* ssp. *cremoris,* and *Leuconostoc citrovorum.*

Cultured sour cream is an extremely viscous product with the flavor and aroma of buttermilk and a fat content of 12 to 30 percent. The microbiological aspects pertaining to the quality of cultured cream resembles more or less those of cultured buttermilk.

### Kefir

Kefir is an acidic, mildly alcoholic, slightly foamy product made from standardized whole, low-fat, or skim milk that has been pasteurized and undergone acidic and alcoholic fermentation. Kefir is the most popular cultured product in the former Soviet Union, and is also produced in small amounts in Czechoslovakia, Poland, Sweden, and other Eastern European countries. It is manufactured using porous polysaccharide structures called *kefir grains*. Microorganisms in kefir grains include lactococci, leuconostocs, and lactobacilli, as well as yeasts and acetic acid bacteria. The final product contains 0.01 to 0.1 percent ethanol and 1 percent titratable acidity. The gross composition and calorific value of the product are very similar to milk, except that about one quarter of the 5 percent lactose might have been converted to lactic acid. This conversion can be beneficial to lactose-intolerant persons by providing lactase, the enzyme in short supply in lactose-intolerant individuals. Kefir is a highly nutritious drink suitable for inclusion in special diets as well as for treatment in gastrointestinal disorders.

### Kumiss

Kumiss is an effervescent, acidic, alcoholic, fermented, milky white/greyish liquid made primarily from mare's milk that is richer in albumin, peptones, and amino-acids, and contains more vitamins C, A, $B_1$, $B_2$, $B_{12}$, and several micronutrients as compared to cow's milk. It is one of the most ancient drinks, and is popular throughout Eastern Europe. The name *Kumiss* was derived from a tribe called Kumanes, and the beverage was consumed by Scythian tribes in Southeast Asia and Middle Asia as a food as well as weak alcoholic drink. The organisms responsible for the fermentation are similar to those described for kefir, but they do not develop masses or grains. The major end products are 0.7 to 1.8 percent lactic acid, 1.3 percent alcohol, and 0.5 to 0.88 percent carbon dioxide.

Kumiss is also considered a refreshing therapeutic drink. In the former Soviet Union, it is used for the treatment of pulmonary tuberculosis. More than 50 percent of Russian Sanitoria recommend kumiss for treatment of tuberculosis patients, and the prescribed dose is 1.5 quarts per day for two months. Mare's milk differs from cow's milk in its immunity to *Mycobacterium tuberculosis*. Kumiss is also considered equally effective in the treatment of gastrointestinal diseases, chronic bronchial pneumonia, dry pleurisy, and for people convalescing after the attack of infectious diseases.

### Cheese

Among all fermented dairy products, cheese is the most important and most popular product of the dairy world. An age-old practice, cheese making served as an effective means of preserving milk solids through moisture removal by coagulation. In additon to its high nutritive value, cheese has a longer shelf life. A number of cheese varieties are based on moisture (very hard, hard, semihard, soft), as well as the mode of ripening (bacteria, mold, unripened). The most popular cheese varieties include cheddar, green,

Swiss, mozzarella, ricotta, Roquefort, Camembert, and processed cheeses, etc. A number of starters are deliberately added to milk for initiating the desired fermentation that in turn controls the appearance, body, texture, and flavor characteristics of cheese. The primary functions of these starters are acid and flavor production, eye formation, inhibition of undesirable bacteria, and creation of a suitable environment within the cheese curd during maturation. Secondary functions include coagulation of milk by rennet, stimulating curd shrinkage, suppression of growth of undesirable bacteria, and controlling enzymatic changes during ripening. The cheese starters include lactic starters (Lactococci, Leuconostocs, etc.), as well as nonlactic starters, such as adjunct bacteria (propionibacteria in swiss cheese, *Brevibacterium linens* in brick cheese) and molds in certain mold-ripened cheeses (blue-veined, Camembert, Brie, etc.). Cheese has a high nutritive value and is in great demand because of its use in pizza, etc.

## LACTIC BEVERAGES

During the past few decades, the number of lactic beverages, both milk- and whey-based, have increased considerably. The milk-based beverages include drinking yogurt, acidophilus milk, and alcoholic milk beverages, whereas whey beverages include natural beverages, acidic beverages, and nonalcoholic beverages. In India, a *Lactobacillus acidophilus*-based whey beverage known as Acido-whey is becoming increasingly popular as a refreshing drink with a pleasant taste and aroma. Developed at NDRI, Karnal, the drink possessess strong therapeutic potential with gastric disorders.

## NEW DEVELOPMENTS IN FERMENTED MILK PRODUCTS

With enforcement of the World Trade Organization (WTO) agreement, it has become mandatory for the dairy industry in all member countries to adopt cost-effective, state-of-the-art technologies to produce international quality fermented milks. Faced with market saturation in the third world and stock dumping in advanced countries, dairy organizations that produce traditional fermented products must explore new avenues of product diversification. New trends are becoming apparent with regard to consumer acceptance of fermented milks. The selection of microorganisms used as starters in the manufacture of fermented milks is now based on the interaction with gastrointestinal microflora and metabolic properties. Genetic engineering of microorganisms and new technological possibilities will allow the creation of new fermented milks in which desired properties are emphasized.

New products should be developed and traditional ones should be maintained and improved. Hence, the introduction of new technologies assumes added significance. Other potential areas include special fermentation products, such as probiotic milk foods with immunomodulating activity. These products could receive greater consumer attention as the market demand for value-added fermented products is expected to be very high in the near future. Similarly, *bifidobacterium*-derived fermented products have shown excellent physiological activity in infant digestion metabolism and nutrient utilization. Milk-based formulae with bioactive peptides of immunological significance can be prepared by fermentation process to mimic the biological attributes of breast milk.

## FUNCTIONAL DAIRY FOODS

With growing consumer interest in health care, a "new era" in the food market has recently emerged with increasing emphasis on the integration of foods with medicine. This integration resulted in the concept of *functional foods,* which was inspired by the age-old quote by Hippocrates (c. 460-377 B.C.), "Let food be thy medicine and medicine be thy food." These specialized foods contain components that may enhance health beyond their nutritional value. Many kinds of functional foods are being developed and marketed to consumers to deliver specific health benefits. This concept has broadened the scope of traditional foods by adding new functions. Some other terms used for functional foods include *designer foods, pharmaceutical foods, biofoods,* or *nutraceuticals.* Such foods contain physiologically active components effective in preventing or controlling disease and promoting optimal health. Fermented dairy products can be included in the category of functional foods because of their content of calcium (which can reduce osteoporosis, hypertension, and colon cancer) and other health-enhancing components. The functionality of dairy foods can be enhanced by either adding certain functional components, such as antioxidants, probiotics, etc., or replacing components with more desirable ones. Probiotic dairy foods containing health-promoting bacteria are an important segment of the functional-food market. A variety of health benefits is attributed to specific strains of lactic acid bacteria, such as *Lactobacillus* and *Bifidobacterium,* or foods containing these probiotic cultures. Potential benefits include alleviation of symptoms of lactose maldigestion (lactose intolerance), control of enteric pathogens or antibiotic-associated diarrhea, maintenance of healthy intestinal flora, decreased risk of cancers and heart diseases, and stimulation of host immune systems. However, controlled human intervention studies are required to substantiate the claimed benefits of such functional foods. Recently, a great deal of interest has focused on the health benefits of prebiotics (i.e., nondigestible food ingredients, such as oligosaccharides, that benefit the host by selective stimulation of the growth of probiotic bacteria in the gastrointestinal tract) and synbiotics (i.e., combined effect of prebiotic and probiotic cultures). However, appropriate biomarkers are needed to adequately assess the physiological impact of functional fermented dairy products, such as probiotic yogurt, dahi, cheese, and srikhand.

Fermented milk products continue to be the subject of intensive investigations to further enhance their inherent nutritional and healthful attributes. These products represent an exciting area of commercial interest for the dairy industry. The commercial salability of fermented milks can be expanded dramatically by catering to the needs of different consumer categories. With the growing interest of consumers in health-related foods, the market for fermented milk products has a bright and promising future.

## SUGGESTED READINGS

Batish VK, S Grover, P Pattnaik, and N Ahmed (1999). Fermented milk products. In *Biotechnology: Food fermentation,* VK Joshi and A Pandey, (eds.). New Delhi: Educational Publishers, pp. 781-864.

Fonden R, G Mogensen, R Tanaka, and S Salminen (2000). Culture-containing dairy products—Effect on intestinal microflora, human nutrition, and health—Current knowledge and future perspectives. *Bulletin of IDF* 352:5-30.

Kosikowaski F (1977). *Cheese and fermented milk foods,* Second edition. Ann Arbor, MI: Edwards Brothers Inc., Printers and Distributors.

Robinson RK and AY Tamime (1982). Microbiology of fermented milks. In *Dairy microbiology,* Volume II, RK Robinson (ed.). New Jersey: Applied Science Pub. Ltd.

Yadav JS, S Grover, and VK Batish (1993). *A comprehensive dairy microbiology.* New Delhi: M/S Meteropolitan Book Co. Ltd.

# Fermented Vegetables

Didier Montet
Gérard Loiseau
Nadine Zakhia

## INTRODUCTION

Vegetables are perishable agricultural products, and can be degraded naturally by various microorganisms whose inhibition may occur under some conditions of acidity, presence or absence of alcohol, antibiotics, bacteriocins, high salt concentration, lack of assimilable carbon-based substrates, etc. These conditions are generally created through the multiplication of certain microorganisms growing on vegetables.

Vegetables have low sugar content and neutral pH, providing a natural medium suitable for microbial development. The microbial flora responsible for vegetable degradation can be neutralized and/or inhibited by the organic acids that are produced during vegetable fermentation by lactic acid bacteria. Among these organic acids, lactic acid has been used empirically for this purpose since the sixteenth century. Starter cultures of lactic acid bacteria are increasingly used for initiating vegetable fermentation and controlling end-product quality.

## LACTIC ACID-FERMENTED VEGETABLES

Since the sixteenth century, lactic acid fermentation techniques were developed for stabilizing and improving the nutritional and organoleptic quality of agricultural products. Lactic acid fermentation is small-scale feasible, inexpensive, and does not require additives. It enhances nutritional benefits and confers organoleptic characteristics to the foodstuffs according to the habits and requirements of consumers. This is essentially achieved by the growth of lactic acid bacteria, which gradually convert the easily assimilated carbon substrates of the medium (i.e., sugars) into organic acids, among them the lactic acid that ensures food stability. The lactic acid production lowers the pH value to around 4, which inhibits the growth of spoilage flora and pathogenic bacteria.

In the industrialized countries, the best known fermented vegetables are sauerkraut, olives, and cucumbers. In developing countries and mainly in the Eastern countries, fermented vegetables are considered to be staple foods and represent a large part of the traditional diet. The most often reported fermented vegetables are brassicaceous vegetables, such as cabbages, cauliflowers, broccolis, mustard *(Brassica juncea);* root vegetables, such as carrots, turnips, beetroots, radishes, celeriacs; vegetable fruits, such as cucumbers, olives, tomatoes, peppers, zucchinis, okra, green beans, and green peas; bulbs, such as onions and garlic; vegetable juices, such as carrot, beetroot, or pepper juices, tomato pulp, and horseradish, onion, or beetroot puree; and mixtures of different vegetables or leaves, such as kimchi in Korea, *tsukemono* in Japan, and *mura-tura* in Rumania.

### Pretreatments of Raw Material

Some pretreatments can favor the growth of lactic flora during fermentation. Vegetable washing prior to fermentation reduces the initial microbial count, thus promoting the development of less prolific lactic acid flora. Fragmentation, i.e., cutting vegetables into pieces or shredding, enhances the development of lactic acid flora by facilitating release of the vacuole liquid and the formation of a nutrient-rich, anaerobic medium. Vegetables can also be macerated with pectinolytic enzymes to allow their homogenization prior to lactic fermentation, mainly for the production of cocktails based on lactic acid fermented vegetables.

Some molecules contained in the vegetables may hamper efficient fermentation. In the case of tomato lactic acid fermentation, it is recommended to use very ripe fruits, because the high solanin content of unripe tomatoes might inhibit the growth of lactic acid bacteria. Bean bleaching prior to fermentation is essential to eliminate phaseolin, a glycoside that can inhibit the fermentation. To reduce their bitterness due to a phenolic glycoside called *oleuropein,* olives are often treated by immersion in a 1 to 2 percent sodium hydroxide solution and an alkaline hydrolysis. The oleuropein is then transformed into phenolic aglycone, which can inhibit the growth of lactic acid bacteria and must therefore be eliminated by rinsing.

## Role of the Ingredients Used for Vegetable Fermentation

### Salt

Salting is performed either by adding dry sodium chloride or crude salt to vegetables or by soaking in brine (brining or pickling). In the case of dry salting, salt is added regularly to the successive layers of the product, avoiding high local salt concentrations that could promote yeast development and product damage (e.g., the pink kraut of sauerkraut). The optimal salt concentration depends on the type of vegetable. NaCl concentrations can range from 20 to 80 g/l during fermentation and up to 160 g/l in certain stored vegetables (Table II.2).

The main role of salt is to promote the growth of lactic acid bacteria over spoilage bacteria, and to inhibit the activity of potential pectinolytic and proteolytic enzymes, which can cause vegetable softening and further putrefaction. Salt induces plasmolysis in the plant cells and the appearance of a liquid phase, which creates anaerobic conditions around the submerged product. The mineral salts and nutrients released from the vacuole and plant cells constitute an excellent substrate for lactic acid bacteria. Anaerobic conditions are more effective in the finely cut and shredded plant material. Whole or nonjuicy vegetables are therefore soaked in highly salted brine.

### Other Ingredients Favoring the Microbial Growth During Fermentation

Other ingredients may be used for lactic acid fermentation of vegetables, and have two main roles: (1) they are a potential source of nutrients (e.g., sugars, mineral salts, and vitamins) for the microorganisms responsible for

TABLE II.2. Salt concentration in the most common lactic acid fermented vegetables

| Food | Salt concentration during fermentation (% wt) | Type of salting |
|------|------|------|
| Sauerkraut | 2-3 | dry salt |
| Korean kimchi | 3 | dry salt |
| Cucumbers | 5-8 | brine |
| Green olives | 4-7 | brine |

*Source:* Adapted from Grazie et al., 1986.

fermentation, (2) they restrict the growth of undesirable bacteria by regulating the pH or producing inhibitory agents. Spices have a deciding contribution to the flavor and taste of fermented vegetables.

For vegetables containing few nutrients, such as turnip and cucumber, the addition of sugar can help bacterial growth, thereby accelerating fermentation. For *jaggery* fermentation in India, slightly refined cane sugar called *gur* is added during lactic acid fermentation of sweet turnip. Adding 1 to 2 g of sucrose or *gur* to 100 g of hand-shredded turnip (mixed with 6 g of salt and 6 g of mustard seed) increases the production of lactic acid during fermentation. However, the acidification is much slower at higher (25 g) sucrose contents, which it is attributed to the partial inhibition of lactic acid bacteria growth.

For bitterness reduction, olives often undergo an alkaline hydrolysis and repeated washings prior to fermentation. This lowers their sugar and nutrient contents, which is corrected by the addition of glucose or sucrose (0.1 to 0.2 percent w/w) prior to fermentation. In the preparation of *sajour asin,* a traditional Indonesian fermented cabbage, cooked rice flour is added to improve the metabolism of lactic acid bacteria. Whey is often recommended for use in traditional lactic acid vegetable fermentation processes, because it has a high lactose content—a potential energy substrate for lactic bacteria. It also supplies mineral salts and vitamins necessary for the lactic flora metabolism. Cereal brans are used as carbohydrate sources in various traditional recipes. In Japan, rice bran is used in *tsukemono,* a lactic acid fermented mixture of vegetables and leaves.

### Ingredients with Buffering Properties

Acids or buffer systems (acid + acid salt) are often added to the fermentation medium to promote the growth of lactic acid bacteria over undesirable microbial strains. Neutrophilic pathogenic bacteria can be inhibited by acidifying the brine from the outset, provided that the initial pH value is not below 3.5 to 4.0, otherwise the growth of lactic acid bacteria flora will be inhibited.

For vegetables having a high fermentable sugar content, the fermentation medium must be buffered to slow down the acidification and allow the lactic bacteria to consume all sugars. The lactic acid fermentation of cucumber may be improved by the addition of a buffer system composed of acetic acid and calcium acetate. Moreover, the calcium ions released by the calcium acetate may form a complex with the vegetable pectins, thus protecting them from enzyme hydrolysis, and strengthening the texture of lactic acid fermented vegetables.

## Ingredients with Antiseptic Properties

Spices or aromatic herbs are added to most lactic acid fermentations of vegetables to improve the flavor of the end products. The aromatic compounds of these spices, mainly terpenes and polyphenols, often act as antimicrobial agents, and may have a selective role on the bacteria development during fermentation. Some spices, mainly garlic, cloves, juniper berries, and red chilies, can help inhibit degradation during lactic acid fermentation. Garlic contains so many sulfur compounds with antibacterial properties that, unlike onion, this vegetable cannot undergo lactic acid fermentation alone, but must be combined with other vegetables at ratios not higher than 150 g/kg of vegetables.

Mustard seed is also of interest because it contains allyl isothiocyanate, a volatile aromatic compound with antibacterial and antifungal properties that inhibit the yeast *Saccharomyces cerevisiae*. Adding 6 to 10 g of mustard seed powder to a turnip (100 g) and salt (6 g) mixture could increase lactic acid levels during fermentation. Essential oils, such as thyme, sage, lemon, and dill, are used to inhibit the growth of various yeasts during olive fermentation. Chemical preservatives, such as sorbic or benzoic acid salts, are sometimes used in the industrial production of lactic acid-fermented sauerkraut, olives, or cucumbers.

## The Fermentation Process

### Spontaneous Fermentation

After harvesting, vegetables may present high microbial counts (around $10^5$ to $10^7$ microorganisms/gram), most of which are Gram-negative bacteria and Gram-positive bacilli with spore-forming potential. Some yeasts and molds could also be counted. Lactic acid bacteria are the least prevalent, accounting for less than 0.1 percent of the total microbial population. They are generally Gram-positive, immobile, non-spore-forming, anaerobic, air-tolerant (to some extent), and can ferment sugars, producing lactic acid alone (homofermentative bacteria), or a mixture of lactic acid, acetic acid, $CO_2$, and ethanol (heterofermentative bacteria). They have high requirements for nutrients, such as amino acids, peptides, vitamins, fatty acids, and some minerals. The plant environment is not generally suitable for their development. Nutrients that are crucial for their growth are rendered from the plant medium through salting or the addition of certain ingredients (whey, bran, etc.). The simultaneous growth of prototrophic bacteria supplies the lactic acid bacteria with metabolites that are essential for their multiplication.

The dominant bacteria at the outset of fermentation are resistant to high salt concentrations and are acid-tolerant. A dominant flora sequence over the course of lactic acid fermentation has been identified successively as *Pediococcus, Leuconostoc,* and *Lactobacillus.* The lactic fermentation of vegetables is halted when all sugars in the medium have been consumed due to the inhibition of bacterial growth, through a decrease in the pH level, or an increase in the lactic acid concentration. The bacterial count can reach $10^9$ cells/ml at the end of fermentation. Residual sugars can prompt the growth of acidophilic yeasts, which in turn modify the product through the production of gas or pigments. When fermented vegetables are stored in open vats, postfermentation can be observed following the growth of oxidative molds and yeasts on the surface.

Gram-negative and spore-forming bacteria are inhibited by the progressive medium acidification. These conditions allow the multiplication of lactic acid bacteria followed by a series of other strains. The most reported lactic acid bacteria generally isolated from fermented vegetables are *Lactobacillus plantarum, Lactobacillus brevis, Pediococcus cerevisiae, Leuconostoc mesenteroides,* and *Lactococcus lactis* (Table II.3).

Lactobacilli are able to reproduce and remain relatively resistant to hydrogen peroxide. 125 µg/ml of $H_2O_2$ were required to inhibit an inoculum of $10^4$ cells of lactobacilli/ml, whereas *Staphylococcus aureus* was inhibited

TABLE II.3. Characteristics of lactic acid bacteria isolated from fermented vegetables

| Characteristic | Lactobacillus plantarum | Lactobacillus brevis | Pediococccus pentosaceus | Leuconostoc mesenteroides |
|---|---|---|---|---|
| Morphology | Short to medium rods, usually occurring singly | Short rods occurring singly or in short chains | Cocci occurring singly, in pairs, and in tetrads | Cocci or bacilli usually in pairs |
| Optimum temperature | 30-35°C | 30°C | 35°C | 20-30°C |
| Growth at 45°C | No | No | Yes | No |
| Growth in NaCl 8 % | Yes | No | Yes | No |
| Glucose metabolism | Homofermentative; lactic acid alone | Heterofermentative; lactic acid + $CO_2$ + acetic acid + ethanol | Homofermentative; lactic acid alone | Heterofermentative; lactic acid + $CO_2$ + acetic acid + ethanol |
| Type of lactic acid produced from glucose | DL | DL | DL | D |

*Source:* Adapted from Montet et al., 1999.

by a 4 μg/ml concentration. Some lactic acid bacteria produce antibiotics that are active against Gram-positive bacteria. In addition to organic acids, the heterofermentative lactobacilli produce carbon dioxide, which also has a preservative effect on foods.

## Control of Fermentation Conditions

To control fermentation, conditions must be created that favor the growth of commensal and/or inoculated lactic acid bacteria while excluding other microorganisms. The brine medium must quickly turn anaerobic and remain such to ensure a high quality for lactic acid-fermented vegetables.

Temperature is a critical factor for vegetable fermentation. It affects the acidification rate and promotes the growth of a single microbial species. At an optimal temperature of 18°C, sauerkraut fermentation takes about two months to achieve. At 7.5°C, the same fermentation takes six months. At 30°C, homofermentative bacteria will thrive, thus excessively increasing the acidity of the final product. The artificial acidification of vegetables can enhance their lactic acid fermentation. Adding a mixture of acetic acid and calcium acetate to the brine can reduce the number of enterobacteria.

## Use of Selected Starter Cultures

The characteristics, mainly organoleptic properties, of the fermented products differ depending on the use of selected pure strains or endogenous strains growing spontaneously. Nevertheless, using selected starter cultures meets overall economic, technological, sensorial, and nutritional requirements.

Starter cultures are selected on the basis of the following criteria:

- The rapid and massive establishment of selected strains
- The ability to acidify rapidly the brine
- The strain's homofermentative character to avoid carbon dioxide production
- The capacity for total depletion of fermentable sugars
- The strain's ability to produce (D-) lactic acid only
- The low potential for biogenic amine production
- The rapid sedimentation to obtain a clear brine
- The natural resistance to bacteriocins and bacteriophages
- The potential of strain preservation by drying, freezing, or freeze-drying

## NUTRITIONAL VALUE OF LACTIC ACID-FERMENTED VEGETABLES

### Beneficial Dietary Effects

Lactic bacteria are often considered to be promoters of human health and active in lowering the serum cholesterol level. They also help in preventing tumors through the stimulation of immune responses, inhibition of carcinogenic compounds in the gastrointestinal tract, and reduction of the enzyme activity of fecal bacteria. Colonization of the digestive tract by lactic acid bacteria prevents pathogenic bacteria from attaching to the cell walls. Lactic acid-fermented foods generally modify the intestinal transit of microorganisms by producing inhibitory substances, such as hydrogen peroxide, lactic acid, and acetic acid, and by lowering the pH or breaking down certain enterotoxins.

The lactic acid-fermented vegetables present the same benefits as fresh vegetables, i.e., they are rich in fiber, mineral salts, and vitamins. Moreover, they show an interesting probiotic effect on health due to their transport of living microorganisms and their corresponding metabolites into the intestinal tract. Pasteurizing or adding preservatives after fermentation, which are commonly done during the industrial production of lactic acid-fermented vegetables (e.g., sauerkraut), destroy most of the lactic acid bacteria present, thus canceling any possible probiotic effects.

### Vitamin C Preservation

The high vitamin C content in sauerkraut (about 20 mg/kg) increases during fermentation and then decreases slightly during storage. To limit vitamin C losses, vegetables should be processed immediately after harvesting, when their vitamin C contents are the highest. Cabbage should be placed in brine immediately after shredding to inhibit enzymes that induce oxidation. More recent studies on whole cabbage have shown that its ascorbic acid content decreased during fermentation, leveling off at about 20 to 25 mg/kg at the cabbage core. Little data is available on the vitamin C content in other fermented vegetables. Values ranging from 7 to 19 mg/100 g have been reported for kimchi.

### Mineral Preservation

After ingestion of a meal including lactic acid-fermented vegetables, the total amount of assimilated iron is more than twice that for a meal with an equal proportion of fresh nonfermented vegetables. Iron bioavailability was also reported to be higher in carrots after lactic acid fermentation, but this phenomenon has not yet been explained. It seems that the presence of ascorbic acid or other organic acids is not the only factor involved in enhancing iron assimilation.

### Denitrifying Role of Lactic Acid-Fermented Vegetables

Due to the widespread use of nitrogen fertilizers, high quantities (up to 1 g/kg) of nitrates are sometimes detected in foods. Nitrates are not toxic, but they can be reduced by enzymes into nitrites, which could then be transformed into highly carcinogenic nitrosamines. A reduction of 90 percent of initial nitrate levels in carrots was observed after four days of fermentation in the presence of *Lactobacillus plantarum.*

### Food Digestibility Improvement

During lactic acid fermentation, some indigestible compounds, such as sulfur compounds in garlic or onion, can break down, improving food digestibility.

## Some Negative Effects of Vegetable Lactic Acid Fermentation on the Diet

### Biogenic Amine Synthesis

Biogenic amines are formed in foodstuffs as a result of the microbial decarboxylation of amino acids. In consequence, they may often be found in fermented foods. These amino compounds can confer an unpleasant flavor to the product or even be toxic. Ingestion of certain amines by man can cause headaches, fever, and vomiting—similar symptoms to those of microbial food poisoning. Histidine, ornithine, tyrosine and lysine are the main amino acids that can be decarboxylated. The corresponding biogenic amines are histamine, tyramine, putrescine, and cadaverine, respectively. A minimum histamine level of 1 g/kg in a foodstuff or the consumption of 0.07 to 1 g of histamine per meal is supposed to elicit histamine toxicity.

Some bacteria commonly involved in lactic acid fermentation, such as *Pseudomonas cerevisiae* or *Leuconostoc mesenteroides,* have been found to contain the amino acid decarboxylase, which induces biogenic amine formation. Conversely, other bacteria, such as *Lactobacillus plantarum,* also commonly found in lactic acid fermentations, can limit biogenic amine concentrations in lactic acid-fermented vegetables.

### Synthesis of D(–) Lactic Acid

As stated previously, during lactic acid fermentation of vegetables, the sugars are transformed either into lactic acid alone (homofermentative bacteria), or lactic acid together with acetic acid, ethanol, or carbon dioxide (heterofermentative bacteria). Two different forms or isomers of lactic acid may be thus produced, depending on whether the polarized light rotates to the right L(+) or to the left D(–).

The L(+) lactic acid isomer is absorbed by the intestinal mucus and used as an energy substrate during metabolic activity. On the other hand, the D(–) form is not assimilated and is eliminated by the kidneys in the form of salts, leading to a loss of calcium and magnesium cations. Concentrations of the D(–) lactic acid isomer in lactic acid-fermented vegetables are reported to be generally low. Accordingly, a man weighing 70 kg would need to consume more than 1.5 kg of sauerkraut daily to attain the critical level. Both lactic acid isomers are usually present in homemade or small-scale fermented vegetable preparations. To improve the nutritional value of industrially produced lactic acid-fermented vegetables, research is under way to select bacterial strains producing the L(+) form only.

### SOME RECIPES

#### Sauerkraut

Sauerkraut results from the natural lactic acid fermentation of salted and shredded cabbage. The high nutritive value of sauerkraut is mainly due to its increased digestibility and relatively low vitamin C losses. For at least 150 years, sauerkraut has been homemade as a means to save fresh cabbage and prevent spoilage. At present, the production of sauerkraut has become an important food industry. Industrial sauerkraut processing consists of trimming the mature and sound heads of cabbage to remove the outer green, broken, or dirty leaves. Then the cores are cut by a reversing corer. The head of cabbage is then sliced by rotary knives into long and fine shreds. Salt is sprinkled on the shreds, which are conveyed to fermentation tanks. Spices could also be added. A salt concentration in the range of 2.25 to 2.5 percent is used. Forks are used to uniformly distribute the shreds dumped and squeezed into the vat. Filled to the proper level, the tank is then closed. The shredded cabbage should be completely immersed to favor anaerobic conditions and prevent undesirable darkening and flavor changes.

Within a few hours, the brine is formed and the fermentation has started. This latter is initiated by *Leuconostoc mesenteroides,* a gas-forming species that produces lactic and acetic acids and carbon dioxide. The pH is quickly lowered, thus limiting the activity of undesirable microorganisms and enzymes that might soften the cabbage shreds. The carbon dioxide replaces air and creates an anaerobic atmosphere, which prevents the oxidation of ascorbic acid and helps in maintaining the natural cabbage color. *Lactobacillus brevis, Lactobacillus plantarum,* and sometimes *Pediococcus cerevisiae* start to grow rapidly and add their contributions to the major products, including lactic and acetic acids, carbon dioxide, and ethanol. The optimal temperature for sauerkraut fermentation is 18°C. At this temperature, fermentation is completely performed in three weeks.

### Korean Kimchi

*Kimchi* is the name given to a group of traditional fermented vegetable foods in Korea. It is a popular side dish served at every meal with rice and other dishes. The main ingredient of kimchi is either cabbage or radish, although cucumber might be added. Cabbages are cut and brined in salt solution. Salting of cabbage can be done at 5 to 7 percent salt concentration for 12 h or in 15 percent saline solution for 3 to 7 h. Salting is followed by rinsing and draining. Minor or seasoning ingredients (10 percent w/w of the main ingredient), including garlic, green onions, pepper, ginger, mustard, parsley, sesame grains, and fermented anchovies or shrimps are then added. The mixture is finally allowed to ferment in jars.

The proper combination of minor ingredients has been said to be a key for delicious and palatable kimchi. The most important factors, either for fermentation success or duration, seem to be the salt concentration and temperature. The fermentation duration varies from days (below 20°C) to one month (below 10°C). The pH is 4 to 4.5, with a lactic acid content of 0.4 to 0.8 percent. Vitamins $B_1$, $B_2$, and $B_{12}$ and niacin contents decrease when the kimchi becomes too sour. The texture depends upon the length of fermentation, temperature, and salt concentration. The organisms found in kimchi include anaerobic bacteria, such as *Lactobacillus plantarum, Lactobacillus brevis, Streptococcus faecalis, Leuconostoc mesenteroides,* and *Pediococcus cerevisiae,* and aerobic bacteria, such as *Achromobacter, Flavobacterium,* and *Pseudomonas* species. The main microorganism responsible for kimchi fermentation is *Leuconostoc mesenteroides* and the main acidifying microorganism is *Lactobacillus plantarum.*

## Cucumbers

Salt-brined cucumbers can be used as a fermentation substrate by lactic acid bacteria. Cucumbers are washed and put in a covered tank containing a salted and acidified brine. Both the concentration and chemical composition of the brine play a governing role in the sequence of microorganisms that occur in natural cucumber fermentations. Proper salt concentration exerts a selective effect on natural flora, resulting in the growth of lactic acid bacteria. Too little salt concentration (<5 percent) favors the growth of *Enterobacteriaceae* and lactic acid bacteria. Too much salt (>15 percent) suppresses the lactic acid bacteria and allows the development of halotolerant fermentative yeast.

Use of acetic acid controls the acidification and suppresses the growth of the natural microbial flora. After one day, the brine is buffered with sodium acetate. Buffering serves to eliminate secondary fermentation by yeasts. When the pH is about 4.7, the brine is inoculated with either *Lactobacillus plantarum* or *Pediococcus pentosaceus* or a combination of these organisms for a total cell count of 1 to 4 billion cells per gallon of brined cucumbers.

Maintenance of the structural integrity of cucumbers during fermentation is greatly dependent on chemical and physical properties of the fresh vegetable, including size, maturity, cultivar, and physiology. Bloater damage is the result of gas accumulation inside the cucumber during brine fermentation. Immature cucumbers are normally used for fermentation because of the presence of natural polygalacturonases in the mature vegetables. These polygalacturonases are associated with ripening, and, consequently, the seed area may liquefy during fermentation and storage. At the end of fermentation, salt (16 percent w/w of brine) is traditionally added to the lactic acid fermented cucumbers in order to stop any undesirable bacterial growth during storage.

## SUGGESTED READINGS

De Valdez GF, GS de Giori, M Garro, F Mozzi, and G Oliver (1990). Lactic acid bacteria from naturally fermented vegetables. *Microbiologie-Aliments-Nutrition*, 8:175-179.

Fleming HP (1982). Fermented vegetables. In *Economic microbiology: Fermented foods*, Volume 7, AH Rose (ed.). New York: Academic Press Inc.

Grazia L, P Romano, A Bagni, D Rogglani, and G. Guglielmi (1986). The role of moulds in the ripening process of salami. *Food Microbiology* 3:19-25.

Lee YK and S Salminen (1995). The coming age of probiotics. *Trends in Food Science and Technology*, 6:241-245.

Montet D, N Zalchia, C Mouquet, and G Loiseau (1999). Fermentation fruits and vegetables. In *Biotechnology: Food fermentation*, Volume II, VK Joshi and A Pandey (eds.). India: Educational Publishers and Distributor, pp. 951-970.

Sanders ME (1994). Lactic acid bacteria as promoters of human health. In *Functional foods*, I Golberg (ed.). United Kingdom: Chapman and Hall Inc.

Vaughn RH (1985). The microbiology of vegetable fermentations. In *Microbiology of fermented foods*, Volume 1, BJB Wood (ed.). United Kingdom: Elsevier Applied Science Publishers Ltd.

# Food Additive Production by Fermentation

Rekha S. Singhal
Pushpa R. Kulkarni

## INTRODUCTION

In food processing and preservation, certain chemical substances called *food additives* are used. According to the definition by the European Economic Commission (EEC),

> a food additive means any substance(s) not normally used as a characteristic ingredient of food, whether or not it has nutritive value, the intentional addition of which to a food is for a technological purpose, in the manufacturing, processing, preparation, treatment, packaging, transport and storage of such food results or may reasonably be expected to result in it or its by-product becoming directly or indirectly a component of food.

A list of these additives, classified according to the functions they perform in foods, is presented in Table II.4. With many chemical additives being banned, the need for natural alternatives has increased. Some of these additives are at present produced by fermentation, whereas others have the possibility of being produced in future. Other additives include leavening agents, anticaking agents, aerating agents, release agents, antifoaming agents, flour-treating agents, etc., none of which are produced by fermentation.

## FOOD ADDITIVES OF FERMENTATION ORIGIN

### Acidulants

#### Acetic Acid (Vinegar)

Acetic acid and vinegar are produced from sugar-rich materials by successive anaerobic and aerobic fermentation. The first step involves conver-

TABLE II.4. Functions, examples, and mechanisms of action of some food additives

| Type of food additive | Mechanism of action/function | Examples | Other comments |
|---|---|---|---|
| Preservatives or antimicrobial agents | Interfering with the genetic mechanism of cell division<br>Interference with cellular enzymes of the microorganisms<br>Altering the permeability of cellular membranes of organisms | Benzoate, parabens, sorbates, propionates, nitrites, sulfur dioxide in the form of various salts, nisin* | Choice dependent on product characteristics, such as pH, $a_w$, chemical composition, and type of spoilage, likely to occur in the product |
| Acidulants | Impart a sour taste | Citric, gluconic,* fumaric,* tartaric,* malic,* lactic, and phosphoric, etc. | Choice of the acidulant dictated by the color and flavor of the final product<br>Used extensively in the soft drink industry<br>A mixture of one or more acidulants used to achieve the desired effect |
| Antioxidants | Interrupting the free radical mechanism<br>By being preferentially oxidized<br>By donating a proton or an electron<br>Complex formation with the lipid | Butylated hydroxyanisole, butylated hydroxy toluene, propyl gallate, tocopherols, tert-butyl hydroquinone, ascorbic acid | Delay, retard, and prevent rancidity in fats and other susceptible materials containing unsaturated double bonds, such as essential oils and vitamins<br>Used generally at 200 ppm |
| Antibrowning agents | Inhibit the formation of dark-colored compounds in dried fruits and vegetables | Ascorbic acid, citric acid,* sodium sulfite, etc. | Inhibits browning that could be due to enzymatic or nonenzymatic reactions |
| Emulsifiers | Decreasing the surface tension between two phases | Glyceryl monostearate, sodium stearoyl lactylate, lecithin, sorbitan esters of fatty acids, etc. | Used in food emulsions, such as ice creams, cake batter, mayonnaise, salad dressings, etc. |
| Stabilizers | Aid in stabilizing the emulsions by increasing the viscosity of the aqueous phase | Locust bean gum, guar gum, gum acacia, carrageenan, xanthan,* etc. | Also used for flavor encapsulation, clarifying agent for beer/wine, coating agents in confectionery, etc. |
| Firming or crisping agents | Maintain the texture of vegetable tissues by maintaining water pressure | Calcium salts, such as hydroxide, citrate, phosphate, lactate, and heptonate, etc. | Salt type dependent on the composition of the vegetable/fruit concerned |
| Flavors | Could be due to both volatile as well as nonvolatile components | A diverse group of compounds of natural, semisynthetic and synthetic origin | Some are manufactured by fermentation |

| Type of food additive | Mechanism of action/function | Examples | Other comments |
|---|---|---|---|
| Flavor enhancers | Increase the flavor effect of certain components beyond the limit contributed by the substance itself | Monosodium glutamate, 5'-ribonucleotides,* maltol, etc. | Have little or no flavor value by themselves |
| Food colors | Impart high aesthetic appeal to foods | Could be of natural origin, or derived from synthetic coal tar dyes | Shortened list of permitted coal tar dyes due to rigid specifications |
| Humectants | Pick up moisture from the environment and pass it on to foods | Sorbitol,* mannitol, propylene glycol, and ethylene glycol | Used for preventing out in cakes and dessicated coconuts, which seriously impair its quality |
| Nutrient supplements | | Vitamins, such as A and D, thiamine and niacin; minerals, such as iodine and calcium, essential amino acids, e.g., lysine | To compensate for the nutrients that are lost during food processing |
| Sequesterants | Entrap the metals in their molecular configuration | Ethylene diamine tetraacetic acid (EDTA); hydroxycarboxylic acids, such as citric,* tartaric, and maleic acids, etc. | Often used in conjunction with antioxidants; also used for preventing struvite in fish/shell fish, turbidity in wine, and discoloration of fruits and vegetables |
| Sweeteners | | Natural sweeteners such as sucrose, glucose, and invert syrup; artificial sweeteners such as saccharin, cyclamate, acesulfame K, aspartame, etc. | Targeted toward diabetics, the obese, and those suffering from dental caries |

*Indicates production by fermentation

sion of sugar to alcohol and $CO_2$ through yeast enzymes. The second involves conversion of alcohol to acetic acid by *Acetobacter* sp. that tolerates high concentrations of acetic acid, requires small amounts of nutrients, does not overoxidize the acid formed, yields high production rates, and is phage resistant. The approaches used for fermentative production of vinegar are (1) *open vat method,* in which the fermented juices are exposed to airborne *Acetobacter,* (2) *trickle method,* in which the stock solution is trickled over twigs or wood shavings (or a silicate carrier material that has been recently proposed) to increase the air contact surface, and (3) *bubble method,* a submerged process in which aeration of the bulk liquid is obtained by bubbling air through it. Continuous production of acetic acid by submerged fermentation with continuous removal of acetic acid by electrodialysis, and continuous supply of nutrients solution and ethanol are known.

Immobilized acetic acid bacteria for continuous fermentation have been investigated. An airlift bioreactor that can be run continuously for 460 days using the acetic acid bacteria immobilized on κ-carrageenan gel beads is of particular interest. A two-stage fermentation that can produce more than 20 percent acetic acid has been reported. In this process, the first stage is carried out at normal temperatures (27 to 32°C), whereas the second stage is carried out at reduced temperatures of 18 to 24°C. The raw vinegar contains bacteria that must be filtered off. Clarification of the vinegar is done traditionally by fining and precoat filtration. In large factories, ultra- and microfiltrations are gaining importance. Pasteurization of the vinegar at 75 to 80°C for 30 to 40 min, before or after bottling is also done.

*Citric Acid*

This is well described in "Organic Acids: Production and Application."

*Fumaric Acid*

Although most fumaric acid is produced synthetically recovered as a byproduct in the manufacture of phthalic acid or maleic anhydride, or by the catalytic isomerization of maleic acid, it can also be produced by fermentation of glucose and molasses with certain strains of *Rhizopus nigricans* and *Rhizopus japonicus*. A typical medium consists of 16 percent glucose, 0.1 percent urea, 0.03 percent $KH_2PO_4$, 0.04 percent $MgSO_4.7H_2O$, 0.0044 percent $ZnSO_4$, 0.001 percent ferrous tartarate, 0.05 percent w/v corn steep liquor, and 0.015 percent methanol, in which the organism is incubated at 33 to 35°C for seven days. 0.1 percent *p*-benzoquinone suppresses the formation of side products and is advantageous. *Candida hydrocarbofumarica* yields 80 percent fumaric acid when grown on *n*-paraffins, but is very sensitive to traces of iron, zinc, and manganese. The increasing price and shortage of petrochemicals is expected to revive the biotechnological production of fumaric acid.

*Gluconic Acid*

Fermentative production of gluconic acid depends on the buildup of glucose oxidase in the organism. Earlier fermentation used *Penicillium* species, whereas improved strains of *Aspergillus niger* are used currently in submerged fermentation in recycled media. A high concentration of glucose (110 to 250 g/l), low concentration of nitrogen and phosphorus (in the range of 20 mM), sufficient quantities of trace minerals, such as manganese, a pH of 4.5 to 6.5, and a high aeration rate have been found to be mandatory for successful fermentation, usually carried out at 30°C for less than 24 h. The downstream processing consists of adding calcium hydroxide or carbonate to recover calcium gluconate, which is converted into gluconic acid by suspending in aqueous suspension and treating with stoichiometric quantities of sulfuric acid. Gluconic acid is concentrated to 50 percent for use, or is converted to glucono-δ-lactone by evaporation in a vacuum. Gluconic acid is used in the dairy industry to prevent milk-stone deposition and cleaning of aluminium cans, whereas lactone is used as a slow-acting acidulant in baking powder and in meat processing for sausage manufacture. An alternate process exploits the ability of *Acetobacter suboxydans* to use hydrolyzed starch for the production of gluconic acid.

### Lactic Acid

This is described in "Organic Acids: Production and Application."

### Other Acids

Use of fumarase from cultures of *Lactobacillus brevis* can convert fumarate to malate in 90 percent yield. *Brevibacterium ammoniagenes* immobilized on polyacrylamide gel has been the basis of continuous production of L-malic acid from fumaric acid. However, the simultaneous production of succinic acid, which is difficult to separate from the malate, posed problems. To a certain extent, this was solved by suppressing the formation of succinic acid by adding deoxycholic acid or bile acid in the substrate. A two-stage process, using *Candida hydrofumarica* in the first and *Candida utilis* in the second, that can give a 72 percent yield of L(−)-malic acid from *n*-paraffins has been reported. Possibilities for economic production of L-malate from maleate using maleate *cis-trans* isomerase, identified first in *Pseudomonas* sp. (later in *Alcaligenes* sp. T501) has been discussed. Tartaric acid can also be obtained as a fermentative product of *Gluconobacter suboxydans* when grown on glucose under appropriately manipulated cultural conditions. Bioconversion of *cis*-epoxysuccinic acid into D(+)-tartaric acid by *Acinetobacter, Agrobacterium, Rhizobium,* and *Pseudomonas* has been patented.

## Antimicrobial Agents As Preservatives

### Bacteriocins

Bacteriocins can be introduced into food either as a pure compound, or by use of lactic acid bacteria that secrete bacteriocins. Amongst the many bacteriocins that have been evaluated, nisin is the only one that is commercially exploited. Few reports are available on the fermentative production of nisin. Cultivation of *Streptococcus lactis* in a medium containing whey, 2 to 5 percent potato syrup or glucose, and 20 to 40 percent protein hydrolysate for 18 h at 28 to 30°C is reported to give good titer values for nisin. The procedure requires neutralization of the medium after the fifth hour of fermentation, followed by pH adjustment every hour to 6.5

Among the other bacteriocins reported are inhibitors of Gram-positive bacteria, such as subtilin produced by *Bacillus subtilis;* inhibitors of lactic acid bacteria and *Listeria,* such as pediocin PA1 produced by *Pediococcus acidilactici,* sakacin A by *Lactobacillus sake,* mesenterocin 5 by *Leuconostoc mesenteroides* UL5 and microgard by *Propionibacterium shermanii.* If commercially exploited, these bacteriocins will have to be produced by fermentation.

*Antimicrobial Enzymes*

The use of enzymes as natural preservatives has attracted substantial scientific interest. These function by depriving the organism of a necessary metabolite, by generating a substance that is toxic to the organism, by altering the cell wall permeability, or by working as the "killer enzyme," i.e., by inactivating other enzymes. Enzymes such as lactoperoxidase have antimicrobial property against *Pseudomonas* and *Escherichia coli* only in dairy products, where it is naturally present. It is currently not produced on an industrial scale. To extend its scope to other food systems, microbial alternatives are necessary.

*Lysozymes* are killer agents in bacteria that are active only during cell fission. Currently, they are isolated from milk (13 μg/100 ml) or egg (3.5 percent of egg white on a dry weight basis), and are active against several food-spoilage and pathogenic organisms, such as *Listeria monocytogenes, Campylobacter jejuni, Salmonella typhimurium, Bacillus cereus,* and *Clostridium botulinum.* However, for any significant commercial application, the microbial route is worth examining. Genetically modifying microorganisms to produce lyzosymes by fermentation is a far-sighted approach to this goal.

Many other enzymes, such as halogenating and oxidizing myeloperoxidase, oxidases, lipases, mannanase and chitinase are reported to have antimicrobial properties. Of these, only chitinase from *Aeromonas hydrophila* ssp. *anaerogenes* A 52 is marketed commercially as a very potent antifungal cocktail. DNA-recombinant technology that can develop overproducing strains of chitinase and downstream processes that can recover these enzymes are the need of the hour. Strategies that would preserve enzyme activity at all times, for example, at low water activity and its effectiveness in conjunction with other food components, are areas that need to be addressed before they become a commercial reality. Many of these enzymes are from non-GRAS (generally regarded as safe) organisms.

### Microbial Antioxidants

The use of enzymes that remove oxygen either as active species or by reducing lipid hydroperoxides is an area of active investigation. The only commercial application, however, is the removal of oxygen by use of glucose oxidase in conjunction with catalase. Microbial antioxidants have been isolated from *Aspergillus niger,* which enjoys GRAS status in several countries, and has shown to be effective in preventing off-flavor development in food products, such as fruit juices, mayonnaise, and salad dressings. Other oxygen-scavenging enzymes, such as alcohol oxidase, thiol oxidase, galactose oxidase, pyranose oxidase, and hexose oxidase have been regarded as potentially useful food antioxidants. Galactose oxidase has been purified from the fungus *Dactylium dendroides,* whereas pyranose oxidase can be isolated from a number of basidiomycetes and various algae. Little information on these enzymes is available in the scientific literature.

### Biosurfactants As Emulsifiers

Defined as surface active molecules possessing a mixed hydrophilic/ hydrophobic nature produced by microbial cells, *biosurfactants* are classified as glycolipid surfactants, amino acid-based surfactants, polysaccharide-lipid complex-based surfactants, and proteinlike substances as surfactants, produced by specific organisms. At present, they do not compete with the chemically synthesized emulsifiers. Problems of efficiency of the process, in some cases lack of acceptance of the producer organism and high degree of purification required for food applications, are areas that need to be sorted out before any commercial application. However, their biodegradability, eco-friendly nature, and a novel range of physical properties may suggest potential food applications in the future.

### Microbial Polysaccharides As Stabilizers and Thickeners

The most important example of this class of food additives is xanthan produced by *Xanthomonas campesteris.*

*Flavors*

About 100 compounds can be produced by fermentation, although only a few are produced on an industrial scale due to cost constraints. An interesting example of biosynthetic production of flavors is production of decalactone, which resulted in a drastic cost reduction. Flavor production using immobilized lipase from *Candida cylindracea* in a nonaqueous system has been reported to produce a broad range of esters, including ethyl butyrate (has a pineapple-bananalike flavor), *iso*amyl acetate, and *iso*butyl acetate.

Diacetyl, an important flavor constituent of cultured buttermilk, sour cream, and cultured butter, can be manufactured by fermentation that is based on the bioconversion of citrate by *Streptococcus diacetylactis* and *Leuconostoc citrovorum*. The desirable conditions for this are a pH lower than 5.5, temperature between 20 to 30°C, aeration, presence of citrate and trace amounts of molybdenum, copper, iron, and cobalt. Steam distillation of the fermentation broth, concentration by solvent extraction of the steam distillate, and further separation of diacetyl from acetoin by salting-out chromatography and/or ion-exchange chromatography is required.

Pyrazines provide a nutty flavor noted in various foods. Cultures of *Bacillus subtilis*, when grown in a media containing sucrose, asparaginase, and metal ions (such as magnesium, sodium, potassium, ferrous, manganese and cupric), are known to produce tetramethylpyrazine.

Lactones can be produced in optically pure forms by fermentation. This was first demonstrated with organisms such as *Candida, Saccharomyces, Penicillium notatum, Cladosporium butyricum, C. suaveolens,* and *Sarcina lutea* within 48 h when incubated with glucose and keto acid. An unsaturated lactone, 6-pentyl pyrone, which has a characteristic coconutlike odor, has been produced by *Trichoderma viride,* a soil fungus.

Organisms belonging to the *Ceratocystis* genus and *Kluyveromyces lactis* are known to produce terpenes. The latter grows on lactose as the sole carbon source, and can be propagated on dairy whey. With proper genetic manipulation and optimization of fermentation parameters, the yields of terpenes such as citronellol and linalool can be improved sufficiently.

Solid-state fermentation (SSF) is an attractive technique to produce flavors due to the ease of release of flavors by the microbial membranes and high concentration of productes in the liquid phase. The volatility and low solubility of flavor compounds makes recovery difficult, although technologies such as pervaporation, perstraction, vapor permeation, adsorption by solid extractants, such as charcoal or resin, and supercritical extraction of flavors could alleviate these problems.

## Flavor Potentiators

### Monosodium Glutamate (MSG)

MSG is the most commonly used flavor potentiator. Although it can be isolated from natural sources, such as wheat or corn gluten, fermentative production is more practical. Organisms belonging to the genera *Corynebacterium (C. glutamicum, C. lilium, C. callunae, C. herculis), Brevibacterium (B. divaricatum, B. aminogenes, B. flavum, B. lactofermentum, B. roseum, B. saccharolyticum, B. thiogenitalis B. immariophilum), Microbacterium (M. flavus* var *glutamicum, M. salicinocolum, M. ammoniaphilum),* and *Arthrobacter (A. globiformis, A. aminofaciens)* can produce L-glutamic acid when grown on a variety of carbon sources, such as acetic acid, glucose, fructose, sucrose, and maltose, which can be derived from molasses, starch, and cane or beet sugar. Sugar molasses is an economical feedstock, but requires treatment with penicillin or certain surface-active agents to depress excess biotin activity. The absence of biotin at the end of the active growth phase results in a loss of integrity of the cell wall, culminating in the leakage of glutamic acid in the medium. A sugar concentration below 10 percent, nitrogen sources such as ammonium salts or urea (which also maintains the pH at 7 to 8), minerals such as ferrous and potassium, a temperature of 30 to 37°C, aeration, and agitation also play a crucial role in glutamic acid fermentation. Glutamic acid fermentation from *n*-paraffins has been studied in some depth, but has never been commercialized due to economic reasons. The use of a fed-batch process in the fermentation can increase yields up to 120 g/l of glutamic acid in the media. Microorganisms used for L-glutamate fermentation are usually preserved by lyophilization below −80°C.

Exothermic fermentation causes generation of heat, which can alter the propagation of the producing organism and subsequently the production of glutamic acid. Foam is created by the $CO_2$ that is generated during the fermentation. This is taken care of by using biochemically inert silicon oil as an antifoaming agent. The fermented broth is centrifuged to remove microbial cells and other organic matter, and the clear liquid is concentrated under reduced pressure, followed by adjustment of the pH to 3.2 with hydrochloric acid. The crude crystals of L-glutamic acid are suspended in water and neutralized with sodium hydroxide. They are then decolorized with activated charcoal to obtain a clear liquid that is further concentrated to crystallize MSG crystals. These crystals are separated from the mother liquor and dried for packaging. Continuous production of MSG using a fluidized bed and immobilized bacteria are also reported. Advances in bioreactor technology, DNA recombination, and cell fusion could result in more efficient production of MSG via fermenter technology.

## 5'-Nucleotides

5'-nucleotides originated in Japan, which remains the main source of production. The approaches to the manufacture of inosine monophosphate (IMP) and guanosine monophosphate (GMP) are (1) degradation of the isolated RNA with 5'-phosphodiesterase (5'-PDE) to form 5'-nucleotides, (2) fermentation to produce nucleosides, which in turn are phosphorylated to 5'-nucleotides, and (3) direct fermentation using *Bacillus subtilis, Brevibacterium* or wild bacterial strains, and actinomycetes.

In general, microbial fermentation gives low yields, although strain-selection and strain-improvement technologies such as DNA recombinant technology could improve this. In the preferred route of degradation of the isolated RNA to 5'-nucleotides, microbial RNA (isolated from torula yeast, baker's yeast, or bacteria) is separated and purified chemically, and then treated with 5'-PDE to produce 5'-AMP, 5'-GMP, 5'-UMP and 5'-CMP. 5'-IMP can be produced from 5'-AMP by action of the adenyl deaminase enzyme system from an *Aspergillus* culture, or it can be produced chemically. 5'-PDE can be isolated from *Penicillium citrinum* (also called as nuclease P1) and *Aspergillus* and *Streptomyces* species. Nuclease P1 attacks single-stranded DNA and RNA, and its crude preparation is generally heated to inactivate the unwanted heat-labile enzymes without any loss of nuclease P1 activity. The nucleotides obtained by action of 5'-PDE are separated by ion-exchange chromatography.

### Microbial Colors

These are described in "Pigment Production."

### Humectants

Among this class of food additives, sorbitol is particularly important. Although it is generally produced by catalytic hydrogenation of glucose, it can be produced by fermentation using *Zymomonas mobilis*. The glucose-fructose oxidoreductase of *Z. mobilis* simultaneously oxidizes glucose to gluconolactone and reduces fructose to sorbitol. Process development for simultaneous production of gluconic acid and D-sorbitol using the enzyme system from *Z. mobilis* may become important in the future. A strain of *Candida boidinii* producing D-sorbitol at 8.8 g/l and 19.1 g/l from 10 and 20 g/l fructose has been reported in the literature, and has a higher conversion efficiency than *Z. mobilis*.

## Miscellaneous Food Additives of Fermentation Origin

These include (1) amino acids such as lysine, tryptophan, proline, threonine, and histidine; (2) trehalose as a new dehydrating aid; and (3) microbial enzymes as novel food additives, such as β-glucanase from *Trichoderma* sp., which is used as a filtration aid for mash in the brewing industry by reducing viscosity; acetolactate decarboxylase from *Aerobacter aerogenes* for reducing the fermentation time of beer from five weeks to two weeks by avoiding the formation of diacetyl; sulfydryl oxidase from *Aspergillus niger* to strengthen weak doughs from low-gluten flour; urease from *Lactobacillus fermentum* to reduce the levels of urethane, a carcinogen in sake; α-galactosidase from *A. niger* to modify guar gum to mimic locust bean gum.

## CONCLUSIONS

Process developments in biotechnology, genetic engineering, and reactor design, coupled with efficient and economic downstream processing, could shift the manufacture of food additives from a chemical route to a fermentation route. A heavy input of research is required for the same.

## SUGGESTED READINGS

Branen AL and Haggerty (2002). *Introduction to food additives,* Second edition, AL Branen, PM Davidson, S Salminen, JH Thorngate III (eds.). New York: Marcel Dekker, Inc., pp. 1-9.

Flickinger MC and SW Drew (eds.) (1999). *Encyclopedia of bioprocess technology: Fermentation, biocatalysis, and bioseparation,* Volumes 1-5. New York: Wiley-Interscience, John Wiley and Sons Inc.

Furia TE (ed.) (1972). *Handbook of food additives,* Second edition. Cleveland, OH: CRC Press.

Goldberg I and RA Williams (eds.) (1991). *Biotechnology of food ingredients.* New York: Van Nostrand Reinhold.

Harlander SK and TP Labuza (eds.) (1986). *Biotechnology in food processing.* Park Ridge, NJ: Noyes Publications.

Singhal RS and PR Kulkarni (1999). Production of food additives by fermentation. In *Biotechnology: Food fermentation,* Volume II, VK Joshi and A Pandey (eds.). New Delhi: Educational Publishers and Distributors, pp. 1145-1200.

Whitaker JR and PE Sonnet (eds.) (1989). *Biocatalysis in agricultural biotechnology,* ACS Symposium Series 389. Washington: American Chemical Society.

# Food-Grade Yeast Production

Argyro Becatorou
Costas Psarianos

## INTRODUCTION

Yeast, a living microorganism formed by a single cell, has been known for more than 6,000 years. Such ancient peoples as the Babylonians and Egyptians knew how to utilize wild yeasts to produce wine and beer, as well as bread with improved properties than the flat cakes baked traditionally. The identification of yeast by Louis Pasteur in the nineteenth century initiated the industrial production of yeast for use in the baking and fermentation industries. Today, the production of food-grade yeast is extremely important for both developed and developing countries, not only because yeast is used for the production of bread, the basic component of human nutrition, but as an alternative source of food to cover the demands in a world of low agricultural production and rapidly increasing population. At the same time, the increasing demands for energy and raw materials, as well as the dangers from increased environmental pollution, have made the conversion of wastes deriving mainly from the food processing industry to edible yeast biomass into a main concern for the industry and the scientific community. The impressive advantages of microorganisms for protein production compared with conventional sources (soybeans or meat) have been extensively reported. Microorganisms have short growth times, leading to rapid biomass production, and can grow at very high cell densities (see Table II.5). Biomass production can be continuous, and is independent from climate or geographical

TABLE II.5. Protein produced per day by 1 ton of source

| Source | Protein (kg) |
|--------|--------------|
| Soybean | $10^4$ |
| Bacteria | $10^{16}$ |
| Yeasts | $10^7$ |

area. Yeasts can be valuable as nutritional supplements when conventional sources of protein are not available or their exploitation is uneconomical as far as raw material, operating, and equipment costs are concerned. Cell biomass, also called single-cell protein (SCP), is compressed or dried and can be used as a raw material itself, for further processing, or for the exploitation of the functional and nutritional properties of its proteins.

## YEASTS

### Metabolism

Yeasts are able to metabolize different carbon substrates, but mainly utilize the sugars glucose, sucrose (after hydrolysis into glucose and fructose by the extracellular enzyme invertase), and maltose (after entering the cell with the aid of maltose permease to be split into two molecules of glucose by the enzyme maltase). Maltose produced from starch hydrolysis is the main substrate employed in bread fermentation. In the presence of air (aerobiosis), yeast oxidizes glucose completely, producing carbon dioxide, water, and the energy needed for cell growth. This process (aerobic fermentation) has been traditionally used to produce biomass for human or animal consumption. In limited or no-oxygen conditions, yeast utilizes the sugars to produce only the energy required to keep the cell alive. In this metabolic process, defined by Pasteur as the *fermentation process,* the sugars are transformed into carbon dioxide and alcohol (incomplete oxidation of glucose).

### Applications

Yeasts are the only microorganisms widely accepted as foodstuffs. They are used in various commercial preparations for the alcoholic fermentation of beverages (beer, wine, cider, and distillates); in the health food industry; as food additives, conditioners, and flavoring agents; as sources of high nutritional value proteins, enzymes, and vitamins; and for the production of yeast extracts and autolysates. Yeasts are often taken as nutritional supplements because they are rich in proteins, B-complex vitamins, niacin, and folic acid. They are also used as starter cultures alone or in mixtures with bacteria to conduct controlled fermentations in the food industry for the production of cheese, fermented meat products, sausages, vinegar, pickles, etc. It should be noted that food yeasts are not infectious, although they can (rarely) cause undesirable reactions in yeast allergic consumers.

The most commercially significant yeast is *Saccharomyces cerevisiae,* commonly known as baker's yeast. It has been used for thousands of years to ferment the sugars of must and cereals to produce alcoholic beverages, and in the baking industry to develop or raise dough.

## COMMERCIAL FOOD-GRADE YEASTS

The yeasts *Saccharomyces cerevisiae* as baker's yeast, *Candida utilis* as torula yeast, and *Kluyveromyces fragilis* as whey yeast, when produced on suitable, food-grade substrates (e.g., sugars, ethanol, and lactose), are permitted in many foods around the world.

### Baker's Yeasts and Related Products

The oxygen incorporated during the kneading of dough, is consumed immediately by baker's yeast, producing carbon dioxide and secondary metabolites, affecting the physical properties of dough, and giving bread its characteristic flavor. Fresh baker's yeast consists of approximately 30 to 33 percent dry materials, 6.5 to 9.3 percent nitrogen, 40.6 to 58.0 percent proteins, 35.0 to 45.0 percent carbohydrates, 4.0 to 6.0 percent lipids, 5.0 to 7.5 percent minerals, and various amounts of vitamins. Its composition depends on its type and growth conditions. Fresh baker's yeast can be found in various commercial preparations, in liquid, creamy, crumbled, or compressed form. *Compressed baker's yeast,* packed in blocks of 30 percent moisture, is the most widely used industrial form, and it is produced commercially only by one yeast species, *S. cerevisiae.* Other yeast strains can be used for the production of dry yeast products, such as active dry yeast or instant dry yeast. *Active dry yeast* is a product of dried yeast cells delivered in granular form or in small beads, whereas *instant dry yeast* comes in the form of fine particles that do not require rehydration before use. *Inactive dry yeast* is a nonleavening yeast product that is used for the conditioning of dough properties in baking, involving the reduction of gluten, the acceleration of dough expansion, and the development of characteristic flavor. *Yeast extract* is the product of the enzymatic digestion of the cell constituents by endogenous and exogenous yeast enzymes. It is rich in peptides, amino acids, nucleotides, and vitamins, and is used in pharmaceutical preparations and culture media as a nutritional supplement. It is also used as a flavoring and taste enhancer, making it possible to replace glutamates and nucleotides from many canned foods.

*Sourdough starters* (mixtures of useful bacteria and yeasts), are produced from various strains of yeasts, and are used for the conditioning of dough and the development of special flavor properties. Pure yeast cultures are produced industrially to supply breweries, and are called *Brewer's yeasts*. In brewing, two *Saccharomyces* species are used: *S. carlsbergensis,* which is used for the production of several types of beer with bottom fermentation, and *S. cerevisiae,* which conducts top fermentation. *Inactive brewer's yeast* preparations, made from inactive yeast and other special ingredients, are produced commercially to be used as nutrients to reinitiate or avoid sluggish and stuck fermentations. *Nutritional brewer's yeast,* which is used as a supplement, is an inactive yeast preparation with no leavening power. It is usually made from dried *S. cerevisiae* cells that are wasted after beer making. Brewer's yeast comes mainly in powder form or in flakes and tablets. It is a rich source of protein, providing all essential amino acids. It is also rich in the B-complex vitamins, and it is used as a supplement to increase their intake. Brewer's yeast is a good source of chromium, including a biologically active form known as *glucose tolerance factor* (GTF), and has been studied extensively for its antidiabetic properties, i.e., its ability to lower insulin levels in blood.

*Wine yeasts* are a wide variety of pure yeast cultures, mainly of the genus *Saccharomyces,* and are produced industrially for use in induced wine fermentations, according to industrial demands for fermentation efficiency and productivity. The suitable type of yeast is selected with respect to the geographical area, climate, and type of grapes and the desirable organoleptic quality of the product (taste, aroma, color, tannin and glycerol content, body, etc). Pure yeast cultures are also used to conduct specific types of fermentations, such as bottle fermentation of champagne and sparkling wines, or to reinitiate stuck and sluggish fermentations.

*Distiller's yeasts* are used for the industrial production of alcohol and spirits (brandy, whiskey, rum, tequila, etc). They are usually isolated from industrial fermentations of fruit pulps and beet or sugarcane molasses, and selected according to product demands for flavor, alcohol yield, productivity, and other technological features. In general, distiller's yeasts must show low foam formation activity, high stress tolerance, and yield high alcohol concentrations. They must also form controlled amounts of ethyl esters, aldehydes, fatty acids, and higher alcohols—an important prerequisite for the production of fine quality distillation products.

*Torula yeast* (or candida yeast) is produced by growing *Candida utilis*. It has been produced commercially since World War II, and is used mainly as a nutritional supplement. Food-grade torula yeast is cultivated in mixtures of sugars and minerals, prepared from molasses, cellulosic wastes, or from the by-products of beer. Considered to be a highly digestible nutritious food, it contains 50 to 54 percent protein (rich in lysine, threonine, valine, and glutamic acid), minerals (6 to 7 percent), and vitamins (mainly niacine, pantothenic acid, and B vitamins). It is used as a meat substitute or a food additive in many processed foods.

*Whey yeasts,* which are strains of *Kluyveromyces fragilis,* have been widely studied and applied at an industrial scale for the production of yeast biomass from whey. However, it has been reported that under aerobic conditions, such as those used in biomass production, some *K. fragilis* strains present a mixed-type metabolism of lactose, with intermediate metabolite production (alcohol, aldehydes, esters, etc.) and low yields of biomass.

## RAW MATERIALS IN FOOD-GRADE YEAST PRODUCTION

The raw materials that are used for industrial biomass production are usually waste by-products of agriculture, forestry, and the food industry, and can be classified as conventional (starch, molasses, bagasses, distiller's wash, whey, fruit and vegetable wastes, wood, straw, sawdust) and nonconventional (petroleum fractions and distillates, natural gas, ethanol, and methanol).

### Molasses

The main raw material used for baker's yeast production is a by-product of the sugar industry: molasses. Cane or beet molasses contain 45 to 55 percent fermentable sugars in the forms of sucrose, glucose, fructose, raffinose, melibiose, and galactose. The amount and type of molasses used depend upon the availability of the raw material, the cost, its composition, and the presence of inhibitors and toxins. Different types of molasses are usually blended to a mixture of pH 4.5 to 5.0, because higher pH values may promote bacterial growth. The mixture is clarified, diluted with water, sterilized, and stored in proper tanks. For high-yield yeast production, an addition of extra nutrients in the mixture is also required. These nutrients usually include nitrogen, potassium, phosphate, magnesium, and calcium, and trace minerals such as iron, zinc, copper, manganese, and molybdenum. Vitamins (biotin, inositol, pantothenic acid, and thiamine) might also be required, but usually only thiamine is added to the mixture because all other vitamins and minerals are already present in sufficient amounts in molasses. Molasses contains (in dry mass) 60 percent of fermentable sugar and 40 percent of nonsugar substances, which cannot be utilized by yeast and constitute a significant cause of pollution if they are released into the natural environment. The environmental issue is a major concern for the industry because waste

242 CONCISE ENCYCLOPEDIA OF BIORESOURCE TECHNOLOGY

treatment and utilization raises significantly the operation cost. The nonfermentable substances are usually collected and used as animal feed or as fertilizers, or are subjected to other biochemical treatments.

## Whey

Whey is a liquid waste from the dairy industry, which also constitutes a real threat for the environment because it is produced in large amounts annually and has a large organic load (COD 35,000 to 68,000), demanding large amounts of oxygen for its biodegradation. On the other hand, whey has a significant nutritional value because it contains respectable amounts of proteins, lactose, organic acids, fat, vitamins, and minerals, making its conversion to useful and consumable products a compulsory need. The physicochemical properties of whey at the moment of its production do not allow an easy fermentation of lactose, and the microorganisms that can grow and ferment whey are few. Lactose, the main sugar constituent in whey, can be metabolized only by species of the fungus *Kluyveromyces,* such as *K. marxianus, K. lactis,* and *K. fragilis.* The yeast *S. cerevisiae* cannot utilize lactose because it lacks β-galactosidase and lactose permease. *K. fragilis* is the only strain used for biomass production from whey on a commercial scale.

## Starch

*S. cerevisiae* can utilize starch after converting it to the fermentable sugars glucose and maltose. Other common processes for starch saccharification include gelatinization by heating and enzymatic hydrolysis, but such processes imply a considerable cost and are the main limiting factor in the industrial utilization of starch for biomass production.

## Lignocellulosic Materials

Wastes of agriculture and forestry consist of a complex mixture of cellulose, hemicellulose, and lignin. Their enzymatic conversion to fermentable sugars requires chemical pretreatment, which leads to different polymer fragments. *S. cerevisiae* does not have the required hydrolytic enzymes that vary according to the composition and structure of these polymers. As a result, yeast biomass production on lignocellulosic wastes implies a high economic cost. A solution to this problem could be the use of mixed cultures of *S. cerevisiae* and cellulolytic microorganisms, but this process is today applied commercially only for ethanol production.

## STAGES OF INDUSTRIAL FOOD-GRADE YEAST PRODUCTION

Yeast production generally involves the following stages: propagation, involving a number of fermentation processes as described in the following paragraphs, harvesting, concentration and/or drying, packaging, and shipment. Figure II.7 presents a baker's yeast propagation scheme, involving two batch and two fed-batch fermentation stages.

### Fermentation

For baker's yeast, the principle raw materials are a pure starter culture and a suitably adjusted mixture of molasses. Yeast cells are grown in a series of fermentation bioreactors, which are operated under aerobic conditions to promote yeast growth. In the first instance, cells from a pure yeast culture are grown with molasses in the laboratory and the produced biomass is transferred aseptically in batch mode into the first fermentor, which operates anaerobically. More than one fermentor can be employed in this stage, and ethanol is produced along with cell mass. The next fermentor usually operates in a fed-batch mode with good aeration, and is an intermediate fermentor before the *stock fermentation* stage. The stock produced in the stock fermentor is separated with centrifugation to be used in the next stage: *pitch fermentation*. Both stages operate in fed-batch mode with vigorous aeration and an incremental addition of nutrients. The content of the pitch fermentor is used for pitching the final *trade fermentations*. At the end of the process, the content in the trade fermentors is aerated for an additional time period, and this is called the *maturation stage*. The amount of yeast biomass produced increases from stage to stage. The sequence and number of fermentation stages vary among manufacturers, but the principle of the process remains the same.

### Treatments and Packaging

The yeast in the final trade fermentor is concentrated by centrifugation and finally harvested by a filter press or a rotary vacuum filter until it contains 27 to 32 percent or 33 percent dry cell mass respectively. The pressed yeast is blended with suitable amounts of water and emulsifiers to obtain its familiar, white, creamy appearance. Small amounts of cutting oils are also added (soybean or cottonseed oil) to help extrude and cut the yeast, which is then packaged and shipped as compressed fresh baker's yeast, or dried to form various types of dry yeast. In dry yeast production, different types of

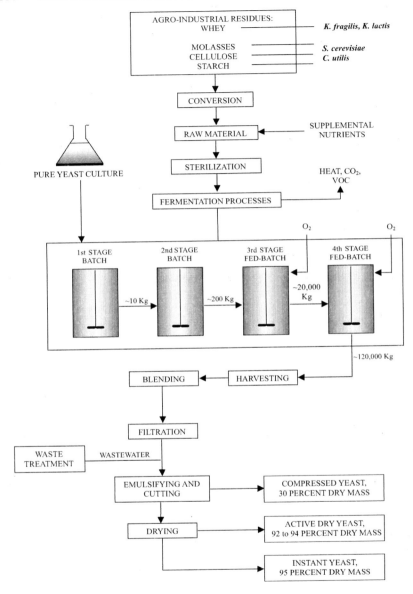

FIGURE II.7. Description of a propagation scheme for the production of food-grade yeast, with respect to baker's yeast, involving two batch and two fed-batch fermentation stages

emulsifiers and oils are used to texturize the yeast. The dried yeast is packed under a vacuum or nitrogen atmosphere. The packaging method varies among manufacturers and depends on the type of yeast product.

## CONCLUSIONS

Today, modern techniques such as DNA recombination, induced mutations, and selection have been employed to obtain new yeast strains with improved properties. Knowledge of *S. cerevisiae*'s genetic potential allows the yeast manufacturer to select or create highly specialized yeast strains according to his or her demands for fermentation efficiency and industrial productivity. For example, it is critical for the modern baking industry that more stable yeast strains be produced which are tolerant in pH and temperature variations in high osmotic pressure and are able to survive preservation, antifungal agents. Also important in terms of productivity and quality is the improvement of industrial strains to solve major problems such as glucose repression on the use of mixed carbohydrate substrates, and the production under aerobic conditions of undesirable by-products such as ethanol and glycerol. On the other hand, genetic engineering has made possible the creation of new yeast strains, with new or enhanced enzymatic properties (e.g., melibiase, invertase, or maltase activity) for maximum utilization of alternative substrates, such as cheese whey from the dairy industry, starch, sugarcane bagasses, sugar-rich virgin grape marc from distilleries, and lignocellulosic materials from forestry and agriculture. This achievement will lead to a solution of the environmental problem arising from the disposal of food-grade wastes with high organic loads. Finally, it will lead to the reduction of yeast production cost by increasing the availability of raw materials and skipping the intermediate traditional methods for their conversion. In the frame of these efforts, new and rapid methods for nuclear or mtDNA analysis have been introduced for the identification of industrial yeast strains, and the design and development of novel aerobic bioreactors is expected to enable an optimal production of yeast biomass with maximum utilization of the raw material, reduction of costs, and a simultaneous reduction of environmental pollution.

## SUGGESTED READINGS

Knorr D (1987). *Food biotechnology.* New York: Marcel Dekker, Inc.
Martin AM (1991). *Bioconversion of waste materials to industrial products.* London and New York: Elsevier Applied Science.

Randez-Gil F, P Sanz, and JA Pietro (1999). Engineering baker's yeast: Room for improvement. *Trends in Biotechnology* 17:237-244.

Rincón AM and T Benítez (2001). Improved organoleptic and nutritive properties of bakery products supplemented with amino acid overproducing *Saccharomyces cerevisiae* yeasts. *Journal of Agricultural and Food Chemistry* 49(4): 1861-1866.

Ringbom K, A Rothberg, and B Saxén (1996). Model-based automation of baker's yeast production. *Journal of Biotechnology* 51(1):73-82.

# Kefir Yeast Technology

Matina Iconomopoulou
Costas Psarianos

## INTRODUCTION

Kefir grains originated from the Caucasus Mountains. Kefir is derived from the Turkish word *kef,* which means "pleasant taste." Kefir is the thick-flowing cream and slightly effervescent fermented milk that is obtained from cow's, goat's, or sheep's milk. It contains 0.8 to 1 percent lactic acid, 0.3 to 0.8 percent ethanol, carbon dioxide, and other flavor products, such as acetaldehyde and acetoin. The alcohol and carbon dioxide, together with small amounts of diacetyl, acetaldehyde, and acetone, contribute to its characteristic refreshing taste. Kefir is produced in large amounts, particularly in Russia, where it accounts for 70 percent of the total amount of fermented milk consumed. In many countries, the popularity of kefir is only slightly less than that of yogurt. It is also well known in Sweden, Norway, Finland, Hungary, Poland, Germany, Greece, Austria, Brazil, and Israel. Fermented dairy products comprise an important segment of the dairy industry. Kefir is being investigated as a new product for wide-scale introduction into the United States, and it is also sold in Japan, although consumption is lower.

## TRADITIONAL PRODUCTION OF KEFIR GRAINS

The traditional process of kefir grain production comes from the Caucasus Mountains. Fresh, raw, full-cream goat's or cow's milk is poured into goatskin leather bags that contain inoculums of kefir grains. The fermentation lasts 24 h at 22°C and the kefir grains are separated from the produced fermented drink (kefir). Afterward they can be washed in clean water and stored moist at 4°C or they can be dried at room temperature for 36 to 48 h. Dried grains retain activity for 12 to 18 months, whereas moist grains lose their activity in eight to ten days.

## MORPHOLOGY OF KEFIR GRAINS

Kefir grains are whitish-yellow clumps. The diameter of each kefir grain is 3 to 20 mm, and together they resemble small cauliflower florets. The kefir grains contain symbiotic, plural lactic acids bacteria and plural yeasts. Using the sparingly water-soluble, but highly swellable polysaccharide kefiran and acid-coagulated casein, each cell is bound to the others. Scanning electron microscopy (SEM) is used for the determination of the microbial content of grains and the observation of the microbial distribution in kefir grains. Yeast colonies grow on the surface and middle of the kefir grain, whereas Lactobacilli grow throughout the grain.

The lactic acid bacteria produce kefiran. The results of nuclear mangetic resonance (NMR) and methylation analysis indicate that the kefiran contains approximately equal proportions of D-galactose and D-glucose residues. It has been suggested that *Lactobacillus kefiranofaciens* is suitable for kefiran production, whereas *Lactobacillus* sp. KPB-167B can grow and produce the capsular polysaccharide with better yield.

Optimum culture conditions for the effective production of kefiran by *Lactobacillus* sp. are pH 5.0 and temperature 30°C. A modified medium containing 10 percent lactose, 5 mM $CaCl_2$, and twofold the original nitrogen sources produces 2 g/L of kefiran in four days. Synergism between the microorganisms of kefir grains is also obtained. In a mixed culture, *Saccharomyces florentinus* supports better survival of *L. hilgardii,* and a significant increase in lactic acid production occurs. At the same time, the growth and alcoholic fermentation of *S. florentinus* are drastically reduced.

## COMPOSITION OF KEFIR GRAINS AND KEFIRLIKE CULTURES

The composition of the mixed kefir culture is variable, according to the origin, climate, storage, temperature, handling, growth media, or the milk used. Typical microflora isolated from kefir grains are divided into four groups: lactobacilli, streptococci, yeasts, and *Acetobacter.* The bacteria are homofermentative and heterofermentative *Lactobacillus, Leuconostoc,* and *Acetobacter.* Kefir has 8.58 log cfu/g lactococci, 8.60 log cfu/g lactobacilli, and 5.09 log cfu/g total yeasts. Typical microflora isolated from kefir grains are shown in Table II.6. The percentages of microbes in kefir grains are lactobacilli 66 percent, streptococci 14 percent, and yeasts 19 percent. Among the isolated yeast from the Iranian kefir grain *Candida kefir, Saccharomyces lactis, Saccharomyces cerevisiae,* and *Saccharomyces fragilis* have been isolated. At least 24 percent of the dry material of the kefir strain

## TABLE II.6. Typical microflora isolated from kefir grains

| Lactobacilli | Streptococci/ Lactococci | Yeasts | Acetobacter |
|---|---|---|---|
| Lb. acidophilus | Enterococcus durans | Candida friedrichii | Acetobacter aceti |
| Lb. brevis | Lc. lactis ssp. cremoris | C. kefir | A. rasens |
| Lb. casei | Lc. lactis ssp. lactis | C. pseudotropicalis | |
| Lb. casei ssp. alactosus | Lc. lactis var. diacetylactis | Kluyveromyces bulgaricus | |
| Lb. casei ssp. rhamnosus | Leuconostoc cremoris | K. fragilis var. marxianus | |
| Lb. cellobiosus | L. mesenteroides | K. lactis | |
| Lb. delbrueckii ssp. bulgaricus | S. lactis | K. marxianus var. marxianus | |
| Lb. delbrueckii ssp. lactis | S. salivarius ssp. thermophilus | Saccharomyces ssp. (delbrueckii, holmii, unisporus) | |
| Lb. fermentum | | Torulapora delbrueckii | |
| Lb. fructivorans | | Torulopsis holmii | |
| Lb. gasseri | | | |
| Lb. helveticus ssp. lactis | | | |
| Lb. hilgardii | | | |
| Lb. kefir | | | |
| Lb. kefiranofaciens | | | |
| Lb. kefirgranum | | | |
| Lb. lactis | | | |
| Lb. parakefir | | | |
| Lb. viridescens | | | |

consists of the capsular polysaccharide. The composition of freeze-dried kefir grains is water 3.5 percent, fat 4.45 percent, ash 12 percent, mucopolysaccharide 45.7 percent, and total protein 34.3 percent.

## *FERMENTATION AND CHEMICAL COMPOSITION OF THE FERMENTED PRODUCT*

Kefir is produced by simultaneously conducting lactic acid fermentation with lactic acid bacteria and alcoholic fermentation with yeasts. A common end product of bacteria is lactate, whereas yeasts are responsible for the alcohol production. Lactate, pyruvate, acetaldehyde, acetoin, and ethanol increase during fermentation. The lactic acid fermentation stops as the pH drops, whereas the alcoholic fermentation may still proceed. Some yeasts assimilate lactose, galactose, and other sugars remaining in the fermented product provided that temperature is appropriate. The subsequent alcoholic fermentation is avoided either (1) by using in combination lactic acid bacteria that do not cause accumulation of galactose and lactose nonfermenting yeast or (2) by selectively using a yeast that is capable of fermenting neither lactose nor galactose. Lactate production rapidly increases between 10 and 15 h of fermentation and is 6.5 mg/g with the completion of the fermentation (in 22 h). Group N streptococci can degrade lactose to galactose and glucose. The glucose can be metabolized by the homofermentative Embden-Meyerhof-Parnas pathway to pyruvate, where 2 mol of lactate are formed per glucose molecule. The residual pyruvate is converted to acetaldehyde and diacetyl. The heterofermentative pathway results in the production of $CO_2$ and lactic acid. Some lactic acid bacteria metabolize the citrate contained in milk to acetoin and diacetyl, but a significant amount remains in the fermented liquid (about 1.4 mg/g). The orotic acid decreases during the fermentation and is used in the synthesis of nucleotides. The hippuric acid is a precursor in the synthesis of benzoic acid and is nullified at the end of the fermentation. *Leuconostoc* and occasionally acetic acid bacteria form flavor products. *L. brevis* can produce $CO_2$, acetate, acetoin, and diacetyl especially.

The diacetyl concentration is related to the fermented milk type because the citrate level is different for each milk and this compound is important during the synthesis of the diacetyl. *Lactobacillus delbrueckii* mainly produces acetaldehyde, and when the starter culture contains this microorganism, the final concentration of acetaldehyde increases to 0.96 µg/g. This amount is low because acetaldehyde is converted to ethanol by alcohol dehydrogenase. Ethanol is the main product of yeasts and increases significantly after 15 h of fermentation. In a parallel way, the heterofermentative *L. kefir* can produce ethanol and $CO_2$. Compared with kefir produced by starter cultures, traditional kefir has a higher alcohol content with a final concentration of about 4 µg/g. Acetoin production is 25 µg/g. The acidity of kefir produced by kefir grain increases to 1.4 percent with 3.0 percent $CO_2$, whereas kefir from starter cultures has lower acidity and $CO_2$.

## *PARAMETERS AFFECTING THE FERMENTATION*

Kefir production is possible by using the starter cultures of native microbial strains, and the quality of produced kefir can be affected by various ratios of starter cultures. Although the product contains more or less similar acidity, carbon dioxide, fat, sugar, protein, and riboflavin, the taste is not as good as kefir made by kefir grain. Cultures with 3 percent bacteria (different ratios of *Lactobacillus: Streptococcus lactis* and *L. mesenteroids*), 2 percent yeast, and 0.5 percent acetic acid bacteria are used as starter cultures for kefir production. It is difficult to justify the use of individual pure cultures in commercial production because it is not easy to keep cultures pure and unchanged, especially kefir in which the grains yield the proper acidity and effervescence. Although the parameters of color, smell, viscosity, and carbon dioxide are not affected by various ratios of starter cultures, flavor and acidity are affected. Kefir produced with kefir grain is more desirable than kefir produced with starter cultures. The kefir grains are generally stable and easily transferred from batch to batch.

## KEFIR PRODUCTION

The prepared milk is heated in the heat exchanger to 70°C, and is then homogenized and pasteurized at 85°C for 30 min. Pasteurized milk is cooled to the fermentation temperature of 20 to 25°C (usually 22°C). The milk is seeded with kefir cultures 2 to 10 percent (w/v) and fermented in the ripening vessel for 18 to 24 h until the pH reaches to 4.6 to 4.4. After incubation, the kefir grains are removed via sieving. The grains can be reused in subsequent starter culture preparation or be washed well with cold water and added to a new production batch (Figure II.8). With each subsequent incubation, the size of the kefir grains increases slightly. The kefir is cooled to 7 to 12°C and filled either into glass bottles or plastic beakers. It can be used for consumption or left to postripen at 7°C for 24 to 48 h. The closure of the bottles permits carbon dioxide to escape, and a significant amount of the alcohol is lost.

For larger production, the fermented product is used as a bulk starter culture after removal of the grains. Wet or freeze-dried grains or kefir starter cultures can be used as bulk starter culture also. Kefir produced traditionally or by selected kefir microflora can be described as being an effervescent, refreshing fermented milk beverage with a pleasant, distinctive taste and flavor. Among its prevalent organoleptic characteristics are its clean (lactic) acid taste, soft alcoholic flavor, and smooth, creamy texture. In the case of a synthetic medium, kefir grains can be cultured by the use of a liquid medium containing, for example, peptone, yeast extract, malt extract, glucose, lactose, an inorganic substance, etc., and more particularly, a liquid medium containing a vegetable juice, such as tomato juice, or a fruit juice, such as orange and grape. The kefir grains can be also used to ferment other types of mediums, such as soy, seed, or nut milk.

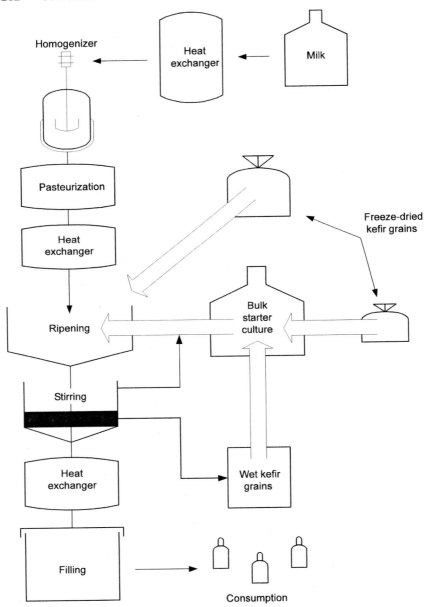

FIGURE II.8. Manufacture of kefir grains and kefir

## PRESERVATION OF KEFIR GRAINS

The live organisms of kefir grains are removed from the fermented product because the excessive acid production will gradually damage them. Acid production is inhibited by refrigeration, but the grains lose their activity after about ten days. The grains grown in the process of kefir production can be dried at room temperature and kept at cold temperature (4°C). When kefir grains are washed with clean, cold water and dried on cloth or paper for two days at room temperature, they can then be stored in a dry, cool place for well over a year and still stay active. For longer preservation, they can also be freeze-dried. Upon sterilization, freeze-dried kefir grains are to be supplemented with yeast preparation showing the lowest survival in the course of freeze drying. A mixture of 20 percent sucrose solution and starch appears to be the most efficient dispersing agent to protect yeast in the freeze-drying process.

Procedures that involve heat, such as sterilizations by autoclaving (e.g., exposure at 110°C for 3 min), or exposure to irradiation (e.g., 5 KGy) and high pressures (e.g., 400 MPa for 5 min) may damage both bacteria and yeast species and deactivate kefir grains. The microbial counts in deactivated kefir may be as low as 0.59 log cfu/g$^{-1}$. Sterilization of kefir by exposure to suitable conditions of heat, pressure, and/or irradiation can deactivate the kefir grains without affecting product quality.

## KEFIR GRAINS AND KEFIR AS PROBIOTICS

For thousands of years microorganisms have been used for the production and preservation of foods through fermentation. Ancient peoples, such as the Babylonians, Egyptians, and Greeks, realized the benefits of fermentation, and foods containing lactic acid bacteria (yogurt, kefir, kumis) were associated with positive effects on human health. Kefir grains and kefir drink are classified as probiotics because they contain microorganisms that are able to survive the gastrointestinal tract and beneficially influence health by changing its microflora. The microorganisms in kefir have been associated with longevity in the Caucasus region, and have been demonstrated to be nonpathogenic. On the contrary, milk inoculated with grains can suppress the growth of pathogens such as salmonella or shigella. Kefir has been used for the treatment of tuberculosis, cancer, and gastrointestinal disorders, and for a variety of conditions, including metabolic disorders, atherosclerosis, and allergic disease. Specific cultures isolated from kefir have also shown to bind to mutagenic substances, such as indole and imidazole.

The specific effects mentioned previously may not be demonstrated in all produced kefirs due to the significant role of the composition of the kefir culture.

## CONCLUSIONS

Today, pure cultures of lactic acid bacteria and yeasts that occur in kefir grains are used for the production of a commercial kefir drink. The manufacturing process enables the dairy industry to produce a product of consistent quality. The starter cultures typically used are mainly mixtures of aerobic and anaerobic *Lactobacillus* spp., *Lactococcus* spp., *Streptococcus thermophilus, Leuconostoc* spp., and yeasts in the ratio 24:24:21:14:16 respectively.

Kefir yeast has been used recently as a convenient culture to treat whey for biomass production. This single-cell protein (SCP) production will presumably decrease the organic load of the polluted whey and produce a new livestock feed for animals. Moreover, the biomass that is produced can ferment whey anaerobicaly for the production of a raw material to produce an alcoholic drink. In this case, the whey liquid effluent of the dairy industry becomes not a liquid waste, but a raw material for the food industry.

### SUGGESTED READINGS

Garrote G, A Abraham, and G De Antoni (1997). Preservation of kefir grains, a comparative study. *Food Science and Technology* 30(1):77-83.

Macrae R, RK Robinson, and MJ Sadler (1993). Kefir. *Encyclopaedia of Food Science, Food Technology, and Nutrition.* London: Academic Press.

# Molecular Methods for Microbial Detection and Characterization for Food Safety

Suresh D. Pillai
James M. Totten

## INTRODUCTION

Ever since Antoni van Leeuwenhoek (1632-1723) discovered animalcules, humans have been intrigued by microorganisms and microbial populations. To this end, improved microscopes, culture methods, and molecular methods were developed. If one were to analyze the groundbreaking developments in microbiology, it would be evident that these developments were very closely linked to key improvements in microbial detection and characterization technologies. The ability to detect and characterize specific microbial populations has played a significant role in improving public health and agricultural production, optimizing industrial processes, and in safeguarding environmental quality.

The term *molecular methods* encompasses both immunological and nucleic acid-based methods. However, for purposes of this chapter the term will be restricted to nucleic acid-based methods only. Since the late 1980s development of polymerase chain reaction (PCR) technology, a virtual "explosion" of nucleic acid-based techniques, have enabled faster, more sensitive, and more specific detection of microorganisms. Because the basic PCR technology and its varied applications have been the subject of a number of books, review articles, and research articles, an in-depth discussion of that technique will not be attempted here. This chapter deals primarily with improved amplification and probe technologies that have been developed for detection and characterization in the last couple of years, and are the subject of extensive optimization trials and evaluations. The objective of this chapter is to highlight the unique features of some of these molecular methods so that possible applications in food safety and environmental quality can be envisioned.

## DETECTION

Molecular detection methods can be broadly divided into amplification-based and probe-based methods. The primary difference between these two categories is that in the former, a particular target DNA or RNA sequence is enzymatically amplified, whereas in the latter, a particular target or nucleotide sequence is directly detected using DNA hybridization based on Watson-Crick base-pairing principles. A recurring theme in some of the newer methods is the integration of both the amplification and probe technologies into the same method.

### *Target Amplification Methods*

#### *Conventional PCR Technology*

A number of significant improvements have occurred in the basic technique, so much so that this method has found numerous applications in almost all fields of biological sciences. A variety of PCR kits are now commercially available for the detection of specific pathogens. PCR-based kits for the detection of *Salmonella* sp., *Listeria* sp., and *Escherichia coli* 0157: H7 are now available. A salient feature of these kits is the ease of their use—all necessary reagents are lyophilized into a tablet form within the reaction tube. All that is required is the addition of a known volume of sample and placement in a temperature-cycling instrument. The availability of these kits has been of significant value in detecting pathogens in foods and the environment. Current versions of these kits also include automated gel-electrophoresis modules, thereby reducing the potential for human errors and laboratory-based contamination that can lead to invalid PCR results.

#### *Real-Time Quantitative PCR Method*

The method is also referred to as the fluorogenic 5' nuclease assay or the TaqMan probe technology. The primary difference between this version of the PCR method and the conventional PCR method is that oligonucleotide probes along with the primers are used in the process. More important, the PCR product formation is detected during the course of the reaction in contrast to the conventional process, in which the product is detected at the end of the reaction. Thus, the PCR product is detected in "real-time" as compared to the "end-point" detection in the conventional PCR process. A schematic representation of the process is shown in Figure II.9.

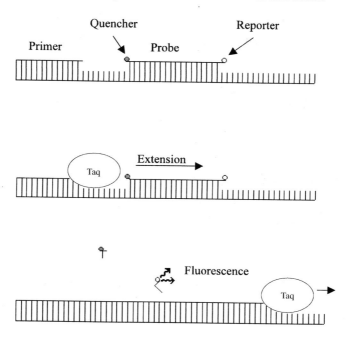

FIGURE II.9. Schematic representation of the real-time PCR assay

In this method, the 5' nuclease activity of the AmpliTaq Gold DNA polymerase to cleave the TaqMan probe off the target sequence is exploited. The
TaqMan probe contains a reporter dye at the 5' end and a quencher dye at the
3' end. Under normal conditions, when the probe is intact, the fluorescence
from the reporter dye is quenched by the quencher dye. When the 5' end of
the probe is cleaved by the DNA polymerase, fluorescence results, which is
then detected by the instrument and quantified using sophisticated algorithms. Because the fluorescence measurements take place during the exponential or logarithmic phase of the amplification, it is possible to quantitate
the formation of a specific PCR product. Suitable standard curves have to be
prepared and run alongside the experimental samples for absolute quantifi-
cation. The primers and the TaqMan probes confer additional detection
specificity as compared to the conventional PCR process. Since the assay
relies on real-time detection product formation and involves detecting fluorescence detection, this assay is more sensitive than the conventional end-
point assay. In addition, because this assay does not involve any post-PCR

product handling, the issue of PCR contamination is also significantly reduced. However, this assay requires very specialized instrumentation.

In addition to the use of TaqMan probes, the assay can also be performed using the SYBR Green 1 Double-Stranded Binding Dye. However, when this dye is used, DNA melting curve analysis needs to be performed to confirm the authenticity of the PCR product. The use of the dye can also result in cost savings as compared to using the TaqMan probes. One limitation of the real-time assays, especially those that involve TaqMan probes, is the need to rely on rather short target regions for optimal results.

Recent improvements and modifications of the TaqMan probes and primers include the Amplifluor and Scorpion primers. In the Scorpion primer-based approach, the specially designed Scorpion primers anneals to the heat-denatured target (Figure II.10). The Taq polymerase then synthesizes a complimentary copy of the target sequence. Once the double-stranded target is heat denatured, the 5' end of the Scorpion primer snaps

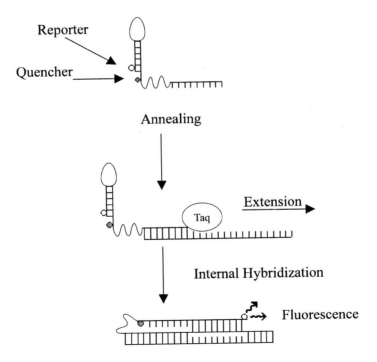

FIGURE II.10. Schematic representation of the Scorpion primer-based PCR assay

back to anneal to the target. This annealing of the primer results in fluorescence that is detected and quantitated as the cycling proceeds.

Other amplification protocols do not necessarily involve the use of the Taq DNA polymerase. One of the first non-PCR amplification protocols developed is called the transcription-based amplification system (TAS). It involves the sequential involvement of reverse transcriptase (formation of cDNA), followed by RNA polymerase, which catalyzes the synthesis of multiple copies of the original RNA template. Further improvements in the TAS protocol resulted in the development of the 3SR (self-sustaining sequence replication) amplification technology. The particular improvement in this method over TAS is the use of RNase H, which replaced heat denaturation of the RNA-DNA duplexes. Because heat denaturation is typically not involved in 3SR, this amplification can be conducted under isothermal conditions, thereby alleviating the need for specialized instrumentation. However, these methods require extensive post-amplification steps, which are cumbersome and can lead to contamination errors.

### Probe Amplification Methods

The Qβ replicase (for amplifying RNA probe molecules), the ligase chain reaction (LCR) and the branched probes are methods that have been developed to amplify probe molecules already hybridized to target sequences. The basic principle behind the Qβ replicase system is to produce RNA probes that can anneal to the target of interest and serve as substrates for the Qβ replicase, which can replicate the RNA probe molecule. The RNA probe is hybridized initially to the target sequence, and all unbound probe molecules are washed off or removed by treatment with RNase. When the Qβ replicase is added, only those probe molecules hybridized to the target will be amplified many times over to facilitate detection of the target sequence.

Ligase chain reaction is a highly specific and sensitive technique that can be used to differentiate DNA target sequences that differ by as little as one base pair. In LCR, probe pairs are designed so that their ends abut one another at the site of the target region. If the base pair at the site matches the nucleotide at the 3' end of the upstream primer, the adjoining probes will anneal if DNA ligase is available. Currently, a thermostable ligase is used in LCR amplifications to mimic an amplifcation analogous to PCR. It has been shown that LCR can be used to detect as few as 10 CFU per reaction of *Listeria monocytogenes* in conjunction with a nonisotopic PCR-coupled LCR.

## Direct Probe Methods

Conventional DNA probes are still being used widely in the clinical and food industries. However, these procedures can be time-consuming, and the detection sensitivity is not as high as the amplification-based approaches. However, given the advances in genomics in recent years, improved nucleotide sequence information is currently available, which in turn has facilitated the design and synthesis of oligonucleotide probes that are extremely specific and sensitive.

## Reverse Sample Genome Probing

A primary drawback of the conventional probe approach is the need to have multiple hybridization filters for each of the different probes that are employed. However, alternate hybridization formats such as reverse sample genome probing, which allows multiple targets to be detected simultaneously, have been reported in the literature. In this approach, probes against the various target organisms are affixed to membranes and the sample that is being screened is labeled and used as the template.

## DNA Microarrays

Considerable progress has been made in the use of DNA microarrays as detection tools. DNA microarrays can be used to screen hundreds and thousands of specific sequences. Although the basic principle is based on the conventional Watson-Crick base-pairing principles, the ability to immobilize thousands of DNA sequences on extremely small matrixes is a significant breakthrough. The DNA sequences can be affixed to the matrixes using either robotic technologies or lithographic processes. The target DNA sample is labeled with a radioactive or fluorescent marker and the microarray is exposed to the labeled sample. Hybridization at the various locations can be detected and the results analyzed. DNA microarrays can be used for the rapid detection of specific nucleotide sequences, as well as to detect the temporal and spatial patterns of gene expression. The ability to screen hundreds of targets makes DNA arrays attractive for use in monitoring environmental and food samples for pathogens. However, given the low concentration of target organisms in environmental and food samples, some initial enrichment using either culture-based amplification or genetic amplification is required for effective detection.

## CHARACTERIZATION

Major advances have occurred in methods that are available to characterize microbial populations. Presently, it is possible to characterize the microbial populations from natural and man-made ecosystems, even when these populations are nonviable or cannot be cultured. Many PCR- and non-PCR-based methods are available for this purpose.

### PCR-Based Fingerprinting Methods

PCR-based fingerprinting methods, such as BOX-PCR and ERIC-PCR, are available to identify the genetic relatedness of multiple bacterial isolates. These methods are based on using primers that are designed to anneal to specific reiterated gene sequences within the genomes of eubacteria. The resulting amplification fingerprint is captured digitally, electronically analyzed, and the genetic relatedness of the isolates can be determined. The utility of these methods to identify the sources of the various isolates (i.e., animal, human, wildlife, domestic pets) is currently a major research focus. The key advantage of using these methods is that they are relatively easy to perform, the published amplification conditions are relatively robust, and the methods are reproducible. The reagents and protocols for these methods are now commercially available.

### PFGE-Based Fingerprinting

Pulse field gel electrophoresis (PFGE) is based on the restriction enzyme digestion of the entire bacterial genome using specific restriction enzymes. The large restriction fragments are resolved using an electrophoresis under specialized conditions to generate a fingerprint. Since the fingerprint is based on the entire genome, this approach of strain characterization is extremely sensitive and reproducible. PFGE is the current worldwide gold standard for isolate characterization. It is used as the primary molecular method by the U.S. Centers for Disease Control and Prevention for tracing the sources of disease outbreaks. The specific protocols and reagents of PFGE have been rigorously standardized, and multiple laboratories around the country use this method to characterize bacterial strains related to disease outbreaks. The fingerprints from the various laboratories are electronically linked via PulseNet, a network of public health laboratories in the United States, allowing quick comparisons of outbreak strains.

## *Denaturing Gradient Gel Electrophoresis (DGGE)*

DGGE is used often to identify the different populations present within a microbial community. The process involves extraction of nucleic acids from the entire microbial community, PCR amplification of all the 16S sequences present with the extracted community, and resolving the various 16S sequences under denaturing gel-electrophoresis conditions. The unique aspect of this method is that the denaturing electrophoresis conditions can resolve nucleotide differences that differ by even a single base pair, even when they are of the same size on conventional gels. The different fragments from the gel are excised and sequenced. The sequence information is then compared to the GenBank database to identify the organisms present within the microbial community.

## *CONCLUSIONS*

Despite the rapid development of these methods, issues related to specificity, sensitivity, costs, and regulatory approval are still paramount and must be carefully considered. The need to use molecular methods should be based on a careful consideration of the overall objective, the potential target copy numbers, the matrix in which the intended target is present, the possible cross reactivity with closely related organisms, and budgetary constraints to hire trained individuals and purchase and maintain the required instrumentation.

The specificity of the primers and the probes has to be rigorously tested. They need to be verified using pure culture preparations of closely related species and appropriate spike tests with different matrices. Studies have shown that although the primers and probes may not show any nonspecificity in pure culture samples, the specificity can be compromised once a natural sample is used. Differences in the ionic conditions between pure cultures and natural samples may result in mispriming of probes and primers. Although these changes cannot always be predicted using pure cultures, appropriate matrix spike tests can help overcome these problems. The sensitivity of these methods has also been shown to be influenced by the sample matrix. Sample constituents could negatively influence the enzymatic activities with the result that the detection sensitivity could be impaired in a natural sample.

Molecular methods such as gene amplification are often expected to solve problems associated with conventional detection methods. For example, the detection of enteric viruses in source water and drinking water is of critical importance to the drinking water industry. Currently, tissue-culture-based systems are capable of detecting enteric viruses, however, these methods are time-consuming and expensive. Gene amplification-based methods would appear to be capable of overcoming these shortcomings of tissue culture. However, lingering issues remain with the use of gene amplification methods and problems associated with interpreting the molecular data. Because the levels of enteric viruses in source waters are generally low, large volumes of the sample have to be concentrated and purified prior to gene amplification. Moreover, only very small aliquots of the sample can be added to the final reaction mixture, and so a negative PCR result should be carefully analyzed. Alternatively, the issue of detecting naked viral nucleic acids not contained within a viable or infective virus particle is still problematic in interpreting molecular data. To overcome some of the limitations associated with sensitivity and nonviability of targets, some of the commercial PCR-based detection kits for bacterial pathogens employ an initial enrichment step.

Without a doubt, the use of molecular methods calls for trained individuals in the laboratory to carry out the tasks and interpret the results. Such individuals have to be adequately trained to avoid cross contamination. In conventional culture plate-based methods, a contaminant can be readily detected. However, it is virtually impossible to detect contamination in molecular methods. The individuals in the laboratory have to be trained so that they understand the numbers and types of negative and positive controls that must be routinely run along with the samples to adequately analyze the results. The susceptibility of molecular methods to laboratory contamination requires that detailed and rigorous quality assurance and quality control programs also be established in the laboratory. Thus, it is necessary to adequately maintain the instrumentation involved in these methods so that the results are trustworthy.

Molecular methods have significantly improved our ability to detect and characterize microbial pathogens with an extreme level of specificity and sensitivity in a variety of matrixes. However, despite these inherent advantages, molecular methods may not totally replace the conventional culture- and immunological-based methods of pathogen detection and characterization. Although molecular methods allow for faster and more accurate detection and characterization, they carry with them an increased need for trained personnel and internal quality control to insure accuracy and proper interpretation of results.

## SUGGESTED READINGS

Barany F (1991). The ligase chain reaction (LCR) in a PCR world. *PCR Methods Applications* 1:5-16.

Guatelli JC, TR Gingeras, and DD Richman (1989). Nucleic acid amplification in vitro: Detection of sequences with low copy numbers and application to diagnosis of human immunodeficiency virus type 1 infection. *Clinical Microbiology Review* 2:217-226.

Lakowicz JR (1983). Energy Transfer. In JR Lakowicz (ed.), *Principles of fluorescent spectroscopy.* New York: Plenum Press, pp. 303-339.

# Mushroom Production

Dan Levanon
Ofer Danai

## INTRODUCTION

Mushrooms have been used as food, spices, and medicine for thousands of years. Even today remarkable amounts of mushrooms are collected every year from the wild, and are available in markets all over the world. The majority of these mushrooms are saprophytic fungi, whereas some are mycorhizal fungi. Saprophytic fungi play an important role in nature by participating in the recycling of organic matter. They play a dominant role in the mineralization of plant residues and animal wastes back to $CO_2$, water, and other minerals. Their ability to biodegrade lignocellulose is important because it enables the recycling of organic carbon from stable organic material. In the past ten years, it was demonstrated that the lignocellulolytic enzymes of mushrooms are also capable of biodegrading the synthetic organic waste materials known as *xenobiotics*.

Mushroom production as "agrothechnology" was developed due to the increase in demand for mushroom consumption and decrease in amounts collected from the wild. The increased demand since the 1980s led to the industrialization of production methods to enhance productivity. Nevertheless, mushroom production was and still is a controlled organic-waste recycling process. In this process, the substrate is selected and prepared to meet the nutritional and ecological needs of the grown fungus and to prevent development of competitors and parasites. In the past ten years, production methods have developed and changed rapidly, but the principles of substrate selection, preparation, and utilization by the fungus remain the same, although they are achieved by more mechanized and sophisticated technology.

265

## THE MUSHROOM PRODUCTION INDUSTRY:
## PAST AND PRESENT

Mushroom production started in the Far East (China and Japan) during the seventh century. Since then, more and more fungal genera were adopted for artificial cultivation. More than 15 fungal genera are cultivated routinely in Far East countries and used as food, spices, and medicine. European mushroom production developed during the seventeenth century in France with the production of *Agaricus bisporus,* also known as *champignon de Paris* (white button mushrooms). The production of this fungus spread worldwide. It is still the most popular mushroom in Western countries.

At present, world production of mushrooms is estimated to be 4 to 5 million tons annually. The most popular mushrooms come from the genera *Agaricus, Pleurotus, Lentinus, Volvariella, Auricularia,* and *Flammulina* (in order of production volume). Of these, *Agaricus bisporus* is produced and consumed mainly in Western countries, whereas the others are produced mainly in Far Eastern countries. Some differences exist between the two groups:

1. In substrate preparation methods
2. With fruit body production methods

*A. bisporus* mushrooms grow naturally in soils with high organic matter content and need relatively low C:N ratio and nitrogen in their organic forms. Their artificial production is based on the use of composts made of manure (horse manure and straw as a first priority). All other fungi are natural lignocellulose degraders, and are therefore grown on uncomposted plant wastes, mainly wood debris and different kinds of straws. Fungi can grow on natural plant material which contains high C:N ratio. This difference in substrate origin and preparation led to the development of two different concepts of mushroom production, as will be discussed later. Several trends are common to the mushroom industry around the world.

1. The production volume of mushrooms has experienced continued (fast) growth since World War II.
2. Mushroom production becomes more and more mechanized in larger production units, mainly in industrial countries where labor is expensive.
3. Market trends lean toward increased shares of fresh mushrooms and decreased demand for processed products.
4. Interest has increased in mushrooms as health foods (nutraceuticals) due to their nutritional and health features.

The mushroom industry today is placed in many countries among the leading horticultural industries, and its growth is correlated with the increase in the standard of living. Industries, such as the following, support the highly developed mushroom industry:

1. Raw material producers and suppliers—substrates (mainly compost), inoculum (spawn and casing inoculum), casing materials (peat moss and lime), chemicals (pesticides, etc.)
2. Machinery equipment and growing rooms producers—the entire technology for compost and mushroom production, including environmental control in producer buildings
3. Processing and marketing industry—production of industry processed mushroom products

Of these industries, the inoculum (spawn) industry is a unique biological industry. It includes

1. selection and breeding of the mushroom strains;
2. preservation of "gene banks" of mushroom species and strains;
3. production of spawn in which mushroom mycelium is grown on cereals, mostly rye and millet grains. The colonized grains covered with the fungal mycelium serve as inoculation units when they are mixed into the substrate for mushroom cultivation.

The main duty of the spawn industry is selection and maintenance of stable commercial strains to supply the needs of mushroom growers. This industry developed the use of pure cultures of mushroom species and later adopted the use of hybrid strains.

## COMPOST-BASED MUSHROOM PRODUCTION

As mentioned previously, the production of *Agaricus* spp., mainly *A. bisporus* (white button mushroom), is based on the use of compost. Although few other species of *Agaricus* and fungi of other genera are also grown on compost, *A. bisporus* comprise more than 95 percent of the production on composted substrates. Therefore, this chapter deals with the production of *A. bisporus*. This mushroom is grown all over the world using methods that differ in sophistication, mechanization, capital investment, etc.

## Substrates

Most substrates are organic wastes or by-products. The traditional main ingredient in composts was horse manure. Due to the unavailability of this manure in several countries, composts based mostly on combinations of cereal straws and poultry manure were developed. In order to ensure production of suitable compost, standard chemical, physical, and biological parameters must be defined during the production process. These parameters are used in a quality control system during the composting process to ensure that the needed compost is produced. Such quality control measures for compost production are used routinely in northern Israel. They include optimal values of the following parameters: humidity percent, pH, C:N ratio, $NH_4$-N, ash, and total N content, which are measured during critical stages of compost production and mushroom growing. If the analysis of these parameters shows differences from the optimal values, specific measures are taken to improve compost quality. The rationale behind the entire composting process is to produce a substrate for *A. bisporus* that will be selective in order to meet its nutritional needs and retard growth of competing fungi and bacteria.

## Technology

Methods of compost production have changed markedly in recent years for two reasons:

1. Environmental legislation has forced composting facilities to eliminate bad odors, flies, contaminated water, etc.
2. Technological advances in production have led to higher efficiency (mainly in the growing rooms by using phase 2 and phase 3 compost) and larger production volumes.

Substrate preparation (composting) in the mushroom industry can be divided into three stages:

1. Phase 1: Mixing, prewetting, wetting the raw materials (manure, straw, gypsum, etc.) and composting at temperatures up to 80°C. In the past, this phase was conducted in open, long windrow piles (2 m wide by 2 m high) that were turned frequently to ensure uniformity and aerobic conditions. Today, this phase is conducted either in bunkers or indoor tunnels. Bunkers are usually 7.5 m high and 8 m wide with aerated floors. Air is blown through the compost, ensuring better

uniformity of temperature and oxygen content in the pile. The compost is transferred from one bunker to another every four to seven days, and the process lasts fourteen to twenty days. Indoor tunnels are operated in basically the same way, but have the advantage of isolated walls and a roof that provides complete uniformity in temperature and oxygen content. Usually the compost is kept in the same tunnel for the entire process. The product of this phase is known as *green compost*.

2. Phase 2: This phase starts with pasteurization of the compost at 60°C for a number of hours ("peak heating"), followed by reduction of the temperature to 45 to 48°C for a few days for "conditioning." It is completed and ready for spawning when the $NH_3$ in the air is reduced to below 5 ppm and pH values are lower than 7.7. This was once done in the growing rooms, but today it is done mainly in bulk in indoor pasteurization tunnels. The bulk process ensures temperature and oxygen uniformity throughout the compost, enhancing control of pests. The bulk process is shorter than before (about six days), thereby reducing the loss of organic matter. The product of this phase is known as *pasteurized, spawned,* or *phase 2* compost.

3. Phase 3: The mushroom mycelium grows until the compost is fully colonized (the "spawn run"). At this stage, the compost is very sensitive to contamination by competitors that are harmful to the mushroom mycelium. In the past, this phase was conducted in shelves, trays, or bags in the growing room, but today it is mostly conducted in bulk in tunnels. Under these conditions, the mycelium enjoys a more uniform temperature, producing more uniform growth. The colonized compost is delivered to the growing rooms in closed containers, and is known as *full grown* or *phase 3* compost. As mentioned previously, all of these phases are needed to ensure the production of selective compost for mushroom cultivation.

Fruit bodies formation is induced after the "full-grown" compost is cased by "casing soil." A peat moss and lime mixture is often used as the main component of the casing material. The casing material must fit the following requirements: sufficient water-holding capacity to serve as a water reservoir for the growing mushroom crop; good structure, notably porosity, to maintain gas exchange between the compost surface and the air of the growing rooms; pH values between 7.3 and 7.8; low presence of soluble ions (electrical conductivity). Casing materials must also be clean of soil pests and pathogens, therefore pasteurization (heat or chemical treatments) is usually needed. Some association between casing microflora and mushroom mycelium supports the latter's transition to the formation of fruit bodies. Therefore, pasteurization must be limited in order to avoid elimination of beneficial microorganisms (Levanon et al., 1988). A shortage of peat moss has led to a (continuing) search for an alternative raw material that could serve as casing soil. The mushroom production research group at Migal has developed an alternative casing material based on the solid fraction of digested sludge from thermophilic anaerobic digestion of cattle manure. Other ideas for alternative casing include recycled, spent mushroom composts, recycled shredded paper, etc., but the use of alternatives is limited.

Modern mushroom production takes place in growing buildings equipped with atmosphere control systems. The growing rooms are built of materials for temperature insulation. Temperature, air relative humidity, and air $CO_2$ content are controlled using heating and cooling systems with computerized control. The average conditions during mushroom growing include: comparatively high compost temperature, $CO_2$ content, and relative humidity (26°C, >3000 ppm, 90 percent, respectively) during mycelium growth in compost (spawn run) and in the casing soil, followed by a decrease of these values to enhance fruit-body development (16°C, 1,000 ppm, 84 percent, respectively). The length of the mushroom growing cycle is about 10 to 11 weeks, including 2 to 2.5 weeks of the "spawn-run," which occurs mainly in bulk in tunnels.

Most of the mushrooms are handpicked as closed cups in three to four flushes. Mechanical harvesting is used in mushroom production only for industrial processing, and these are mainly open cups. Mushroom yields are often calculated a "biological-efficiency," which is determined by *fresh* weight of the mushroom yield divided by the *dry* weight of the compost, at the beginning of the cropping cycle.

## LIGNOCELLULOSE-BASED MUSHROOM PRODUCTION

Edible fungi that utilize lignocellulose as their substrate belong to the group of "white-rot" fungi. Their ability to degrade lignocellulose is based on the lignocellulolytic enzymes that they produce. With these enzymes, such fungi grow naturally, mainly on wood and straws of several plants. Of these mushrooms, we will discuss, as an example, the genus *Pleurotus,* which is second to *Agaricus* in production volume worldwide. The *Pleurotus.* sp. known as oyster mushrooms are produced in great amounts, especially in east Asia. Since 1970, they became more popular in Europe, and their production increased in several countries, such as Italy, Spain, and Hungary. They are cultivated on wood debris, straws of several crops (e.g., wheat, barley, rice, cotton, etc.), and the agricultural wastes of industries (e.g., sugar, corn, olives, coffee, bananas, etc.).

## *Substrates*

Because the mushrooms under consideration are wood-degrading fungi, their substrates contain a high lignocellulose content. Lignocellulosic materials are the most common organic wastes of forest-related industries (timber, paper, etc.), agriculture, and gardening. To make use of these wastes or their associated by-products for the cultivation of mushrooms, their compatibility with the nutrient requirements of the fungus must be determined. Standard chemical, physical, and biological parameters have been defined to facilitate the study of potential suitability of substrates for *Pleurotus* spp. cultivation. In our work on the possibility of using cotton straw as a substrate, we adapted methods employed for the chemical analysis of feed for ruminants (Silanikove et al., 1988). Using these analytical methods, we monitored humidity, electrical conductivity (EC), and pH values of the fresh substrate, and the ash, nitrogen, lignin, cellulose, and hemicellulose contents in the dry matter. These parameters were recorded at several stages of the growth cycle of the fungus on cotton straw. Optimal values for each parameter at every stage of the cultivation cycle were determined based on yield results. Biological assays for the definition of optimal substrates include recording the growth rate of the fungal colony on the lignocellulosic material, as measured by colony diameter and quality, observed in terms of the density of mycelial biomass.

According to our experience, fast and complete colonization of the substrate by the mycelium is a key requisite for a good yield. Although such observation is based partly on subjective scaling of the biomass, it adds an important component to the measurement of fungal/substrate compatibility. Such analysis is routinely conducted in surveys of different agricultural wastes from different countries to determine their suitability for *Pleurotus* production. These parameters have guided our continuous efforts to identify the most suitable substrates for the cultivation of *Pleurotus* spp. on the assumption that accurate analyses can provide the data on which to base the preparation of the substrate to suit fungal requirements.

## *Technology*

The technology used for the cultivation of oyster mushrooms in eastern Asia is mainly the same technology used for the cultivation of all other wood-degrading edible fungi. It is based on the use of small substrate units

(1 to 2 kg) in plastic bags for the cultivation process. The advantage of this technology is that the heat treatment (sterilization or pasteurization in a semiopen autoclave) is done in small units, ensuring uniformity of temperature in the substrate. The main disadvantage of this technology is the high demand for human labor due to the small growing units. Therefore, in countries where human labor is more expensive, technology that uses bigger substrate units was developed. The cultivation process includes these stages:

### Substrate Collection, Transportation, Storage, and Processing

The machinery for crop harvesting could be adapted to the collection of straws to be used as substrates for mushroom production. We used a forage harvester to collect cotton straw and cut the stalks to 2 to 5 cm long pieces. Transportation could be expensive due to the high volume:weight ratio of the substrate, so chopping and compacting before transporting is recommended.

Storage is also an important aspect of the production cycle. Mushroom production units plan their work to continue throughout the year to ensure continuous supply to the market, whereas the raw materials for the substrate for *Pleurotus* cultivation are usually grown as seasonal crops. Storage facilities are therefore essential to the maintenance of the year-round supply of prepared substrate. To minimize the loss of material, storage facilities should be kept shaded and dry in most climates. Because our chopped cotton straw contained 60 percent moisture, it was impossible to store it raw. Drying it in the rainy season would involve the use of special ovens, which would be very expensive. After considering other possibilities, we produced ensiling material. The results were promising. We found that compacting the pile and covering it with PVC sheeting created anaerobic conditions, leading to a decrease in the pH to 5.5, as with the ensilage of green cereal forages (e.g., corn and wheat). The chopped cotton straw was preserved by ensiling it in suitable condition for a year.

The process was scaled up by storing the cotton straw in farm facilities originally built for cereal silage. The cotton straw silage was successfully used as a substrate for the commercial cultivation of *Pleurotus* spp., and was also found to be equally suitable for *Lentinus edodes*. Although this is only an example of substrate handling, it contains all the aspects that should be taken into consideration when developing successful *Pleurotus* cultivation. The preparation of the substrate continues with a short composting period, which raises the pH to alkaline levels (8.0 to 8.5) in cotton-based substrates. This pH value is suitable for *Pleurotus*, but retards the growth of other fungi in the substrate. The substrate is then transferred to indoor tunnels for pasteurization. The temperature is raised to 60°C for 12 hours followed by a cooling period.

## Cultivation

Inoculation (spawning) is done in combination with filling 20 to 30 kg plastic bags with substrate. The bags are perforated to ensure air movement into the growing mushroom mycelium. In an effort to minimize the use of costly human labor, we have developed larger growing units of up to 400 kg of substrate that can be moved by fork lifts. The filled bags inoculated with 1 to 2 percent "spawn" are transferred to incubation rooms. The optimal temperature for mycelium growth is around 27°C. The bags create an environment of high $CO_2$ content around the growing mycelium that enhances the mycelium's growth rate and defend it from incoming pests. Fast and uniform mycelium growth is essential to eliminate other molds that are competitors and parasites to the growing mycelium.

After the substrate is fully colonized, the bags are moved to mushroom growing rooms. The atmosphere for the low-temperature species is controlled to 18°C, with a relative humidity of 85 to 90 percent. The $CO_2$ content is reduced to 600 to 1,500 ppm, and a light intensity of 8 to 100 lux is set for 8 to 12 hours each day. The bags are either perforated to enable the growing fruit bodies to develop or completely taken off. The mushrooms are picked in three to four flushes and the entire growing cycle is about 60 days. The main species of *Pleurotus* that are used for production in Western countries are *P. ostreatus* and *P. pulmonarius,* whereas high-temperature species, such as *P. abalonus* and *P. cystidosus,* which can produce fruit bodies at temperatures up to 30°C, are more popular in the Far East (China especially).

## ENVIRONMENTAL ASPECTS

The mushroom industry is often regarded as problematic from the point of view of environmental quality. This attitude is due mainly to its use of manures, operation of open composting yards, and uncontrolled disposal of spent mushroom substrates (SMS). Such operations have the potential of creating environmental nuisances, such as bad odors, water pollution, and the proliferation of flies and other mushroom pests.

Today, environmental aspects should be taken into careful consideration as an important aspect of production activity. Increased mushroom production sometimes takes place near urban centers, close to markets. In such areas, environmental awareness is most important, since dense population's pockets of unsanitary conditions render them particularly sensitive to environmental quality and dangerous to public health.

Environmental considerations must take into account the entire cycle of mushroom cultivation and substrate utilization. Only a production scheme based on this realization can ensure that the outcome will be an environmentally friendly system. This cycle involves the collection, transportation, storage, and processing of wastes to be used for substrate, the sowing, cultivation, and harvest of the mushrooms, and the disposal of SMS. When all of these stages are conducted properly, the operation will not only be environmentally safe, it will be beneficial to the environment. We offer, as an example, the use of cotton straw for the cultivation of *Pleurotus* spp. (Levanon et al., 1988). Cotton straw is a problematic waste product of cotton cultivation, due to its high lignin content and the fact that it can carry pests over from one season to the next. It is often chopped and plowed deep into the soil. In some countries it is even burned, causing air pollution. We have developed its use as an economically viable substrate for the production of fungi. Its SMS can be used as nutritious feed for ruminants (cattle, sheep, and goats), whose droppings, in turn, further provide organic manure for use in agriculture.

Composting facilities are known to cause environmental nuisances. Emission to the air of volatile compounds and leachates containing composting residues are the main factors requiring special attention. Air, water, and soil pollution by agriculture and industrial wastes are causing growing concerns that give rise to accelerating environmental legislation. In industrial and densely populated countries, composting activities are strictly regulated. In several such countries, indoor composting is becoming mandatory as the ultimate solution to the problem of odors, especially near populated areas. This mainly affects composting for the production of *Agaricus* spp. The producers of compost for this mushroom are forced to invest in indoor facilities to comply with new environmental regulations.

After mushroom cultivation is complete, the substrates are usually pasteurized, i,e., "cooked out" to avoid pathogens, and are considered to be spent mushroom substrates. In a symposium on the beneficial use of SMS derived from the cultivation of *Agaricus* spp., a number of options were demonstrated (Wuest et al., 1994):

1. As an organic amendment for container-media combinations, for example as a substitute for peat moss. The demand for such material is growing, in proportion to the increased use of disconnected media in agriculture, especially horticulture. SMS is used for this purpose increasingly.
2. As an organic fertilizer for agriculture and horticulture.

3. As a primary component for the reconstruction of wetlands. These wetlands had been designed to remediate water that had been downgraded by drainage from mines. The organic content of the SMS serves to support the development of flora and fauna in the wetland, but also absorbs heavy metals from the polluted water.

4. As a stabilizing organic soil amendment on severely disturbed sites. These include abandoned strip-mine culm banks, excavation sites, roadsides (especially in mountainous areas), and urban multiuse green spaces.

5. In visits to *Pleurotus* farms in Italy, we observed the use of SMS in composting agricultural wastes, both as a bulking agent in composting organic municipal waste and sewage sludge, and as a substrate for *vermicomposting,* a process in which the organic substrate serves as a nutrient for soil worms. In the latter case, the substrate is transformed to *vermicompost,* a high quality additive to container media for ornamental pot plants.

6. The SMS of wood-degrading edible fungi can be used as an animal feed. Our experience is with cotton-straw SMS after cultivation of *Pleurotus* spp. In this case, the SMS is used for the feeding of beef cattle, and its nutritional value is comparable to cereals hay.

7. White-rot fungi have the ability to degrade xenobiotic compounds— organosynthetic chemicals used in industry, agriculture, transportation, and households. Among these are toxic pesticides and other compounds that pose a danger to human health and environmental quality. The pollution of water, air, and soil by such chemicals is one of the most common threats to the stability of the environment. The nonspecifics, exocelluar enzymes that enable white-rot fungi to degrade their substrate, especially lignin, are also able to degrade or transform organosynthetic pollutants. Masaphy et al. (1999), studied the ability of *Pleurotus* to degrade pesticides in liquid and soiled-state fermentation. It was demonstrated that in liquid cultures, *P. pulmonarius* transformed and detoxified herbicides of the triazine group. These are the most commonly used herbicides, and their residues contaminate water sources all over the world. Further studies with SMS of *Pleurotus* on cotton straw demonstrated the potential to use this ability for biological filtration of water and air.

## *CONCLUSIONS*

Mushroom production is a fast-growing industry worldwide, especially since 1990. Fresh mushrooms are consumed in increasing amounts in industrial countries, and their popularity is due to their taste and nutritional value. In developing countries, mushrooms are important sources of proteins. The production of mushrooms is based on utilization of organic substrates. These are mainly plant wastes and manure that are recycled via this industry. Therefore this industry could be considered environmentally friendly by utilizing problematic waste materials. On the other hand, the mushroom production cycle itself, and especially composting, could cause soil, water, and air pollution. The pressure of environmental legislation is forcing the mushroom industry in industrialized countries to move into indoor production facilities. At the same time competition in the growing market and high labor costs create the need for bigger and more mechanized production units with full atmosphere control. Mushroom production today is becoming a more sophisticated mechanized industry due to the growing competition in the market. Nevertheless, the industry is still based on the same biological principles discussed in this chapter.

## SUGGESTED READINGS

Danai O and D Levanon (2000). Selection of substrates for mushroom cultivation and spawn production. In *Mushroom genetic resources for food and agriculture*, JE Labarere and UG Menini (eds.). Bordeaux, France: FAO publication.

Levanon D, O Danai, and SD Masaphy (1988). Chemical and physical parameters in recycling organic wastes for mushroom production. *Biological Wastes* 26: 341-348.

Masaphy S, Y Henis, and D Levanon (1999). Physiological and biochemical aspects of fungal transformation of chloro-s-triazine. *Recent Research and Development in Microbiology* 3:161-173.

Masaphy S and D Levanon (1992). The effect of lignocellulose on ligno-cellulolytic activity of *Pleurotus pulmonarius* in submerged culture. *Applied Microbiology and Biotechnology* 36:828-832.

Silanikove N, O Danai, and D Levanon (1988). Composted cotton straw silage as a substrate for *Pleurotus* sp. cultivation. *Biological Wastes* 25:219-226.

Wuest, PJ, D Levanon, and Y Hader (1994). Environmental, agricultural, and industrial uses for spent mushroom substrates. *Proceedings from the Spent Mushroom Symposium*. Philadelphia: American Mushroom Institute.

# Nutraceutical Production and Use

### Sudip Kumar Rakshit

## *INTRODUCTION*

It is known that diet and food play a role in health besides providing energy and supporting growth. However, with new scientific methods it is now possible to determine the exact function of some the components of food. Evidence from epidemiology, clinical trials, and modern nutritional biochemistry underlines the connection between diet and health. At the same time, it is becoming more popular and common to modify one's diet to reduce the risk of developing chronic diseases. Food companies have thus sought to fulfill consumers' appetites for products derived from foods that could be used to promote good health. The result has been the development and marketing of a growing spectrum of products called *nutraceuticals* and *functional foods.*

All foods have functions of nutrition, taste, aroma, etc. However, since the 1990s, the term *functional food* has taken a different implication. It is applied to food that provides an additional physiological (and in some cases a sensory) benefit. The term includes ingredients that aid specific body functions in addition to being nutritious. On the other hand, the term *nutraceutical* is more specific. The term is a combination of the words *nutrition* and *pharmaceutical.* This implies that such substances should have both these characteristics. The best-known description of the term *nutraceutical* is that it should be a bioactive compound that, when included in the diet, improves health beyond the traditional nutrients it contains. Such ingredients may have to be added externally. A number of food products that have traditionally been used for good health are being drawn into these markets. The extraction, separation, and refinement of the bioactive substances they contain is the focus of considerable research.

## MINERAL FORTIFICATION OF FOODS

This is one of the earliest forms in which the nutritive value of foods has been improved. Starting with calcium and iron fortification, a number of other minerals such as magnesium and selenium, are now being considered. Products are being developed in a number of innovative ways. Binding calcium to milk proteins has been found to increase the calcium composition manifold. Calcium salt of glycerophosphoric acid increases calcium's bioavailability and has a low impact on taste, color, or odor. Calcium in this form has been incorporated into beverages, dairy products, cereals, infant formulas, candies, chewing gum, energy bars, and nutritional supplements. Other forms of calcium that have obtained FDA approval in the United States for food fortification include carbonates, citrates, oxides, phosphates, pyrophosphate, chlorides, lactates, and sulfate.

Selenium is being studied with great interest because of its possible value in health. Present in large quantities in Brazil nuts, for example, selenium functions as an antioxidant and a component of another antioxidant glutathione peroxidase. Along with vitamin E, it is supposed to help maintain levels of coenzyme Q in the heart muscle. The latter, responsible for energy metabolism, is an important cofactor, deficiencies of which would lead to reduced production of energy in the heart and other muscles leading to serious health problems. Selenium has also been said to have a life-extension possibility to HIV-positive individuals. In addition, a connection between selenium deficiencies and certain deadly viruses appears to exist.

Zinc is said to be essential for normal growth, appetite, and immune function. Blood cells are said to become more fragile when deprived of this element. However, the latter problem can be overcome by supplementation of vitamins C, vitamin E, and beta-carotene. Zinc lactate produced by fermentation of sugars has been incorporated in a number of products. Another important mineral, magnesium, could be successfully supplemented in the form of magnesium phosphate. In this way both magnesium and phosphate can be added together.

## NUTRACEUTICALS FROM PLANT SOURCES

*Phytochemical* is a term that emphasizes the plant source of most protective and disease-preventing compounds. A great deal of supporting evidence from epidemiological, in vivo, and in vitro studies indicates that plant-based diets reduce the risk of chronic diseases and cancer. The risk of cancer is reduced by half for people whose diets are plant-based, compared to those whose diets come from other sources. Some of the common sources of phytochemicals and their sources are mentioned in the following paragraphs.

Soy is a source of high-quality protein, as assessed by its protein digestibility corrected amino acid score. However, it is also found to play a preventive role in cardiovascular disease, cancer, osteoporosis, and the alleviation of menopausal symptoms. Soybeans contain a group of phytochemicals rich in isoflavones, which may reduce the risk of several cancers, including breast, lung, and prostrate cancer. Genistein and daidzein are isoflavones that are considered to be phytoestrogens because they look and act like estrogens. The former, in particular, acts as an anticancer compound, interfering with enzymes important for cancer growth and preventing blood supply to the tumor. Several classes of anticarcinogens, including protease inhibitors, phytosterols, saponins, phenolic acids, and isoflavones, are also present in soybean.

Oats have long been known to be multifunctional foods. They reduce total and low-density lipoprotein (LDL) cholesterol, thereby reducing the risk of coronary heart disease (CHD), and have an effect on glucose metabolism and gut function. In addition, they promote weight loss, enhance physical performance and mood, improve immune status, and enhance antioxidant protection.

Garlic is widely reported for its medicinal properties. Its health benefits include cancer chemoprevention, antibiotic, antihypertensive, and cholesterol-lowering properties. These properties are attributed to its water-soluble sulfur-containing elements. In its intact form, the substances present in garlic are inactive, and are converted to the active form called *allicin* upon crushing. These substances are further spontaneously broken down to many other effective forms. The cardioprotective effects are more likely due to its cholesterol-lowering properties and consequent antihypertensive effects.

Broccoli and other cruciferous vegetables, such as cabbages, cauliflower, and Brussels prunes, have high anticarcinogenic properties that are attributed to a group of glycosides called *glucosinolates* stored within the cell vacuoles. Indole-3-carbinol is supposed to reduce cancer, especially breast cancer, by modulating estrogen metabolism. Antioxidants have now been recognized as an important ingredient in food because they offer a variety of health benefits. They are involved in neutralizing free radicals, which damage DNA molecules and lead to cancer, and retard the effects of aging, particularly loss of memory and motor cells. A number of antioxidants are available in fruits, vegetables, and plant sources.

One of the most well-known antioxidants is beta-carotene, present in large quantities in carrots. These compounds are supposed to help reduce the risk of cancer and enhance the immune system. Other members of the carotenoid family with great potential for such activity include alpha-carotene, lycopene, xanthin, and capsanthin. Vitamin E is also an antioxidant, which helps prevent disease by preventing oxygen in the blood from combining with LDL cholesterol. Oxidized LDL is one of the major causes for plaque in the arteries. The American Heart Association recommends taking vitamins from a variety of foods rather than from supplements. Similarly, vitamin K is necessary for the synthesis of prothrombin and other blood-clotting factors in the liver.

Folic acid reduces the risk of birth defects when consumed in adequate quantities by women in early pregnancy. This resulted in the FDA ruling requiring all enriched grains to be supplemented with folic acid. Epidemiological studies have shown that citrus fruits have a protective role against a number of cancers. Although vitamin C can be obtained from lemons, limes, and grapefruits, it has been shown recently that another group of phytochemicals called *limonoids* are responsible for real cancer prevention benefits.

In general, it is well known that vitamins are organic food substances found only in living things, that is, plants and animals. With few exceptions, the body cannot manufacture or synthesize vitamins. They must be supplied in the diet or in dietary supplements. Vitamins are essential to the normal functioning of our bodies. They are necessary for our growth, vitality, and general well-being. Vitamins cannot be assimilated without ingesting food. Vitamins help regulate metabolism, help convert fat and carbohydrates into energy, and assist in forming bone and tissue.

Lycopene present in tomatoes contributes to the reduction of several cancers, including prostrate and digestive tract cancer. Lycopene gives the red color to tomatoes and is said to be twice as powerful as beta-carotene. It has been claimed that lycopene is the most efficient quencher of singlet oxygen in biological systems. Suprisingly, it is said to be more effective when the tomato is consumed in the processed form, as in sauce, paste, and ketchup, than from raw tomato. Lycopene is found to be better absorbed by the body when tomato products have been heat processed.

Wild blueberries contain high levels of anthocyanins, antioxidant flavonoids that are responsible for the intense blue color of the berries. It has been shown that proanthocyanins inhibit an enzyme involved in the promotion stage of cancer. Similarly, cranberry juice has been found to be useful in the treatment of urinary tract infections. The juice is found to have compounds that inhibit adhesions of pathogenic or harmful organisms to the uroepithelial tissue, thus preventing infection. Pyruvates naturally occur in fruits, vegetables, wines, and some types of cheese. They are being studied for their weight loss capacities and their abilities to increase or maintain muscle mass and speed up energy production.

Fibers aid bowel movement and the prevention of cancers. A number of fibers are available commercially at present. However, the fortification of foods with fibers gives products a sandy texture, increased viscosity, or bad taste and odor, which reduces the pleasure of eating. Acacia gum, a fiber that overcomes this problem, does not alter the taste and texture of the food in which it is incorporated.

Polyphenols present in tea as well as in coffee, red grapes, kidney beans, prunes, raisins, and red wine, show anticarcinogenic, antioxidant, antibacterial, and antiviral action. Catechins and aflavins contribute to the antioxidant properties of tea. Tea is also associated with lowering serum cholesterol and triglycerides, and improves LDL: HDL ratios, which in turn have a positive impact on the heart. Red wine appears to be particularly beneficial in reducing the risk of heart attacks. This became apparent when it was found that a negative relationship exists between wine intake and death from heart disease in 18 countries. Although alcohol itself is said to have the positive effect of increasing high-density cholesterol in the blood, the so-called French Paradox is more likely due to flavonoids. The phenolic content of red wines is 20 to 50 times higher than white wines due to the incorporation of the skins into the fermented grape juice. These phenolics prevent the oxidation of LDL, a critical reaction during atherogenesis. Resveratrol found in the skin of grapes has been shown to have estrogenic properties, leading to the benefits in heart care. However, the consumption of red grape juice or alcohol-free wine is recommended to avoid the negative effects of alcohol.

Many sterols are present in the unsaponifiable fraction of rice-bran oil. Crude rice-bran oil contains 2 percent or more of gamma-oryzanol, which belongs to a group of ferulate esters and is known to have high antioxidant properties. Ferulate esters have been known to have a number of abilities, such as a positive cholesterol metabolism, inhibition of platelet aggregation, increase in fecal bile acid excretion, and control of nerve disorders and disorders of menopause. They can be retained in the oil by a nonconventional refining procedure, or they can be extracted and added back to the oil or other functional foods. Tocotrienols are similar to vitamin E and have powerful antioxidant capacity, preventing cardiovascular disease and some forms of cancer. They are stripped from the rice-bran oil in the deodorization step and can be recovered by further fractionation.

## FISH, MARINE, AND DAIRY PRODUCTS

Fish oils have long been known to have a positive effect on health. The so-called omega-3 (n-3) fatty acids are present in fish oils in the highest quantities. Fish-eating communities (e.g., Denmark and Japan) have a markedly decreased incidence of coronary artery disease. Eskimo communities likewise have a reduced incidence of coronary artery disease despite their heavy consumption of whale blubber. This may be explained by the replacement, in part, of arachidonic acid by omega-3 (n-3) polyunsaturated fatty acids (PUFA) in the cell membranes, and the resultant changes in the functional properties of the prostaglandins derived from these.

It has been suggested that dietary omega-3 polyunsaturated fatty acids, such as eicosapentaenoic acid (EPA) and docosahexaenoic acid (DHA), may provide one of the best means of primary prevention of coronary artery disease through their effects on plasma lipids and platelet function. Of equal importance is the possible secondary prevention of progressive coronary artery atherosclerosis and peripheral vascular disease through similar mechanisms (i.e., cholesterol concentration, blood viscosity, and platelet aggregability). Omega-3 polyunsaturated fatty acids also may have a role in the treatment of specific illnesses (i.e., lupus, hypertension, and immune problems). In large doses, PUFA are known to have an ameliorative effect on hypertension, inflammatory, immune, and other diseases. It is also said to have an effect on brain function and memory.

Existing sources of dietary omega-3 PUFA are completely limited to fish and other marine animals (e.g., seals, whales), rare plants, and commercial extracts of whole fish as a liquid or encapsulated oil. Most land animals and vegetables have extremely low concentrations of EPA and DHA. Furthermore, fish and other marine animals seem to be acceptable and easily available only to coastal fishing communities with a long history of consuming fish as food. Most other populations find fish to be both too expensive and less appealing in terms of taste when compared to land animal meats. As daily dietary supplements, fish oils have an unacceptable taste and flavor. Incorporation of omega-3 long chain PUFAs is not simple, because these ingredients are highly susceptible to oxidation, leading to fishy flavors and aromas in the product.

In response to these shortcomings, researchers are attempting to create alternative foods that can provide a significant source of omega-3 PUFAs without necessitating the consumption of fish or fish oils. Methods have been developed to increase the concentration of omega-3 PUFAs in poultry and eggs. The method involves administering an effective amount of either preformed omega-3 PUFA or a metabolic precursor thereof to poultry.

*Microencapsulation* is a process in which small amounts of liquids, solids, or gases are coated with materials that provide a barrier to undesirable environmental and chemical interactions until release is required. Microencapsulation masks tastes, flavor, and odors, provides protection against oxidation, and puts active ingredients into free-flowing powder for ease of handling and incorporation in dry food systems. This technique has been used successfully to incorporate PUFAs into foods. A number of products, including infant foods, have PUFAs, popularly DHA, included in them without any change in sensory characteristics.

Milk fat is known to be the richest source of conjugated linoleic acid, a potential anticarcinogen. It also contains sphingomyelin, butyric acid, and ether lipids, which have cancer-fighting attributes.

## HERBAL SOURCES

The list of beneficial bioactive compounds from herbs is very large, and their identification and use continues to grow. An extract of *Ginko biloba,* which improves cognitive performance and social functioning of patients suffering from Alzheimer's disease, is being studied currently. Bioactive compounds are supposed to improve blood circulation to the brain and may be used as a potential treatment for hardening of arteries and oxygen deprivation. Other such botanicals include ginseng, which reduces stress and fatigue; echinacea, which supports a healthy immune system; hawthorn, which helps efficiency heart function; valerian, which promotes restful sleep, etc. Depending on their solubility, herbal compunds are used in sport drinks, juices, tea, etc.

## REQUIRED CHARACTERISTICS FOR NUTRACEUTICALS

The factors that need to be taken into account when formulating foods containing functional or nutraceutical ingredients are safety, stability, bio-availability, and organoleptic qualities. When the source of the compound is from a natural source, it is unlikely that it would have a negative effect on health. However, dosage is an important factor when concentrated forms of these products are supplemented into so-called health foods. Stability of the added bioactive compound is an important consideration in the process. For example, as discussed earlier, the main problem with the use of polyunsaturated fatty acids in foods is their easy oxidation. Methods to preserve and extend their useful characteristics are important considerations. The bio-availability of the nutrient is of prime importance. An added nutrient must be in a chemical form that can be effectively absorbed and utilized by the body. The food product matrix certainly has an effect on this. Fibers, for example, are known to bind many minerals, reducing the availability of the latter for absorption. Finally, the organoleptic character and sensory qualities have to be maintained so that customers consider it to be a food rather than medicine.

## CONSUMER CONCERNS AND THE FUTURE

Not all food foods available in the market deliver everything they promise. Nutraceuticals foods have to be regulated without unduly compromising the rights of consumers. Products with proven physiological benefits should be allowed into the market. The regulatory environment should fairly and responsibly permit the promotion to consumers of food and drug products that have been shown by valid scientific evidence to improve health. To benefit consumers, health claims should be supported by information that is clearly stated, substantiated, truthful, not misleading, and not likely to lead to harm.

A substantial increase in the variety and volume of nutraceutical/functional foods is expected with scientific developments. Raw material composition can be enhanced by genetic modification. Instead of reducing risks, the new products will aim to prevent disease and even cure ailments efficiently. Functional foods will be designed to help vulnerable and risk groups of specific problems. Foods to reduce the effects of aging, improving physical and mental performance and moods, are to be expected in the years ahead.

## SUGGESTED READINGS

Garcia DG (1998). Omega-3 long chain PUFA nutracueticals. *Food Technology* 52(6): 44-50.

Hasler CM (1998). Functional foods: Their role in disease prevention and health promotion. *Food Technology* 52(11):63-70.

Sadler MJ and M Satmarsh (eds.) (1998). *Functional foods: The consumer, the product, and the evidence.* Cambridge, UK: The Royal Society of Chemistry Information Services.

Sloan AE (2000). The top ten functional food trends. *Food Technology* 54(4):33-62.

# Prebiotics and Probiotics

Sudip Kumar Rakshit

## INTRODUCTION

Many of the first generation functional foods involved supplementation and fortification of foods with vitamins and minerals. More recently the concept has moved toward an exogenous food additive consisting of microorganisms that could have a positive effect on gut micro flora besides carrying other positive immunological and pharmaceutical attributes. This has led to considerable research in the area of prebiotics and probiotics.

The word *probiotic* is derived from Greek, and means "for life." By definition, it is a viable microbial food or feed supplement that beneficially affects the host animal's health by improving its intestinal microbial balance. Probiotics are thus friendly, beneficial, or healthy organisms that inhabit the intestinal tract and help maintain health while fighting illness and disease.

A *prebiotic* is a nondigestible food ingredient that beneficially affects the host by selectively stimulating (by fermentation) the growth and/or activity of one or a limited number of useful bacteria in the colon. Food ingredients classified as prebiotics must not be hydrolyzed or absorbed in the upper gastrointestinal tract, need to be a selective substrate for a limited number of colonic bacteria, must alter the microbiota in the colon to a healthier composition, and should induce luminal or systematic effects that are beneficial to host health. In addition to simulating the indigenous bacteria to grow, prebiotics may also produce compounds beneficial to the host. Fermentation of prebiotics to small-chain fatty acids (SCFA) is central to many proposed mechanisms for health effects provided by prebiotics.

In a pure culture, most species of probiotics are adapted to the utilization of nondigestible oligosaccharides, but many other bacteria are also capable of metabolizing them. Clearly, these studies of pure bacteria are of limited use unless their results are supported by the results of studies using mixed cultures. Indeed, as many components of the gut microbiota as possible should be measured to indicate a true prebiotic effect. Simple in vitro stimulation of probiotics, such as bifidobacteria, are insufficient to demonstrate effects on gut microorganisms. In vivo studies, possibly with human volunteers, are necessary for confirming this. As we age, the healthy bacteria in the gut have a tendency to diminish. A typical diet high in protein and carbohydrates contributes to this reduction. We can also encourage healthy bacteria by supplementing our diets with prebiotics.

Probiotics have been used for centuries as food preservatives and natural sources to promote good human health without specific knowledge of their active ingredients or how they work. A real understanding of how probiotics function began when Nobel Prize-winning Russian physiologist Élie Metchnikoff (1845-1916) introduced his theory of intoxication. He stated that the main cause of aging is "toxicants" formed by intestinal putrefaction and fermentation, and suggested that drinking beverages such as yogurt containing lactic acid bacteria would prevent aging. Lactobacilli suddenly attracted world attention.

Since Metchnikoff, a great deal of research and clinical trials have been conducted, but his theory of eternal youth has repeated a cycle of disappearing for a time and then returning again to public notice with the issue never really being resolved in either a scientific or practical sense. Recently, thanks to remarkable advances in microbiology and intestinal bacteriology, it has been made clear that certain lactobacilli, especially those of *Lactobacillus* and *Bifidobacterium* genera, have high mucus membrane chemical affinity and play important roles in human health. The mechanism of action of these organisms has since been proved to be not only the action of the organic acids they produce, but also due to some bacteriostatic compounds they produce.

## IMPORTANCE OF PROBIOTICS

Pathogenic bacteria can cause intestinal microflora imbalances and lead to illness and disease. Although human beings usually start life with a relatively healthy intestinal tract, the factors that break the balance are lifestyle and climate, environmental factors such as poor diet (excessive alcohol, sugar, fat, meat, antacids, etc.), aging, medication (antibiotics), and illness, including bacterial infections, stress, etc. A reduction in the number of friendly bacteria allows pathogenic bacteria to take hold and cause problems. While curing other diseases, antibiotics could lead to a reduction in the number of viable, useful organisms. This often leads to diarrhea in such cases. Supplementing our diets with an effective probiotic repopulates the intestinal tract with friendly strains to reverse this trend, improve intestinal health, and help guard against disease.

Almost 500 different species and 100 trillion total bacteria exist in the 25- to 35-foot-long gastrointestinal tract. This complex and highly adapted community provides the host resistance to pathogens. Because the native microorganisms are so well adapted to the environment, it is difficult for microorganisms, including pathogens, to colonize in the lumen. Friendly and pathogenic bacteria form a delicate and constantly changing balance as they compete to take hold and remain viable. The general functions of the beneficial microflora in the gut include energy salvage, modulation of cell growth and differentiation, antagonism against pathogens, immune simulation, innate immunity against infections, production of vitamins, reduction of blood lipids, etc. Some common symptoms of this imbalance include flatulence, constipation, and/or diarrhea. Acute inflammatory reactions cause diarrhea and can be due to a number of bacterial genera, including *Salmonella, Campylobacter, Yersinia, Aeromonas, Clostridium,* and *Escherichia.* If this imbalance is left untreated, the symptoms can become chronic, as in irritable bowel syndrome, and can compromise the immune system and lead to other serious illnesses. The consumption of probiotic organisms could help overcome these problems.

## *PROBIOTIC ORGANISMS*

Prevention of illness by a well-maintained microflora balance is accomplished by a method referred to as *competitive exclusion.* The friendly bacteria take up positions known as *enteric sites,* therefore preventing the pathogenic bacteria from establishing themselves. Probiotic organisms are generally, though not exclusively, lactic acid bacteria. They include a number of *Lactobacillus* and *Bifidobacterium* species. These Gram-positive lactic acid-producing organisms make up a major part of normal intestinal microflora in humans and animals. Lactobacilli have been considered especially beneficial bacteria in their ability to aid in the breakdown of proteins, carbohydrates and fats in food, and help in the absorption of necessary elements and nutrients, such as minerals, amino acids, and vitamins required for humans and other animals to survive. They are strictly fermentative, aero-tolerant, anaerobic organisms that can survive very low pH levels.

Bifidobacteria appear in the stool of infants a few days after birth and increase in number thereafter. They predominate in the colons of breast-fed babies, and account for more than 95 percent of culturable bacteria, and protect against infection. In formula-fed babies, on the other hand, more putrefactive intestinal flora are present. Bacteria are characterized by higher pH, lower redox potential, and the presence of ammonium and amines in the feces. In adults, bifidobacteria number $10^8$ to $10^{11}$ colony-forming units

(CFU) per gram. Their numbers reduce with age. They are nonmotile, nonsporulating, Gram-positive rods with varying appearance. Strains of *Streptococcus* have also been used as probiotics for human consumption. Other probiotics used in animals include *Bacillus subtilis, Pediococcus pentosaceus, Enterococcus faecium, Saccharomyces cerevisiae, Asperigillus oryzae,* and *Torulopsis* sp.

Lactic acid-producing bacteria are a popular choice of microbes in intestinal modifications. This is partly due to their historical usage. Lactobacilli and lactococci have long been used for the production of foods containing fermented milk (cheese and yogurt) without harm to the consumer. Also, large-scale cultures of these organisms have already been developed by the diary industry. Despite being lactic acid producers and intestinal colony formers, their use as human probiotics is curious because they are not numerically dominant in the digestive system and are even absent in a large majority of humans. On the other hand, when present in the intestinal tract, members of the genus *Bifidobacterium* are consistently more numerous, and hence are increasingly being used as probiotics.

Attempts are being made to develop organisms with superior abilities to adhere to intestinal walls, displace pathogenic bacteria, and absorb harmful compounds. However, probiotics are not known to permanently colonize hosts, and hence would have to be ingested regularly for many health promoting properties to persist.

## DESIRABLE CHARACTERISTICS

The problem of choosing criteria for the in vitro selection of organisms to be used as health-promoting, probiotic ingredients in food and pharmaceutical preparations was apparent even in the original work of Metchnikoff. In the late 1990s, a consensus was reached by scientists on some criteria. These include

1. ecological origin,
2. tolerance to the hostile conditions of the stomach and the small intestine (specifically acid and bile conditions),
3. ability to adhere and colonize the colon intestinal surfaces,
4. antagonistic relationship toward carcinogenic and pathogenic microorganisms,
5. genetic stability with no plasmid transfer mechanism,
6. capacity to produce organic acids and other biologically active compounds in the gastrointestinal tract,

7. contribution to the nutrition of the host animal by synthesizing essential nutrients that become readily available to the host,
8. capacity to digest dietary substances that the host is physiologically ill-equipped to utilize,
9. avirulent nature devoid of metabolic characteristics that would compromise the health of the host, and
10. reproducibility and viability during processing and storage.

Of primary importance is that the organism should have a history of being safe, and this may be most likely when it is of human origin. Although these criteria have been used to select probiotic lactobacilli, some doubts still remain. A critical rethinking of selection criteria seems necessary in order to improve the process of developing better probiotics.

## BENEFITS OF PROBIOTIC CONSUMPTION

Probiotic supplements that have been studied and accepted are those that bring about significant health benefits. The potential benefits suggested in the literature include antimicrobial effects inhibiting intestinal and food poisoning pathogens through the production of acids and other bacteriocines, improvement of gut function by normalizing microflora balance, reducing constipation and improving intestinal mobility, enhancement of the immune system through the production of secretory immunoglobulins, reduces diarrhea duration, including infantile, traveler's, and antibiotic-induced types, reduction of serum cholesterol concentration, management of diabetes and prevention of osteoperosis, improved nutrition through the enhanced production breakdown of vitamins, minerals, and amino acids and their absorption through the intestinal walls, normalization of the capability of cells, cleansing blood, making it cleaner and freer of toxins, reduction in blood pressures and allergies, stimulation of phagocytosis by peripheral blood leukocytes, modulation of cytokine gene expression, have an adjuvant effect, regression of tumors and repression of potentially harmful microbial enzymes associated with colon cancer, reduction in carcinogen or cocarcinogen production, growth promotion in rats and poultry, and reduction in lactose intolerance through the consumption of *L. acidophilus*-containing products. Although many studies indicating the advantages of consuming probiotics seem promising, a large amount of work is being carried out to substantiate these claims.

## SOURCES OF PREBIOTICS

Prebiotics basically consist of nondigestible fibers. Chief among these fibers are inulin, fructooligosaccharides and to a smaller extent galactooligosaccharides. These low molecular weight carbohydrates occur naturally in artichokes, onions, chicory, garlic, leeks, soybeans, specific herbs and roots, and to a smaller extent in cereals. Other oligosaccharides, such as raffinose and stachyose are present in peas and beans. A number of such oligosaccharides are also being produced industrially.

Inulin is a long-chain oligosaccharide (degree of polymerization of 30). The acknowledged effects of the prebiotic inulin are improved bowel functions, due mainly to the increase of fecal bulk; improved bioavailability of minerals; reduction in the risk of osteoporosis; improved fat metabolism; triglyceride-reduction; reduction of the risk of colon cancer, etc.

Some prebiotics are synthesized and obtained from dairy sources (lactulose, lactosucrose, and lactitol), and fall under the broad category of oligosaccharides (fructooligosaccharides and maltooligosaccharides). Nondigestible oligosaccharides have been developed since the 1980s as low-calorie, low-carcinogenic, sucrose substitutes for use as bulking agents in food. When the effects of these substances were investigated, it was found that some of them have the potential to selectively increase the population of bifidobacteria. These oligosaccharides have three to ten sugar moieties, and are produced enzymatically, either through the hydrolysis of larger polymers or by the synthesis from smaller sugars using transglycosylases. Such sugars are also obtained from soybean by extraction. Disaccharides such as lactulose and lactitol, used predominantly as drugs for the treatment of chronic constipation and hepatic encephalopathy, have also found to have many of the required characteristics of prebiotics.

In the large bowel, starches that have escaped small intestinal digestion (resistant starch) are fermented by the resident microflora. Resistant starches are of different types depending on their inaccessibility, high amylose content, retrograded forms produced during processing, and chemically modified starches. In the past resistant starch was not classified as a prebiotic because, in addition to bifidobacteria, many other bacterial species were found to ferment this starch. However, because of its capacity to act as a good carrier as it passes through the intestine, its role as prebiotic in symbiotic applications is highly likely.

Evidence for the cancer-preventing properties of probiotics and prebiotics is derived from studies on fecal enzyme activities in animals and humans, inhibition of genotoxicity of known carcinogens in vitro and in vivo, and suppression of carcinogen-induced preneoplastic lesions and tumors in laboratory animals. Some of these studies indicate that combinations of probiotics and prebiotics (synbiotics) are more effective.

## MODEL SYSTEMS

Several fermentor models have been used to test the growth and substrate utilization of different types of probiotics. This helps in the assessment of prebiotics and tests their performance in vitro. However, to test the effectiveness and mechanism of action of these organisms, animal tests are a necessary next step. Most of the animals used in these tests differ from humans in the relative size of the gut compartment, in the presence or absence of bile secretions, in coprophagic habits, and in the nature of their microbial population in the gut. Consequently, although animal models are valuable for probiotic research, data on health efficacy in humans also require scientifically valid human tests. This includes clinical tests with volunteers, epidemiological studies, and anecdotal studies. For proven health efficacy, such proof will be needed for new generation probiotics to meet consumer demands. Collaborative work with commercial companies producing probiotics and health care specialists are certainly needed for this.

## CONCLUSIONS

The screening of a prototype strain from nature with all the desirable probiotic characteristics is expensive and has small chance of success. It is difficult to imagine how probiotics could influence host biochemistry if they are not able to colonize the digestive tract for a sufficiently long period. Rapid and accurate methods are thus required for the detection and enumeration of specific bacterial strains to confirm that such strains administered as probiotics survive and replicate in appropriate regions of the digestive tract. Identification of these strains by morphology or serological methods or other classical approaches would be extremely difficult because of their inherent lack of precision and labor intensiveness. This limits their effectiveness for analyzing a large number of individuals. Molecular biology techniques that could be used for reliable differentiation of bacterial strains are plasmid profiling, ribosomal RNA differentiation, pulsed field gel electrophoresis, repetitive extragenic palindromic elements, nucleic acid probes, etc. Also, recombinant DNA technology could be used to inactivate genes that encode undesirable attributes while encoding desirable characteristics into the probiotic culture.

The development of efficacious strains by molecular genetic technologies will lead to a conceptual change in the use of probiotics. Instead of trying to bring about a balance in the microbial flora in the intestine, the aim will be to colonize the recipient with genetically modified organisms that could become an internal source of molecules with specific immunological or pharmacological activity. In the former, an immunizing strain would be developed genetically so that cells can synthesize an immunogen characteristic of a particular intestinal pathogen. When exposed to this strain, the intestinal mucosa will secrete specific IgA antibodies even before the pathogen is consumed. This will give immunity to the host against possible pathogens. For the latter, it would be possible to develop modified delivery strains that would be used to deliver in situ molecules of biological activity to specific levels of the intestinal tract. Public fear of genetically modified organisms will have to allayed before such organisms are used in foods.

The prevention of disease by probiotics has been recognized by most societies. Probiotic product development is thus a major area of research interest. Although effective probiotics have scientifically proven benefits, some confusion exists amid the wide range of supplements available and the claims made for them. Some of these products are not as effective as projected, resulting in consumer disappointment. Fundamental knowledge of intestinal bacteria and their interactions with one another and with their human or animal host is a prerequisite for successful probiotic research and development.

## SUGGESTED READINGS

Conway PL (1995). Microbial ecology of the human large intestine. In *Human colonic bacteria,* GR Gibson and GT Macfarlane (eds.). Boca Raton, FL: CRC Press Inc.

Sanders ME (1999). Probiotics. *Food Technology* 53(11):67-77.

Tannock GW (ed.) (1999). *Probiotics: A Critical Review.*Wymondham, UK: Horizon Scientific Press.

Wang, XD and SK Rakshit (2000). Iso-ologosaccharide production by multiple forms of transferase enzyme from *Aspergillus foetidus. Process Biochemistry* 35:771-775.

Ziemer CM and GR Gibson (1998). An overview of probiotics, prebiotics, and synbiotics in the functional food concept: Perspectives and future strategies. *International Dairy Journal* 8:473-479.

# Single-Cell Protein

Chundakkadu Krishna
Murray Moo-Young

## INTRODUCTION

The term *single-cell protein* (SCP) refers to dead, dry cells of microorganisms, such as yeast, fungi, bacteria, and algae, grown on different carbon sources for their protein content. Carol Wilson used the term for the first time in 1967 to replace less aesthetic terminology, such as *petroprotein* and *microbial protein*. Because the majority of the microorganisms used for SCP are unicellular, the protein content from them is called single cell protein. These cells also contain some other nutrients such as vitamins, fats, minerals, etc.

In the 1930s, the less developed areas of the world, such as Asia, Africa, and South America, were the exporters of grains to the developed countries, but toward the later half of 1940, a reverse trend was observed, due mainly to the higher rate of growth of the world's population in less-developed countries. This led to a protein mortgage, and the scarcity of protein-rich food from plant and animal sources, despite tremendous advancements in traditional crop-growing methods and improved crop varieties, forced mankind to search for alternative protein sources that can either replace or lessen the burden on conventional, but expensive protein sources, such as soymeal or fishmeal.

In the 1960s, the idea that SCP can help less-developed countries tackle problems associated with food shortages, specifically protein shortages, was gaining momentum among research scientists. This prompted cultivation of microorganisms on a large scale, which resulted in the development of SCP technology for livestock and human consumption. It has been estimated that a single-cell fermentor covering one-third of a square mile could yield enough protein to supply 10 percent of the world's needs. SCP technology for food production was developed over the last 100 years, but large-scale commercial production was developed only after World War I. The greatest production was carried out in Germany. After World War II, growth of fungi in submerged cultures for the production of antibiotics led to investigation on the potential of microfungi as flavor additives to replace mushrooms.

## NEED FOR MICROBIAL PROTEIN PRODUCTION

The use of microbes as a food source may not be acceptable to some people, but the idea is certainly an innovative way to solve global food scarcity. The main source of protein for human consumption is the agricultural sector, which uses large areas of land, but in return provides only low levels of production per unit area. Climatic factors greatly influence per capita production, and rapid progress in the area of plant biotechnology has given some hope that it will fill the gap of total dependency on conventional agricultural practices to cope up with the increasing demand for plant proteins. The scenario is none too comfortable regarding animal protein as well. The majority of animal protein-consuming countries depend on each other to meet the requirements. The main source of protein, marine and terrestrial fauna, is vulnerable to fluctuations in climatic conditions, as well as to deteriorating hydrological conditions due to water pollution.

The cultivation of microorganisms for protein has many advantages, such as high protein content, high ratio of surface area to volume, small doubling time, high growth rate, and flexibility in the use of substrates. Other advantages of SCP over conventional protein sources are that it is independent of land and climate, works on a continuous basis, can be genetically controlled, and causes less pollution. Because of the small doubling time of cells, the productivity of protein production from microorganisms is greater than that of traditional proteins.

## SOURCES

A large number of microorganisms, such as algae, fungi, yeast, and bacteria are used for SCP production. These organisms are selected on the basis of certain criteria, such as their ability to utilize a range of carbon and nitrogen sources, moderate growth conditions, tolerance to pH, temperature, and mineral concentrations, resistance against viral infection, nontoxicity, nonpathogenicity, acceptable nutritive value of the cell biomass, etc.

Among algae, *Spirulina* is used most extensively. This alga has a high nutritional value due to its large filamentous cells, and is resistant to bacterial degradation, making storage convenient. Similarly, biomass from *Chlorella, Senedesmus,* and *Dunaliella* are also being used in large-scale SCP production. The major problems associated with SCP from algae are their foul odor and tastelessness.

Many fungal species, such as *Aspergillus, Fusarium, Candida, Chaetomium, Trichoderma, Torulopsis, Penicillium, Geotrichum,* etc., are considered to be good candidates for SCP production due to their wide range of substrate utilization and ability to withstand fluctuating abiotic conditions. Moreover, fungal biomass can be recovered easily by filtration. Their slow growth and proneness to bacterial contamination are the major disadvantages. A recent trend in SCP production is the exploration of fungal species for bioconversion of lignocellulosic wastes.

Many strains of *Saccharomyces, Candida, Torulopsis,* and *Kluyveromyces fragilis* are used in biomass production. Of late, the methylotrophic yeast *Pichia pastoris* has emerged as an excellent microorganism in the production of SCP.

Different species of bacteria are also used in SCP production, including *Bacillus, Lactobacillus, Cellulomonas, Alcaligenes, Pseudomonas, Aeromonas,* etc. However, the success rate of those species has not been very encouraging. Mixed cultures of bacterial strains have shown better results with better stability and resistance to contamination.

## SUBSTRATES

A variety of substrates have been utilized to grow microorganisms for SCP production. Carbon dioxide and sunlight are the main factors required for optimal growth of algae. Fungal species are cultured on different substrates, mainly wastes, such as sulfite waste liquor, prawn shell wastes, dairy wastes, whey, molasses, etc., which provide carbon and nitrogen for growth. Lignocellulosic wastes have varying composition of hemicellulose, cellulose, and lignin. Based on the dominant component, specific fungi are used for biomass production. For bacteria, a variety of substrates, such as C1-C4 compounds, agricultural, animal, and fruit processing wastes, methane, methanol, etc., are used for cultivation.

## NUTRITIONAL ASPECTS OF SCP

The nutritional value of SCP varies depending upon the kind of microorganisms and substrates used for production. For assessment of the nutritional value of SCP, factors such as nutrient composition, amino acid, protein, carbohydrate, and lipid profiles, vitamins and nucleic acid contents, as well as palatability, allergies, and gastrointestinal effects are taken into consideration, in addition to undertaking long-term feeding trials, and studies on toxicological effects and carcinogenesis. Moreover, protein efficiency ratio (PER = weight gain in grams by the organisms/protein intake in grams), biological value (BV = retained nitrogen/absorbed nitrogen), net protein utilization (NPU = retained nitrogen/food nitrogen intake × 100), and/or protein digestibility value (PDV) are also considered for assessing nutritional aspects of SCP.

Algae are rich in proteins (40 to 60 percent), fats (5 to 20 percent), and vitamins A, B, C, D, and E, and they also contain mineral salts (7 percent), chlorophyll, bile pigments, and fiber, but have a very low nucleic acid content (4 to 6 percent). Algal proteins, though easily digestible, are assimilated less efficiently in comparison to animal proteins. The overall protein concentration is lower in fungi than in yeast and bacteria, but fungal biomass has high RNA contents in addition to substantial amounts of *N*-acetyl glucosamine. Fungi contain the B-complex group of vitamins, and the amino acid composition is reasonably high, but lipid contents are low. Dry yeast has about 50 percent protein, which resembles soy, and about 20 percent nonprotein material. Yeast proteins are easily digestible compared to those from bacteria. Yeast contains lysine, thiamine, biotin, riboflavin, niacin, folic acid, choline, etc., but are deficient in methionine. However, yeasts grown on molasses have a high concentration of methionine. The majority of microorganisms have well-balanced amino acid compositions. The amino acid composition of *Aspergillus niger* is well balanced and on par with the standards prescribed by the World Health Organization (WHO). Bacterial protein is similar to fish protein, and has higher protein levels, certain essential amino acids, and methionine when compared with algae and fungi. The crude protein content is around 80 percent of the total dry weight. The nucleic acid content, especially RNA, is very high in bacterial protein. The essential amino acid composition of different *Lactobacilli* appears comparable to the Food and Agriculture Organization (FAO) reference protein.

In general, SCP products contain approximately 50 to 70 percent crude protein, which is calculated as N × 6.25. Although SCP products are deficient in the amino acid methionine, they are a good source of vitamins, especially vitamin B. Before using an SCP as a consumption item, its nutritive values need to be clearly defined, such as the exact amount of energy obtained for metabolic processes, crude protein content, acceptable nucleic acid level, presence of essential amino acids and minerals, fatty acids, vitamins, trace elements, etc.

## LIMITATIONS

Although algae are excellent nutrition sources, some limitations exist for human consumption. The most important is the presence of the algal wall, whose digestibility is impaired because humans lack the cellulase enzyme and hence cannot digest the cellulose component of the wall. This problem does not arise when algae used as feed for cattle, because cattle have cellulose-degrading symbiotic bacteria and protozoa in their rumen. Two other factors are unacceptable coloration and disagreeable flavor. Moreover, elaborate methods and preparations are required to eliminate contamination.

The presence of mycotoxins in certain fungal species is a major hindrance to their use, because these toxins are known to produce many allergic reactions, diseases, and liver cancer in humans and animals. The high cost of bacterial SCP is restricting its industrial production considerably. Harvesting bacterial protein is costly due to its smaller cell size, and hence they have to be flocculated to create more solid slurry prior to centrifugation. High nucleic acid content is yet another limiting factor and cause for concern. A high content can cause an increase in the concentration of uric acid by 100 to 150 mg/g RNA in urine. A balanced relationship between the amount of consumable SCP with the required amount of nucleic acid is to be ascertained to make it acceptable for human consumption because natural plant and animal proteins do not pose this problem. Mineral level is yet another factor, which should be, tested both for nutritional and toxicological significance, as potassium level in SCP is reported to be low as compared to conventional foods.

A comparison among algae, fungi, and bacteria based on components indicates that bacteria have high true proteins, total nitrogen, fats, methionine, mineral salts, and nucleic acids. When acceptability is measured in terms of the growth rate, substrate used, and absence of contaminants and toxins, algae and fungi have an edge over bacteria. Nucleic acid levels are safer in algae, and fungal SCP is rich in lysine. However, among all SCP sources, yeast has attained global acceptability. Among algae, *Spirulina* and *Chlorella* are the most favored candidates.

## FACTORS AFFECTING SCP PRODUCTION

SCP production is a very complex and costly process. Production is greatly influenced by the kind of microorganisms used, technical feasibility, and cost effectiveness. Factors such as temperature, pH, humidity, oxygen requirement, carbon and nitrogen sources, composition of the medium, quality of chemicals and fermentation, and, most important, fermentor design play important roles in SCP production. Heat generation associated with biomass production during microbial growth of thick cultures necessitates cooling devices, which add to the cost of the product, and hence thermophilic microorganisms are often recommended for commercial production of SCP. Normally, the optimum temperature is 40 to 60°C, with a pH between 6.0 and 7.2.

## COMMERCIAL PRODUCTION OF SCP

Different processes for SCP production are being employed. In Scandinavian countries, the potato-processing industry produces wastewater with substantial amounts of carbohydrates. *Candida utilis,* cocultured with *Endomycopsis fibuliger,* which breaks down the starch to a simple sugar monomer, uses this carbohydrate for growth and this process is referred to as the "Symba Process." It has been found to be very efficient in potato-processing industries. The final product, "Symba Yeast," contains about 45 percent of protein in addition to vitamins. Another SCP, mycoprotein, developed by Rank Hovis McDougall Ltd., United Kingdom, uses a strain of *Fusarium* to produce SCP. For the production of a human-grade SCP named Probion, developed by Hoechst-Uhde, Germany, *Methylomonas clara* on methanol was tried, but the process was not scaled up. The Norprotein process of Norsk Hydro in Norway uses *Methanomonas methanolica,* the Mitsubishi Petrochemical Co. Ltd. process in Japan uses *Pseudomonas* sp., and the Sanraku-Ocean Co. Ltd., process uses *Methylomonas* sp. The Pruteen process of Imperial Chemical Industries (ICI) of United Kingdom, for feed grade SCP had been using *Methylophilus methylotrophus.*

## ALTERNATIVE SOURCES OF SCP PRODUCTION

### SCP from N-Alkanes

Yeast cells were probably the first to be harvested commercially but their overall production was very low. In the 1960s, however, a large number of microorganisms and substrates were screened and evaluated for SCP production. In the late 1950s, British Petroleum (BP) became interested in the growth of microorganisms on *N-alkanes,* which constitutes the wax fraction of gas oils for treating. British Petroleum used two yeasts, *Candida lipolytica* and *C. tropicalis,* and built two plants in France and England. The product was called Toprina, for which $NH_3$ was used as nitrogen base with Mg ions to increase yields. Although no signs of carcinogenicity or toxicity were observed, opposition from many countries by environmental groups prevented its marketing as a human food supplement, and it was decided to label the product as an animal feed. Japan became the first country to ban petrochemical proteins. In 1977 Italy stopped SCP production from alkanes altogether due to the increase in oil prices. Although Imperial Chemical Industries (ICI) in the United Kingdom produced Pruteen as animal feed, escalating oil prices in the international market forced the closure of their plants.

### SCP from Methane

Methane is cheap, abundant, and does not have the toxicity problem that alkanes do. In addition to being a constituent of North Sea gas, it is also produced during anaerobic digestion. Because methane contains the most highly reduced form of carbon, high yields are attained. *Methylomonas* and *Methylococcus* are the two important genera utilizing methane as a carbon source. Nitrates or ammonium salts serve as N sources. The most extensive work was carried out by Shell in the United Kingdom, involving the process of methane oxidation by stable mixed cultures of methane utilizing Gram-negative rods, a *Hyphomicrobium* sp., and two Gram-negative rods: *Acinetobacter* and *Flavobacterium*. Commercialization of the product and all developmental activities were indefinitely postponed because of the low prices of soybeans and maize, potential of many countries for expanding existing protein sources, and the difficulty in applying Shell's sophisticated process in developing countries.

### SCP from Methanol

ICI is credited with developing the most advanced process technology for the production of SCP from methanol using the bacterium *Methylophilus methylotropha* and ammonia as the nitrogen base. Although the product, Pruteen, contained 72 percent crude protein and was considered to be a balanced protein, it could not compete with soy and fishmeal, and hence the engineering success became an economic disaster.

### SCP from Ethanol

Yet another casualty was Torutein, an ethanol-based product from Amoco in the United States. Nestlé Alimentana (Switzerland) and Esso Research and Engineering (United States) also tried to produce SCP from ethanol. Although Torutein had 52 percent protein and was marketed as a flavor enhancer of high nutritive value and a replacement for meat, milk, and egg protein, it could not compete with soy.

## SCP from Lignocellulose

The lingocellulosic wastes, mainly from agriculture, forestry, and horti-culture constitute the most abundant substrates for SCP, but the necessity of pretreatment to break down the complex polysaccharide weighs against the production cost. Pretreatment with some physical or chemical methods be-comes essential because the lignin, hemicellulose, and cellulose (LHC) complex is tough to unravel and does not allow easy accessibility of en-zymes in enzymatic hydrolysis of the lignocellulosics. The Waterloo pro-cess, developed at the University of Waterloo, Ontario, Canada, is based on the cellulolytic fungus *Chaetomium cellulolyticum,* and utilizes agricultural wastes, such as crop residues of straw, corn stover, and bagasse, animal ma-nure, and forestry residues, such as wood sawdust and pulp mill sludges. At present, the only economical utilization of lignocellulosic wastes is in mushroom production.

## SCP from Other Renewable Resources

Beet and cane molasses have been used for yeast biomass production since 1939. Many other renewable and food-processing wastes, such as sug-arcane bagasse, wastes from paper mills and sugar syrup industries, fruit-processing wastes, wheat bran, starch wastes, wastes from meat-processing industries, sulfite liquor wastes, activated sewage sludge, etc., are used in SCP production. Microbial biomass has been produced commercially from whey since the 1940s in the United States and many European countries. Among the several processes that have been described (Sico, 1996), the Vi-enna process and the Bel process stand out. In order to improve the nutri-tional characteristics for consumption, methionine-enriched mutant *Kluy-veromyces lactis* and *Candida intermedia* are being used.

## OPTIMUM SCP PRODUCTION PARAMETERS

Substrate, yield, and nutritive value in terms of proteins and vitamins dic-tate the cost of the final product. The microorganism and substrate used for the fermentation determine the yield of the process. Among yeasts, *Candida tropicalis* and *Yarrowia lipolytica* were found to be the most effective for SCP production on diesel oil as the sole carbon source. Culture conditions, pretreatment of substrates, nutrient supplementation, types of fermentation processes, and strain improvement can, individually or in combination, alter the final SCP composition. Several fungal cultures produced double the amount of crude protein on alkali-treated rice straw when compared with untreated straw.

Genetic engineering techniques are also used for improvement of SCP production. *Pseudomonas methylotrophus* was considerably improved by ICI through genetic engineering and physiological development. The use of genetic engineering is not restricted to the design and production of microbes with high protein yield alone, but also for the improvement of downstream processing in the postfermentation stage. It is used in the production of "designer" or recombinant proteins of high nutritive value and their subsequent purification. Specifically designed tags or modification of sequences with target-gene products are used for efficient recovery of native and modified proteins. Suppression or elimination of protease activity in the cells can also achieve improvement of protein recovery. Mutants with modified gene sequences can be isolated and used for this purpose. Recombinant DNA technology can be used to isolate mutant genes that can produce high amounts of amino acids, such as glutamate, tryptophan, and phenylalanine, in addition to high protein yields. Through recombinant techniques, such genes were combined and then incorporated into an organism with a wide substrate range. Unstructured logistic models were also applied to stimulate the kinetic process of SCP batch cultures with yeast to increase the productivity of SCP.

Since the late 1980s, solid state fermentation (SSF) has generated interest because of the need to reduce manufacturing costs from wastes by applying process engineering principles and techniques. This includes simplicity in operating the Koji fermentor, simultaneous saccharification, fermentation of lignocellulosic substrates, and release of concentrated hydrolytic enzymes in the medium during growth. Although SSF has many advantages over submerged fermentation, substrate particle size, moisture level, and C:N ratio are critical factors of SSF.

## TOXICITY

The major problems associated with SCP for human consumption are their very high concentrations of 4 to 20 percent nucleic acids against the allowed concentration of 2 percent, allergies, threat of carcinogenic compounds carried along with different sources of substrates, gastrointestinal disturbances, and the presence of toxic heavy metals, chemical residues, microbial toxins, pathogens, etc. The problem that occurs from the consumption of proteins with high concentrations of nucleic acids is the high level of uric acid, which may lead to kidney stone formation and gout. Uric acid accumulates in the body due to lack of the uricase enzyme in humans. Removal or reduction of nucleic acid is possible through chemical treatment with NaOH, treatment with 10 percent NaCl, and thermal shock.

Toxins are secondary metabolites produced by certain fungi and bacteria during growth. In general, algae do not produce harmful toxins. The toxicity of SCP products must be evaluated and assessed before marketing the product.

### *Mycotoxins*

Prominent among mycotoxins are fungal toxins, which include aflatoxins of types B1, B2, G1, and G2 from *Aspergillus flavus,* citrinin from *Penicillium citrinum,* tricothecenes and zearalenone from *Fusarium* species, and ergotamine from *Claviceps* species. Aflatoxins have been linked to human liver cancer. Ochratoxins are also important mycotoxins. Of the five metabolites in this group, ochratoxin A is the most abundant, and the metabolites are found to occur in *Aspergillus* and *Penicillium* species, causing damage to the liver and kidneys. With about 80 types, trichothecenes are yet another group among mycotoxins that cause dermal toxicity and many hematopoietic problems.

Removal of mycotoxins is a challenging task, and research has focused on aflatoxins. Ammoniation has been the most successful method. Molecular biology techniques have also been exploited for detoxication. Research on molecular dissection and elimination of genes responsible for mycotoxin synthesis is fast developing. Techniques of cloning, probing, sequencing, transcript mapping, gene disruption, etc., have been employed to isolate the aflatoxin pathway clusters. Studies that identify the molecular determinants regulating mycotoxin production are promising rational control strategies. It is heartening to note that detoxication of SCP from fungal sources is a possibility, although research is still in the initial stages.

### *Bacterial Toxins*

Bacterial toxins are either endotoxins or exotoxins. Exotoxins are secreted by G(+) bacteria into the surrounding media, whereas endotoxins are an integral part of the cell walls of G(−) bacteria. Exotoxins do not produce fever, but cause generalized symptoms and lesions. Endotoxins, on the other hand, produce fever. Because these toxins are part of the cellular components, their removal is somewhat difficult.

## USES OF SCP

In addition to proteins, SCPs are also rich in carbohydrates, fats, and minerals. The market acceptability of SCPs as animal feed, as supplements to human food, or as flavor enhancers depends on extensive tasting before their use. SCPs produced on natural substrates are considered safer than those produced on hydrocarbons and related substrates. Nutritional value is of prime importance if SCPs are used as feed or food, whereas functional properties such as fat binding and water binding, emulsion stability, dispensability, gel formation, etc., count when used as ingredients. Microbial proteins have a majority of these properties, and are being used in many other foodstuffs as additives, raising their overall protein values. The products from yeasts are used as protein and vitamin supplements in canned foods, bakery products, cheese, sausages, beverages, etc. Microbial proteins are also used as flavor enhancers and in improving the texture of baked foods. So far, only mycoprotein from *Fusarium graminearum* has been considered acceptable for human consumption. A sizable part of the European market is dominated with SCP, such as Toparina and Pruteen for animal feed despite their high prices and the added fear of unknown effects of microbial cellwall components and its chemicals.

The Protein Advisory Group (PAG) of the UN and the International Union of Pure and Applied Chemistry (IUPA) has prepared systematic guidelines for feeding trials in animals. The extensive trials conducted on Toparina and Pruteen have qualified these protein products for use in animal feed, and no reports of any toxicological problems with these proteins have been made to date.

## SOCIOECONOMIC PROBLEMS AND COST EFFECTIVENESS

The selection of microorganisms, their maintenance, growth, and harvesting of protein, etc., are common constraints. Socioeconomic problems include availability of substrates, general fear of eating microbes, culture maintenance, power supply, cost, need for specialized equipment, environmental contamination, processing of final product for marketing, etc. The cost of SCP is dependent on carbon and nitrogen sources, and it is this high cost that has prevented the large-scale inclusion of SCPs in animal feed and human food. Moreover, large-scale production plants of SCP are capital intensive, and although several oil companies have developed large-scale plants, escalating oil prices have affected the economic feasibility of these plants, and many are on the verge of closure.

## CONCLUSIONS

The development of SCP was the beginning of biotechnology, initiated by oil companies because they could risk developing an expensive product that had no real expected profit. To explore the potential of SCP to its maximum extent, it should be produced with human consumption in mind. However, people fear that microbial genes cloned into crops will enter the human system and lead to diseases. Their fears have to be alleviated, for which there should be more fundamental studies on the utilization of SCP as human food. Today, in most countries where market forces operate, SCP cannot compete with soy, alfalfa, or fishmeal because of its high cost. Development of genetically improved microorganisms with improved substrate conversion efficiencies, coupled with high productivity and better stability characteristics having lower cost of separation methods may lead to reduced production costs. In the wake of considerable advancement in biotechnology, SCP production stands as the best alternative to supplement the requirements of food and feed-grade protein, vitamins, and amino acids.

## SUGGESTED READINGS

Anupama and P Ravindra (2000). Value-added food: Single cell protein. *Biotechnology Advances* 18:459-479.
Bhalla TC, H Gajju, and HO Agrawal (1999). In *Biotechnology: Food fermentation,* Volume II, VK Joshi and A Pandey (eds.). New Delhi: Educational Publishers and Distributors, pp. 1003-1022.
Goldberg I (1985). *Single cell protein.* Germany: Springer-Verlag.
Gowthaman MK, C Krishna, and M Moo-Young (2001). Fungal solid state fermentation—An overview. In *Applied Mycology and Biotechnology,* Volume I, *Agriculture and Food Production,* GG Khachatourians and DK Arora (eds.). The Netherlands: Elsevier Science, pp. 305-352.
Moo-Young M (1977). Economics of SCP production. *Process Biochemistry* 12(4): 6-10.
Sico MIG (1996). The biotechnological utilization of cheese whey: A review. *Bioresource Technology* 57:1-11.

# Vitamin Production by Fermentation

Rekha S. Singhal
Pushpa R. Kulkarni

## INTRODUCTION

Vitamins are essential constituents of food that are required in trace quantities and cannot be synthesized completely in the body. Their deficiency has been associated with certain diseases. Vitamins are classified by their activity, as well as their solubility as fat-soluble (vitamins A, D, E, and K) and water-soluble vitamins (members of the B group and vitamin C, also known as ascorbic acid).

All vitamins can be extracted from natural sources. However, fat-soluble vitamins are often produced commerically via synthetic processes. Among the water-soluble vitamins, vitamin $B_2$ (riboflavin) and vitamin $B_{12}$ (also known as cyanocobalamin, which due to its extremely complex structure precludes chemical synthesis and requires 70 steps) are produced by fermentation. For ascorbic acid, one of the steps in its synthesis uses the biosynthetic ability of microorganisms. Microbial production is commercially feasible for some vitamins, such as vitamin $B_{12}$. Microbial production of vitamin $B_1$ (thiamine), vitamin $B_6$ (pyridoxine), biotin, folic acid, and pantothenic acid is commercially possible.

## MICROBIAL PRODUCTION OF VITAMINS

### Vitamin C or Ascorbic acid

Vitamin C is manufactured commercially by Reichstein-Grussner synthesis, which uses D-glucose as the starting material. D-glucose is hydrogenated catalytically to D-sorbitol at elevated temperature and pressure using a nickel catalyst, and then fermented with *Acetobacter suboxydans* in sterile solutions in the presence of large amounts of air. The fermentation oxidizes D-sorbitol to L-sorbose, which is subsequently isolated by crystallization, filtration, and drying. Although other organisms, such as *Acetobacter xylinum* and *Streptomyces* species can also ferment D-sorbitol to L-sorbose, *Acetobacter suboxydans* remains the organism of choice because it gives L-sorbose in yields more than 90 percent. Sterilization is required to prevent contamination, both in batch or continuous fermentations. Large-scale fermentations are carried out at pH 5 to 6 at 30 to 35°C.

L-Sorbose is then converted to bis-*O*-isopropylidene-α-L-sorbofuranose in >90 percent yield on reaction with acetone and excess sulfuric acid at low temperatures in the presence of ferric chloride or perchloric acid as catalysts. This substance is then oxidized at elevated temperatures in diluted sodium hydroxide in the presence of nickel chloride or palladium-carbon as catalysts. After completion of the reaction, the mixture is acidified to bis-*O*-isopropylidene-2-oxo-L-gulconic acid, which on treatment with hydrochloric acid gas in a water-free chloroform-ethanol mixture gives ascorbic acid in 80 percent yield. The crude product is filtered and purified by recrystallization from diluted ethanol. This is shown schematically in Figure II.11. Efforts to reduce production costs by optimizing and shortening various reaction routes have been attempted. These include a combination of chemical and microbial reaction sequences, direct chemical oxidations, enzymatic catalysis, use of genetically modified organisms or plant tissues, and cofermentations. Reichstein synthesis still predominates commercial production, although reports of a single-step fermentation to 2-keto-L-gluconic acid are believed to have reached commercial scale. Single-step fermentation is summarized as follows:

- A novel process developed for the synthesis of ascorbic acid involves the use of a genetically engineered strain of *Erwinia herbicola* that contains a gene from *Corynebacterium* sp. This organism converts glucose into 2-keto-L-gluconic acid, which can be converted by acid or base to ascorbic acid.
- Fermentative production of 2-keto-L-gluconic acid from L-sorbose using *Pseudomonas, Bacillus, Gluconobacter,* and other organisms is available in patented literature. Single- as well as mixed-culture fermentations using improved bioengineering techniques have been reported. Yields as high as 86 percent have been reported with a mixed culture of *Pseudogluconobacter saccharogenes* and *Bacillus megaterium* when the culture medium is supplemented with rare earth elements. Purification techniques decrease the yield to about 70 percent. Better results with D-sorbitol as the starting material have been patented. A single-step fermentation of D-sorbitol or L-sorbose to 2-keto-L-gluconic acid could enable economic production routes of ascorbic acid.

- Production of 2,5-diketogulonic acid from D-glucose by several species of *Acetobacter, Gluconobacter,* or *Erwinia* and subsequent reduction (chemically or microbiologically) to 2-ketogulonic acid has been suggested as intermediate steps for the manufacture of ascorbic acid. Yet another method that converts glucose (40 g/l) to 2-keto-L- gluconate (20 g/l) involves cloning of a gene encoding 2,5-diketo-D-gluconate reductase from *Corynebacterium* sp. into *Erwinia citreus*. Plasmid cloning of the genes encoding L-sorbose dehydrogenase and L-sorbosone dehydrogenase from *Gluconobacter oxydans* back into the same organism yields a strain that can convert 150 g/l D-sorbitol to 13 g/l 2-keto-L-gulonate.
- Enzymatic hydrolysis of pectic acid to D-galacturonic acid followed by catalytic reduction of the aldehyde group to L-galactonic acid and further transormation of the same to L-ascorbic acid by fermentation with *Candida* sp. is another approach toward the manufacture of ascorbic acid.
- Direct synthesis of ascorbic acid from D-glucose can be achieved by mutagenized microalgae of the *Chlorella* species. Although the yields are low for industrial feasibility, the L-ascorbic acid enriched culture is useful as an aquaculture fish feed or as a feed additive.

### Riboflavin

Riboflavin is produced both by chemical synthesis as well as by fermentation. Initial attempts at commercial production of riboflavin used *Clostridium acetobutylicum,* which is inoculated into a sterilized carbohydrate-containing mash, adjusted to pH 6 to 7, and later buffered with calcium carbonate. This yielded only 70 mg/l of riboflavin. Later, the yields improved to about 49 mg/l on inoculation of several *Candida* sp. in a low-cost synthetic medium. Organisms assimilating ethanol and lactose were developed in this process. Other efforts at microbial production of riboflavin have been made with an aerobic culture of *Pichia guilliermondii* on a medium containing n-$C_{10}$ to $C_{15}$ parrafins. Several patents that utilize other *Pichia* sp. using hydrocarbon sources are available, although the yields are much lower than that available presently. Similarly, patented information using *Torulopsis xylinus, Hansenula polymorpha, Brevibacterium ammoniagenes, Achromobacter butrii, Micrococcus lactis,* and *Streptomyces testaceus* is available in the scientific literature.

At present, microbial producers of riboflavin involve two yeastlike molds, *Eremothecium ashbyii* and *Ashbya gossypii,* which synthesize it at levels greater than 20 g/L. *A. gossypii* is cultivated in corn steep liquor, and

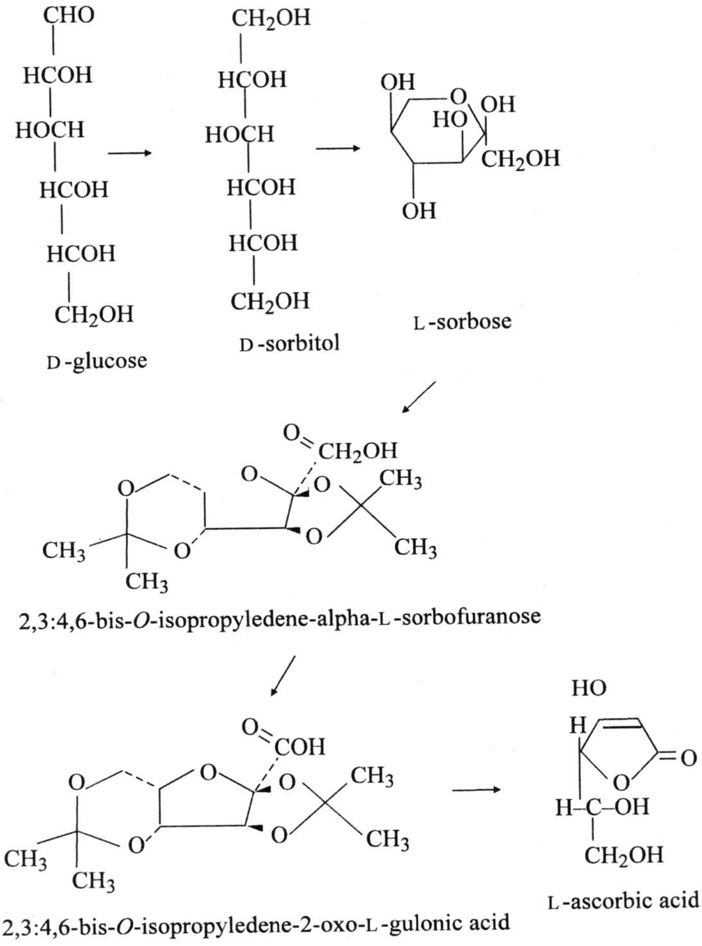
D-glucose
D-sorbitol
L-sorbose
2,3:4,6-bis-*O*-isopropyledene-alpha-L-sorbofuranose
2,3:4,6-bis-*O*-isopropyledene-2-oxo-L-gulonic acid
L-ascorbic acid

FIGURE II.11. Synthesis of L-ascorbic acid

excess vitamin $B_2$ is recovered from the medium. It makes 40,000 times more vitamin $B_2$ than it needs for its own growth. This is mainly due to the metabolic role of iron on the production of riboflavin. Iron has no repressive effects on the production of vitamin $B_2$ by these organisms, whereas it severely inhibits riboflavin production by low and moderate overproducers such as *Clostridia* and *Candida*. In most organisms, iron represses almost all of the enzymes in the biosynthesis of riboflavin. In addition, riboflavin itself inhibits the first enzyme of the pathway, GTP cyclophydrolase II. Chelating agents such as 2,2'-dipyridyl are recommended to control the iron content. Processes using *Candida* sp. or recombinant strains of *Bacillus subtilis* that produce up to 20 to 30 g/L riboflavin are now available. In a sterile aerobic submerged process, high yields are obtained within a few days with good aeration and stirring at temperatures below 30°C.

Downstream processing consists of separating the biomass, and evaporation and drying of the concentrate to obtain an enriched product containing up to 80 percent riboflavin. Companies such as Archer Daniels Midland (ADM) in the United States and BASF in Germany produce riboflavin by fermentation.

### Vitamin $B_{12}$ (Cyanocobalamin)

Recovery of vitamin $B_{12}$ from spent liquors of streptomycete antibiotic fermentation has been known for a number of years, e.g., streptomycin production by *Streptomyces griseus*, neomycin by *S. fradiae,* and chlorotetracycline by *S. aureofaciens*. However, these processes are no longer economical.

A proportion of vitamin $B_{12}$ is used for the synthesis of other cobalamins. With an increase in demand for this vitamin, separate fermentations were developed.

More than 100 processes using microorganisms belonging to the genera *Propionibacterium, Bacillus, Corynebacterium, Arthrobacter, Rhodopseudomonas, Protaminobacter, Streptomyces, Rhodospirillum, Actinomyces, Selenomonas,* and *Nocardia* for fermentative production of vitamin $B_{12}$ are available in literature and patents. Although some of these organisms utilize carbohydrates as the carbon source, *Corynebacterium, Arthrobacter, Pseudomonas,* and *Nocardia* utilize hydrocarbons. Others such as *Pseudomonas* and *Protaminobacter* utilize methanol. These organisms not only differ with respect to the substrates required for fermentation, they all produce low levels of $B_{12}$. Only five to ten processes using different organisms are practiced worldwide.

### Fermentation Using Propionibacterium

Vitamin $B_{12}$ is produced industrially by *Propionibacterium shermanii* or *Pseudomonas denitrificans,* which make about 50,000 to 100,000 times more vitamin $B_{12}$ than needed for their own growth. Resistance to cobalt has been used for selection of higher-producing mutants. All fermentations produce a mixture of methyl-, hydroxo-, and adenosylcobalamin, isolation of which is tedious. Hence, the workup is usually carried out after the corrinoids are converted to the cyano form by the addition of cyanide. The main factor governing the production of vitamin $B_{12}$ is feedback repression. The production is done in fermentors, which are filled with the production medium in which the bacteria grow. The fermentor is inoculated from a preculture that comes from a working cell bank. The strains used for commercial production are generally improved by a strain development program to improve productivity. Improved characteristics include high productivity, high growth rate, improved nutrient utilization, higher tolerance to starting and end materials, or improved genetic stability. These fermentations are quite tedious, but can be eased out if characteristics connected with improved production are targeted. For example, in the production of vitamin $B_{12}$, mutants with reduced catalase activity are desirable because they have reduced porphyrin synthesis. This is desirable because porphyrin and vitamin $B_{12}$ have a common precursor in their biosynthesis. Hence, strains with reduced catalase activity could be selected and tested further for $B_{12}$ productivity.

The *Propionibacterium* process is the oldest fermentation process for the production of $B_{12}$, and *P. shermanii* and *P. freudenreichii* are the preferred species. With *P. shermanii*, a two-step fermentation is carried out as follows:

1. The fermentation is carried out initially under anaerobic conditions in the absence of the precursor, 5,6-dimethylbenzimidazole. These conditions are necessary because *Propionibacterium* is an anaerobic organism that grows and produces $B_{12}$ poorly in the presence of oxygen. It also allows the accumulation of the intermediate, cobinamide.
2. Cobinamide is converted subsequently to vitamin $B_{12}$ when the culture is aerated and dimethylbenzimidazole is added. The biosynthesis of $B_{12}$ is inhibited by the $B_{12}$ itself, i.e., feedback inhibition. This can be avoided by using the two-stage fermentation process described previously. This approach not only reduces the time of fermentation, but also yields more than 150 mg/L $B_{12}$.

## *Fermentation Using* Pseudomonas

Fermentation with *Pseudomonas denitrificans* is carried out under low oxygen conditions because higher levels of oxygen oxidize the intracellular environment, which represses formation of early enzymes in the pathway. Strain development programs using mutagenic agents, such as UV radiation and nitrosomethylurea, have increased the production from 4 mg/L to 150 mg/L in eight steps. In this fermentation process, production of $B_{12}$ parallels the growth of the organism, which converts the glucose to carbon dioxide and consumes the oxygen in the process. The culture needs to be aerated in the logarithmic phase, although care has to be taken to limit the oxygen concentration in the medium. Here, dimethylbenzimidazole, as a precursor of $B_{12}$, is added to the fermentation medium. Glutamate in the medium is also known to improve yields.

Vitamin $B_{12}$ overproduction is dependent on betaine addition, which is the key to the fermentation. Its mechanism is not completely understood. Sugar beet molasses contains a significant amount of betaine, and is therefore used in industrial fermentations. Production levels have reached 150 mg/L.

## Media Formulation and Downstream Processing

Microbial production of $B_{12}$ is generally carried out under submerged culture. It is associated mostly with the cellular material. Centrifugation yields a sludge that releases the vitamin on dispersion in a minimum amount of water, water-alcohol, or water-acetone upon heating.

Media formulations for the production of $B_{12}$ include raw materials, such as soybean meal, fish meal, corn steep liquor, meat extract, casein hydrolysates, etc. Typical media composition for the production of $B_{12}$ by *Propionibacterium* and *Pseudomonas* sp. is shown in Table II.7. The amount of cobamide produced intracellularly is proportional to the cell yield. The addition of carbohydrate and ammonium hydroxide to the fermentation medium is known to increase the yield of vitamin $B_{12}$. The steps in down-

TABLE II.7. Typical media composition for the fermentative production of vitamin $B_{12}$

| *Propionibacterium* sp. | | *Pseudomonas* sp. | |
|---|---|---|---|
| Glucose | 120 g | Sugar beet molasses | 105 g |
| Corn steep liquor | 80 ml | Sucrose | 15 g |
| Glycine | 5 g | Betaine | 3 g |
| $NH_4NO_3$ | 3 g | Ammonium sulfate | 2.5 g |
| $MgSO_4.5H_2O$ | 0.5 g | Magnesium sulfate | 0.2 g |
| $Na_2MoO_4$ | 10 mg | Zinc sulfate | 0.08 g |
| Calcium pantothenate | 5 mg | 5,6-Dimethylimidazole | 0.025 g |
| $CoCl_2.6H_2O$ | 0 mg | Tap water | 1 L |
| Dimethylbenzimidazole | 20 g | | |
| Tap water | 1 L | | |

stream processing are summarized in Figure II.12. The biomass is separated by centrifugation to obtain a cell mass concentrate, which is then dried. Alternatively, the entire contents of the fermentor can be concentrated or spray dried. Cell lysis by heating the centrifuged cell mass in an aqueous solution, or by other methods to get the corrinoids, are often resorted to. Corrinoids are converted to $B_{12}$ or cyanocobalamin by the addition of KCN, usually in the presence of sodium nitrite and heat. The $B_{12}$ solution is clarified subsequently by filtration, treatment with zinc chloride, and then precipitated out by the addition of tannic acid or cresol to give a product of 80 percent purity that is suitable for use as an animal feed additive. For the greater purity that is required for pharmaceutical use, the clarified solution is extracted with organic solvents, such as cresol or carbon tetrachloride, and then with water and butanol, followed again by organic solvents. In addition, adsorption processes, such as ion exchangers, aluminium oxide, or activated carbon can be used. Pure $B_{12}$ is obtained by crystallization after the addition of organic solvents, such as phenol and water.

### *Biotin*

D-biotin, a vitamin required for human health care, is an animal feed additive, and is also required for the production of metabolites such as L-lysine and other L-amino acids. D-biotin is produced mainly by chemical synthesis, although efforts to manufacture it economically using microorganisms are being made by several research groups.

The main problem in the fermentative production of biotin is the feedback repression caused by acetyl-CoA carboxylase biotin and synthetase. In addition, biotin 5-adenylate also acts as a corepressor. Strains of *Serratia marcescens* obtained by mutagenesis, selection for resistance to biotin antimetabolites, and molecular cloning produce up to 600 mg/L of biotin in the presence of high concentration of sulfur and ferrous ion. Recently, genetically modified *Escherichia coli* and *Bacillus sphaericus* have proven to be a richer source of natural biotin, and yields up to 230 mg/L have been obtained in fermentor charges. To seriously compete with the stereo-specific total chemical synthesis, biotin concentration of at least 1 g/l must be attained. These require sustained research and development efforts.

### CONCLUSIONS

Vitamins and related compounds, such as coenzymes, are used in foods, feeds, cosmetics, and pharmaceutical preparations. These high-value biochemicals are produced in low concentrations, even in optimized fermenta-

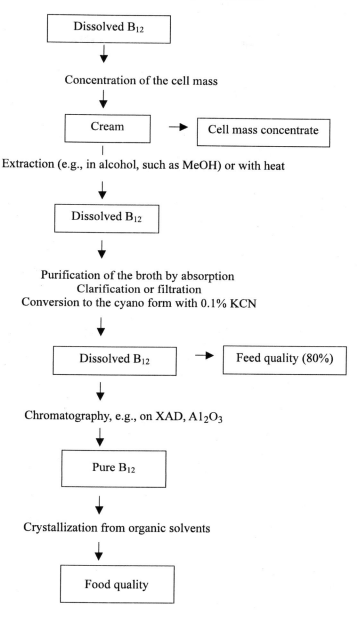

FIGURE II.12. Downstream processing of vitamin $B_{12}$

tions. Recovery and purification of these biochemicals is a complex process, and involves a number of operations. Considerable research needs to be done in recovering these biochemicals from the fermentation broth with a minimum number of steps. Also, implementation of novel recovery techniques, such as extractive fermentation and membrane technology, needs to be investigated.

## SUGGESTED READINGS

Demain AL (1999). Metabolites, primary and secondary. In *Encyclopedia of bioprocess technology: Fermentation, biocatalysis, and bioseparation,* Volume 3, MC Flickinger and SW Draw (eds). New York: Wiley Interscience, John Wiley and Sons Inc., pp. 1713-1732.

Elvers B and S Hawkins (eds.) Vitamins. In *Ullman's Encyclopedia of Industrial Chemistry,* Volume A 27, Fifth completely revised edition. Weinheim, Germany: VCH Verlagsgesellschaft GmbH, pp. 443-613.

Grayson M (ed.) (1984). Vitamins. In *Kirk-Othmer encyclopedia of chemical technology,* Volume 24, Third edition. New York: Wiley Interscience, John Wiley and Sons Inc., p. 226.

# Xanthan Gum Production

Maria Papagianni

## INTRODUCTION

Many microorganisms synthesize large quantities of polysaccharides under a wide variety of conditions. Polysaccharides are usually thought to play specific roles, either as storage compounds, structural compounds, or, in the case of extracellularly produced polysaccharides, as mediators in the interaction of the microorganisms with their environment. Exopolysaccharides (EPS) either remain attached to the cell surface or are found in the extracellular medium in the form of amorphous slime. In both natural and manmade environments, EPS play a major structural role in *biofilms,* the normal habitat of many microbial communities, in which varying numbers of prokaryotic and eukaryotic microorganisms grow while attached to solid-liquid interfaces.

Extracellular microbial polysaccharides are of major interest commercially as members of a class of water-soluble polymers or gums that are used as thickening, gelling, or suspending agents or protective colloids. Several such microbial polysaccharides are now widely accepted products of biotechnology, whereas others are in various stages of development. The production of gums for commercial use by fermentation, compared to extraction from plants and seaweeds or chemical synthesis, offers several advantages, such as continuous production in reliable quantities and qualities and modification of the structure and properties of the original exopolysaccharide by manipulating the fermentation parameters, which increases the value and extends the range of their applications. Included in this category are xanthan, dextran, gellan, and many others that have found various food and non-food applications. Despite the wide range of applications, the penetration of microbial polysaccharides into the water-soluble polymer market has been slow, due to the high capital and energy costs that tend to make microbial gums less cost-effective when compared to most other water-soluble polymers. The costs and times associated with obtaining approval for the use of novel gums in foods are also very high. The screening and selection of new microbial gums of commercial interest is difficult because of the poor understanding of the complex chemical and physical nature of polysaccharides, their relationships to the end-use applications, and the marked effect of impurities on polymer performance. Although we now have a better idea of the relationships existing between structure and function, it is still difficult to predict which microbial polymers will prove worth developing. Two products have proved to be valuable—bacterial cellulose and hyaluronic acid—despite the fact that both were already available from nonbacterial sources. Another example of biological properties that have led to polysaccharide applications can found in the range of fungal 1,4-β-D-glucans, which have proven to be potent immune-system modulators, a property that is still poorly understood. Thus, despite their potential advantages, xanthan, and to a lesser extent dextran, are sold in significant quantities at present, although many other microbial gums are attracting interest.

## GENERAL PROPERTIES

A combination of properties, with their ability to modify the rheology of solutions, makes most of these biopolymers multifunctional compounds in the end-use application. These properties are determined by their chemical composition, molecular structure, molecular weight, and distribution. Some polysaccharides, such as dextran and scleroglucan, are neutral, whereas others, such as xanthan and gellan, are acidic. Acidic polysaccharides are polyelectrolytes, and they possess carboxyl groups from uronic acids and/or pyruvate residues. They often contain side groups, such as pyruvate, succinate, acetate, lipid-type components, and inorganic ions, whose degree of substitution greatly affects the polymer's properties. The conformation of the molecules in solution is affected by the ionic strength, pH, and the concentration of the polysaccharide itself. Acidic polysaccharides are generally more affected by the presence of cations in solution. Divalent cations can cross-link polysaccharide chains to produce strong gel structures.

## XANTHAN

Xanthan gum is produced by the Gram-negative bacterium *Xanthomonas campestris*. It is a hetero polysaccharide with a primary structure, as shown in Figure II.13. The presence of acetic and pyruvic acids in the molecule produces an anionic polysaccharide. The pyruvate and acetate content depends on the bacterial strain, culture conditions, and processing of the polysaccharide. Commercial production of xanthan gum began in early

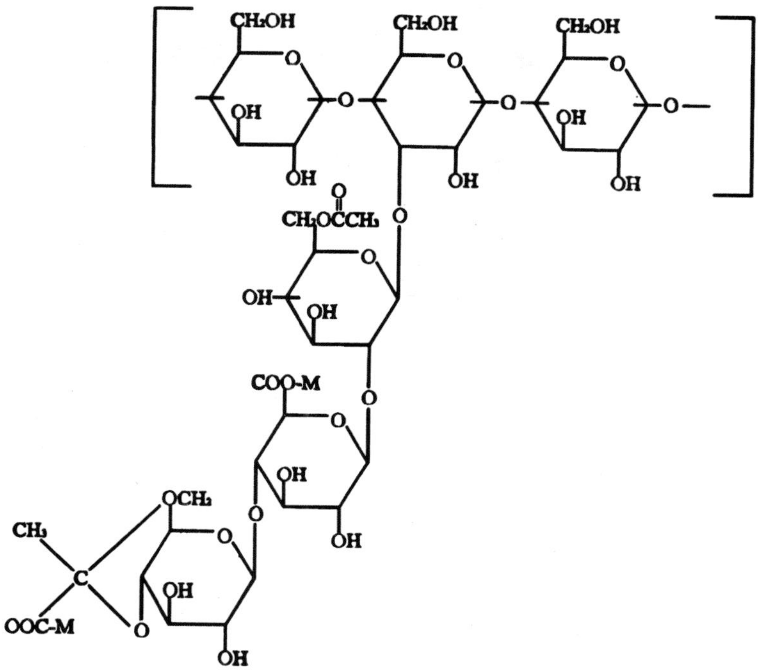

FIGURE II.13. Structure of the exopolysaccharide xanthan from *Xanthomonas campestris*

1964. Today, it is the most important commercial polysaccharide, with an annual production of around 20,000 tons. It is widely used for stabilization, suspension, and viscosity control in the food industry. Its properties are also exploited in a wide variety of applications in the chemical and cosmetics industries, as shown in Table II.8.

## *GELLAN*

Gellan is a linear heteropolysaccharide whose repeating unit consists of two glucose units, one glucuronic acid unit, and one rhamnose unit arranged as follows:

→3)–β–D–Glc–(1→4)–β–D–GlcA–(1→4)–D–Glc–(1→4)–α–L–Rha–(1→

TABLE II.8. Properties and established applications of xanthan gum

| Main functions/properties | Usage |
| --- | --- |
| Emulsion stabilizer | Salad dressings, mayonnaise, ice cream, sauces |
| Syneresis inhibitor | Dairy products, sauces, frozen food |
| Adhesive | Icings, glazes |
| Foam stabilizer | Beer |
| Thickening agent | Sauces, syrups, soups, fillings |
| Swelling agent | Meat products, bakeries |
| Viscosity controller | Aqueous flowables for agricultural applications, water-based paints, printing pastes, oil-drilling muds |
| Flocculant | Water clarification, fruit juice processing |
| Lubricant | Rust removal, texture coatings |
| Gelling agent | Explosives, jelled anodes preparations |
| Encapsulation | Flavorings, pharmaceuticals |
| Temperature and pH stabilizer | Food and technical applications |
| Suspending agent | Chemicals, sprays, liquid animal feed |

As with xanthan, gellan is an acidic polysaccharide produced by the bacterium *Sphingomonas paucimobilis*. Gellan was developed by CP Kelco Inc., and it is currently marketed as Kelcogel and Gelrite. Gellan has approval in the United States and the European Union for food use as a gelling, stabilizing, and suspending agent for a wide range of foods on its own or in combination with other water-soluble polymers. Gellan forms thermoreversible gels that give good flavor release and are stable over the wide pH range found in food products. As Gelrite, it offers various advantages over traditional agar for microbiological applications because it resists enzymatic degradation and forms strong gels at low concentrations.

## *DEXTRAN*

Dextran is an $\alpha$-glucan with various linkages, the predominant being the $\alpha$-(1→6), depending on the producer microorganism. It is produced by many Gram-positive and Gram-negative bacteria, with *Leuconostoc mesenteroides* most usually employed in commercial processes. Unlike most EPS, which are synthesized intracellularly, dextrans are produced from sucrose by the extracellular enzyme dextran sucrase, which acts on sucrose polymerizing the glucose units and releasing fructose into the medium. Control over the activity and mode of action of the enzyme can be achieved by manipulating the process conditions, producing a wide variety of dextran types. Dextran was the first commercial polysaccharide and has been manufactured by the Pharmacia company for almost 50 years. Dextrans have many clinical and laboratory applications, and are also used in the food industry.

## SCLEROGLUCAN

Scleroglucan is a neutral polysaccharide produced by several fungal species, including *Sclerotium* and *Schizophyllum* species. Its main chain is composed of $(1\rightarrow3)$-β-D-linked glucose residues, to which $(1\rightarrow6)$-β-D-glucosyl residues may be attached with varying degrees of frequency. Scleroglucan's solubility varies and depends on the structure of the molecule. Solutions of scleroglucan are pseudoplastic, and their viscosity is not greatly affected over a wide temperature and pH range, nor is it affected by the presence of salts. However, scleroglucan is susceptible to degradation by a number of different enzyme preparations. Scleroglucan is used as a stabilizer for drilling muds, latex paints, printing inks, and seed coatings.

## BIOSYNTHETIC MECHANISMS AND PRODUCTION KINETICS

The biosynthetic process leading to most extracellular polysaccharides comprises five distinct steps: synthesis or transport into the cell of the basic sugar components as 1-phosphate esters of sugars, activation of monosaccharides through formation of sugar nucleotides and modification to other derivatives, assembly of the activated sugars or derivatives on a long-chain isoprenoid lipid carrier and simultaneous addition of non-sugar groups, and transport and release from the lipid carrier to the environment.

These pathways are controlled by several mechanisms, such as substrate uptake mechanisms, substrate competition for the synthesis of other polymers by the cell, chain elongation, and release control mechanisms. Biosynthesis of levans and dextrans differs, because it does not involve multienzyme systems, activated sugars, and lipid carriers. The synthesis of levans and dextrans is an entirely extracellular process and it involves the polymerization of an oligosaccharide in the substrate with the controlled action of polymerases, which directly provides carbon and energy.

Understanding and controlling the important environmental variables affecting EPS biosynthesis can be used advantageously in the design of a successful process. The goal is to achieve the maximum substrate conversion efficiency and overall process productivities, as well as to obtain the desirable polymer structure. The specific rate of EPS formation may be either independent of the growth rate (non-growth-associated product formation) or it may increase with increasing growth rate (growth-associated product formation), or it may decrease during the production phase, as in the case of xanthan (partly growth-associated product formation), depending on the producer microorganism and the growth-liming substrate.

Changes in growth conditions affect the process kinetics and efficiency, as well as the fine structure of the produced exopolysaccharide. Process variables, such as the temperature and pH, dissolved oxygen and agitation intensity, and the source and levels of the carbon substrate, play an important role in fermentation productivities. However, the type of the observed responses varies between microorganisms and reflects the variety of specific in situ roles played by different exopolysaccharides. Although the basic structure of most exopolysaccharides does not generally change with growth conditions, the content of groups attached to the basic structure and the molecular weight of the produced molecules can vary widely. Variations in acyl or ketal groups can have a dramatic effect on the rheological behavior of the polymers and their subsequent effectiveness in various applications. For example, the pyruvate content of xanthan can be varied from almost 0 to 8 percent by altering the growth media and the agitation intensity in the bioreactor. The application of xanthan for improved oil recovery by polymer flooding and the injectivity may depend mainly on the degree of pyruvilation due to xanthan precipitation or adsorption on the soil. The molecular weight of these polymers is another important factor critical for intrinsic viscosity and the thickening properties exhibited. During the course of a xanthan batch fermentation, polysaccharides of different molecular weights are formed and the variation can be higher during growth and determined by the oxygen transfer rate during the nongrowth phase. In chemostat experiments, the xanthan molar mass increases with increased specific growth rates. Studies on alginate production by *Azotobacter vinelandii* showed the molecular weight to depend on dissolved oxygen levels, medium composition, and pH.

## FERMENTATION

Figure II.14 shows the process steps for microbial gum production. All commercial-scale polysaccharide formation processes are aerobic. As indicated previously, the choice of growth conditions determines the substrate conversion efficiency, productivity, and product quality. However, industrial fermentation processes must be designed in a way that the overall rate, efficiency, and product concentration are ultimately constrained by the heat and mass transfer capability of the bioreactor, so as to make maximum use of the provided energy. In EPS fermentations, the product concentration, through its effect on broth rheology, has a strong feedback effect on the heat and mass transfer capability of the bioreactor, and thus is of primary concern in scaling up operations. To increase oxygen transfer, hot air is sparged through the medium with high levels of aeration. The main contributor to the rheological behavior of microbial polysaccharide cultures is the product itself dissolved in the continuous liquid phase. The main rheological feature of these cultures is their extreme viscosity, even at low product concentrations, in addition to shear thinning or pseudoplastic behavior. As the product concentration increases in batch culture, both viscosity and pseudoplasticity increase. Other types of rheological behavior can also be observed, e.g., first normal stress differences and yield stresses in xanthan fermentations, and viscoelastic behavior in alginate broths.

Temperature is an important parameter in polysaccharide synthesis. In general, the optimum temperature for growth is the same for product formation. All commercial polysaccharide-producing microorganisms are mesophiles. The optimum pH for the synthesis of polysaccharides of bacteria is 6 to 7.5, whereas the optimum for polysaccharides from fungi is 4 to 5.5. Many microorganisms have strict requirements for certain elements, such as calcium, potassium, magnesium, and phosphorus. Iron, copper, and zinc may also be necessary. Depending on the microbial species, certain minerals can inhibit product synthesis. Production of microbial polysaccharides is generally favored by a high carbon/nitrogen ratio in the medium. The nitrogen source is the growth-limiting substrate, and its concentration is set to produce the required biomass levels. An additional carbon source may be added after growth cessation (fed-batch culture). Continuous cultures are less frequently employed in polysaccharide fermentations.

## PRODUCT RECOVERY

The recovery and further processing of microbial gums follows closely the technology used in the processing of other water-soluble polymers, such as plant and algal gums. The main steps of the recovery process (Figure II.14) are deactivation and/or removal of cells, precipitation of the polymer, dewatering, drying, milling, and blending. The specific purification method used is determined by the end use of the gum and the process economics. For example, the use of xanthan in enhanced oil-recovery requires removal of cells that may clog up the porous oil-bearing rock. However, commercial processes for the production of food-grade xanthan do not involve cell

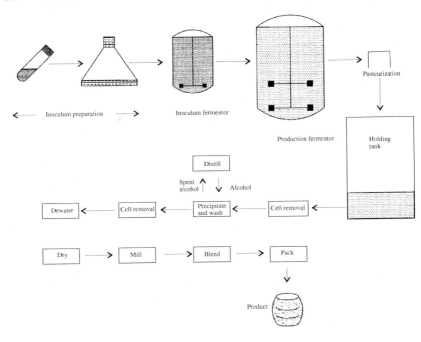

FIGURE II.14. Process outline for production of microbial gums

removal, and the bacteria are rendered nonviable by pasteurization. Cell removal is required when the presence of cells affect the product performance, appearance, or toxicology. The final product is either a powder or a concentrated solution. Numerous methods have been developed to deactivate, lyse, or remove cells from the fermentation broth. Treatment could be chemical, mechanical, or thermal. Care should be taken to avoid product degradation, especially during thermal treatments. The method of choice depends on the biopolymer, e.g., chemical treatment of xanthan at elevated pH can cause depyruvilation of the product. The increased temperature reduces the broth viscosity and eases the removal of insolubles by filtration or centrifugation. When enzymes are used, they must be removed from the medium.

Precipitation of the biopolymers is achieved by decreasing the solubility of the dissolved colloid using methods such as water-miscible nonsolvents, salts addition, or concentration by evaporation. The favored method for the primary isolation and purification of microbial gums is precipitation using water-miscible nonsolvents, such as alcohols. The U.S. Food and Drug Administration regulations on food-grade xanthan gum prescribe the use of isopropanol for its precipitation. The lower alcohols (methanol, ethanol, isopropanol) and acetone, which are nonsolvents for the polysaccharide, can be added to the fermentation broth not only to decrease the solubility until phase separation occurs, but also to wash out impurities, such as colored components, salts, and cell debris. The cost of alcohol for recovery, the cost of distilling spent alcohol, and the solvent-handling losses contribute significantly to the total cost of production. The amount of alcohol necessary for the precipitation of xanthan is dependent on ionic strength and independent of gum concentration. This makes the production cost very sensitive to the product concentration in the fermentation broth. Thus, bioprocessing strategies leading to higher product concentrations would significantly reduce the variable cost of alcohol recovery per weight of product.

Once the polymer is obtained as a wet precipitate, it is dried, milled, and packed. The precipitate is dried in dryers, under vacuum or with forced circulation of air. The final moisture content of most commercial-grade polysaccharides is about 10 percent. The dried product is milled to a predetermined particle size to control dispersibility and hydration rates. Care must be taken throughout the recovery process, because exposure to excess heat and mechanical stress may result in product modification or even degradation. Finally, the dried and milled product is packed into containers with low permeability to water to avoid water retention and hydrolytic degradation.

## SUGGESTED READINGS

Garcia-Ochoa F, VE Santos, JA Casas, and E Gomez (2000). Xanthan gum: Production, recovery, and properties. *Biotechnology Advances* 18:549-579.

Giavasis I, LM Harvey, and B McNeil (2000). Gellan gum. *Critical Reviews in Biotechnology* 20(3):177-211

Papagianni M, SK Psomas, L Batsilas, SV Paras, DA Kyriakidis, and M Liakopoulou-Kyriakides (2001). Xanthan production by *Xanthomonas campestris* in batch cultures. *Process Biochemistry* 37:73-80.

Sutherland IW (1998). Novel and established applications of microbial polysaccharides. *TIBTECH* 16:41-46.

Sutherland IW (2001). Microbial polysaccharides from Gram-negative bacteria. *International Dairy Journal* 11:663-674.

# PART III:
# INDUSTRIAL BIOTECHNOLOGY

# Alcoholic Fermentation

## Bacterial Alcoholic Fermentation

K. Chandraraj

P. Gunasekaran

### *INTRODUCTION*

Ethanol can be produced either by chemical synthesis or by a biological fermentation process. Chemical synthesis is based on the oxidation of ethylene under specialized conditions of temperature and pressure. The biological process of alcohol production is based on the growth of microorganisms on sugars in an anaerobic environment, and this process is called *fermentation*. Wine, beer, and alcohol production are well-known examples of fermentation.

### *ETHANOL BY FERMENTATION*

#### *Microorganisms*

Traditionally, yeast strains belonging to the genera *Saccharomyces* and *Kluyveromyces* are used in the production of ethanol from sucrose by fermentation. Several bacterial strains such as *Zymomonas mobilis, Clostridium* sp., *Thermoanaerobacter ethanolicus,* and *Zymobacter palmae* are known to produce ethanol and were considered for use by the alcohol fermentation industry. Among them, *Z. mobilis,* a Gram-negative anaerobic ethanologenic bacterium, is widely studied for use in the production of ethanol from glucose, fructose, and sucrose. It uses the Entner-Doudoroff pathway instead of Emden-Meyerhoff pathway for growth. *Zymomonas mobilis* has been demonstrated to be the potential candidate for ethanol fermentation rather than the yeast *Saccharomyces cerevisiae* because of its attractive features, such as high rate of substrate consumption, high rate of ethanol production, high volumetric ethanol productivity, high ethanol yield, lower

327

biomass yield, no requirement of controlled supply of oxygen during fermentation, and amenability to genetic manipulation.

## Substrates

Sugars are the only source for the fermentative production of ethanol. Traditionally used yeast and bacterial strains efficiently convert glucose and sucrose to ethanol. The major raw materials for ethanol production are corn, potato, barley, tapioca, and sugarcane. Most of the raw materials are subjected to acid or enzymatic hydrolysis and subsequently used for alcohol fermentation. Molasses, a sugar industry by-product, is widely used as substrate in yeast-ethanol fermentation. However, molasses is not a good medium for bacterial fermentation because of its heavy metal content which inhibits bacterial growth. To date, alcohol is produced on a large scale from corncob in the United States and from sugarcane juice in Brazil. However, these raw materials are not economical; therefore, the search for an alternative raw material is necessary for low-cost/high-volume production of ethanol. Plant biomass is one of the promising substrates that is a renewable resource and is rich in polymers of hexoses and pentoses. Unfortunately, a suitable microbial strain is not currently available to efficiently produce ethanol from plant biomass.

# FACTORS AFFECTING ETHANOL FERMENTATION

## Substrate

In the ethanol fermentation process, the final ethanol concentration depends on the initial sugar concentrations. Economic analysis of the ethanol fermentation process demands a high concentration of ethanol with substrate conversion close to 100 percent so that the cost of the distillation is reduced. However, the high concentration of sugar affects the bacterial growth and increases the lag period. *Zymomonas mobilis* strains grow well in a medium containing 20 to 40 percent (w/v) glucose and 46 percent (w/v) sucrose and produce a high concentration (>8.5 percent w/v) of ethanol. Increase in the initial concentration of sucrose affects the kinetic parameters, including specific growth rate ($\mu$), specific biomass yield ($Y_{x/s}$), specific rate of ethanol production ($q_p$), and specific ethanol yield ($Y_{p/s}$). *Zymomonas mobilis* utilizes 0.5 to 4.5 percent of the carbon source for biomass buildup in fermentation, and the remaining carbon source is used for only ethanol production. *Zymomonas mobilis* produces 20 percent less ethanol in sucrose fermentation compared to glucose, due to the formation of levan and sorbitol as by-products. When fructose is used as a substrate, about 9 percent of the carbon source is used for the by-product formation, but from a glucose medium, less than 4 percent of the carbon source is accounted for in the by-products. Therefore, glucose is considered to be the ideal substrate for fermentation. The by-product formation during fermentation depends on the temperature, pH, aeration, and method of cultivation.

### Temperature

Strains of *Z. mobilis* grow between 25 to 40°C, with optimum growth at 30°C. The ethanol yield, biomass, and specific kinetic parameters of ethanol fermentation are at their maximum at 30°C and were reduced at temperatures above 30°C. The elevated temperatures affect the composition and structure of the cytoplasmic membrane. The concentration of phospholipids is decreased when *Z. mobilis* is grown at 40°C, leading to the loss of integrity of the membrane. Furthermore, the elevated temperature results in the accumulation of ethanol within the cell, which has a significant effect on the viability of the cells. Addition of $Mg^{2+}$ to the medium improves the ethanol yield from 38 percent to 76 percent in fermentation of *Z. mobilis* at 40°C.

### Ethanol

An interest in the production of high concentrations of ethanol prompted several studies on the effect of ethanol on the producing organisms. Addition of ethanol to the growing culture resulted in the inhibition of growth and the reduction of ethanol production. In general, an ethanol concentration greater than 6 percent has an inhibitory effect on the growth of the producer strain. Most strains grow in the presence of 5.5 percent ethanol in the medium. Twelve strains of *Z. mobilis* are able to grow in the presence of 10 percent ethanol added to the growth medium. Similar to the elevated temperature, the ethanol concentration also has a significant effect on the composition of the cell membrane. Increase in permeability of the membrane in the presence of a high concentration of ethanol led to the leakage of co-factors necessary for the activity of several enzymes. Hopanoids have an even greater influence on the membrane properties. During growth of *Z. mobilis* in the presence of a high concentration of ethanol, the 1,2,3,4-tetrahydroxy pentane 29-hopanoid (thph) is the major hopanoid, and it represents a major part of the total lipids. A significant level of *cis*-vaccenic acid is produced in the presence of a high concentration of glucose in the medium.

## pH

All strains of Z. *mobilis* grow at a pH range between 3 and 7. About 20 strains of Z. *mobilis* studied so far could grow at pH 3.5. Traditionally, the pH values 5 to 6.5 are used for the growth of Z. *mobilis,* although the strains could grow at pH values lower than 5.0. Because the strains could grow at a low pH, the contamination risk can be reduced considerably. Optimization of fermentation conditions, including temperature and pH levels, results in ethanol production without any by-products in sucrose fermentation.

## *Oxygen*

Most strains of Z. *mobilis* grow under anaerobic conditions, and oxygen has a negative effect on ethanol production by Z. *mobilis.* Aeration induces the production of by-products including acetate, acetaldehyde, and lactate. Moreover, oxygen has an inhibitory effect on substrate consumption and growth. At low concentration of substrates, the rates of growth and biomass yield are independent of the presence of oxygen. On the contrary, a high concentration of substrates decreased the growth parameters ($\mu$ and $Y_{x/s}$) in the presence of oxygen. Ethanol yield in the aerobic conditions was 25 percent less than the ethanol yield produced under anaerobic conditions. This suggests that Z. *mobilis* does not require controlled addition of oxygen, an advantage in ethanol production.

## KINETICS OF ETHANOL FERMENTATION

Preliminary studies of the production of ethanol by Z. *mobilis* in continuous fermentation using >10 percent (w/v) glucose showed substrate conversion of 80 percent due to the ethanol inhibitory effect on the strain. When the substrate is 10 percent (w/v), the ethanol production ranges from 96 to 98 percent of the theoretical yield. At a dilution rate less than 0.1 h, sucrose is completely utilized without the formation of the by-product levan, and the theoretical ethanol yield is 98 percent. When the dilution rate is more than 0.1 h, sucrose and residual sugars such as glucose and fructose are accumulated in the culture medium, accompanied by the formation of levan. At a dilution rate less than 0.1 h, fructooligomers and sorbitol are formed from sucrose.

## *PROCESS IMPROVEMENT*

For efficient large-scale production of ethanol, the fermentative microorganism should exhibit the desirable characteristics, including capacity to metabolize various substrates, high rate of growth and ethanol production, maximum efficiency of substrate conversion, tolerance to high concentration of substrate and ethanol, and tolerance to high temperatures. It is almost impossible to obtain a strain with all of these characteristics. Therefore, it is necessary to select suitable strains with at least some of the desirable characteristics and then genetically manipulate the strains and/or improve the process conditions so that maximum productivity of ethanol can be obtained. The processes involving immobilized cell reactors, cell recycling reactors, and vacuum fermentation reactors are some of the operational modes that improve ethanol productivity. Genetic engineering approaches should be employed to increase the rate of substrate utilization and the ethanol production and thermotolerance of the producing organisms.

Among *Z. mobilis* strains, two strains, namely ZM1 and ZM4, are used by several groups of researchers for process optimization and genetic engineering studies. A final ethanol concentration of 10 to 12.5 percent (w/v) with >80 percent substrate conversion is obtained in batch fermentation using 20 percent (w/v) substrates. Although in many cases the ethanol yield is considerably high, the productivity is poor. To improve ethanol productivity, several investigators have attempted various types of processes that are different from batch fermentation. Batch fermentation with a high concentration of substrate causes the bacterial cells to take nearly 30 percent of the fermentation time for adaptation, resulting in lowered ethanol productivity. This can be avoided by adding the substrate gradually, which results in increased productivity. Ethanol productivity of >5 g/l per h with ethanol yield and substrate conversion close to the theoretical value can be achieved by the progressive addition of substrates in batch fermentation. Another method of reducing the time for culture adaptation is by using the culture repeatedly in batch fermentation. In this type of process it is necessary to recover the culture at the end of fermentation, and the biomass can then be used for the subsequent fermentation. For such a process, immobilized cells or flocculent cells are recommended. Flocculent strain ZM401 produced 7.3 percent ethanol from 15 percent (w/v) glucose in four successive fermentations with an ethanol productivity of 50 g/l per h. Similarly, with the use of immobilized cells in repeated batch fermentation, it is possible to obtain ethanol productivity of 15 g/l per h for six successive fermentations with 10 percent (w/v) fructose as a substrate. It is also necessary to recall that an ethanol concentration of >6 percent (w/v) has an inhibitory effect on the metabolic activity of the producer strains.

Studies on the ethanol production in a continuous-culture technique have shown that an ethanol concentration greater than 98 percent of the theoretical value could be obtained from the substrate concentration at <10 percent (w/v) and the dilution rate at <0.13/h. When the dilution rate is >0.15/h, the concentration of ethanol decreased and the rate of substrate consumption became less than the dilution rate. Under those conditions, the ethanol productivity could be less than or equal to the productivity of the batch fermentation. The ethanol productivity in the continuous-culture system can be significantly increased by cell recycling and using flocculent strains and immobilized cells. In the case of flocculent cells, the biomass may be accumulated inside the reactor or may be accumulated with the use of an external recycler. The biomass of the free cells may be concentrated with the use of centrifugation or a membrane filtration system.

A two-step process has been developed to produce ethanol at a concentration higher than the inhibitory concentration (6 percent [w/v]). In the first step, biomass and ethanol at <5 percent (w/v) are produced; in the second step, fermentation is carried out to produce ethanol at a concentration >10 percent (w/v). In another method involving three steps, cells at a high concentration are employed in the immobilized form, which resulted in ethanol productivity of 108 g/l per h with 98 percent substrate conversion.

## ETHANOL FROM RENEWABLE RESOURCES

Ethanol production by *Z. mobilis* from defined media with glucose, fructose, or sucrose has been well studied. However, the use of renewable resources, including agricultural residues for ethanol production by *Z. mobilis* has been studied to a limited extent. Molasses, the conventional substrate for ethanol production by yeast, is not a good substrate for *Z. mobilis,* because the substrate contains a high concentration of salts. Deionized molasses and sugarcane juice have been successfully used for fermentation by *Z. mobilis* with relative substrate consumption of 60 to 99 percent. In contrast to molasses, cellulose, inulin, and starch could not be used as substrates for the growth of *Z. mobilis* because the strain does not produce any polysaccharide hydrolytic enzymes. Therefore, cocultivation of cellulolytic or amylolytic organisms with *Z. mobilis* is considered to be a potential approach for ethanol production from polysaccharides, but the limitations in these processes are the lower ethanol tolerance level of the hydrolase-producing organism and sensitivity of the hydrolases to the high concentration of reducing sugars formed during the fermentation. The microbial conversion of plant sugars would lead to continuous and large-scale production of ethanol at a low cost. Hence, development of economically feasible new fermentation processes is necessary. The previously mentioned microorganisms are not efficient in producing ethanol from sugars other than sucrose. Therefore, development of new microorganisms capable of efficiently converting the spectrum of plant sugars that are abundant and renewable is necessary. Toward this direction, the bacterium *Escherichia coli* has been genetically engineered to produce ethanol from glucose and xylose by introducing the genes *pdc* and *adh* from *Z. mobilis* encoding pyruvate decarboxylase and alcohol dehydrogenase, respectively, which are key enzymes for ethanol production. On the other hand, *Z. mobilis* has been modified to metabolize xylose by introducing the genetic machinery for xylose metabolism. Nevertheless, these recombinant *E. coli* and *Z. mobilis* strains are not suitable for industrial production of ethanol directly from plant biomass.

## ETHANOL AS AN AUTOMOBILE FUEL

Hazardous pollutants are emitted from transportation-fuel combustion. Environmentally-friendly, nonpolluting automobile fuels to replace conventional fossil fuels need to be developed. Some options include methanol, ethanol, propane, natural gas, and hydrogen as gasoline additives or fuel. Among them, ethanol is projected to be the future transportation fuel due to various technical advantages: Ethanol serves as an oxygenate (gasohol [E10] prevents carbon monoxide and ozone emission), an octane booster (to prevent early ignition, or "engine knock"), and an extender of gasoline; pure ethanol can be used as an alternative to gasoline.

## CONCLUSIONS

Today, *S. cerevisiae* is widely used in the industry for ethanol production. However, *Z. mobilis* has been demonstrated to be the most promising potential bacterial strain for ethanol production on a pilot scale. The substrate range is limited to sucrose for both *S. cerevisiae* and *Z. mobilis*. Though attempts are being made to isolate a novel ethanologen possessing better substrate conversion capability than these two strains, the modern recombinant technology is quite promising to improve the existing strains. *Zymomonas mobilis* is advantageous over *S. cerevisiae* for strain improvement because of its amenability to genetic manipulation. In recent years, an *E. coli* laboratory strain has been transformed into ethanologen by recombinant technology using genes from *Z. mobilis*. Therefore, the future of ethanol fermentation technology will rely heavily on genetically modified bacterial strains.

## SUGGESTED READINGS

Bothast RJ, NN Nichols, and BS Dien (1999). Fermentations with new recombinant organisms. *Biotechnology Progress* 15:867-875.

Dien BS, NN Nichols, PJ O'Bryan, and RJ Bothast (2000). Development of new ethanologenic *Escherichia coli* strains for fermentation of lignocellulosic biomass. *Applied Biochemistry and Biotechnology* 84-86:181-196.

Gunasekaran P and K Chandra Raj (1999). Ethanol Fermentation Technology—*Zymomonas mobilis*. *Current Science* 77:56-68.

Ingram LO, PF Gomez, X Lai, M Moniruzzaman, BE Wood, LP Yomano, and SW York (1998). Metabolic engineering of bacteria for ethanol production. *Biotechnology and Bioengineering* 58:204-214.

# Fruit-Based Alcoholic Beverages

Vinod K. Joshi
Somesh Sharma
Shashi Bhushan
Devender Attri

Fruits—possessing refreshing characteristics and appealing sensory and nutritional qualities—have been employed to produce a variety of alcoholic beverages, such as fruit wines and brandies. The word *wine* is historically associated with fermented products of grapes. Wines from fruits other than grapes are called "fruit wines." Wines have been consumed since human settlement in the Tigris-Euphrates River basin, when they were used as therapeutic agents. The Rig Vedas, the sacred scriptures of Hinduism composed between 1500 and 900 B.C., also mentioned the medicinal value of wine. The actual birthplace of wine is unknown, although it is known that wines were prepared by the Assyrians by 3500 B.C. Cider (or sicera) fermentation has been practiced for over 2,000 years and was a common drink at the time of Roman invasion of the British Isles in 55 B.C. Essentially, wine is a transformation of juice by yeast during fermentation, involving a series of biochemical reactions. Wine making has developed from a haphazard, ill understood, and risky process into the well-defined scientific discipline "enology."

Wines are preferable to distilled liquors for their stimulatory and healthful properties. Moderate consumption of low levels of alcohol has been associated with lowered mortality from not only all coronary heart diseases (CHD) but also other diseases. These beverages are regarded as an important adjunct to the human diet. Alcoholic beverage production from fruits other than grapes is discussed in the following sections.

## QUALITY FACTORS AND COMPOSITION OF WINES

The quality of wine is determined primarily by the composition and quality of the raw material used and the vinification practices followed. These factors include the specific fruit variety; stage of harvest and maturity of the fruit; total sugar, acid, phenols, pigments, nitrogenous compounds, etc., in the fruit or the must; additives such as nitrogenous compounds, pectin esterase, sulfur dioxide, or other preservatives; fruits yielding pulp or juice; yeast strains and other vinification practices; postfermentation operations (especially the length of maturation); and the method of preservation employed. The fruits or their concentrates (apple wine, cider, and vermouth) constitute the most important raw materials. Spices and herbs or their extracts are employed to prepare fortified wines such as vermouth. Sugar is the second-most important raw material dictating the cost of production of these beverages. Almost all the non-grape fruits, their juices, and extracts (Table III.1) are low in sugar but have high acidity and must be ameliorated to produce a table wine. Even when the sugar level is satisfactory, the high

TABLE III.1. Sugar and acid contents of some of the fruits that could be used in wine making

| Fruit | Total sugar (% of fresh weight) | Major sugars (% of total) | | | Acid (% major acids) | | |
|---|---|---|---|---|---|---|---|
| | | Fructose | Glucose | Sucrose | Citric | Malic | Tartaric |
| Apple | | | | | | | |
| Cooking | 8-10 | 55 | 20 | 25 | 0.9-1.4 | – | 90 |
| Eating | 10-13 | 55 | 20 | 25 | 0.4-0.9 | – | 90 |
| Apricot | 6-7 | 10 | 20 | 70 | 1.1-1.3 | 25 | 5 |
| Banana | 18 | 20 | 40 | 40 | 0.3-0.4 | 20 | 70 |
| Blackberry | 5-6 | 50 | 45 | 5 | 0.9-1.3 | 50 | 50 |
| Black-currant | 5-8 | 55 | 35 | 10 | 3.0-4.0 | 90 | 10 |
| Cherry | 9-13 | 55 | 40 | 5 | 0.4-0.6 | 10 | 90 |
| Elderberry | 10-13 | 45 | 45 | 10 | 0.8-1.3 | 85 | 15 |
| Goose-berry | | | | | | | |
| Cooking | 4-6 | 45 | 45 | 10 | 1.4-2.00 | 50 | 50 |
| Dessert | 8-9 | 45 | 45 | 10 | – | – | – |
| Grape | 15-22 | 50 | 50 | – | 0.4-1.3 | – | 20 |
| Orange | 9-10 | 25 | 20 | 55 | 0.8-1.1 | 90 | 10 |
| Peach | 8-9 | 10 | 10 | 80 | 0.5-0.8 | 25 | 75 |
| Pear | 9-11 | 65 | 25 | 10 | 0.2-0.4 | – | 90 |
| Pineapple | 12 | 10 | 20 | 70 | 0.8-1.3 | 80 | 20 |
| Plum | | | | | | | |
| Cooking | 6-8 | 20 | 55 | 25 | 1.4-1.7 | – | 95 |
| Dessert | 9-11 | 15 | 40 | 45 | – | – | – |
| Raspberry | 6-7 | 40 | 40 | 20 | 1.4-1.7 | 75 | 25 |
| Redcurrant | 5 | 45 | 55 | – | 2.0-2.5 | 85 | 15 |
| Strawberry | 5-6 | 40 | 40 | 20 | 0.6-1.5 | 90 | 10 |

acidity demands dilution, consequently requiring addition of sugar to the must. For brandy, a cheaper source of sugar might be the cost-determining factor.

Yeast growth in wine fermentation is influenced by a number of factors including composition of juice, clarification of juice, addition of sulfur dioxide and/or other preservatives, temperature of fermentation, inoculation of juice or pulp, and interaction with other microorganisms. Although *Saccharomyces cerevisiae* can grow over a wide temperature range (0 to 45°C), the favorable temperature is between 22 and 27°C. The fermentation temperature greatly influences the production of aroma-active compounds, because at higher temperatures more loss of volatile compounds results, while at lower temperatures more entrainment of alcohol by $CO_2$ takes place.

Different microorganisms belonging to molds, yeast, and bacteria are involved in wine making. In addition to damaging the fruits, molds can affect the flavor of wine by their growth on the cooperage. However, molds, being aerobic, cannot grow in wine due to the inhibitory effect of ethanol and the prevailing anaerobic conditions. Yeasts are important microorganisms associated not only with the production but also the spoilage of wine. Although the yeast strains of *S. cerevisiae* predominantly carry out the alcoholic fermentation of fruit juices, others, known as wild yeasts, may spoil the wine. Some of these wild yeasts secrete toxins affecting the fermentation, causing them to be called "killer yeasts."

Slow or incomplete alcoholic fermentation is a chronic problem for the wine industry, and the premature termination of alcoholic fermentation is known as stuck fermentation. Several factors have been held responsible for impacting fermentation rate and leading to stuck and sluggish fermentation, including nutrient limitation, ethanol toxicity, organic and fatty acid toxicity, presence of killer factors or other microbially produced toxins, cation imbalance, temperature extremes, pesticide/fungicide residue, microbial competition, poor enological practices, excessive $SO_2$ use, excessive must clarification, and lack of agitation. The wine making process could be seen as the product of enzymatic transformation of fruit juices. Enzymes could be contributed by the juice or yeast or could be added exogenously. A number of enzymes, such as pectinases, oxidoreductase, proteases, glycosidase, and lipoxygenase, play a significant role in grape wine making.

Many advancements have been made in the production of wines from grapes, including conventional bioreactor systems, thermovinification, continuous wine making, improved design of fermentation vessels, etc. The conventional vessles for wine making in a batch system were traditionally barrels or vats made of wood or cement. These vessels have been now replaced with well-designed stainless steel fermentors of various shapes, such as barrel, vat, cylindroconical, cylindrical, spheroconical, and tower. In designing a suitable bioreactor to conduct wine fermentation, it is essential to understand the physiology of yeast, because the entire process of wine making depends upon its activity, either as natural or controlled inoculum.

A typical wine contains ethyl alcohol, sugars, acids, higher alcohols, tannins, aldehydes, esters, amino acids, minerals, vitamins, anthocyanins, and fatty acids in addition to minor constituents such as methanol and flavoring compounds. Quantitatively, ethyl alcohol is the most important component present in all alcoholic beverages and is associated with the stimulating and intoxicating properties of these beverages. Alcoholic beverages are distinguished based on their quantity of ethyl alcohol. Sugars of different types in wines include hexoses, sucrose, trioses, and pentoses. Dry wines have very low or almost negligible sugar, while sweet/dessert wines may contain considerably higher quantities. Acids are significant in maintaining pH, balancing the sugar level, and helping flavor development. Grapes and apples contain tartaric and malic acid, respectively, as major acids, but in wine acetic acid is responsible for acidity. Fruit wines have pigments derived from the fruits themselves. Methyl alcohol is also found in alcoholic beverages, and its quantity is influenced by the type of fermenting agent, the temperature, and the raw materials used. Naturally fermented alcoholic beverages contain abnormally high levels of methanol, which arises from hydrolysis of pectins. Fruit brandies have higher levels of methanol than do the grape brandies, and methanol quantity needs to be reduced to keep its content within the safety limits.

Among the minerals, K, Ca, Na, and Mg are the major elements present in wines that play an important role in alcoholic fermentation, being used by yeast for its metabolism. Trace elements (Fe, Cu, Mn, Zn) are significant for the normal alcoholic fermentation and growth of yeast, by taking part in the oxidation reduction system. The zinc content of wines (which normally occurs as the result of contact with galvanized iron utensils) should not exceed 5 mg/L (legal limit and threshold for astringent taste). Normal levels of Cu, Mn, and Zn in wines are not toxic.

Biochemically, higher alcohols constitute an important component of wine. The color and taste of wines depend upon the total amount and properties of the phenolics of wine. Using the biochemical characteristics, quality-defining values, called the "RSK value," have been developed for wine. Esters are another indispensable component influencing wine quality, imparting the fruity flavor to wines. Normally, the amount of esters increases with enhancement in maturation periods.

## TECHNOLOGY OF FRUIT WINE PREPARATION

### Apple

Cider is a low-alcohol drink produced by fermentation of apple juice and is known by different names around the world, such as cidre (France), sidro (Italy), sidra (Spain), and Apfelwein (Germany and Switzerland). It can be sweet or dry, soft (1 to 5 percent alcohol) or hard (6 to 7 percent alcohol), and sparkling (with low sugar and $CO_2$) or still (without $CO_2$). The optimum temperature for cider fermentation ranges from 64 to 69°F (15 to 18°C). Various factors influence fermentation, such as the apple juice (variety, maturity, fresh or juice concentrate), other ingredients (sugar, amelioration with acid, yeast nutrients), $SO_2$ concentration, yeast strains (natural or inoculated strains), fermentation temperature, fermentor design and operation, maturation, and processing factors. $SO_2$ controls the microorganisms in the must and prevents the enzymatic browning of the juice.

Stainless steel tanks are used today for fermentation of cider, although traditionally barrels of oak were used for this purpose. A temperature of 4°C for bulk storage of cider is desirable. After fermentation, the cider is racked and filtered. After aging and clarification, the cider is pasteurized at 60°C for 20 to 30 minutes or preserved with $SO_2$.

Wine is another product made from apple juice by alcoholic fermentation (alcohol content 11 to 14 percent). Amelioration with sugar or juice concentrate is essential. Similar to cider, natural fermentation is also practiced, but pure culture of the yeast *S. cerevisiae* is necessary to make wine of predictable quality. Addition of ammonium salts to the fermenting solution reduces the higher alcohol production in wine due to nondegradation of amino acids of the must. Bitterness is related to fermentation conditions in apple wine, particularly yeast nutrients. To prepare table apple wine (11 percent alcohol), apples are washed, grated, and pressed to extract juice, which is ameliorated to 24°Brix and fermented with *S. cerevisiae* (at 5 percent). To hasten clarification, 0.25 percent pectinase enzyme is added.

Sparkling wine is produced by secondary fermentation of apple wines (5 to 6 percent ethanol content) under normal pressure, resulting in alcohol levels of 9 to 10 percent by volume. Sparkling apple wines are also prepared by carbonation in either a tank or bottle by secondary fermentation of base wine. A clear juice is obtained by pectinase enzyme treatment prior to rough filtration and amelioration to 16 percent solids. It is fermented at 25°C for four days and chilled to −1.7°C to stop fermentation. Hydrolyzed autolysate favorably affects the secondary fermentation of apple wine and is considered suitable to be a nitrogen source for secondary fermentation of apple wine at 40 mg/l concentration.

An aperitif wine known as vermouth can also be prepared, and the process includes preparation of the base wine, herb and spice extract making, fortification and sweetening, blending with the extract, and finally maturation. The best product contains 15 percent alcohol, 2.5 percent spice extract, and 4 percent sugar.

## *Pear*

To prepare perry (fermented pear juice), the fruits are grated and pressed in a rack and cloth press. The juice, with original total soluble solids (TSS) of 14°Brix and 0.25 percent acid, is ameliorated to 21°Brix and 0.5 percent citric acid along with 100 ppm $SO_2$. The fermentation is carried out with a pure wine yeast culture. The wine is allowed to settle after the completion of fermentation, racked, and finally clarified using bentonite and preserved by pasteurization. It can be sweetened, fortified, or blended with other fruit wine, if needed. Perry having 5 percent alcohol, 10°Brix, and 0.5 percent acid was most acceptable. The procedure includes raising the TSS to 20°Brix, addition of diammonium hydrogen phosphate (DAHP) (0.1 percent), and carrying out the alcoholic fermentation at 22±1°C by addition of yeast culture (5 percent). Addition of different sugar sources influences the fermentation behavior and sensory quality of perry.

## *Coconut*

The alcoholic beverage obtained by the natural fermentation of coconut palm inflorescence sap is known as toddy. The sap is traditionally collected in clay pots, sterilized by inverting over a flame for five minutes, and allowed to ferment in open pots for up to two days. During this period, microorganisms from the atmosphere enter the clay pots and multiply in the palm sap, which contains 15 to 18 percent sucrose and yields about 7 percent ethanol.

## *Plum*

Plum wines are quite popular in many countries, particularly Germany and the Pacific coastal states. The fruit gives wine of appealing color and acceptable quality. For wine preparation, to every pound of plum one liter of water is added, followed by addition of starter culture. The mixture is allowed to ferment for eight to ten days before pressing. Addition of pectolytic enzyme before fermentation facilitates this pressing by increasing the yield of juice and hastening wine clarification. Additional sugar is added to the partially fermented juice, depending on the type of wine required (table or dessert). Aging, filtration, bottling, and processing are similar to those processes for any other wine. Another method specifies that the plum fruits should be fully ripe, diluted with water in a 1:1 ratio (whole-fruit basis), added with 0.3 percent pectinol, 150 ppm $SO_2$, and sugar to raise the TSS of the must to 24°Brix. It is fermented into wine. The quality of plum wine can be improved by raising the sugar content of the wine to 12°Brix. The use of sodium benzoate instead of potassium metabisulfite (KMS) gives a wine with better color and sensory qualities. Plum fruit, being acidic and pulpy in nature, needs dilution of the pulp with water, but a yeast such as *Schizosaccharomyces pombe* can be employed as a biological deacidifying agent in addition to the use of *Saccharomyces cerevisiae* var. *ellipsoideus* to produce alcohol. The deacidification of the plum must by this yeast is independent of sugar content of the must but is adversely affected by higher concentrations of ethanol, 2.5 pH, and $SO_2$ content of more than 150 ppm, while addition of ammonium sulfate enhanced the malic acid degradation.

Sparkling plum wine, like champagne from grapes, is well known and is produced by secondary fermentation in closed containers, such as bottles or tanks, to retain the carbon dioxide produced. Plum base wine treated with sodium benzoate was considered better for sparkling wine preparation than wine treated with KMS. In preparation of sparkling plum wine, 1.5 percent sugar, 0.2 percent diammonium hydrogen phosphate, *S. cerevisiae* (UCD 595 [Pasteur Champagne yeast]) gives a better product.

Vermouth of commercial acceptability can be made from plum similar to grape vermouth. The spice extract contributes to the increase in total phenols, esters, and aldehyde content. The best product contains about 15 percent alcohol and is sweet in nature.

### Kinnow

An effective method of wine making from kinnow, a type of mandarin orange, includes the use of cyclodextrin or Amberlite XAD-16 which reduces considerably the extent of bitterness in the wine by degrading limonin and naringin.

### Peach

Peach fruit has less acid than plums or apricots, but being pulpy, it needs dilution with water. The method for making peach wine consists of dilution of the pulp in the ratio of 1:1, raising the initial TSS to 24°Brix, and adding pectinol and DAHP at the rate of 0.5 and 0.1 percent, respectively. To this,

100 ppm of $SO_2$ is added to control undesirable microflora. Treatment of wines with wood chips of *Quercus* gives wine the best sensory quality.

### Strawberry

Strawberry wine (Table III.2) of good quality has the appealing color of premium rose wine. In one method, the juice is ameliorated to 22°Brix by the addition of cane sugar added in stages, e.g., 25 percent of the total sugar is added to prepare the must and the rest is added during fermentation. However, addition of sugar after fermentation dilutes the alcohol level. The must is mixed with 1 percent ammonium phosphate, and the fermentation is initiated by addition of 5 percent yeast culture at a temperature of 16°C. The juice is transferred to the jar, and the fermentation is continued until 0.1 to 0.2 percent reducing sugars are obtained. After the completion of fermentation, it is racked, bottled, and stored in the dark. Treatment with enzymes (mainly pectinases) inhibits polymerization and increases color extraction and color density in strawberry wine. Juice yield, which is affected by addition of pectic enzyme, is an important cost consideration for wine production, as the price of berry juice is quite high.

### Apricot

Wine is made from both the cultivated and wild apricot. The method for wild apricot consists of diluting the pulp in the ratio of 1:2, addition of DAHP (0.1 percent) and 0.5 percent pectinol, and fermentation with *Saccharomyces cerevisiae*. In cultivated apricot wine preparation, the extrac-

TABLE III.2. Composition of strawberry wine

| Components | Percentage (%) |
|---|---|
| Total soluble solids (°B) | 8.1-9.7 |
| Total sugars (%) | 0.6-1.7 |
| Reducing sugars (%) | 0.124-0.135 |
| Titratable acidity (% citric acid) | 0.63-0.73 |
| pH | 3.18-3.26 |
| Ethanol (%) | 9.2-11.5 |
| Higher alcohols (mg/l) | 151-169 |
| Volatile acidity (% A.A) | 0.025-0.032 |
| Esters (mg/l) | 78.3-102.4 |
| Phenols (mg/l) | 126.8-144.7 |
| Anthocyanins (OD/ml of wine) | 0.104-0.152 |

tion of pulp either by the hot method or by addition of enzymes and water to the fruit could be adopted. The hot method of pulping refers to heating the apricot fruits with 10 percent water by cooking in a pressure cooker until pressure develops, followed by pulping in a suitable pulper. Dilution of pulp in the ratio of 1:1 with addition of DAHP (0.1 percent) and 0.5 percent (liquid pectinase), raising the initial TSS to 30ºBrix, makes wine of superior quality.

### Pineapple

Pineapple juice has only 12 to 15ºBrix, so its sugar content is raised by the addition of sugar up to 22 to 23ºBrix to produce a wine having 12 to 13 percent alcohol. The wine is preserved by pasteurization but can be fortified and sweetened. Because the flavor of pineapple is not stable, oxidation can occur easily.

## SPOILAGE OF WINE

Wine can have defects from both microbial and nonmicrobial causes. The latter defects include those due to metals or their salts, enzymes, and materials employed in wine clarification. Wine spoilage by microorganisms could occur in three stages of the wine making process. The first is the raw material, such as the grapes, plums, peaches, or other fruits, which can be contaminated with molds, yeasts, acetic acid, or lactic acid bacteria. The second stage is fermentation, in which the wild yeast or microorganisms from the winery equipment may spoil the wine, even in inoculated fermentation with wine yeast. Similarly, if the wine is not stored properly, it may develop microbiological defects, which constitutes the third stage of microbiological spoilage. Microbiological spoilage manifests itself in altered sensory qualities, such as taste and aroma. The susceptibility of wine to microbial spoilage depends on acidity, sugar content, alcohol content, accessory growth substances, tannin concentration, sulfur dioxide amount, storage temperature, and air availability. If these factors are taken care of, the wines do not spoil but instead will improve in the quality during storage.

## FRUIT BRANDY: THE TECHNOLOGY OF PRODUCTION

The term *brandy* is applied to the distillate obtained from wine or any other fermented fruit juice or residue thereof. According to the U.S. Standard of Identity, a brandy should be produced at not less than 190 proof and bottled at not less than 80 proof. A fruit brandy is a product prepared from fermented juice, i.e., plum brandy from plum wine. The distillation is carried out in a copper still in two steps. The first distillation results in a wine of 28 percent alcohol by volume, while the second results in alcohol levels of 70 percent by volume. The brandy is stored in new oak barrels.

## Apple

Apple brandy, or "applejack," was a commercial product of colonial and nineteenth-century America, but at present its production is quite small. In France, apple brandy known as calvados, with 45 percent alcohol, is produced in Normandy. Apple brandy is produced by a double-pot still distillation of the hard cider. For making quality apple brandy, fresh, mold-free, ripe apples are used for fermentation, and distillation after clarification has been recommended. Continuous columns are mostly used to produce apple brandy commercially. Distillation of apple wine under reduced pressure (600 mm Hg) decreases the methanol content in the brandy. Apple brandies produced in the United States are aged with oak chips for a very short time.

## Plum

Plum brandy is highly prized for its distinctive flavor, and its generic name is slivovitz. The method of making plum brandy is similar to that of grape. The aroma components of an experimental brandy include aliphatic fatty acids, free acids, free fatty acids, aromatic acid, esters, alcohols, ethyl acetate lactone, and unsaturated aliphatic aldehydes.

## Peach

Peach brandy is prepared in a manner similar to any fruit brandy. The dried peach, however, does not make a good brandy. The type of sugar used in peach must influences the quality of peach brandy, as does the type of wood chips employed during maturation.

## Wild Apricot

To make wild apricot brandy, the wine is distilled. The product is treated with slightly roasted oak wood chips during maturation to impart color and flavor.

## CONCLUSIONS

Research and development for different types of wines, such as vermouth, sparkling wine, sherry, and brandy, from non-grape fruits is scanty. Despite the efforts made and described here, a large number of research gaps remain for more elaboration in the future. It could be a fruitful area of future research.

## SUGGESTED READINGS

Amerine MA, HW Berg, RE Kunkee, CS Qugh, VL Singleton, and AD Webb (1980). *The technology of wine making,* Fourth edition. Westport, CT: AVI.

Joshi K (1998). *Fruit wines.* Nauni, Solan, India: Dr YSP University of Horticulture and Forestry.

Joshi VK, SK Chauhan, and S Bhushan (2000). Technology of fruit-based alcoholic beverages. In *Post-harvest technology of fruits and vegetables,* Volume II, LR Verma and VK Joshi (eds.). New Delhi: Indus Publication Co, pp.1020-1101.

Joshi VK, DK Sandhu, and NS Thakur (1999). Fruit based alcoholic beverages. In *Biotechnology food fermentation,* Volume II, VK Joshi and A Pandey (eds.). New Delhi: Educational Publishers, pp. 648-744.

# Fuel Ethanol Production
# from Renewable Biomass Resources

James Chukwuma Ogbonna

## FEEDSTOCKS—INTRODUCTION

The energy crisis in the 1970s highlighted the risks of depending solely on nonrenewable fossil fuels. Consequently, many projects investigating the production of alternative energy sources, including production of ethanol from renewable biomass resources, were started in various parts of the world. Even with stabilization in crude oil supply and prices, the interest on ethanol fuel production has been sustained to an extent by environmental issues. Because carbon dioxide produced from ethanol combustion is recycled by plants, use of ethanol as a fuel source does not contribute to global warming. Furthermore, during combustion of ethanol, there is no soot emission, the $SO_X$, $NO_X$, and CO emissions are very small, and the octane value is very high. Ethanol is now mixed with gasoline in various ratios to produce *gasohols* or *ethanol blends,* which are currently used in many countries, especially Brazil and the United States.

Ethanol can be produced from many biomass materials, but the potential for use of these materials as feedstock for industrial/large-scale ethanol fuel production depends on their cost, their abundance/availability, their carbohydrate contents (ethanol yield), and the ease by which they can be converted to ethanol.

## RENEWABLE BIOMASS MATERIALS USED
## FOR ETHANOL PRODUCTION

The choice of feedstock has a decisive effect on the cost of ethanol production, since the cost of raw materials currently represents up to half of the total ethanol production costs. For simplicity, one can classify the various biomass materials used for ethanol production into (1) sugar materials, (2) starch materials, and (3) lignocellulosic materials.

## Sugar Materials

Various sugar crops such as sugarcane, sugar beet, fodder beet, Jerusalem artichoke, and sweet sorghum have been extensively investigated as feedstock for fermentation alcohol production. They can be converted to ethanol in a single process, and productivities as high as 60 g/l per h have been reported with yields of up to 99 percent. Theoretically, 51.4 g of ethanol and 48.8 g of $CO_2$ are produced from 100 g of glucose ($C_6H_{12}O_6 = 2C_2H_5OH + 2CO_2$). However, in practice, part of the glucose is used for the growth of the microorganisms, hence the yield is usually lower. The energy content of the produced ethanol is 95 percent of that in the sugar used. Although in some countries, such as Brazil, most of the ethanol is still produced from sugarcane, the future prospect of sugar crops as feedstocks for large-scale ethanol fuel production is considered low because of their high costs. The noncrystallizable residue (molasses) remaining after sucrose purification from sugar crops is more widely used for industrial ethanol production. However, although molasses is comparably cheap, the supply is tied to sugar processing industries; due to demand for molasses from other sectors, the price has been going up gradually in many countries. Depending on the concentration, fermentation may be slow due to high osmolality. Addition of invertase is reported to be effective in lowering the osmolality and restoring the rate of ethanol production from molasses.

Although sucrose is the main sugar component of most sugar materials, there are still trace amounts of other sugars such as glucose, fructose, and raffinose. Some of the currently used strains can ferment both sucrose and glucose to ethanol. For example, it has been reported that *Zymomonas mobilis* can covert fructose, sucrose, and glucose to ethanol. However, for maximum ethanol yield from sucrose, invertase is added to reduce levan and sorbitol accumulation. The concentrations of other sugars in sugar crops are usually negligibly small. Consequently, very high ethanol yields can be obtained with a single strain of the currently used microorganisms.

## Starch Materials

Ethanol is now produced on an industrial scale from various starch crops as well, such as grains (corn, wheat, barley, etc.), potatoes, sweet potatoes, cassava, and sago. The importance of each of them as feedstock for ethanol production varies from region to region. In the United States, for example, most ethanol is produced from corn, while in France and China, ethanol is produced mainly from wheat and sweet potatoes, respectively. As cheaper alternative sources, damaged agricultural products such as deformed, discolored, or partially softened tubers, and discolored, broken, cracked, insect-damaged, or chalky grains can also be used, but the fermentation efficiency and ethanol yield from such materials would depend on the extent of the damage.

Unlike sugar materials, starch materials must first be hydrolyzed to sugar before they are converted to ethanol. A few strains of microorganisms capable of direct conversion of starch to ethanol have been isolated. For example, some strains of *Schizosaccharomyces pombe, Saccharomyces uvarum, S. carlsbergensis, S. bayanus,* and *S. diastaticus* can produce ethanol from starch. However, with these strains, the ethanol productivity and yields are usually low. Thus, most processes for ethanol production from starch materials consist of two steps: hydrolysis of starch to fermentable sugars and conversion of the sugars to ethanol. The hydrolysis step involves liquefaction and saccharification processes, each requiring a specific enzyme. This can be done using living cells or some enzyme preparations. The microbial strains most widely used for starch hydrolysis include *Aspergillus niger, Aspergillus oryzae, Aspergillus awamori,* and some species of *Rhizopus.* To facilitate enzymatic hydrolysis, the starch is often pretreated by heating it at a high temperature (~140°C), in some cases under acidic conditions. This high-temperature treatment also helps to reduce contamination risks but consumes a lot of energy. Heating at temperatures below gelatinization temperature (~60 percent) and under low pH (~pH 2) has also been investigated. Acid hydrolysis can also be used, but this can lead to formation of inhibitory products such as levulinic acid and formic acid. Some microorganisms that can hydrolyze raw starch have been isolated, and efforts are currently being made to develop processes for efficient ethanol production from raw starch without heat treatment.

Hexoses, especially glucose, are the main sugar products of starch hydrolysis. Depending on other components of the starch material as well as on the method used for the hydrolysis, some non-hexose sugars are also produced. The relative proportion of such sugars are usually small so that most ethanol production strains, such as *Saccharomyces cerevisiae, Zymomonas mobilis,* and *Candida brassicae,* are able to convert the starch hydrolysate into ethanol with high yields.

### Lignocellulosic Materials

Many cheap and abundant lignocellulosic materials can be converted to ethanol, thus the prospect of lignocellulosic materials as feedstock for fermentation ethanol production is very high. Examples of abundant lignocellulosic materials include hardwood, softwood, forest residues, municipal solid wastes, and agricultural residues such as rice straws, wheat straws, corn straws, and corn stovers. However, with the present technology, it is still very difficult to hydrolyze them to fermentable sugars because they are composed of mainly cellulose, hemicellulose, and lignin. Processes for ethanol production from lignocellulosic materials involve three steps: pretreatment (including delignification), hydrolysis, and fermentation.

*Pretreatment*

Various physical methods such as milling (hammer milling, ball milling, fluid energy milling, colloid milling), heat treatment, and irradiation, as well as chemical methods such as ozonation, alkali (usually NaOH), or acid (phosphoric acid, sulfuric acid, $SO_2$, etc.,) are used to pretreat lignocellulosic materials before hydrolysis. Usually combinations of physical and chemical methods are more effective than a physical or chemical method alone. For example, the lignocellulosic materials are usually soaked in an acid or alkali solution before heating at various temperatures. Although it is known that lignin does not chemically inhibit cellulase, it limits access of the enzyme to cellulose. Thus delignification treatments such as treatment with sodium hydroxide or hydrogen peroxide or oxygen delignification have been investigated. Oxygen delignification entails suspending the lignocellulosic material in an alkaline solution (e.g., 0.8M NaOH), heating to about 80°C, and sparging with molecular oxygen.

These pretreatments help to break down the wood structure and enlarge the pore sizes, making it easier for penetration of the hydrolysis enzymes. It is difficult to remove all the lignin, but the residual lignin is partially lumped together, making it easier for the enzymes to access the cellulose. The hemicellulose is hydrolyzed to sugars and other by-products, but cellulose is usually not affected. Furthermore, various volatile and nonvolatile compounds inhibitory to enzyme hydrolysis and fermentation are generated. The nonvolatile compounds inhibit the processes more than the volatile compounds. After the treatment, it is neutralized, filtered, washed with water, dried, and milled before hydrolysis.

*Hydrolysis*

Hydrolysis of cellulose in the lignocellulosic materials after pretreatment can be achieved by enzymatic treatment, dilute acid treatment, or concentrated acid treatment.

*Enzymatic hydrolysis.* This involves mixing the pretreated material with enzyme preparation and incubating at a given temperature for a certain period of time. The enzyme can be a single or a mixture of different enzymes. The enzymes may be either purified or crude, and microorganism(s) can also be used for simultaneous enzyme production and hydrolysis. The amount of enzyme varies, depending on the nature of the raw material and the type of enzyme used. The incubation temperature depends on the temperature characteristics of the enzyme. Cellulases are the most thoroughly studied enzymes used for hydrolysis of lignocellulosic materials. They are usually produced by aerobic fungi, *Trichoderma* species, but some other aerobic microorganisms such as *Cellulomonas, Bacillus, Microbispora, Pseudomonas, Rhizopus niveus,* and *Thermomonospora,* as well as anaerobic species such as *Clostridium* sp., *Ruminococcus* sp., and *Micromonospora,* are also known to produce lignocellulose hydrolyzing enzymes. Some strains, such as *Clostridium thermocellum* and *Neurospora crassa,* can convert cellulose and hemicellulose directly into ethanol. Some criteria used for selection of cellulose hydrolyzing strains include their enzyme production ability, ability to reduce the viscosity by hydrolyzing the pentosans, low temperature optima (in case of simultaneous saccharification and fermentation [SSF] processes), and low pH optima (to avoid contamination).

*Dilute acid hydrolysis.* This is a two-step process. In the first step, the hemicellulose fraction is converted to sugars and by-products using steam and dilute acid (sulfuric acid, mineral acids, or sulfur dioxide). This is similar to pretreatment, but the temperature is lower (130 to 190°C) and the treatment time is longer (10 to 30 minutes). The second step also involves treatment with dilute acid and steam, but the temperature is higher (190 to 265°C) and the treatment time is very short (a few seconds). The hydrolysis products are treated with either lime or sodium sulfite (to neutralize the pH and remove the inhibitory substances) before fermentation.

*Concentrated acid hydrolysis.* The feedstock is dried to below 10 percent moisture and soaked in concentrated acid. Usually hydrochloric acid or anhydrous hydrofluoric acid is used, but sulfuric acid can also be used. The hydrolysis is usually done at relatively lower temperatures for 5 to 60 minutes. There are variations in the temperature, pressure, time, and other detailed procedures. A major disadvantage of concentrated acid treatment is that a large quantity of acid is used, thus there is a need to recover and reuse the acid.

*Hydrolysis products.* The hydrolysis products depend on the feedstock as well as on the method of hydrolysis. The major products include hexose sugars (mainly glucose), various pentose sugars such as xylose and arabinose, and various inhibitory by-products such as acetic acid, furfurals, and sugar acids. A major disadvantage of acid hydrolysis is the high concentration of various inhibitory substances in the hydrolysis products. Also, when acid is used for hydrolysis, other problems arise, including rusting of the fermentation vessels, reduced yield due to sugar modification, the need to neutralize the sugars before fermentation, and environmental problems.

*Fermentation*

Fermentation is the conversion of sugar in the hydrolysis products into ethanol. Examples of cell strains used for fermentation of sugars to ethanol include *Saccharomyces cerevisiae, Candida brassicae, Zymomonas mobilis, Pichia stipitis, Schizosaccharomyces pombe, Clostridium* sp., and *Bacillus macerans*. The strain used depends on the composition of the hydrolysate and the process. Temperature tolerance (especially for SSF processes), ethanol tolerance, resistance to the inhibitory products, oxygen tolerance, fermentation rate, ethanol yield, and ability to grow and ferment under low pH are the major criteria used for strain selection. The hydrolysis products of lignocellulosic materials contain a very high amount of pentose sugars that cannot be fermented by the most widely used strains of *Saccharomyces cerevisiae* and *Zymomonas mobilis*. To increase the overall yield, the pentoses must be fermented to alcohol. Some species of *Candida, Pichia stipitis, Clostridium thermohydrosulfuricum, Bacillus macerans, Pachysolen, Monilia,* and *Fusarium* can ferment D-xylose to ethanol. Unfortunately, some of the pentose-fermenting strains are not efficient in fermenting hexose sugars. Thus, a mixed culture of efficient hexose fermenters and pentose fermenters is desirable for efficient ethanol production from hydrolysis products of lignocellulosic material. However, some strains cannot be cultured together. For example, *Pichia stipitis* has a killer action against *Saccharomyces cerevisiae*. Thus, care must be taken for selection of the strains for the mixed culture systems.

## *FEEDSTOCKS—CONCLUSIONS*

Ethanol yields from some feedstocks are summarized in Table III.3. The data are the representative values reported in literature or obtained in the author's own laboratory and are based on the gross weight of the unprocessed raw material. The actual yields depend on the carbohydrate contents and their forms in the feedstock. Even for a given feedstock, the form and contents of carbohydrates vary depending on the crop or plant line. Therefore, the Table III.3 data should be regarded as only approximate values. The choice of feedstock should be based not only on the potential ethanol yields but also on the productivity (the ease with which they can be converted to ethanol) and ethanol production costs. There are no reliable data for comparison of ethanol productivity from the various feedstocks. The reported

TABLE III.3. Examples of feedstocks for fuel ethanol production

| Feedstock | Yield (L-ethanol/kg-feedstock) | Comments |
|---|---|---|
| Sugarcane | 0.07 | Expensive, but the process is simple and cheap. Yield is based on fermentation of the sugar only. Higher yield can be obtained if the bagasse is also hydrolyzed and fermented. |
| Molasses | 0.3 | Relatively expensive, but the process is simple and cheap. Yield varies greatly depending on the composition, especially on the concentration of sugar. |
| Sweet potatoes | 0.17 | Cheap and easy to hydrolyze. The low yield is mainly due to high water content of the tubers. |
| Cassava | 0.15 | Cheap but difficult to hydrolyze. The low yield is due to the thick outer skin and large content of fibers that are difficult to be hydrolyzed by starch-hydrolyzing enzymes. |
| Corn | 0.4 | Cheap and relatively easy to hydrolyze, this is currently the main feedstock used for ethanol production in the United States. |
| Rice | 0.45 | Expensive but relatively easy to hydrolyze, this is currently used mainly for Japanese sake production. |
| Wheat | 0.42 | Cheap and relatively easy to hydrolyze, this is used in France for fermentation ethanol production. |
| Rice straw | 0.27 | Very cheap but difficult and expensive to hydrolyze. |
| Newspaper | 0.43 | Very cheap but difficult and expensive to hydrolyze. |
| Wood | 0.25 | Very cheap but difficult and expensive to hydrolyze. Softwood is more resistant to hydrolysis than hardwood. |

productivities vary greatly depending on the process used. However, the trend is that higher productivities are reported for sugar crops, followed by starch materials, while the cheapest and most abundant lignocellulosic materials are more difficult to hydrolyze, resulting in much lower productivities.

## PROCESS STRATEGIES—INTRODUCTION

In the first half of this chapter, the potential of various feedstocks for ethanol production was discussed. However, the feasibility of using any of the feedstocks for large-scale ethanol production depends on the availability of efficient technology. From relatively expensive sugar materials, ethanol can be efficiently produced using a very cheap and simple technology. However, the technologies for conversion of starch and, especially, lignocellulosic materials to ethanol are relatively complex and expensive. In this part, various strategies used for ethanol production from these feedstocks are discussed.

## PROCESSES FOR ETHANOL PRODUCTION FROM SUGAR MATERIALS

Fermentation processes used for ethanol production from sugars can be classified into batch, fed-batch, and continuous fermentation processes.

### Batch Fermentation

This is the "traditional," simple method for ethanol production. The microorganism is simply inoculated into the sugar solution, sometimes supplemented with some nitrogen sources. Ideally, the culture parameters such as the temperature and pH are controlled, but depending on the strain used and the prevailing climatic conditions, relatively high productivity can be obtained without controlling the culture conditions. Usually the initial sugar concentration ranges from 11 to 17 percent, but much higher sugar concentration can be used, depending on the ethanol tolerance of the strain. The productivity can be significantly increased by recycling (reusing) the cells. At the end of each batch, the cells are separated by centrifuge, and the cell sediment is disinfected by addition of sulfide or other disinfectants. However, the process of centrifuging the whole culture broth is expensive, and repeated-batch process can be done by replacing only a certain percentage of the culture broth with a fresh medium at the end of each batch process. In this case, however, the rate of fermentation is relatively lower because of the lower cell concentration at the beginning of each batch. The optimum ratio of the culture broth to be replaced varies depending on the feedstock, the cell strain, and the culture conditions, especially the temperature and the aeration rate. Because the batch process is very simple and cheap, it is the most widely used process today. However, it is labor intensive, and because the cells are exposed to very high sugar concentration at the initial stage and to a very high ethanol concentration at the final stage, the productivity is relatively low.

### Fed-Batch Fermentation

The fed-batch process is used to obtain a very high ethanol concentration while avoiding the long lag phase that is sometimes observed when a high initial sugar concentration is used. The fermentation is started with a low sugar concentration (usually less than 10 percent), and concentrated sugar solution is added either continuously or intermittently until the desired ethanol concentration is reached. As in the case of batch fermentation, repeated fed-batch processes can be done by replacing a certain percentage of the culture broth with a fresh medium at the end of each fed-batch. This process is repeated until the rate of fermentation decreases due to decrease in cell viability. Aside from high productivities obtained with this process, the high ethanol concentration means a significant reduction in the cost of distillation. However, the advantage of fed-batch processes can be realized only if an ethanol-tolerant strain is used.

### Continuous Fermentation

In a continuous process, concentrated sugar solution is continuously fed into the bioreactor at a desired rate and fermented broth is pumped out of the bioreactor at the same rate. At a steady state, the broth volume, the sugar, and the ethanol concentrations are constant. The high ethanol concentration and low sugar concentration at the steady state help to minimize contamination risks. However, if not well managed, contamination can still be a problem during long-term operation. Although very high productivity can be achieved, at a dilution rate resulting in the maximum productivity, the residual sugar concentration would be high with consequent decrease in ethanol conversion efficiency. Furthermore, with free cells, the dilution rate has to be maintained lower than the specific growth rate of the cells to avoid washout. This problem can be avoided either by using a membrane to retain the cells inside the reactor or by immobilizing the cells. These techniques also help to maintain high cell concentration, to increase the volumetric productivity, and thus to reduce the required reactor volume per unit of product. Results of various studies suggest that for a given volume of ethanol produced, the capital investment cost (mainly due to reduction in the volume of fermenter required) and the production costs (due to lower labor cost and higher productivity) are much lower than those of batch processes. However, the extent of cost reduction depends on the scale of production and the ability to integrate the fermentation with the pretreatment and distillation processes.

### *Cell Immobilization*

Cell immobilization can be achieved by entrapment of the cells in polymer materials such as carrageenan, alginate, agar, agarose, pectin, polyacrylamide, and gelatin. However, some of these materials are very expensive, and it is often very difficult and expensive to produce a large amount of entrapped cells for large-scale applications. Furthermore, some of them are very unstable and fragile for long-term operations. Cells can also be immobilized by colonization of porous particles, such as porous diatomaceous earth, borosilicate glass beads, silica gel particles, and porous ceramic beads/plates. Cell adhesion to some synthetic support materials, such as stainless steel mesh and synthetic cellulose materials, or to lignocellulosic materials, such as jute fabric, sawdust, sugarcane bagasse, wood chip/shavings, rice husk, cotton fibers, and straw, have also been investigated. Immobilization by cell colonization or cell adhesion is simple, but most of the carriers have a nonuniform and unsuitable structure for preparation of stable fixed beds. Furthermore, the amounts of immobilized cells are low, and the immobilized cells are susceptible to physical properties of the broth (pH, ionic strength, etc.). Also, shear stress due to aeration, agitation, gas evolution, and liquid flow can lead to sloughing of the cells. They are thus not suitable for fluidized-bed bioreactors.

Advantages of cell immobilization include process stability, repeated use of the cells, high volumetric productivity (due to higher cell concentrations and operation at dilution rates higher than the specific growth rate of the cells), and increase in the thermostability of the cells. However, to use immobilized cells for ethanol production, the immobilization carrier should be cheap, the immobilization method should be simple, it should be easy to prepare large amounts of immobilized cells for large-scale production, and the immobilized cells should be stable over a long period of time. Among the lignocellulosic materials, loofa sponge seems to meet these requirements. It is a very economical and excellent carrier for immobilization of both flocculating and nonflocculating cells. Immobilization can be achieved by inoculation of the seed culture into a bioreactor containing a fixed bed of loofa sponge. A very high cell concentration of more than 10 g cell/g sponge can be achieved, and the immobilized cells are stable for a very long time. Either cylindrical or sliced loofa sponge can be used for bed construction. When a cylindrical form is used, the immobilized cell concentration is relatively lower (about 4.5 g cell/g sponge), but the three central cavities in the sponge facilitate mass transfer. In a packed-bed reactor with a cylindrical loofa sponge (Figure III.3), the broth flow is very similar to that of an airlift reactor with multiple draft tubes.

## PROCESSES FOR ETHANOL PRODUCTION FROM STARCH AND LIGNOCELLULOSIC MATERIALS

### Separate Hydrolysis and Fermentation Processes (SHF)

Traditionally, hydrolysis and fermentation processes are done in separate steps using either a single reactor or a number of bioreactors in series. The hydrolysis step can be done with purified enzymes, crude enzymes, or microorganisms. High hydrolysis rates and sugar yields can be obtained by using suitable enzymes. However, the enzymes may be expensive, leading to increase in the overall cost of ethanol production. Immobilization of the enzymes permits their repeated use, but immobilization also leads to additional costs. The use of microorganisms for simultaneous enzyme production and hydrolysis is more economical, but the need to maintain the cells in an active state makes process optimization more difficult. The optimal conditions for cell growth and enzyme production are often different from the optimal conditions for hydrolysis.

In a batch process, the feedstock is mixed with the enzyme or inoculated with the hydrolyzing microorganism(s) and incubated for a desired period of time. After hydrolysis, the enzymes or the microorganisms are inactivated (usually by heating) and the ethanol-producing microorganism is inoculated. Continuous sequential hydrolysis and fermentation can be achieved by connecting the hydrolysis tank to the fermentation tank. The feedstock is fed continuously to the hydrolysis tank, and the hydrolyzed broth is continuously pumped into the fermentation tank. However, it is necessary to retain the biocatalyst (enzymes or microbial cells) inside the hydrolysis tank. This is achieved either by immobilization or by equipping the effluent port with a membrane so that only the filtrate is passed into the fermentation tank. A major disadvantage of this process is that the enzyme activity is inhibited by the produced sugars (feedback repression) so that it is often difficult to obtain a very high concentration of sugars. Consequently, the final ethanol concentration is usually low, and most of the strains of microorganisms used for hydrolysis also use the produced fermentable sugars for growth and by-product accumulation with consequent decrease in ethanol yield. However, these problems do not arise in the case of acid hydrolysis.

## Simultaneous Hydrolysis and Fermentation Processes

The simultaneous hydrolysis and fermentation process entails inoculating the enzyme-producing microorganism(s) (or the enzyme) and the ethanol producing microorganism(s) at the same time so that the produced sugars are simultaneously converted to ethanol. Because the produced sugars are immediately converted to ethanol, the problem of feedback inhibition is avoided. Contamination risk is also low since the sugar concentration is very low throughout the process. In general, the productivities and yields reported for this method are higher than those reported for the SHF process. Furthermore, less enzyme is needed because glucose inhibition is avoided. This method is widely used for production of Japanese sake and shochu. The hydrolysis enzyme preparation (koji) is produced by solid-state cultivation of *Aspergillus* sp. on rice or wheat grains. The koji is mixed with steamed rice or mashed sweet potatoes, and the yeast cells are inoculated. In the simultaneous hydrolysis and fermentation processes, however, recycling of the biocatalysts is very difficult when free cells or free enzymes are used. This problem can be avoided by immobilizing the biocatalysts. The biocatalysts can be immobilized separately and mixed together in the same bioreactor or coimmobilized within one carrier. Another problem is that the optimal conditions (especially temperature and pH) for hydrolysis are often different from those for fermentation. The temperature optima for most hydrolysis enzymes are often much higher than those for most fermenting microorganisms. The use of thermophilic or thermotolerant strains of fermentation microorganisms can help to overcome this problem.

### High-Gravity Fermentation

In simultaneous hydrolysis and fermentation processes, usually 11 to 18 percent dissolved solids concentration is used and 5 to 9 percent ethanol is produced. Higher concentrations of substrates are required to produce higher ethanol concentrations and thus reduce the cost of distillation. It has been estimated that the unit cost of distilling 12 percent ethanol is about 40 percent lower than the cost of distilling 6 percent ethanol. However, higher substrate concentration leads to slow or stuck fermentation due to inhibition by high ethanol concentration and/or inhibition at high osmotic pressure. Ethanol can be efficiently produced from high dissolved-solid concentrations by supplementing with nutrients such as yeast extracts, ergosterol, and oleic acid. In that case, ethanol concentrations as high as 15 percent can be produced. However, for such high ethanol concentration, a longer fermentation time is generally needed. To avoid ethanol inhibition, it is necessary to maintain a low temperature with a consequent decrease in fermentation rate. Thus, this high-gravity fermentation is recommended only if the cost savings from distillation are enough to compensate for the decrease in productivity. There is also a need to use ethanol-tolerant strains and to maintain high cell concentration. For high-moisture/high-fiber crops and pulpy feedstocks in which it is difficult to separate the suspended components from the fiber due to high viscosity, solid-state fermentation can be employed.

## BIOREACTORS

The simplest and most economical bioreactors used for ethanol production are the nonaerated and nonagitated open tanks. These types of reactors are commonly used for production of sake and shochu. They are mixed using wooden paddles once or twice a day to release the trapped carbon dioxide gas. However, the fermentation rates are usually very low, and it often takes up to two weeks or more to obtain broth with about 10 percent ethanol. Aerated stirred-tank bioreactors (Figure III.1) or aerated bubble-column bioreactors are also used. The rates of fermentation obtained with these types of bioreactors are much higher than those obtained with nonaerated tanks. However, they are more expensive and the running costs are often higher due to energy used for agitation and aeration.

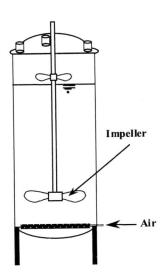

FIGURE III.1. Continuous stirred-tank bioreactor

For immobilized cells, fluidized-bed bioreactors can be used. The amount of immobilized particles has to be relatively small to enable good fluidization (Figure III.2). The hydrodynamic stress generated by aeration, agitation, and collision among the immobilized particles, as well as between the immobilized particles and the walls of the bioreactor, can lead to dislodging of the immobilized cells and, in the case of polymer beads, to the breakage of the beads. Thus, the durability of immobilized preparations in these types of bioreactors is often short. The mass transfer rates are high, but due to lower cell concentrations, the productivities are relatively low. Packed-bed bioreactors are much more stable since the hydrodynamic stress is low. The cell loading is usually very high, leading to high volumetric productivities. However, depending on the type of carriers used and the structure of the bed, intraparticulate cells can lead to blocking of the beds with consequent channeling of the nutrients. The mass transfer rates are usually much lower than those in fluidized beds, thus they are not suitable for simultaneous enzyme production and hydrolysis by aerobic microbial strains. Nevertheless, it has been demonstrated that cylindrical loofa sponge can be used to construct fixed beds with high mass transfer capacity (Figure III.3). An external loop reactor is used to facilitate culture broth circulation, especially during cell immobilization. However, after cell immobilization, it is not necessary to circulate the broth through the loop. Such fixed beds are very effective for aerobic enzyme production and hydrolysis. In the case of lignocellulosic

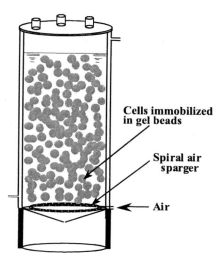

FIGURE III.2. Fluidized-bed bioreactor with cells immobilized in gel beads

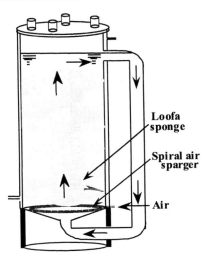

FIGURE III.3. External loop bioreactor with cells immobilized in cylindrical loofa sponge. This bioreactor was developed in the author's laboratory for ethanol production from sugar beet juice.

feedstock, the loofa sponge has to be protected from cellulases. This can be achieved by acetylation of the loofa sponge or by coating it with materials such as paints.

The simultaneous enzyme production, hydrolysis, and fermentation process needs a special type of bioreactor, since the enzyme production requires an aerobic condition while ethanol production is more efficient under anaerobic condition. An example of a bioreactor for simultaneous aerobic and anaerobic processes is shown in Figure III.4. The aerated riser column is used for enzyme production while the nonaerated downcomer column is used for ethanol production. To increase the oxygen transfer rate in the riser column, a cylindrical loofa sponge can be used for bed construction. However, a sliced loofa sponge can be used for construction of the fixed bed in the downcomer column. Without the broth flow control valve, increasing the aeration rate increases the rate of broth circulation between the two columns. Under this condition, the dissolved oxygen concentration in the downcomer column increases, with consequent increase in the yeast growth rate but decrease in ethanol production rate and yield. On the other hand, at a low aeration rate, the dissolved oxygen concentration in the riser column is low with subsequent decrease in enzyme production. By equipping the reactor with a broth flow control valve and optimizing the frequency and duration of the valve opening, the riser column can be maintained under aerobic

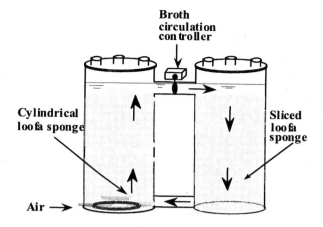

FIGURE III.4. Circulating aerobic-anaerobic bioreactor with cells immobilized in loofa sponge. This bioreactor was developed in the author's laboratory for simultaneous enzyme production, raw cassava starch hydrolysis, and ethanol fermentation.

conditions while the downcomer column is maintained under anaerobic conditions. When this reactor was used for simultaneous hydrolysis of raw cassava starch and ethanol production, the enzyme productivity, rate of starch hydrolysis, ethanol productivity, and yield were very high and stable over a long period of time.

## *PROCESS STRATEGIES—CONCLUSIONS*

With the present technology, the cost of ethanol production is not competitive with the current prices of gasoline. Bioenergy is still less than 5 percent of total energy used in most countries, and aside from a few countries such as Brazil, ethanol is only a small percentage of the total bioenergy. Even in the United States (the highest ethanol-producing country), ethanol makes up only about 1 percent of the total gasoline used. Because the costs of sugar crops are high, development of efficient systems for ethanol production from lignocellulosic materials is more promising. However, there is still a need to optimize the pretreatment step and to improve the efficiency of enzyme hydrolysis to replace the use of expensive and environmentally unfriendly acid hydrolysis. This can be achieved by screening and developing strains that produce high titers of cellulase and then using them to develop efficient processes for enzyme production and hydrolysis. For efficient SSF, there is a need to improve the thermostability of the ethanol-producing strains and to develop strains that can efficiently ferment both hexose and pentose sugars, or, still better, strains that can ferment cellulose directly to ethanol. However, technology development and improvement alone may not be enough to make ethanol fuel competitive with the current prices of gasoline, at least in a very near future. Therefore, energy policies that consider environmental issues and the nonrenewable nature of petroleum are needed before ethanol can be generally used as an alternative liquid fuel.

## SUGGESTED READINGS

Lynd LR (1996). Overview and evaluation of fuel ethanol from cellulosic biomass: Technology, economics, the environment, and policy. *Annual Review of Energy and the Environment* 21:403-465.

Moreira JR and J Goldemberg (1999). The alcohol program. *Energy Policy* 27: 229-245.

Ogbonna JC, H Mashima, and H Tanaka (2001). Scale up of fuel ethanol production from sugar beet juice using loofa sponge immobilized bioreactor. *Bioresearch Technology* 76:1-8.

# Grape-Based Alcoholic Beverages

Ronald S. Jackson

## INTRODUCTION

Grapes *(Vitis vinifera)* have been fermented for millennia to produce wine. In contrast, only in the past 500 years has distillation been perfected sufficiently to transform wine into brandy. Correspondingly, the evolution of fortified wines is even more recent. In the past few decades, production has outpaced consumption (Table III.4). This has led to serious overproduction in some countries, requiring the conversion of wine into industrial alcohol. Other than as a means of draining Europe's infamous "wine lake," grapes are not an economical source of producing industrial alcohol.

Wines have traditionally been classified into three major categories: still, sparkling, and fortified wines. Figure III.5 summarizes the basic steps in their production.

Still table wines possess an alcohol content that can vary from 7 to 14 percent. The alcohol comes from the fermentation of grape sugars—glucose and fructose. Mature grapes contain from 16 to over 30 percent sugar, depending on the cultivar and fruit maturity. In some jurisdictions, cane or beet sugar can be added to fermenting grape juice to increase the wine's alcohol content. If the wine possesses a clearly noticeable effervescence, the wine is categorized as sparkling, whereas if distilled alcohol is added to the wine, it is classified as fortified. Fortified wines typically possess alcohol contents between 16 and 24 percent.

## TABLE WINES

In most instances, grapes begin their transformation into wine following crushing. In only a few instances are the fruit exposed to an extended period of anaerobiosis before crushing. In the absence of air, respiration soon consumes all the available oxygen and energy metabolism shifts to fermentation. As ethanol production reaches about 2 percent, the cells die and alcohol production ceases. Thus, the treatment, called carbonic maceration, is not an important means of generating alcohol. Its principal benefits are the production of a unique, fresh, fruity bouquet in a wine that matures rapidly

TABLE III.4. Wine production and consumption statistics over about 30 years for several major wine-producing countries

| Country | Wine production (hl.10³) | | | | | | Wine consumption (hl.10³) | | | | | |
|---|---|---|---|---|---|---|---|---|---|---|---|---|
| | 1971-1975 | 1976-1980 | 1981-1985 | 1986-1990 | 1991-1995 | 1998 | 1971-1975 | 1976-1980 | 1981-1985 | 1986-1990 | 1991-1995 | 1998 |
| Argentina | 22,778 | 24,597 | 20,463 | 19,914 | 15,588 | 12,673 | 19,472 | 21,711 | 20,188 | 17,804 | 15,720 | 13,552 |
| Australia | 2,498 | 3,655 | 4,025 | 4,285 | 4,810 | 7,415 | 1,312 | 2,066 | 3,011 | 3,297 | 3,212 | 3,644 |
| Chile | 5,052 | 5,655 | 6,600 | 4,135 | 3,326 | 5,475 | 4,141 | 5,283 | 5,142 | 3,456 | 2,350 | 2,300 |
| France | 68,742 | 67,259 | 67,462 | 64,641 | 52,886 | 52,671 | 54,886 | 51,567 | 46,161 | 41,715 | 37,310 | 35,500 |
| Germany | 8,085 | 7,832 | 9,799 | 10,012 | 10,391 | 10,834 | 12,545 | 14,911 | 15,903 | 18,389 | 18,641 | 18,970 |
| Italy | 69,557 | 74,619 | 72,146 | 65,715 | 60,768 | 54,188 | 60,515 | 51,328 | 46,301 | 36,621 | 34,693 | 32,000 |
| Portugal | 10,326 | 9,475 | 9,076 | 8,455 | 7,276 | 3,621 | 7,495 | 7,686 | 7,951 | 5,889 | 5,800 | 5,000 |
| Spain | 32,189 | 33,832 | 33,964 | 33,519 | 26,438 | 30,320 | 25,837 | 23,319 | 19,681 | 17,402 | 15,439 | 15,500 |
| United States | 13,223 | 16,538 | 17,710 | 18,167 | 17,619 | 20,450 | 13,259 | 16,143 | 20,305 | 20,845 | 18,406 | 20,800 |
| World | 313,115 | 326,046 | 332,586 | 303,976 | 261,985 | 258,459 | 279,354 | 284,346 | 280,476 | 239,889 | 223,057 | 223,787 |

Source: Data from OIV, 1991; Dutruc-Rosset, 2000.

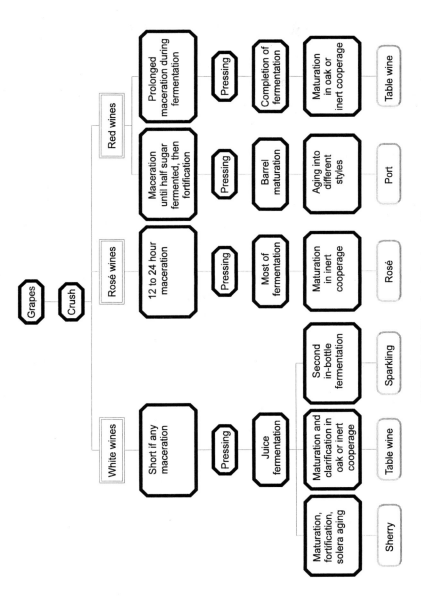

FIGURE III.5. Flowchart of wine making

(can be consumed within a few weeks of production). Examples are Beaujolais nouveau and vino novello.

Crushing liberates the juice, starts the liberation of flavorants from the skins, and inoculates the juice with indigenous yeasts and bacteria. Although several of these can initiate fermentation, *Saccharomyces cerevisiae* (the principal wine yeast) soon dominates and completes fermentation. Consequently, *S. cerevisiae* produces most of the flavorants that typify the majority of wines. Once alcoholic fermentation is complete, lactic acid bacteria may induce malolactic fermentation. It converts one of the major grape acids (malic acid) to lactic acid. This increases the wine's pH and reduces its perceived acidity.

It is at this point that the differentiation between red, rosé, and white table wines begins. If the must (juice, seeds, and skins) comes from red grapes, the temperature is brought to between 20 and 25°C. Fermentation commences almost immediately. For reds, fermentation generally goes to completion in the presence of the seeds and skins (pomace). However, if the fermenting juice is separated from the pomace (pressed) within 12 to 24 hours, a rosé results. White wines can be produced from red grapes if the juice is uncolored (as usual) and is separated from the pomace immediately after crushing.

Most white wines are produced from nonpigmented (white) grapes. Typically, the juice is left in contact with the seed and skins for 6 to 24 hours. This exposure (maceration) enhances flavor extraction from the skins and pulp. Maceration typically occurs at about 10 to 15°C and in the presence of a moderate amount of sulfur dioxide. Sulfur dioxide retards the initiation of fermentation. After maceration, pressing separates the juice from the pomace. Fermentation is often conducted at about 15°C.

Fermentation may occur spontaneously or may be induced by the addition of a yeast inoculum. In either case, yeasts derived from the grapes and winery equipment are present. In spontaneous fermentation, a diverse collection of indigenous yeasts initiate fermentation. However, as the alcohol content rises above 2 percent, most wild yeasts become inactive or die. Fermentation subsequently occurs under the action of one or a few related wine yeasts. Although *Saccharomyces cerevisiae* is most frequently involved, *S. bayanus* and *S. uvarum* may be dominant under special conditions, notably the second fermentation in sparkling wine production or during the fermentation of very sweet juice. Surprisingly, these wine yeasts are poorly represented in the grape skin flora. They come primarily from winery equipment. Although some wine makers prefer spontaneous fermentation, the modern trend is to add a particular strain. Inoculation has several advantages. It not only reduces the risks of off-odor production (by undesirable wild yeasts) but also gives the wine maker increased control over the types of flavors possessed by the wine. This is particularly important when grapes possessing little unique (varietal-derived) aroma are used. In such situations, most of the wine's fragrance comes from yeast-derived metabolites.

Frequently, alcoholic fermentation is followed by malolactic fermentation. Its reduction of wine acidity and perceived sourness is particularly valuable in cool climatic regions. Here, even mature grapes may be overly acidic. In warm to hot climatic regions, malolactic fermentation is often discouraged because the grapes may be low in acidity. Any further reduction would give the wine a flat taste, reduce its color intensity and stability, increase its susceptibility to oxidation, and enhance the likelihood of microbial spoilage. Although malolactic fermentation diminishes acidity, it can also significantly influence the wine's bouquet. This is one of the principal reasons why producers frequently inoculate their wines (when desired) with a particular strain of lactic acid bacterium—usually a variety of *Oenococcus oeni*. This both speeds the onset of malolactic fermentation and gives the wine maker another control over the wine's attributes.

After the completion of fermentation, the young wine is stored under cool (~10°C) anaerobic conditions. The absence of oxygen is essential to avoid oxidation and limit the action of spoilage bacteria. Storage typically occurs in stainless steel or wooden cooperage. Wines possessing little distinctive fragrance are usually stored in inert cooperage to retain their mild aroma and bouquet. In contrast, wines possessing a distinctive or pronounced varietal flavor are frequently matured in oak cooperage. Oak donates its own fragrance that may highlight the wine's varietal aroma. The nature and intensity of the oak flavors depend on the oak species, the method of seasoning, cooperage production method, cooperage size, and the duration of contact.

Although storage protects the wine from oxidation and may enhance flavor development, its principal function is to promote maturation and clarification. Maturation involves an incredible range of organic chemical reactions. Some reduce undesirable fermentation odors (e.g., hydrogen sulfide), whereas others favor the production or release of desirable aromatics from the wine. In addition, dead and dying yeast cells (in the sediment) release compounds such as mannoproteins. These help bind aromatic compounds, slowing but prolonging their release. Maturation also includes poorly understood phenomena that lead to the blending (harmonizing) of its constituents.

In addition to maturation, physical and physicochemical reactions promote wine clarification and stabilization. These include physical reactions such as sedimentation. The wine is periodically removed (racked) from yeast, bacteria, and grape cell remnants that sediment. Physicochemical reactions include the polymerization of tannins and proteins. As these polymers enlarge, they precipitate. To enhance polymerization and sedimentation, the wine is often fined near the end of maturation. Fining involves the addition of one or more compounds, for example oak-gall tannins, beaten egg whites, or bentonite (a form of montmorillonite clay). Clarification also involves crystallization phenomena. This is particularly valuable in removing the excessive amounts of potassium bitartrate commonly found in young wine. If these salts are not removed, they may form visible crystals in bottled wine. Consumers have often mistaken these harmless salt crystals as splinters of glass. To encourage early crystallization, most wines are chilled to below 0°C. After several days (or weeks) the crystals are removed by filtration. Filtration (or centrifugation) may also be used to speed clarification. This is particularly valuable when the wine is bottled before natural sedimentation has achieved adequate clarification.

Before bottling, different lots of wine are usually selectively combined to make a final blend. These may come from similar or dissimilar batches of wine. Blending minimizes the sensory deficiencies that occur in almost every sample. After a short stabilization period, the wine is given a final fining before bottling. Bottling typically occurs under sterile conditions in the absence of oxygen.

After bottling, the wine is allowed to rest or age before shipping. This may last from a few weeks to several years. Prolonged aging at the winery is much less common than in the past and has primarily become the prerogative of the purchaser. Aging is of clear benefit only for premium wines that require several years to "smooth," or develop their traditional fragrance. For the majority of wines, aging is of value only if the consumer prefers the complex subtlety of an aged bouquet (that may develop) to the more fruity, varietal aroma of the young wine.

## SPARKLING WINES

Sparkling wines begin their production similar to most white table wine. One of the more significant differences, however, occurs shortly after harvesting. Instead of crushing, whole grape clusters are placed directly in large presses. Slow pressing releases the juice with a minimum of pigment, tannin, or flavor extraction. This is particularly important when the juice is derived from red grapes. No maceration period precedes juice inoculation and the initiation of fermentation.

Following clarification, wines from different sites and/or grape varieties are combined to produce the *cuvée*. Blending creates the characteristics that typify the brand being produced. If a rosé is desired, a small amount of light red wine is added to the cuvée.

The principal attributes of a sparkling wine develop during its second fermentation and subsequent maturation. The second fermentation produces the carbon dioxide that gives the wine its effervescence. Because the cuvée does not possess fermentable sugars, these are added in quantities sufficient to produce the desired amount of carbon dioxide. Inorganic nutrients and a yeast inoculum are also added along with the sugars. In the standard method *(méthode champenoise)*, the mixture of sugar, nutrients, yeast, and wine is dispensed into thick bottles for the second fermentation. The bottles are sealed with metal crown caps.

Fermentation occurs slowly, typically taking several weeks or months. On completion, the bottles are cooled to about 10°C and matured for one to three years (occasionally longer). It is during this period that the subtle bouquet that characterizes sparkling wines develops. Mannoproteins dissolve out of dead yeast cells as well. These probably prolong the slow release of bubbles after the wine has been poured.

On completion of maturation, the bottles are periodically shaken over a period of several days to weeks. This moves the yeasts to the neck of the bottle (positioned upside down). Subsequently, the bottles are chilled and the neck immersed in a freezing solution. As the wine in the neck freezes, it encases the yeasts. When the bottle is inverted and the cap removed, the yeast and ice plug is ejected. Immediately after, the level of the wine is adjusted, sweetening added, and the traditional cork closure inserted. After a short rest period, the wine is ready for release.

## FORTIFIED WINES

Fortified wines come in many styles, the most common of which are sherry, port, and vermouth. All derive their enhanced alcohol content from the addition of distilled spirits, derived either from wine or other fermented products. The steps in their production are briefly outlined in this section.

Vermouth is the oldest of fortified wines, having its origin in the herb-flavored table wines of antiquity. Current versions are made from white grapes. If red, the color comes from the addition of non-grape pigments. The flavor attributes of the different vermouth brands come from the use of proprietary combinations of up to fifty or more herbs, roots, seeds, bark, or other plant products. These may be steeped either in the fortified wine (usually about 18 percent alcohol) or in distilled spirit before being used to fortify the wine. Depending on the style, vermouth may be sweet or dry. Some sugar is always added to vermouth to partially mask its marked bitterness.

By comparison, sherries form a much more complex set of fortified wines. Although produced elsewhere, the most extensive range comes from southern Spain (Andalusia), where the style evolved. Spanish sherry development follows either the fino or oloroso process.

Both sherry styles start out as dry white wines. Stylistic differentiation begins both in the vineyard and winery. The more subtle (fino) sherries come largely from grapes grown in the primarily chalky soils around Jerez de la Frontera. The grapes are also pressed more gently to extract fewer tannins. Wines designed for oloroso production often come from less preferred sites and may be crushed and pressed less gently.

After fermentation (at about 20 to 25°C), the wine is clarified for several months. The next step is fortification. For fino production, fortification raises the alcohol content to about 15 percent. In contrast, wines intended to develop into an oloroso are fortified to about 18 percent alcohol. The wine is placed in barrels containing about 500 liters (butts). For fino production, the butts are usually left 20 percent empty. The young fortified wine is called the *añada*. The *añada* is the first step in the fractional blending *(solera)* system (Figure III.6) that characterizes Spanish sherry production. Each subsequent step is called a *criadera*. The last in the sequence is termed the *solera*. In fractional blending, about 20 percent of the wine is transferred from one *criadera* to the next (older) *criadera*. The wine so removed is replaced by an equivalent volume from the next youngest *criadera*. The process continues through all *criadera* stages until the youngest receives wine from the *añada*. Wine removed from the last *criadera (solera)* is blended with wine from other lots of *solera*-aged wine. Blending generates the attributes that traditionally characterize a particular brand. The number of *criaderas* in a *solera* system, the frequency of transfer, and the level of filling direct the wine's evolution into either major category—fino or oloroso.

In fino production, wine is transferred several times a year, and there may be up to 20 *criaderas* in each solera. Leaving the butts partially empty (20 percent ullage) provides the surface over which a crust of yeasts *(flor)* can form. Its development is aided by fortification of the *añada* wine to 15 to 15.5 percent alcohol. At this concentration, the chemistry of the cell wall changes, giving yeasts the ability to float on the wine. The yeast crust limits oxidation of the wine as well as metabolizes some of the aldehydes formed during the wine's partial oxidation. Frequent wine transfer helps maintain *flor* growth throughout the many *criaderas* that constitute a fino *solera*. Maturation of a fino sherry frequently takes about five years.

In contrast, the number of *criaderas* in an oloroso *solera* may be as few as three, transfers occur infrequently, and the butts are filled completely. *Flor* development is prevented by fortifying the *añada* wine to 18 percent alcohol. Evolution of an oloroso may take up to ten years.

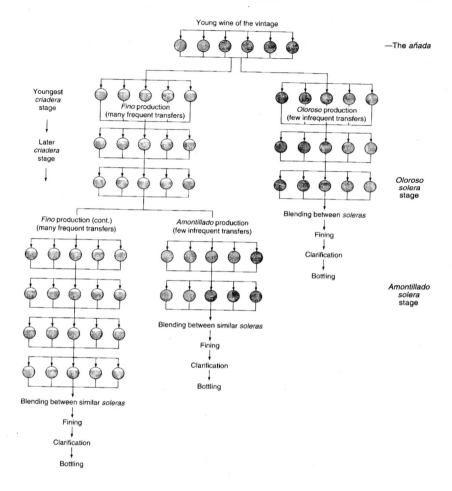

FIGURE III.6. Flowchart for the production of fino, amontillado, and oloroso sherries. Shading indicates whether the butts are kept full or partially (~20 percent) empty. (*Source:* Jackson, 2000. Reproduced by permission.)

A somewhat intermediate style, called amontillado, begins its development as a fino sherry. However, after several years under *flor,* the butts are filled to the top and the frequency of transfer slows to that of an oloroso. As appropriate for its evolution, amontillado sherries have attributes reminiscent of both a fuller-bodied fino and a lighter oloroso. When maturation and final blending are complete, the wine may be darkened (with boiled wine concentrate) and/or sweetened (as appropriate for the brand). All sherries are initially dry.

Port wines also come in a wide diversity of styles, differentiated primarily by their means of maturation. Although white ports are produced, red versions are more common. The production of red port begins like most red table wines. The most noticeable modification is the intense mixing of the fermenting juice with the seed and skins. This accelerates the extraction of pigments and tannins from the pomace. When yeast activity has consumed about half the sugars, the ferment is fortified to about 18 percent alcohol. This rapidly suppresses fermentation, conserving most of the residual sugars in the juice. Pressing separates the partially fermented juice from the pomace.

The wine is stored in oak or inert cooperage for several months or years, depending on its quality and the intents of the cellar master. The majority of port is processed to generate ruby port. It is a blend of many different wines derived from a diversity of grape varieties, frequently from several vintages. The wine is permitted to receive slight oxidation during its typical two-year maturation. Bottling occurs after clarification and fining. Better-quality wines may be aged similarly for many years, usually in small oak cooperage. During prolonged maturation, the ruby color fades to a tawny shade, and the fruity fragrance is replaced by a more subtle complex bouquet. Such wines are called tawny ports.

Superior quality wines are often blended only within a single vintage, and consequently are generically called vintage ports. The most prestigious is simply called vintage port. They are bottled within two years and are only lightly fined before bottling. Because such wines are often bottle-aged for 20 years (or more), they typically deposit considerable sediment. Thus, opening and decanting must be done carefully to avoid resuspending the sediment. Late-bottled vintage ports are similar but are aged in large cooperage for several years and carefully clarified before bottling. This usually occurs late in the fourth year following production. They have many of the same sensory traits that have made vintage ports famous. However, they are ready for consumption when released and do not develop sediment.

## BRANDY

Brandy is the oak-aged condensate of distilled white wine. Partially immature grapes are preferred because of their acidity, freedom from off-flavors, and minimal varietal aroma. Most of the desired flavor attributes come from fermentation by-products. Thus, careful attention to yeast strain is important to generate the desired bouquet. It is also important that the strain synthesize little acetic acid or sulfur dioxide. Fermentation of the wine follows standard techniques, except that the juice is separated from the pomace almost immediately after crushing. Distillation preferably occurs shortly after fermentation so that the yeast-derived fruit esters are at their maximal concentration. They generate much of the traditional fruitiness of brandy. That early distillation provides little time for clarification is unimportant because yeast sediment is typically added to the wine before distillation. Yeast-cell remains are the principal source of fatty acid esters. They not only contribute to brandy's traditional flavor but also extend the release of its bouquet. Fusel oils (higher alcohols) are another important group of fermentation by-products concentrated during distillation. These typify all distilled beverages.

Depending on the type of still employed, either superheated steam or direct exposure to fire (Figure III.7) induces vaporization of the wine's alcohol and other aromatics. Finer brandies are often produced in stills that permit the separation of different fractions as they condense along plates or tubes in the still. Early and late fractions are rarely incorporated into brandy due to their aldehydic odors or sharp chemical taints. The maximum tem-

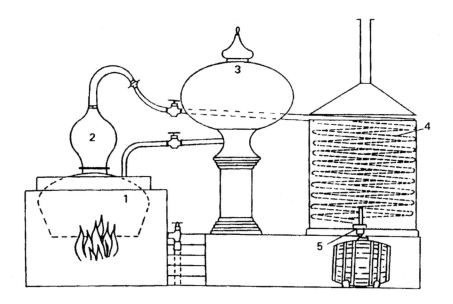

FIGURE III.7. Schematic drawing of a pot distillation system: (1) boiler, (2) reflux condenser, (3) preheater, (4) cooling coils, (5) effluent port. (*Source:* van den Berg and Maarse, 1993. Reproduced by permission.)

perature to which the wine is exposed during distillation also affects the brandy's characteristics. For example, pot stills (using direct exposure to flame) generate a more complex set of heat breakdown products (from amino acids and sugars) than do those using superheated steam. Heating also helps liberate various aromatics bound in nonvolatile sugar complexes.

The retained fractions are aged in oak barrels for many years. During maturation, the alcohol content slowly diminishes and the rough attributes of the young brandy mellow. In addition, tannins and breakdown products of oak lignins contribute to the brandy's traditional color, as well as donate vanilla-like essences. To avoid the incorporation of a marked oak flavor, most of the barrels are old (having been used repeatedly in brandy maturation). After maturation, blending creates the features typical of each brand.

## WINE USE

Wine use is defined more by tradition (habituation) than any other factor. For example, the predominate use of red wines in southern Europe reflects the need for tannins (extracted simultaneously with red pigments). They compensate for the preservative characteristics missing due to their generally higher pH. In contrast, in more northern (cooler) regions, red grapes seldom produce sufficient pigment (anthocyanins) to make a red wine. In addition, ripe white grapes often retain sufficient acidity to limit most microbial spoilage. Hence, white wines have generally been produced (and preferred) in north-central Europe. Nevertheless, there is some logic to traditional views on wine-food combination.

The principle guiding most food-wine combinations is similar flavor intensity. Because flavor intensity is often related to color intensity, red wines often combine particularly well with red meats, whereas white wines tend to pair well with fish and poultry. Nevertheless, pale red wines can often substitute for white wines, whereas intense white wines can pair well with some red dishes. As the name implies, table wines have evolved for pairing with meals. The bitter to acidic characteristics that typify most red and white wines, respectively, become more mellow when taken with food (bind with proteins that softens their bitter, astringent, and/or sour attributes). The misappropriation of dry table wines as an aperitif is a harmless aberration seen primarily in the New World. In Europe, sweet to semisweet wines are used in this situation. In contrast, sparkling wines seem ideally suited to their standard role as a celebratory aperitif. Attempts by the champagne industry to convince consumers that sparkling wines combine well with most meals seem doomed to failure.

Although dry fortified sherries can also act as ideal aperitifs, most fortified wines are decidedly sweet. Correspondingly, they are generally taken after meals and occasionally substitute for dessert. The high alcohol content, pronounced flavors, and partially oxidized character provide them with an ability to retain their character for weeks or months after opening. This is desirable because their intense character generally means that only part of a bottle is consumed upon opening.

Brandies are even more resistant to spoilage or character loss than fortified wines. They are taken in even smaller quantities, often being more sniffed than drunk.

## SUGGESTED READINGS

Amerine MA, HW Berg, RE Kunkee, CS Ough, VL Singleton, and AD Webb (1980). *The technology of wine making.* Westport, CT: Avi.

Amerine MA and VL Singleton (1977). *Wine—An introduction.* Berkeley: University of California Press.

Dutruc-Rosset G (2000). The state of vitiviniculture in the world and the statistical information in 1998. *Bulletin O.I.V.* 73:1-94.

Jackson RS (2000). *Wine science: Principles, practice, perception,* Second edition. San Diego, CA: Academic Press.

Jackson RS (2002). *Wine tasting: A professional handbook.* London: Academic Press.

Johnson H and J Halliday (1992). *The vintner's art.* New York: Simon and Schuster.

Office International de la Vigne et du Vin (OIV) (1991). The world viticultural situation in 1990. *Bulletin O.I.V.* 64:894-954.

van den Berg F and H Maarse (1993). Brandy and cognac—Brandy and its manufacture. In *Encyclopedia of food science, food technology and nutrition,* Macrae, R Robinson and M Sadler (eds.). London: Academic Press, pp. 450-453.

# Malted Barley, Scotch Whiskey, and Beer

## G. H. Palmer

## *INTRODUCTION*

Malt is the product of germinated cereals (Figure III.8). Barley is hard, while malt is soft or friable. Malt contains more enzymes than barley. Barley malt can be described as either "green" or kilned. Green malt is not dried and can contain about 40 to 45 percent moisture; kilned malt is dried and can have a moisture content of about 5 percent. Green malt contains more enzymes than kilned malts. Different temperatures (60 to 230°C) can be used to produce malts of different moistures and colors. Although any cereal grain can be malted, barley is the preferred cereal for making the malts.

### *Scotch Whiskey and Beer*

Malted barley has been found in ancient Egypt. The samples found were about 3,000 years old. Herodotus (450 B.C.) mentioned images of the goddess Isis brewing with barley that date to 1960 B.C. Although barley malt was used in ancient Egypt to make beer, sorghum and millet malts were used in other parts of Africa to make a particulate brew called opaque beer.

The beginning of Scotch whiskey is lost in antiquity. However, in 1494 the Exchequer Roll of Scotland recorded that "eight bolls of malt" were required by Friar John Cor, "wherein to make aqua vitae." Present law dictates that only malted barley can be used to make Scotch malt whiskey. Scotch grain whiskey can be made using about 80 to 90 percent unmalted types of grain, e.g., maize or wheat, and 10 to 20 percent of malt. The malt figure is not fixed, but no extraneous enzymes can be added to the process to assist sugar production from the cereals used. The small quantities of malt added must effect the conversion of a very large quantity of starch into sugars. If extraneous enzymes are used, the grain spirit cannot be called Scotch but can be used to produce gin or vodka spirits.

Today, of the 70,000,000 cases of Scotch whiskey sold worldwide, 95 percent are blended whiskeys and 5 percent are malt whiskeys. United Distillers are the largest producers at about 23.6 million cases per year. Present Scotch whiskey sales per region are as follows: Europe 40 percent, Asia 16

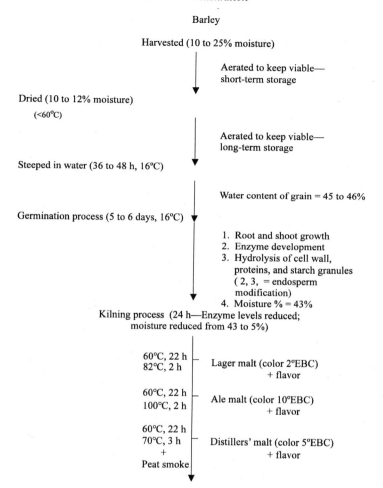

FIGURE III.8. Malting process (including handling of barley)

percent, North America 14 percent, Latin America 14 percent, United Kingdom 11 percent, duty free 2.5 percent, and Africa 2.5 percent. However, beer is the more popular drink. Beer consumption in Europe and the Americas is about 460 and 480 million hectoliters, respectively. Although the figures for Asia and the Pacific are about 390 million hectoliters, it is projected that this figure will exceed that of Europe or the Americas by 2010. Africa and the Middle East have the lowest consumption figure of about 70 million hectoliters per year. To put these production figures into company perspective, Anheuser-Busch is, by far, the largest brewing company in the world, producing about 170 million hectoliters of beer per year. About 77 percent of this volume is produced in the United States. In contrast, malt sales worldwide constitute about 14 million tonnes. The largest malting company in the world is Cargill, producing about 1,300,000 tonnes of malt each year. However, three other malting companies each produce over 1,000,000 tonnes, per year. About 51 percent of malt is produced in Europe, 21 percent in North America, 16 percent in Asia and Africa, 6 percent in South America, and 4 percent in Australia. Of the total production of malt, brewing takes 94 percent, distilling about 4 percent, and 2 percent is used for the production of biscuits, cakes, bread, beverages, and special foods. Except in countries such as Germany where the Reinheitsgebot is applied strictly to the production of beer for local consumption, malt, unmalted cereals, sugars, and syrups are the ingredients of over 80 percent of the beers produced in the world. Of these ingredients, malted barley is the major raw material.

## MALT PRODUCTION

There are two kinds of malting barleys, *Hordeum distichon* and *Hordeum vulgare*. The former has a two-rowed ear of grains, while the latter has a six-rowed ear of grains. Two-rowed and six-rowed barleys may be spring or winter. This means that spring barleys are planted in the spring (March) and winter barleys are planted in the winter (September). In terms of brewing and distilling preferences, two-rowed spring and winter barleys are preferred. In the United Kingdom, malting barleys are given quality ratings: grade 1 is poorest and grade 9 is the best. Quality ratings are based on the rate of extract development during malting, disease resistance, and factors that promote grain yield such as standing power of the plant in the field. All malting barleys are named and are morphologically distinct. It takes about ten years to breed a new malting barley. To date, no genetically modified cereals are knowingly used in the production of beer or Scotch whiskey.

The hot water extract is the most important component of malted barley and is linked to alcohol production and yeast nutrition. Malt extract can vary between 75 and 82 percent for "standard malts." Malt extract is composed mainly of partly degraded starch, sugars derived from amylolytic degradation of starch, large molecular weight soluble proteins, polypeptides, peptides and amino acids, minerals, vitamin B, and hydrolytic enzymes. The malting process is designed to cause enzymic solubilization of the starch, protein, and cell wall food reserves of the starchy endosperm.

# THE MALTING PROCESS

## Steeping, Germination, Kilning

Barley of the desired quality is selected based on variety, malting grade, soundness of structure, grain size, and germination potential. Pregerminated or heat-damaged grains, or grains infected by pests or microorganisms that develop in storage, are unacceptable. Fungal infection can produce mycotoxins. *Fusarium* is especially unacceptable because it is regarded as being responsible for the production of deoxynivalenol (DON), which is involved in gushing or fobbing of beer. DON levels in barley are assessed by appropriate testing kits. Microbial material is reduced in the grain during steeping. Formaldehyde at low concentrations (0.1 ppm) in the steep water can reduce microbial infection but is a banned chemical. Calcium hydroxide at low concentrations in the steep will extract polyphenols from the malt, thereby reducing the astringency of the beer. Limited steeping can leave an excess of polyphenols in the grain, which can contribute to beer astringency and beer haze. Malting barley is expected to germinate to about 98 percent in specific tests of the Institute and Guild of Brewing (London), European Brewery Convention (EBC) (Continental Europe), or American Society of Brewing Chemists (United States). The production capacities of malting plants vary from about 25 tonnes to about 500 tonnes per batch and, as described in the following sections, contain storage, drying, steeping, germination, and kilning units. The malting process is set out in Figure III.8.

## Enzyme Development

The physiological mechanisms of malt modification and extract development have been studied in great detail. Vigorous steeping washes the grain and encourages it to germinate. The germinated grain produces the plant hormone gibberellic acid, which is transported from the embryo to the aleurone layer. This transport is primarily to the dorsal surface of the grain. As a result, more endosperm-degrading enzymes are produced on the dorsal side of the malting grain, causing the pattern of enzymic modification of the endosperm to be asymmetric. Gibberellic acid stimulates the aleurone to produce enzymes such as $\alpha$-amylase, limit dextrinase, endo-$\beta$-1,3-1,4-glucanase, endoprotease, and pentosanases. Other enzymes develop, in the absence of gibberellic acid, in the aleurone layer and the starchy endosperm. These enzymes assist in the hydrolysis and release of other endosperm substrates. They are $\beta$-glucan solubilase, endo-$\beta$-1,3-glucanase, $\beta$-amylase, carboxypeptidase, lipase, and phytase. During malting, the solubilase and endo-$\beta$-13-glucanases release nonstarch polysaccharide materials, such as $\beta$-glucans, from the endosperm cell walls. These $\beta$-glucans are broken down by the endo-$\beta$-1,3-1,4-glucanases. Pentosanase attack on the endosperm cell walls is limited. The endoproteases hydrolyze and solubilize proteins, and the carboxypeptidases release amino acids, described analytically as $\alpha$-amino nitrogen or free amino nitrogen. Starch degradation is limited during malting and is effected by $\alpha$-amylase.

### Endosperm Modification

Ideally, during malting, about 90 percent of the endosperm cell wall should be degraded and about 40 percent of the proteins should be solubilized. About 10 percent of the starch (mainly small starch granules) is degraded and contributes to what is described as malting loss. In general, the action of these enzymes should release optimal hot water extract from the mashed malt. If the protein content of the barley is high (e.g., 2.0 percent nitrogen), then a lower starch extract will be achieved than if the nitrogen of the barley was 1.7 percent. Extracts, which have high levels of fermentable sugars and high levels of $\alpha$-amino nitrogen, are best derived from malting barleys that have about 1.5 percent to 1.6 percent nitrogen. There is a general principle that the higher the barley nitrogen, the lower the (starch) extract. Recent studies suggest that injudicious blending of barley or malt of different proteins and modifications can cause mashhouse and beer filtration problems, which are linked to inadequate enzymic breakdown of $\beta$-glucans and proteins. Because enzyme levels of malt are not correlated with endosperm modification, it would seem that the structure of the starchy endosperm might retard or encourage enzymic action in the endosperm during malting. Steeliness (high nitrogen) and mealiness (low nitrogen) are examples of these kinds of structural differences. Limited proteolysis during malting is associated with limited breakdown of $\beta$-glucan during malting. Protein breakdown during malting is therefore important for malt modification and extract development. The production of amino acids is important for yeast performance during fermentation. However, excessive proteolysis can destroy the potential of beers to form foam. The control of proteolysis during malting and mashing is therefore very important.

During malting and brewing, malt-derived fatty acids can be oxidized by lipoxygenases or oxygen to produce flavor compounds such as aldehydes, ketones, organic acid, and alcohols. Some aldehydes, such as *trans*-2-nonenal, are associated with the staling of beer. Amino acids react with sugars, especially during kilning, to produce melanoidin compounds. Reductones are also formed. These reductones can produce furans, pyrroles, thiophenes, and pyrazines. Reductones can act as antioxidants, thereby limiting the oxidation of lipids by oxygen. Many of these reactions combine to give color to the malt and help to form its distinctive nutty, roasted, malty flavor. Temperature effects during kilning reduce the levels of enzymes such as β-amylase, endoprotease, limit dextrinase, and endo-β-1,3-1,4-glucanase. These enzymes are particularly sensitive to heat, and a significant amount of their activities are lost during kilning.

### Distiller's and Brewer's Malts

Distiller's malts differ from brewer's malts in many ways. Both types of malts are analyzed by the recommended methods referred to previously. Kilned distiller's malts are subjected to additional analyses such as fermentable extract, fermentability, sulfur dioxide, and spirit yield. Friability is a physical test of malt modification. Friability results below 90 percent mean that some troublesome undermodification could exist in the malt sample. Modification is caused by enzyme hydrolysis of endosperm substrates during malting. A well-modified malt gives optimal brewer's extract. Extract is determined, as described by the Institute of Brewing Methods, by extracting a fixed amount of milled malt (50 g) in a specified volume of hot water (e.g., 515 ml, 65°C) for one hour. Some extract determinations are carried out at two temperatures, 45°C and then 65°C, over a period of two hours. Factors that influence enzymic modification of the endosperm and promote extract development are barley variety, aleurone activity, cell wall structure, total nitrogen, corn size, and duration of malting and mashing conditions. Gibberellic acid can be added to the malting grain to increase enzyme production, which accelerates endosperm modification and extract development. In the past, the barley abrasion process was used extensively in the United Kingdom. It was developed to accelerate enzymic modification of the endosperm and to improve the rate of extract development. Abrasion deliberately damaged the pericarp and allowed gibberellic acid to enter the distal nonembryo end of the grain. The activation of the distal parts of the aleurone layer, at the beginning of malting, caused the grain to malt from both ends simultaneously. This process showed that *uniform* production of endosperm-degrading enzymes is an important aspect of malting quality. Gibberellic acid is applied at very low concentrations (0.1 to 0.25 ppm). It is used worldwide, but because of legal requirements, it is not used in the production of distiller's malt or malts made in Germany for the production of beers consumed locally.

In addition to the three kinds of malts shown in Figure III.8, there are also special malts. These malts contain no enzymes and have strong or dark colors because they are kilned only at high temperatures, >80 to 230°C. These malts or their extracts are used mainly in brewing to add color and flavor. Barley malt contains about 3 percent lipids, mainly in the embryo and aleurone layer. During malting, lipids are hydrolyzed to give fatty acids. Some of these fatty acids are unsaturated and can become oxidized during the brewing and distilling processes. In brewing, the products of fatty acid oxidation can cause accelerated staling of beer. Phytin is present in the aleurone layer of barley and barley malt. It is hydrolyzed during malting by phytases, which develop in the aleurone layer. A wide range of phytin-derived compounds are extracted from barley malt during the mashing operation. These compounds range from inositol to intermediate inositol phosphate compounds to phosphates. Released phosphates react with calcium compounds present in the mash to form calcium phosphate. The resulting increase in hydrogen ions acts to maintain the mash pH at about 5.2. This pH is buffered by the amino acids of the extracted malt. Collectively, the enzymes of the malt work well at this pH. The carcinogenic compound nitrosodimethylamine (NDMA) can be produced during kilning from the reaction between nitrogen oxides and hordenine of the embryo of malting barley. Burning of sulfur can control this reaction during kilning. Indirect kilning, in which exhaust gases are not passed through the malt, can also reduce the development of NDMA.

## MALT SPIRIT AND GRAIN SPIRIT PRODUCTION

### Milling and Mashing

Malt is milled mainly in four-roll mills for malt whiskey production. The grist (flour) is mashed with soft water (low in bicarbonates) at 63 to 64°C. Liquor:grist ratio is about 4:1. There are two types of starch granules in barley malt, large (25 µm) and small (1 to 5 µm). The small starch granules are only 10 percent of the total weight of starch granules in the starchy endosperm. During malting, about 50 percent of the small starch granules are degraded by α-amylase. Mashing is carried out mainly in infusion vessels which have deep grist beds (ca 5 feet). Wort is separated (run off) by gravity flow. In some modern vessels rakes are present. These deep bed infusion vessels are called semi-lauters. Rakes are used to cut the mash bed to assist wort separation. During mashing, the large starch granules, which constitute 90 percent of the starch in the grain, are gelatinized at about 62°C. The gelatinized starch is hydrolyzed to sugars and dextrins by the combined actions of α-amylase and β-amylase. Limit dextrinase is associated with an inhibitor and has very limited activity during mashing. β-Amylase is responsible for most of the maltose produced. Proteins are hydrolyzed to produce more polypeptides, peptides, and α-amino nitrogen. About 70 percent of the protein products found in the extracted wort were produced during the malting process. Vitamins (e.g., B vitamins) and minerals (e.g., potassium, phosphate, magnesium) are also extracted into the wort. This "first" wort is run off after a mashing period of one to two hours. The mash bed is then washed two or three times with water at 70°C, 80°C, and 90°C. The sugary worts from the 63 to 64°C mash and 70°C and 80°C mash bed washings are pooled to give a wort (wash) of specific gravity 1.060 (ca 15 percent sugar). The weak wort from the 90°C washing contains very little sugar and is used to restart the mashing process at 63 to 64°C.

The sugar composition of distiller's malt worts is in the order of fructose 1 percent, glucose 10 percent, maltose 46 percent, maltotriose 15 percent, maltotetraose 10 percent, sucrose 5 percent, and dextrins 13 percent. Levels of free amino acids range from 250 to 300 mg/l and constitute 25 percent of the soluble proteins. Minerals include potassium (550 mg/l), phosphate (500 mg/l), and magnesium (100 mg/l). Organic acids include citrate (170 mg/l), malate (60 mg/l), and pyruvate (8 mg/l). Important trace elements such as zinc (0.15 mg/l) and manganese (0.15 mg/l) are also present. The total fatty acids in the wort, from the 3 to 3.5 percent lipids originally present in the malt, are only about 10 mg/l.

In contrast, the production of the worts in grain distilleries involves the hammermilling of malt and then similar milling of wheat or maize to produce a flourlike grist. This nonmalt grist is cooked at 105°C. The cooking temperature is about 145°C if the grains are not milled. The cooked cereals are cooled, and then the milled malt is added to produce a mash at about 63°C. Green malt (milled by attrition milling) or kilned malt is used at 9 to 10 percent of the total grist. Some grain whiskey distillers use larger quantities of malted barley. The mash tun for malt whiskey production usually holds about 8 to 10 tonnes of malt. The grain distiller's mash can hold as much as 16 to 18 tonnes of grain and malt grist. Grain whiskey worts (washes) are extracted in a similar manner to malt whiskey worts. Sugar compositions of the worts are similar, but the α-amino nitrogen levels are much lower, at about 110 to 120 mg/l. The higher level of carbohydrate (starch) materials may encourage the yeast to produce high levels of fusel oils (higher alcohols), which are later reduced in quantity (as feints) during distillation.

## Fermentation

Malt whiskey and grain whiskey worts (washes) are cooled to about 20°C. These are transferred to separate fermenters. Yeast is often added as a slurry. Brewer's and special distiller's ($M_3$) yeasts are used together at about $20 \times 10^6$ cells per ml, which starts to ferment worts, which are about 86 percent fermentable. After about 48 hours, the fermentation is completed and 7 to 8 percent of alcohol is produced. During this period the temperature has increased from about 20°C to about 30°C. During fermentation the activities of lactic acid and acetic acid bacteria are kept to a minimum because they can reduce alcohol production. Lactic acid bacteria may add flavor compounds, some unacceptable, to the wort (wash). However, the main regulator of alcohol production and flavor is the actively growing yeast. Sugars and amino acids are absorbed in sequence because of yeast's permease regulatory system. The carbon dioxide from the fermenters of grain distilleries is collected, purified, and sold primarily to the brewing and soft drink industries.

## Distillation

The fermented wort (wash) from an all-malt mash, for malt whiskey production, is transferred to an onion-shaped copper wash (pot) still. The wash is boiled and a 20 percent alcohol condensate is collected. This condensate is transferred to an onion-shaped copper spirit (pot) still. The early condensate (fore shots) and the late condensate (feints) are collected and redistilled. The middle condensate (or cut) of about 68 percent alcohol is collected. This condensate is the Scotch whiskey spirit and is diluted to 63.5 percent alcohol and matured in oak barrels for a *minimum* of three years before it can be called Scotch malt whiskey. It is during maturation that the transformation of Scotch whiskey spirit to Scotch whiskey takes place. All malt distilleries contain pairs of wash and spirit stills. Both stills are made of copper and are unique in terms of shape, size, and reflux properties. Therefore, each pair of stills will produce a whiskey that is unique. Every malt distillery has a unique pair of stills and therefore produces a unique whiskey. It is worth noting that during boiling in the wash still, proteins from undermodified malts can cause "burning on" which reduces the efficiency of the still. Therefore, even after malting and mashing, malt modification is important.

The Coffey still, for grain spirit production, also contains internal sections of copper. Copper is critical for Scotch whiskey production. It reduces the content of sulfur compounds and ensures that the spirit is clear. Scotch malt whiskey spirit is usually double distilled. However, in a few distilleries a triple distillation process is used. The distillation of the fermented wash, in a grain distillery, is carried out in a Coffey still. The Coffey still is comprised of rectifier and analyzer columns. The fermented wash (wort) of 7 to 8 percent alcohol is piped into the rectifier and heated. It is then transferred to the analyzer where it is moved down against a flow of steam that pushes off alcohol and other volatile compounds. These are returned to the rectifier where higher alcohols (feints) are removed and sold to the perfume industry. The grain spirit is taken off higher up the column at the spirit plate at, by law, no more than 94.8 percent alcohol. The grain spirit is also diluted to 63.5 percent and is matured in oak barrels for a minimum of three years. Grain spirits contain lower-level flavor compounds than malt spirits but carry distinct flavors that are important in blending operations. During the distillation process, ethylcarbamate can be produced. This compound, like nitrosamines, is found in minute quantities of parts per billion but is regarded as unacceptable because of possible carcinogenic properties. Control of this compound is effected by selecting barley varieties that have very low precursor levels.

### *Maturation*

Maturation of Scotch whiskey reduces the initial pungency of the product and determines the age claim found on bottles of Scotch whiskeys. The age claim relates to the youngest age of the different whiskeys in the bottle. Therefore, a bottle of blended Scotch may have as many as forty whiskeys in the blend. However, although some of these whiskeys may be 30 years old, if the "youngest" of the whiskeys is ten years old, then the bottle must be labeled ten years old or no age claim can be made. During maturation, the inner burned carbon surface of the barrel absorbs unpleasant sulfides and aldehydes but releases pleasant sugars, tannins, vanillin (from burned lignin), sherry flavor, and lactones. As the maturation proceeds, a 2 percent loss (the angels' share) of alcoholic materials from the barrel occurs. Thus, a 12-year-old whiskey, starting at 63.5 percent alcohol at the beginning of maturation, may have only 58 percent alcohol at the end of maturation. After maturation the whiskeys are "vatted" (malt whiskeys) or blended (malt and grain whiskeys) before filtering cold, then diluted to 40 or 43 percent alcohol before bottling. The only permitted additive to Scotch whiskey is alcohol caramel which, *if required*, can be used to ensure that a particular brand of whiskey is of the expected color. Color is derived naturally from the barrels.

American bourbon barrels are used only once (by law) to mature bourbon before they are used to mature Scotch malt whiskey spirit. Spanish sherry barrels are also used. Sizes are limited by law. Maximum barrel size permitted is 700 liters. First-fill barrels impart greater color and flavor than second-, third-, or fourth-fill barrels. Although Scotch whiskey can be made only in Scotland, Scotch whiskey can be sent abroad for blending with other spirits, but the final product cannot be called Scotch whiskey. Many whiskey enthusiasts now buy Scotch whiskey at full strength (58 to 60 percent alcohol), unfiltered from the barrel. Such whiskeys can form a white haze when water is added. Scotch whiskey ages in the barrel. The time the whiskey spends in its bottle does not add age to the whiskey. It is an established tradition that water added to Scotch whiskey increases its aroma. This style of drinking or nosing helps to distinguish between different brands of Scotch whiskeys. However, if preferred, any other drinks (such as soda or cola) or other materials (such as ice) can be added to Scotch whiskeys.

### Generic Types of Scotch Whiskeys

In general, each malt distillery (there are about 90 malt distilleries) produces an average of about two million liters of malt whiskey spirit each year. In contrast, there are about six grain distilleries, each producing an average of about 30 million liters of alcohol per year. A *single malt* whiskey is produced in one distillery. A *pure malt* whiskey can be a single malt or a mixture of malt whiskeys. Here, pure means *of one kind.* All blended whiskeys contain a wide range of complementing malt whiskeys and specific quantities of selected grain whiskeys. In marketing terms, the word pure cannot be used with blended whiskeys because blends contain two kinds of whiskeys, *pure single malt whiskeys* and *pure grain whiskeys.* Pure is a description of type and does not relate to quality or preference. Quality means that the product meets the expectations and approval (in terms of repeat sales) of the customer.

## BEER PRODUCTION

### Mashing

Beers in Nigeria are being made using mainly unmalted sorghum and maize grains, and low-malt beers are selling well in Kenya and Japan *(happoshu).* In the absence of malt, yeast food and/or proteolytic enzymes are required to provide yeast with the nutrients it needs to ferment to expectations. Although German beers and some Greek, Dutch, and Austrian beers are made using 100 percent malted barley, most beers in the world are made from an average of about 80 percent malt. Cereals are added to the mash tun, and sugars and syrups are added to the wort kettle where hops are boiled.

The unmalted cereals used are mainly maize, rice, barley, wheat, and sorghum. Sugars (sucrose) are derived from sugarcane and sugar beet plants, and syrups are made mainly from enzyme hydrolyzed starches of maize or wheat. The starches of maize, rice, and sorghum gelatinize above 70°C, and because mashing (starch conversion) is usually carried out at about 63 to 65°C, small endosperm pieces of these cereals are cooked at about 100°C. About 5 percent of malt or heat-stable industrial amylases are added to liquefy starch during the cooking operation. Like in the grain distilling process, the cooked starch materials are cooled and then mashed with malt at 63 to 65°C. The main starches of wheat and barley gelatinize at about 58°C and 62°C, respectively.

Specialized "precooked" adjuncts can be prepared from wheat, barley, maize, or rice. These are called torrefied or micronized grains or flaked cereal products. These products are more soluble than malt because the starch is gelatinized. During production, whole wheat, barley, or rice grains or endosperm pieces of maize are heated or micronized (at 140°C) to gelatinize starches. These heated products are then rolled into flakes or left as popcorn-like grains. Torrefied, micronized, or flaked cereals do not require cooking. Torrefied or micronized grains are milled with malt. Flaked cereals are added directly to the mash tun.

In all-malt mashes, the malt is milled and mashed and the operation is similar to that described for all-malt distiller's mashes. Brewing liquor should be low in bicarbonates (temporary hardness) to reduce a drift toward alkalinity of the wort. Alkaline worts can extract polyphenols from the grist and increase astringency in derived beers. Added or natural calcium sulfate (gypsum) confers permanent hardness to the brewing liquor and contributes to the pleasant slaking effect of the beer. Calcium stabilizes $\alpha$-amylase and reacts with phosphate to help produce a wort pH of about 5.2.

Brewing mashing systems are more varied and more complex than mashing systems used by distillers. Both brewers and distillers use the traditional (British) infusion (deep grist-bed) mashing systems, in which the malt is mashed and the wort is run off (separated) from a single large vessel. Brewers also use decoction (continental) mashing systems in which the grist of all-malt or malt and cooked adjuncts are mixed and then specific quantities are removed, boiled, and returned to the original vessel during the mashing period. This process helps to gelatinize starch and to raise the mashing temperature from 45°C or 55°C (proteolytic rests) to about 64°C, the temperature at which starch conversion occurs. Extra protein breakdown occurs during the "protein rest" at 45 to 55°C.

After mashing, the entire mash is transferred to a filter vessel, called a lauter tun, which has a thinner filtration bed (ca 18 inches) than the infusion system, and filters faster. The alternative mashing system to the decoction system is the programmed mashing system in which temperature changes during mashing are similar to those in the decoction system but are effected by internal heating systems. Separation of the wort is also effected by a separate lauter system. Unlike the infusion system which combines mashing and filtration, the lauter system is a dedicated wort separation system and has rakes to assist wort separation. Recently, lauter tun systems are being replaced, in some breweries, by the mash filter system. After mashing, the entire mash is placed into a multichamber/membrane filter system. The mash-filter bed is thinner (ca 4 inches) than the corresponding bed of the lauter tun. Filtration is faster and extract yield is higher, but undermodified cell walls and proteins from malts or cooked cereals can impede filtration. Sometimes external β-glucanases are added to facilitate filtration (wort separation). In general, as the milled grist gets finer as a result of milling in four-roll, six-roll, or hammer mills, the mash bed gets thinner and filters faster. These changes follow Darcy's filtration equation. However, it should not be overlooked that mash beds are compressible and that undermodified cell walls are sticky and can block mash beds irrespective of the viscosity of the wort, particle size, and bed depth.

In brewing mashing systems, hot water is used at the end of the mashing to sparge (wash) the mash bed (at about 75 to 80°C) to ensure that all sugars and amino acids produced during mashing are extracted into the worts. Malt enzymes are very heat labile, and some brewers add commercial enzymes such as endo-β-glucanase, α-amylase, and neutral proteases to carry out the mashing process (where mainly cereal adjuncts are being used) or to facilitate it (where a combination of malt and adjuncts are being mashed). The small starch granules gelatinize in the mash at a higher temperature (80°C) than large starch granules (62°C) and may release starch into the wort during sparging at temperatures which approach 80°C. At this temperature amylolytic enzymes are no longer active. Such starch materials can cause haze in beers. The spent cereal residues of brewer's mash tun, distiller's mash tun, wash stills, and Coffey stills are usually sold as wet products or processed into dried animal feed. Undergraded β-glucans in the spent grains from the mash can limit dewatering and drying during animal feed production. These feeds can have high yeast and copper content and may not be suitable for certain animals.

## Hops

After mashing, brewer's worts (at about 1.050 specific gravity) are boiled with hops. Boiling converts α-acids of hops into iso-α-acids. The iso-α-acids are bitter. Other bittering compounds (oxidized β-acids) and flavorsome hop essential oils are also extracted during wort boiling. Some hops of high aroma characteristics can have low bittering potential. The converse can also occur. $\alpha$-Acids, $\beta$-acids, and essential oils are extracted during wort boiling or by chemical solvents or liquid carbon dioxide from yellow lupulin glands located on bracteoles of the hop cone. Pellitized hop cones and isomerized hop extracts are now in popular use. Specific reactions between certain hop compounds (tetrahydro-iso-$\alpha$-acids or $\beta$-acids) and hydrophobic proteins in the beer can improve foam potential. Boiling also concentrates the wort, removes unwanted flavor compounds, develops beer color, coagulates proteins that may form haze, inactivates enzymes, and sterilizes the wort. Isomerized hop extracts are also used to bitter beer. When beer is exposed to sunlight a mercaptan flavor develops because of changes to the isomerized bitter compounds in beer. Brown bottles can reduce this deleterious effect. Sunlight-insensitive (i.e., reduced iso-$\alpha$-acid) compounds of hops can eliminate this effect. Before the use of hops for bittering, the barks of various trees, fruits, herbs, and seeds were used as bittering compounds. In 1700 the English parliament decreed that only hops should be used as bittering compound in beer. Curiously enough, one major distinction between ale and continental beer in the fifteenth and sixteenth centuries was that ale was made without hops.

The percentage fermentability of brewer's worts is about 75 percent, which is lower than that of distiller's worts (86 percent), because boiling inactivates malt enzymes from brewer's mashes that continue to produce sugars during distiller's fermentation. Some brewers ferment at low gravities (e.g., 1.050 or 1.048 = 12° Plato). Others ferment at higher gravities and dilute the beer with low-oxygen water before packaging. However, beers fermented at high malt content and gravities and diluted do not always match similar products produced at lower gravities. High percentages of malt (or low percentages of carbohydrate) tend to give high levels of esters. The components responsible for this effect are not known. Conversely, low contents of malt in the grist can result in beers that have low ester levels. Worts can be concentrated by evaporations to produce malt syrups containing 80 percent solid material. Such malt syrups can be added to the wort kettle to increase the malt component of the wort. In general, malt syrups are popular in both the food and brewing industries and, among other uses, they can be added to the worts of high-adjunct mashes as a substitute for malt.

### Maturation and Filtration

After wort boiling, the wort is cooled. Precipitated proteins and spent hop material are removed by whirlpool separation or centrifugation. Lager yeast *(Saccharomyces carlsbergensis)* or ale yeast *(Saccharomyces cerevisiae)* is added at about $10^7$ cells per ml, depending on the type of beer being made. After primary fermentation (ca 5 days) at different temperatures (<10°C lager; >10°C ales) most of the yeast is removed. A wort of specific gravity of 1.050 can produce a beer of about 5 percent alcohol. Brewer's yeast usually has a high viability at the end of fermentation and can be reused or sold to distillers. Ale yeast is suitable for distilling. Lager yeast is unsuitable because off-flavors are produced. In marked contrast, distiller's yeast is almost inviable after fermentation and is destroyed in the stills. New fermentations in every distillery require new yeast. During brewing and distilling fermentations, the pH levels fall from about 5.2 to about 4. Beer pH is therefore acidic and will not support the successful development of pathogenic bacteria.

Beers can be conditioned (stored) at low temperatures (5 to 8°C) and can be fined to remove excess yeast and proteins. Fined beer is clearer than unfined beer but still contains small residues of yeast. Isinglass is a popular fining. It is produced from the swim bladders of certain saltwater fishes. In contrast, finings used in the wort kettle to assist protein precipitation are derived from Irish moss (carragheen). Beers, especially lagers, are matured for weeks at low temperatures (−1° to −2°C). During maturation polyphenols react with proteins to further clarify the beer (lagering). Papain is a protease that reduces the haze effects of proteins. Silica gel and tannins can be added to eliminate the involvement of proteins in haze formation by precipitating them. Chill haze is haze that forms when the beer is chilled but disappears when it is warmed. Permanent haze does not disappear when the beer is warmed. Sugar/syrup adjuncts are usually added to the copper during the boiling of the hops. However, priming sugars (50 percent fructose plus 50 percent glucose—similar to hydrolyzed sucrose) or partly fermented worts (krausened) can be added during conditioning to assist secondary fermentation or later to increase sweetness of the beer. Proteins precipitated by tannins or silica gels are removed from beers during filtration or centrifugation. Excess polyphenols, from hops or malt, that could cause further protein precipitation in packaged beer and cause haze are removed prior to beer filtration by adding polyvinylpyrrolidone (PVPP). Polyphenols derived from hops are called tannins; those from malt are called anthocyanogens. In some ales, hop cones or hop oil extracts are added to barrels of beer to add an aromatic "dry hop" character. Conditioning and maturation are used not only to clarify the beer prior to filtration but also to improve stability (shelf life), flavor, and aroma potentials of beers. Maturation in oak barrels during distilling is also carried out to improve the flavor potentials of Scotch whiskeys.

Undergraded β-glucans from undermodified malts, which can cause wort separation problems in the mash tun and slow down beer filtration, can, like starch residues, contribute to nonbiological hazes of packaged beers.

Incidentally, biological hazes can be caused by wild yeasts or bacteria. Wild yeasts do not flocculate readily and will produce off-flavors. Some wild yeast will use lysine to grow; brewing yeasts will not grow on this essential amino acid. The β-glucan-related hazes can be controlled by either improving malt modification or applying commercial β-glucanases. Kieselguhr (diatomaceous earth) is dosed into beers to facilitate beer filtration. The clarified beer is packaged at the appropriate levels of dissolved oxygen and carbon dioxide. Nitrogen can be used in ales and stouts to form a more stable foam. Beer is usually sold either in barrels, after fining, in an unfiltered, unpasteurized (conditioned) form or in filtered pasteurized forms, in barrels, bottles, cans, or kegs. Beer and Scotch whiskey are quality-branded products that endeavor to meet the expectations of the customer. Quality is a very important part of product image, where quality can be defined as meeting the expectations of the customer.

### Beer Flavor

This general outline of the malting process and allied processes of distilling and brewing show that malted barley is still the primary raw material used in the production of Scotch whiskey and beer. It provides yeast not only with general nutrients such as sugars, from which alcohol is produced, but also with essential nutrients such as amino acids, minerals, and vitamins, which allow the yeast to form complexes of flavors described as, e.g., estery, alcoholic, musty, sour, acidic, spicy, phenolic, oily, sulfury, fatty, grassy, floral, fruity, roasted, smokey, malty, nutty, dry, sweet, astringent, stale, and fresh. Flavors and aromas in beers and Scotch whiskeys are experienced together by the customer and defy meaningful chemical analyses. It would therefore be unwise to change the "expected" sensation of flavors and aromas of a successful brand of Scotch whiskey or beer. Lagers are lighter in color than ales because ales are made from more highly kilned malts. Associated with this higher color are reductones, which enable ales to be more stable, in terms of oxidation and staling, than lagers.

As is the case for Scotch whiskey, caramel compounds are sometimes used to achieve the desired color of dark beers. Lagers usually contain distinct compounds such as dimethyl sulfide (DMS). The latter is derived from the malt precursor, $S$-methylmethionine, which develops during malting and kilning. Lagers tend to have lower sugar contents than ales because of more extensive secondary fermentation and maturation. Pilsner-type lagers usually have a dry taste combined with higher bitterness than corresponding lager beers. Ales usually have lower carbonation and higher levels of salts, such as calcium sulfate. Combined with these differences are the different flavors, aromas, and bitterness values imparted by different hops and different wort boiling regimes. Special malts of a wide range of colors (e.g., 15 to 1500°EBC) can be used instead of caramel in beer to increase color, add flavor, and make very dark beers, such as stouts. Roasted barley is used in some beers and stouts. Despite the virtues of pure all-malt beers or Scotch malt whiskeys, it should not be overlooked that the "lighter" products, such as blended Scotch whiskeys and part-malt beers, dominate the market worldwide. In this regard, it would appear that *flavor balance* is a more important aspect of drinkability than flavor optima. Two of the primary benefits derived from using unmalted adjuncts are that malt/adjunct beers exhibit subtle balances between flavor and aroma and that they have fewer proteins than all-malt beers. This enables them to have greater stability and longer shelf lives.

Cereals, especially barley malt, are natural ingredients of Scotch whiskeys and beers. Niche-market products, such as fruit beers and low alcohol or alcohol-free beers (made by limited fermentation or alcohol removal), will expand but are unlikely to dominate a market led by lagers, ales, and stouts. A better understanding of the science of these raw materials will improve processing technology in the grain, malting, brewing, and distilling industries, in which quality has always been maintained by innovative research and development.

## CONCLUSIONS

The ancient technologies of malting, distilling, and brewing are based on the controlled biological function of raw materials such as malted and unmalted cereals, hops, and yeast. Over many centuries these industries have developed, through both trial and error and research, the production techniques required to optimize quality, efficiency, and profitability. In many ways, the success of the malting, distilling, and brewing industries has been based on the concept that quality and efficiency can be sustained only by a sound understanding of the biotechnology principles that control process operations. It is therefore imperative that this successful approach not be damaged by the view, in some quarters, that research is not an essential part of industrial production. The dynamic nature of the raw materials of malting, distilling, and brewing and the changing needs of the customer demand that the knowledge base of these industries continues to develop.

## SUGGESTED READINGS

Bamforth CW (1999). The science and understanding of the flavor stability of beer: A critical assessment. *Brauwelt International* 17:98-110.

Bathgate GN (1989). Cereal science and technology. In *Cereals in Scotch whisky production,* GH Palmer (ed.). Scotland: Aberdeen University Press, p. 243.

Hough JS (1985). *The biochemistry of malting and brewing.* Cambridge: Cambridge University Press.

Jacques KA, TP Lyons, and DR Kelsall (1999). *The alcohol text book,* Third edition. United Kingdom: Nottingham University Press.

Lyons TP (1999). Production of Scotch and Irish whiskies: Their history and evolution. In *The alcohol text book,* Third edition, KA Jacques, TP Lyons, and DR Kelsall (eds.). United Kingdom: Nottingham University Press, p. 137.

Palmer GH (1989). *Cereal science and technology, cereals in malting and brewing.* Scotland: Aberdeen University Press.

Palmer GH (1992). Sorghum—Food, beverage and brewing potentials. *Process Biochemistry* 27:145.

Palmer GH (1997). Scientific review of Scotch malt whiskey. *Ferment* 101:367.

Palmer GH (1999). Achieving homogeneity in malting. In *Proceedings European Brewing Congress, Cannes.* De Bibk br Leider Press, pp. 323-363.

# Thermotolerant and Osmotolerant Yeasts for Alcoholic Fermentation

L. Venkateswar Rao
M. Sridhar

## INTRODUCTION

There has been a considerable upsurge of interest in thermophillic and osmophillic microorganisms because of their potential industrial applications. Yeasts are ubiquitous in nature. Most of the industrially used strains are mesophilic, therefore ethanol production in hot climates is not economically viable. This is largely due to the high energy input required to maintain the temperature of the fermentation process between 25 and 30°C to prevent thermal killing of yeast cells, which reduces the fermentation efficiency.

During ethanol fermentation, about 140.2 calories of heat is released per gram of glucose fermented, although the quantity of heat released varies with different substrates. For example, fermentation of pentoses results in the release of larger quantities of heat than hexoses. This problem becomes more complicated as the substrate concentration increases, which causes a rise in the temperature of the fermentation medium (generally above 40°C) to an extent that it becomes intolerable for growth and activity of yeasts. This results in incomplete fermentation, which generally occurs at temperatures above 35°C (it varies depending on the strain). In some alcohol production industries this overheating problem is partially overcome by spraying cold water on the fermentor walls, which adds to the production costs. In the absence of cooling, heat can be removed from the fermentor in two ways, through walls of the vessels by conduction and radiation or by evaporation caused by evolution of carbon dioxide gas saturated with water. In many fermentations, the rise in temperature is controlled by the use of energy-intensive heat exchangers or by circulating cooling water through coils suspended in the medium.

For cooling water to be effective, the water temperature must be substantially colder than the operating temperature of the fermentor, which adds to the refrigeration costs to cool the water. In large-scale operations, as the size of the fermentor increases, the amount of surface area available for heat transfer per unit volume decreases. This decrease in heat loss necessitates more substantial investments for cooling. Another way to minimize this problem is to operate the fermentor at high temperatures, providing a greater driving force for heat removal and minimizing the cooling costs.

## NEED FOR THERMOTOLERANT AND OSMOTOLERANT YEASTS IN THE ETHANOL INDUSTRY

One key objective in any fermentative process is to reduce energy requirements and production costs. In addition, yeast strains normally used in industrial processes have limited osmotolerance, and for this reason alcohol fermentations are carried out at relatively low sugar concentrations (usually 20 percent w/v or lower). High initial sugar concentration results in loss of sugar transport activity, producing less ethanol. High ethanol productivity and reduced energy demand are the two important aspects of most alcoholic fermentation research. This can be achieved by the use of thermotolerant and osmotolerant yeasts.

Yeasts that grow or ferment at or above 40°C are called thermotolerant yeasts. Thermotolerant yeasts help in decreasing or minimizing distillation and mixing costs and by increasing growth and productivity rates. Osmotolerant and thermotolerant yeasts reduce the risk of contamination and also make product recovery very easy. Thermotolerant yeasts are especially attractive in tropical countries where ambient temperature ranges from 30 to 45°C. They can also be used in leavening process in the baking industry; in addition, they can be used for efficient simultaneous saccharification and fermentation of cellulose by cellulases because the temperature optimum of cellulase enzyme is close to the fermentation temperature of thermotolerant yeasts. In this regard, thermotolerant yeasts would be advantageous in many warmer regions of the world where cooling costs are expensive. This is exemplified by the fact that many of the selections for thermotolerant yeasts have been conducted in countries such as India, South Africa, Cuba, the Philippines, etc. Osmotolerant yeasts can be used for growing and fermenting in high initial sugar concentrations in the preparation of Ayurvedic medicines such as Osavas and Aristas.

In spite of the potential advantages of thermotolerant and osmotolerant yeasts, only few reports have described the successful selection and isolation of thermotolerant and osmotolerant yeasts suitable for ethanol production on a large scale. Although there are some references in the literature to yeasts having the ability to grow at temperatures higher than 40°C, there have been very few reports of yeasts capable of fermenting at these high temperatures. This is mostly due to lack of exploration in this area. There are no true thermophilic yeasts, although some species are definitely more thermotolerant and osmotolerant than others.

## EFFECT OF TEMPERATURE ON THE GROWTH AND FERMENTATION OF YEASTS

The rate of alcohol production increases with temperatures up to 40°C, but the growth coefficient of *Saccharomyces* species increases steadily up to 30°C and then marginally increases up to 36°C. In fact, for most species the optimum temperature for fermentation is shown to be 5 to 10°C higher than that for optimum growth. This is because of the optimum activity of alcohol dehydrogenase at these temperatures. Some yeasts capable of growing at temperatures up to 37°C are often referred to as thermophilic, while others which have a $T_{max}$ of >45°C are sometimes described as being only thermotolerant. Watson and Cavicchoii (1983) define thermophilic yeasts as those that have a minimum temperature for growth of 20°C and no restriction on the maximum temperature for growth. In general, *Saccharomyces* species are less thermotolerant than *Kluyveromyces* and *Candida*. There are some reports on successful selection and isolation of *Kluyveromyces* and *Candida* strains having good thermotolerance, although they have less ethanol tolerance than *Saccharomyces cerevisiae,* which is the industrially used strain for ethanol production.

## MEDIA SUPPLEMENTATION FOR ENHANCED OSMOTOLERANCE AND THERMOTOLERANCE

The optimum temperature for growth and fermentation of thermotolerant and osmotolerant yeasts depends on several factors. Because ethanol toxicity is increased at high temperatures, it seems quite possible that supplementation of the media with skim milk powder, Tween 80, monoolein, unsaturated fatty acids, sterols, inorganic ions, and vitamins increases the fermentation efficiency of thermotolerant yeasts. It was shown that percentage of unsaturated fatty acids in cells supplemented with Tween 80 was 66 percent. Cells supplemented with linoleic acid contained 73 percent of unsaturated fatty acids. By supplementing molasses with potassium, phosphorus, magnesium, and manganese, an increase of 13 to 20 percent alcohol yield was obtained by thermotolerant *Kluyveromyces* sp. at 40°C.

Supplementation of the medium with calcium was found to protect cells against glucose-induced leakage, suggesting the effect of it on cytoplasmic membranes. Recently it was shown that zinc ion was more important in maintaining the structural integrity of yeast alcohol dehydrogenase. By addition of ascorbic acid in the medium, the amount of ethanol produced increased by 2 percent (w/v). The basis for enhanced ethanol production on inclusion of ascorbic acid is unknown.

Addition of fatty acids and sterols increased ethanol production and ethanol tolerance at elevated temperatures. Addition of vegetable oils, linseed oil, and cotton seed oil has stimulated growth and increased both thermotolerance and ethanol tolerance of *Saccharomyces cerevisiae*. They alter the membrane composition and structure in a favorable manner, thereby reducing the harmful effects of high temperature. Because yeasts cannot synthesize unsaturated fatty acids under anaerobic conditions, osmotolerance and thermotolerance could be achieved by supplementation of the media with unsaturated fatty acids such as oleic acid, linoleic acid, palmitic acid, etc. Because high temperatures lower oxygen solubility, it is possible that yeasts require a greater amount of exogenous fatty acids and sterols to grow at elevated temperatures. Enzymes involved in ergosterol synthesis are inhibited at high temperatures; incorporation of media with ergosterol helps in increasing the growth and fermentation at high temperatures. Supplementation of ergosterol or unsaturated sterols in the fermentation medium protects yeast cells against killing by ethanol.

Incorporation of medium with magnesium prolonged exponential growth, resulting in increased yeast cell mass and increased fermentative capacity, possibly because some of the glycolytic enzymes involved in alcoholic fermentations have a requirement for magnesium. Addition of soy flour increased the rate of ethanol production and ethanol yield with *Saccharomyces cerevisiae;* the reason for this may be due to soy flour's abundance of protein (38 percent) and lipid content (28 percent). Supplementation of the medium with fungal mycelium resulted in an increase of ethanol production from 4.9 to 8.3 percent w/v using 25 percent molasses.

## MECHANISM OF OSMOTOLERANCE AND THERMOTOLERANCE

### Heat-Shock Proteins

Heat-shock proteins (HSPs) play an important role in acquisition of thermotolerance and ethanol tolerance in *S. cerevisiae*. Accumulation of denatured proteins in the cell in response to stress caused induction of genes responsible for HSP production. In *S. cerevisiae,* the increased transcription of heat-shock genes following heat shock is mediated by the activation of heat-shock factor (HSF) production.

HSF constitutively binds DNA and undergoes heat-induced phosphorylation with an increase in its transcriptional activity. HSP-104, HSP-90, HSP-70, and HSP-26 are the major heat-shock proteins produced in *S. cerevisiae*. These HSPs, which function as molecular chaperons, play an important role in protein biosynthesis, specifically in the transport, translocation, and folding of proteins. They are not necessarily newly synthesized proteins but rather are constitutively expressed ones that are normally synthesized at a basal rate and whose synthesis is greatly increased in response to stress.

The HSP-70 protein is needed for import of several proteins into the endoplasmic reticulum, chloroplast, and ribosomes. It unfolds the partially folded polypeptide so that it can be translocated through the membrane pore. HSP-70 is localized in the nucleus, mitochondria, and endoplasmic reticulum, is mostly abundant in normal cells, and is localized to cytoplasmic compartments of the cell. A small fraction of it translocates into the nucleus after heat shock. HSP-104 is a strongly induced heat-shock protein that plays a critical role in induced thermotolerance. The major function of this heat-shock protein is to protect, preserve, and recover the function of various protein complexes by maintaining them in a properly folded state.

Another group of HSPs participates in degradation of proteins, because accumulation of denatured proteins following heat shock could be toxic to the cell. The proteins that are to be marked for degradation employ a small, very highly conserved polypeptide called ubiquitin. Although positive correlation exists between the amount of HSPs present and the degree of thermotolerance, exceptions do occur; thus some HSPs are necessary but may not be sufficient for thermotolerance.

Acquisition of thermotolerance is dependent on the stage in the cell division cycle attained by the cells at the time of heat shock. A temperature compensatory mechanism appears to operate in the S-phase, while duration of G2+M phases exhibit a much more pronounced temperature difference. It is interesting to note that there is a cell cycle dependence of heat sensitivity and thermotolerance. Yeast cells also acquire a thermotolerant state in the presence of cyloheximide (25 to 100mg/ml).

### Trehalose

Next to HSPs, the most important compound that plays a role in thermotolerance and osmotolerance of *Saccharomyces cerevisiae* is trehalose. It is a nonreducing disaccharide composed of $\alpha(1,1)$-linked glucose molecules. Trehalose is an enigmatic compound that accumulates in *Saccharomyces cerevisiae* and has been implicated in survival under various stress conditions by acting as a membrane protectant, supplementary compatible solute, or reserve carbohydrate that may be mobilized during stress. During heat stress, trehalose concentration increases in yeast cells parallel to thermotolerance. The protective function of elevated trehalose levels on the machinery that synthesizes heat-shock proteins suggests a "fire brigade" function of trehalose. The final long-term protective effects might then be mediated by the accumulated heat-shock proteins.

A strong relationship exists between intracellular trehalose levels and resistance to osmotic stress. The mutant strains unable to produce trehalose are more sensitive to severe osmotic stress, confirming a role for trehalose in survival. Exposure of yeast cells to temperatures higher than that of the optimum for growth results in enhanced metabolism of trehalose, which prevents protein denaturation and stabilizes the membrane. It protects the membrane from dessication and possibily displaces ethanol in yeast membranes. In so doing it maintains the membrane integrity. Trehalose is synthesized by trehalose synthetase, whihc is encoded by trehalose 6-phosphate synthetase and trehalose 6-phosphate phosphotase genes and a regulatory subunits encoded by TSL-1 and TPS-3. Trehalose increases thermal stability of proteins. Glycerol and trehalose may interact with a lipid membrane, which reduces the amount of leakage from the membrane. It excludes water from the protein surface and thus protects proteins from denaturation in hydrated cells. It was recently shown that HSP-104 and trehalose are required for refolding proteins in the cytosol and also for conformational repair of heat-damaged glycoprotein in the endoplasmic reticulum lumen. The high levels of trehalose produced in response to stress suppress the aggregation of denatured proteins, which prevents their subsequent refolding by molecular chaperons. Synergism between trehalose and some heat-shock proteins plays an important role in acquiring thermotolerance and other stress tolerance in yeasts.

### Fatty Acids

Unsaturated fatty acids such as linoleic and oleic are known to increase membrane fluidity and protect the membrane against high temperatures in yeast. The increased synthesis of saturated fatty acids at high temperatures may provide the correct degree of rigidity required for membrane function under the conditions; however, it may also be responsible for the greater toxicity of ethanol observed at high temperatures. The more rigid membrane caused by the greater amount of saturated fatty acids at high temperatures may prevent intracellular ethanol or truly toxic metabolite from leaving the cell.

The unsaturated fatty acid would provide a more permeable membrane, which could allow intracellular ethanol to leave the cell. Growth of yeast is arrested when a critical intracellular ethanol concentration is reached. This intracellular accumulation is higher at high temperatures. High intracellular ethanol concentration is a consequence of resistance to diffusion through the membrane to the outside. Therefore, at elevated temperatures the rate of ethanol production increases faster than the rate of excretion; furthermore, at high temperatures yeasts become more sensitive to ethanol, which results in poor fermentation abilities at high temperatures.

### *Glycerol*

Yeasts also produce and accumulate intracellularly high levels of glycerol when exposed to osmotic stress in order to balance the osmotic pressure across the cell membrane. Strains that have a reduced ability to produce glycerol are unable to produce any glycerol at all are highly sensitive to hyperosmotic stress. Exponentially grown yeasts cells are more heat sensitive than older stationary cells. High initial cell numbers had greater protective effects at elevated temperatures. This increased thermotolerance with cell numbers is due to release of protective substances from the cell such as non-polar or uncharged hydrophobic amino acids. These thermoprotectors are thought to stabilize the membrane and enhance the thermotolerance of yeast. Recent studies have shown that the primary temperature sensor exists at the level of the membrane. Glycosylated proteins are more thermostable than nonglycosylated ones. Recently it was proposed that thermotolerance was induced in cells of *Saccharomyces cerevisiae* preexposed for ten minutes to mild acid stress in the presence of glucose with HCl at pH 3.5.

## *FERMENTATION ABILITIES OF ISOLATED OSMOTOLERANT AND THERMOTOLERANT YEASTS*

In general, thermotolerant strains are isolated following enrichment techniques. Several strains of *Candida* have been reported to give good ethanol yields at 37, 40, or even 45°C. Yeast strains capable of growth and ethanol production above 40°C have been actively sought, and strains of *Saccharomyces cerevisiae* and *Kluyveromyces marxianus* that could grow up to 34°C with an average ethanol productivity of 75 g/l in synthetic medium containing glucose have been isolated. However, *Kluyveromyces* and *Candida* strains are not as ethanol tolerant as *S. cerevisiae,* although some strains of *Kluyveromyces* sp. were capable of growing at 52°C and producing ethanol at 45 and 50°C. The maximum ethanol yield produced by these strains was 5.7 to 7.0 g (w/v) at 45°C and 5.0 to 5.5 g (w/v) at 50°C, when grown on 14 percent (w/v) glucose. Strains of *S. cerevisiae* were capable of fermenting at 44°C with a maximum ethanol yield of 5.8 g (w/v) using 15 percent glucose.

## APPROACHES FOR OBTAINING NOVEL THERMOTOLERANT AND OSMOTOLERANT YEAST STRAINS WITH GOOD ETHANOL YIELDS

- Thermotolerant yeasts can be obtained by cultivating *Saccharomyces cerevisiae* at progressively higher temperatures and looking for survivors of a gentle heating process, allowing for rapid selection of thermotolerant yeasts.
- More research is needed to screen and select for yeasts capable of fermentation at high temperatures.
- Selection of ethanol-producing strains in a chemostat at higher temperatures might also lead to thermotolerant isolates with good fermentation ability.
- Studies should be conducted on various physiological factors affecting fermentation at high temperatures.
- Temperature-dependent interaction between membrane lipids and proteins should be investigated.
- Efforts to improve the thermal stability of alcohol dehydrogenase enzyme at high temperatures would be more fruitful in improving the thermotolerance of yeasts.
- A complex study of the effect of unsaturated and saturated fatty acids, vitamins, nitrogen sources, sugar type and concentration, pH, ionic strength, cell density, degree of aeration and dissolved oxygen content, age of cells, and hydrostatic pressure on the ability of yeasts to grow or ferment at high temperatures should be explained.
- Though *Candida* and *Kluyveromyces* are more thermotolerant than *Saccharomyces cerevisiae*, improvement of their ethanol tolerance might lead to higher ethanol productivity at elevated temperatures.
- Research efforts should be aimed at cloning structural or regulatory genes responsible for unsaturated fatty acid synthesis.
- The rate of synthesis of HSPs responsible for the acquisition of both thermotolerance and ethanol tolerance should be increased.
- Physiological or genetic changes that increase trehalose accumulation in microbial cells may permit survival at high temperatures and sugar concentrations without the requirement for a rigid membrane.
- Strain improvement studies should be carried out on isolated thermotolerant *S. cerevisiae* strains using both physical and chemical mutagens.

- Protoplast fusion studies should be carried out between superior thermotolerant strains of *Kluyveromyces marxianus* and highly ethanol-tolerant and thermotolerant strains of *S. cerevisiae.*
- Studies on protein folding which leads to increase of thermostability of HSPs should be carried out using novel technologies in genomics and proteomics which will help to address the problems of thermotolerance and osmotolerance of *Saccharomyces cerevisiae.*
- Polyols play a role in osmotic stability of osmophilic yeasts. Efforts should be made to improve or increase the rate of synthesis of polyols in times of need which helps in improving osmotolerance.
- Studies on translational and posttranslational modifications of HSPs (such as phosphorylations and glycosylations, etc.) may help to unravel the functional state of HSPs in thermotolerance.

## CONCLUSIONS

Although ethanol production technology is old and many yeasts are used in industries, research should continue to be carried out to obtain a novel strain of *Saccharomyces cerevisiae* that has superior osmotolerance, thermotolerance, and ethanol tolerance compared to the existing strains, which will tremendously change the scenario of ethanol production in the near future by implementing the previously mentioned strategies. The ethanol fermentation industry is very large, so any small improvement in the efficiency of ethanol production by novel strains would make the process more economically significant.

## SUGGESTED READINGS

Francois J and JL Parrou (2001). Reserve carbohydrate metabolism in the yeast *Saccharomyces cerevisiae. FEMS Microbiology Reviews* 25:125-145.

Kiran Sree N, M Sridhar, LV Rao, and A Pandey (1999). Ethanol production in solid substrate fermentation using thermotolerant yeasts. *Process Biochemistry* 34:115-119.

Schlesinger MJ (1990). Heat shock proteins. *The Journal of Biological Chemistry* 265(21):12111-12114.

Slapack GE, I Russell, and GG Stewart (1985). *Thermophilic bacteria and thermotolerant yeasts for ethanol production.* London, Ontario, Canada: Labatt Brewing Company Limited.

Watson K and R Caviccholi (1983). Acquistion of ethanol tolerance in yeast cells by heat shock proteins. *Biotechnology Letters* 5:683-684.

# Alkaloids, Aflatoxins, and Other Secondary Metabolites: Production Techniques

Javier Barrios-González
Araceli Tomasini
Francisco J. Fernández
Armando Mejía

## INTRODUCTION

Although antibiotics are the best-known secondary metabolites (SM), other such metabolites exist with an enormous range of biological activities (Table III.5). The past two decades have been a phase of rapid discovery of new activities and development of major compounds for use in different industrial fields, mainly pharmaceuticals, cosmetics, food, agriculture, and farming. On the other hand, mycotoxins are dangerous fungal metabolites, so their production must be controlled.

## ALKALOIDS

*Claviceps* species (Figure III.9), the so-called ergot fungi, grow on wild grasses and cereals where they form sclerotia, a latent form that contain pharmacologically active ergot alkaloids. Before recognizing their therapeutic use, ergot alkaloids were known only for their toxic effects, causing mass poisoning in animals and humans over the centuries. The ergot alkaloids were responsible in the Middle Ages for the disease known as "holy fire" or St. Anthony's fire"; these names are surely related to the symptoms: hallucinations, gangrene, cramps, and convulsions.

These alkaloids exhibit a surprisingly wide range of pharmacological effects which are shared in varying degrees by the individual alkaloids. In ergometrine the effect on smooth muscle is enhanced, prompting use in obstetrics as a valuable uterocontractant. Ergotamine has a broader activity spectrum and is primarily used to treat migraine headaches. A chemical modification of ergotoxines enhances α-adrenergic blocking and yields a

TABLE III.5. Microbial secondary metabolites of industrial importance

| Metabolites | Family* | Microorganism | Use |
|---|---|---|---|
| *Pigments* | | | |
| Astaxanthin | Acetyl-CoA Terpenes | *Phaffia rhodozyma* | Food and pharmaceutical |
| Monascin | Acetyl-CoA Terpenes | *Monascus purpureus, M. ruber* | Food, cosmetic, and pharmaceutical |
| *Herbicidal* | | | |
| Bialaphos | Amino acids | *Streptomyces hygroscopicus* | Agriculture |
| *Growth promotant* | | | |
| Monensin | Acetyl-CoA Polyketides | *Streptomyces cinnamonensis* | Growth promoter (livestock) |
| Tylosin | Acetyl-CoA Polyketides | *Streptomyces fradiae* | Agriculture and veterinary use |
| Gibberellin | Acetyl-CoA Terpenes | *Gibberella fujikuroi* | Agriculture (plant growth promoter) |
| *Insecticide and antiparasitic* | | | |
| Avermectin | Acetyl-CoA Polyketides | *Streptomyces avermitilis* | Veterinary and pharmaceutical |
| Milbemycin | Acetyl-CoA Polyketides | *Streptomyces hygroscopicus* | Agriculture, antiparasitic |

*See "Antibiotic Production" in *Part III: Industrial Biotechnology.*

useful agent to treat hypertension. Another modification of ergotoxines shows antagonism with serotonin. Agroclavine inhibits prolactin release. Other natural and semisynthetic ergot alkaloids are being used to treat senile cerebral insufficiency and Parkinson's disease, since these compounds stimulate dopamine receptors.

Ergot alkaloids are SM derived from the shikimate pathway, so their biosynthesis is related to aromatic amino acids. The main biosynthetic precursors are tryptophan, mevalonic acid, and the methyl group of methionine. In ergot alkaloid biosynthesis, the first pathway-specific enzyme, dimethylallyltryptophan synthetase is induced by tryptophan. This biosynthetic pathway is also regulated by carbon, nitrogen, and phosphate sources (phosphate regulation might be mediated through tryptophan). Moreover, it has been shown that dimethylallyltryptophane synthetase is also feedback inhibited by some end products.

The most important commercially produced alkaloids are ergotamine, ergocryptine, ergocornine, ergocristine, ergometrine, and lysergic acid. Dif-

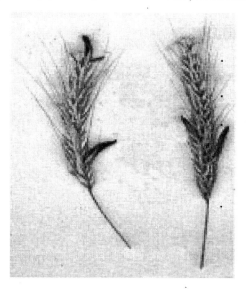

FIGURE III.9. *Claviceps paspali,* sclerotial cells

ferent species of *Claviceps* are used to produce different kind of alkaloids. From approximately the end of the nineteenth century through the first half of the twentieth century, ergot alkaloids were obtained exclusively by inoculating rye flowers with spores of *Claviceps purpurea* and extracting them from field-cultivated sclerotia, which represent an early stage of sexual differentiation and contain 0.1 to 1 percent of alkaloids. Today, ergot alkaloids are produced by submerged fermentation, a more efficient and economical process. However, this technological change has not been easy because in saprophytic conditions, particularly in liquid culture, no sexual reproduction is possible, hence no sclerotia formation occurs. Fortunately, fungal cells, similar to sclerotial cells, can be obtained under certain culture conditions with some strains. In liquid culture, conidia or arthrospores grow out into mycelium, consisting of thin-walled, multinucleated cells (representing vegetative growth) that are not capable of synthesizing alkaloids. In further development to a productive form, in some strains, such as *C. paspali,* mycelial cells become thick-walled. Other strains, especially high alkaloid producers, differentiate toward ovoid cells, which resemble the natural sclerotial cells. In numerous *Claviceps* strains a close parallelism between morphological differentiation, toward sclerotial-like cells, and alkaloid-synthesizing capacity has been established. This is the reason why researchers try to identify conditions to induce differentiation in submerged fermentation. In fermentors, alkaloid yields may exceed 10 percent of the mycelial weight. Like any secondary metabolite, ergot alkaloid submerged-batch fermentation proceeds in two phases: inoculum (7 to 10 days) and production. Production stage takes 12 to 20 days and is carried out in bioreactors of 30,000 liters, using polyols (sorbitol and manitol), organic acids, and low concentrations of glucose to avoid catabolic repression.

Recently, the use of immobilized microbial cells in alkaloid production processes, as used with other SM, was proposed. Solid-state fermentation is another innovative process that has been studied and increased alkaloid production claimed. Commercial impact of ergot alkaloids was increased due to the development of semisynthetic derived alkaloids, which have important pharmacological activity.

Isolation of appropriate species and strains of *Claviceps* was the key to successful commercial submerged alkaloid fermentations. A second important step was genetic improvement of these strains, by mutation and selection, to generate high-yielding strains of particular alkaloid spectra. Relatively few genetic studies of *Claviceps* fungi have been performed, as compared to genetic studies of other commercially important microorganisms. This is probably due to the complex life cycle of the producing fungus. Until recently, genetic manipulation was performed mainly by classical methods of mutation and selection, preferentially using mononucleate conidia as starting material. The development of techniques such as protoplast fusion and recombinant DNA technology has expanded the possibilities to obtain higher-producing strains of industrial interest and to synthesize a novel spectrum of products through interspecies hybrids. The effectiveness of such techniques will increase as basic knowledge of this fungus accumulates.

## AFLATOXINS

Aflatoxins (AF) were discovered during the investigations into the deaths of more than 100,000 turkeys in England in 1960. Brazilian groundnut meal, which contained aflatoxins, was a component of the feeds and was implicated as the cause of the outbreak. The main aflatoxins are $B_1$, $B_2$, $G_1$, and $G_2$. Aflatoxin $B_1$ (AFB$_1$) is one of the most potent hepatocarcinogens known and has been classified by the International Agency for Research on Cancer (IARC) as a group I carcinogen. It is also a teratogen and mutagen, and is thus considered of prime importance in public and animal health. It is a surprisingly strong carcinogen in rats, inducing liver cancer at concentrations in the diet as low as 1 ng/g. Moreover, in rainbow trout a diet containing 0.4 ng/g will cause liver tumors. Epidemiological correlations have been made between AF contamination of the food supply and incidences of human primary hepatoma. Hence, maximum levels of aflatoxins permitted in several products in Canada and the United States are 15 ng/g.

Aflatoxins are SM produced by strains of *Aspergillus flavus* and *A. parasiticus,* and are considered very dangerous mycotoxins because of their potency and abundance. Mycotoxins are usually resistant to most of the treatments used in food processing, such as high temperatures, contributing to their threat to public health. Moreover, these toxins can also reach humans through animal products such as milk or meat. Other important mycotoxins are zearalenone, tricothecenes, patulin, penicillic acid, ochratoxins, citrinin, slaframine, sporidesmin, and sterigmatocystin, which are produced by several different species of fungi, mainly *Aspergillus, Penicillium,* and *Fusarium.* These microorganisms are frequently found as contaminants of grains.

AF have been shown to occur naturally in many agriculture commodities, in particular corn, cottonseed, copra, and nuts. Moreover, aflatoxin $M_1$ is a carcinogenic metabolite found in milk and urine of various animals, including humans, after ingestion of feed or food contaminated with $AFB_1$. Agricultural products can be infected by *A. flavus* or *A. parasiticus* (after injury) while in the field, although toxin development may take place in storage. Maize, groundnuts, and cotton can become contaminated with AT while in the field, under certain weather conditions. For example, groundnuts can be infected during drought conditions. In stored grains, some species of *Aspergillus* grow slowly at moisture contents below 18 percent, increasing general moisture content with their metabolism and thus allowing other fungi to grow. In fact, moisture content is a critical factor for AT biosynthesis. It has been found that when availability falls bellow 16 percent moisture content in maize (or 0.85 Aw), growth of aflatoxigenic fungi is restricted and AT production stops. Hence, it is critical to safeguard store products by storing them at moisture values below this limit (less than 15 percent is recommended).

A modified atmosphere is another strategy that has been employed for this end. It has been reported that artificial atmospheres with less than 0.5 percent $O_2$ inhibit any AT biosynthesis. Fortunately, if the crops are properly stored, at moisture contents and temperatures that do not permit invasion by *A. flavus* or *A. parasiticus,* they will not present any AT hazard.

Aflatoxins are polyketide-derived SM, and studies in liquid medium show that AF synthesis is triggered by the exhaustion of the nitrogen and/or phosphorus source. *Aspergillus flavus* and *A. parasiticus* do not present a sexual stage, displaying only a parasexual cycle. Despite this obstacle for genetic studies, it has been shown that the AT biosynthetic genes in both species are located within a 75 to 90 kb region. The physical order of the genes in the cluster largely coincides with the sequential enzymatic steps of the pathway. Recent reports indicate that the transcription of the genes *nor1, ver1,* and *amtA* is activated by the product of a regulatory gene, *aflR*. Cloning and molecular characterization of AT (and other mycotoxin) biosynthetic genes will help to understand the physiological factors controlling the process. Moreover, this knowledge will also be applied to the development of molecular-based modern detection systems for mycotoxins and mycotoxigenic fungi in food systems. This information could also drive the development of strategies for the biological control of mycotoxigenic fungi and the construction of genetically engineered resistant crop plants.

## *OTHER SECONDARY METABOLITES*

### *Pigments*

Pigments are excellent examples of microbial SM used in the food industry. These compounds are also used in the pharmaceutical and cosmetic industries. In the past, pigments were extracted from plants, but demand increases made these compounds expensive and scarce, which drove a new phase of synthetic pigment production. However, in recent decades concern about the effect of such molecules in human health has turned the interest back to natural pigments, particularly compounds produced by microorganisms These can be divided into carotenoids and *Monascus* red pigments (red mold rice).

Carotenoids are molecules with antioxidant properties, hence they induce many health benefits such as enhancing the immune system, protecting against cancer, and generally contributing to prevention of degenerative diseases. β-Carotene is responsible for the yellow-orange color in legumes and fruits such as carrots, pumpkins, peaches, and sweet potatoes, and it is a precursor of vitamin A. This compound is industrially produced by the fungus *Phycomyces blakesleeanus*. Another important carotenoid is astaxanthin (synthesized by the yeast *Phaffia rhodozyma*), a red-orange pigment responsible for the orange-red color of many marine organisms, including fish, crustaceans, and some birds. It is approved by the U.S. Food and Drug Administration (FDA) as a pigment and is widely used in aquaculture as a feed additive for trouts and salmonid fish (Figure III.10).

Red mold rice (angkak) is the product of a traditional fermentation using cooked rice inoculated with strains of the fungi *Monascus ruber* and *M. purpureus*. Recently, interest in red mold rice is increasing since it is a source of natural pigments. *Monascus* produces six primary pigments (two yellow, two orange, and two red), which are SM derived from the acetyl-

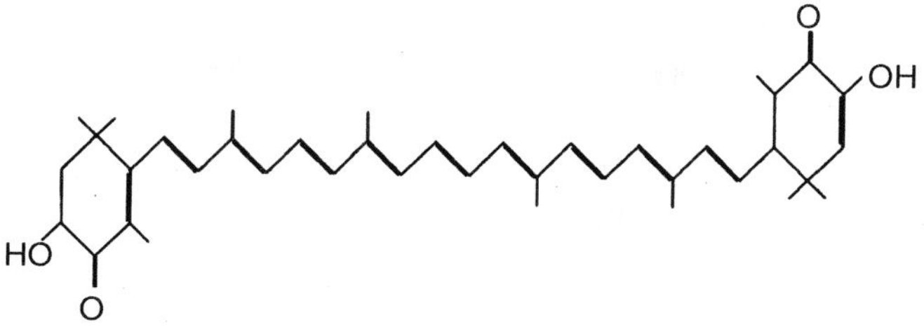

FIGURE III.10. Astaxanthin molecule

CoA-polyketide family (see "Antibiotic Production" in *Part III: Industrial Biotechnology*). On the other hand, microbial SM include bioactive molecules with surprising pharmacological activities (Table III.6). These compounds have found increasing importance in nonantibiotic medical applications.

### Antitumoral

Today, most of the important antiumor compounds used in chemotherapy are microbial products. The search for natural anticancer agents began in the late 1950s and reached its goal in 1964 with the discovery of daunorubicin. This compound proved effective in the treatment of solid tumors and leukemias. In 1969, doxorubicin, a wider-range antiumor agent, was isolated from broths of *Streptomyces peucetius*. Doxorubicin is widely used in chemotherapy and has proven efficiency against breast and ovarian cancers. Moreover, it has remained a mainstay in chemotherapy for more than 35 years. These metabolites are cytotoxic compounds, which are more effective against cells involved in accelerated division (such as cancer cells) than against normal cells. This is why these anticancer agents are considered to be drugs of the past. The desired future drugs are noncytotoxic. This drawback was avoided with the discovery of new antitumoral agents without this toxic effect. Actinomycin D, Taxol, and its derivatives represent these new compounds with novel modes of action (tubulin stabilizers).

### Antichloresterolemics

In 1982 Umezawa showed the enormous potential of microbial enzyme inhibitors as drugs. Today microbial metabolites are being applied to diseases that previously were treated only with synthetic compounds. Statins are a group of microorganism-produced polyketides that greatly impair the

TABLE III.6. Microbial secondary metabolites with nonantibiotic medical application

| Metabolites | Family* | Microorganism |
|---|---|---|
| *Antitumoral* | | |
| Doxorubicin | Acetyl-CoA Polyketides | *Streptomyces peucetius* |
| Mitomycin C | Amino acids-Peptides | *Streptomyces lavendulae* |
| Actinomycin D | Acetyl-CoA Polyketides | *Streptomyces antibioticus, S. parvulus* |
| Bleomycin | Amino acids-Peptides | *Streptomyces verticillus* |
| Taxol | Acetyl-CoA Terpenes | *Taxomyces andreanae,* plants |
| *Antichloresterolemic* | | |
| Monacolin | Acetyl-CoA Terpenes | *Monascus ruber* |
| Lovastatin | Acetyl-CoA Terpenes | *Aspergillus terreus* |
| Pravastatin | Acetyl-CoA Terpenes | *Penicillium citrinum, Streptomyces carbophilus* |
| *Inmunosuppresive* | | |
| Cyclosporin A | Amino acids | *Tolypocladium inflatum* |
| Rapamycin | Acetyl-CoA Polyketides | *Streptomyces hygroscopicus* |
| Ascomycin (FK520) | Acetyl-CoA Polyketides | |
| Tacrolimus (FK506) | Acetyl-CoA Polyketides | several *Streptomyces* species |
| *Antifungal* | | |
| Nystatin | Acetyl-CoA Polyketides | *Streptomyces noursei, S. aureus* |
| Amphotericin | Acetyl-CoA Polyketides | *Streptomyces nodosus* |
| Aspergillic acid | Diketopiperazine-like | *Aspergillus flavus* |
| Aureofacin | | *Streptomyces aureofaciens* |
| Griseofulvin | Acetyl-CoA Polyketides | *Penicillium griseofulvum* |
| Oligomycin | | *Streptomyces diastatochromogenes* |
| *Enzyme inhibitory* | | |
| Clavulanic acid | Amino acids | *Streptomyces clavuligerus* |

*See "Antibiotic Production" in *Part III: Industrial Biotechnology.*

cell synthesis of cholesterol by competitively inhibiting the activity of the enzyme hydroxymethylglutaryl coenzyme A (HMG-CoA) reductase. This is a key enzyme of cholesterol biosynthesis in the liver, the main source of blood cholesterol.

The first hypocholestrolemic agent of this kind was a fungal metabolite discovered in 1976 (compactin). New, more active compounds were isolated later from broths of the fungi *Monascus ruber* and from *Aspergillus terreus.* Lovastatin (also called mevinolin) was approved by the FDA in

1987. This compound and its derivatives, such as pravastatin *(Penicillium citrinum),* are currently used as cholesterol-lowering agents in humans and animals and represent a rapidly growing market of 6 billion dollars per year.

## Immunosuppressive

A few antifungal metabolites also display immunosuppressive activity in humans. Cyclosporin A was the first such compound to be discovered, and it is an intracellular secondary metabolite produced by a filamentous fungus, *Tolypocladium inflatum.* This compound has been used as an immuno-suppressive agent since the mid-1980s and is responsible for the success in the organ transplant field. Sales of this compound reached 1 billion dollars in 1994. Recently two antifungal metabolites of actinomycete origin have been found to possess this pharmacological activity. Tacrolimus and rapa-mycin are not only less toxic that cyclosporin but also show a 100-fold higher immunosuppressant activity. All these compounds suppress the im-mune response by disabling helper T cells by a new mechanism of drug ac-tion. In interaction with an intracellular protein (an immunophilin), they form a novel complex which selectively disrupts signal transduction events of lymphocyte activation.

## Other Enzyme Inhibitors

Widespread use of the beta-lactam class of antibiotics, such as penicillin and cephalosporin, to combat bacterial infections has led to the emergence of bacterial resistant strains. These bacteria produce $\beta$-lactamases, enzymes that disintegrate its $\beta$-lactam ring. Clavulanic acid, a $\beta$-lactamic secondary metabolite from *Streptomyces clavuligerus,* presents a weak antimicrobial effect. However, it can inhibit $\beta$-lactamase activity, so these protective en-zymes miss their target and penicillins are free to act. Acarbose, produced by an actinomycete of the genus *Actinoplanes,* is another enzyme inhibitor. It is used in diabetes and hyperlipoproteinemia.

## Antifungal

Life-threatening fungal diseases have risen dramatically during the past two decades. The most important pathogenic fungi are *Candida* spp., *Aspergillus fumigatus,* and *Cryptococcus neoformans.* Current antifungal drugs are synthetic azoles or natural polyene macrolides such as ampho-tericin B, but these drugs present problems that make them less than optimal for clinical use. Because of the development of resistance to azoles and the toxicity of polyenes, there is a critical need for new antifungal agents that act against new targets. Taking advantage of the sequencing of the entire yeast *(Saccharomyces cerevisiae)* genome, a search for novel targets unique for fungi has been taking place. The screening of microbial SM with these new targets has produced a new generation of very promising antifungal drug candidates such as echinocandins and pneumocandins which are in phase II clinical tests. On the other hand, SM with other important microbial SM are being produced. These could be grouped into antivirals and biopesticides, which include biofungicides, bioinsecticides, bioherbicides, and antihelmintics.

## CONCLUSIONS

Microbial SM are now increasingly being applied to diseases previously treated only by synthetic drugs, e.g., anti-inflammatory and anithypotensive. Moreover, new microbial metabolites are being used in nonmedical fields such as agriculture, with major antiparasitic agents, growth promoters, plant growth regulators, and environmentally friendly herbicides and pesticides. The discovery of SM with these new activities and their development or application as industrial compounds will continue to be an exciting and rapidly expanding field.

This new era has been driven by the strategies to find microbial SM. Older whole-cell assay methods are being replaced by new and sophisticated target-directed, mode-of-action screens. In this way, the activity of culture broths of new isolates is tested in key enzymatic reactions or as antagonists or agonists of particular receptors. This new approach relies on the technological tools of modern molecular biology and on the deepening of the biochemical and molecular details of different diseases or physiological processes.

## SUGGESTED READINGS

Barrios-González J and A Mejía (1996). Production of secondary metabolites by solid-state fermentation. In R El-Gewly (ed.), *Biotechnol Annual Rev. 2.* Amsterdam, The Netherlands, pp. 85-121.

Flickinger M and D Stephen (1999). *Encyclopedia of bioprocess technology: Fermentation, biocatalysis and bioseparation.* New York: John Wiley & Sons, Inc.

Umezawa H (1982). Low molecular-weight inhibitors of microbial origin. *Annual Review in Microbiology* 36:75-99.

# Amino Acid Production

K. Madhavan Nampoothiri

## INTRODUCTION

In recent years a considerable amount of interest has been displayed in various parts of the world for the production of amino acids by fermentation processes. With the major markets in animal nutrition and food additives, the worldwide demand for amino acids is increasing annually by 5 to 10 percent. In comparison to chemical methods, fermentative production of amino acids using microbes has advantages in terms of yielding optically active and biologically required L-form amino acids from cheap carbon and nitrogen sources.

In 1908, researchers determined that the unique flavor-enhancing property of *konbu,* a kelplike seaweed very popular among the Japanese, was due to its L-glutamic acid content. Until the 1950s no appropriate commercial processes for the production of natural amino acids were known except for hydrolysis of wheat gluten, soybean cake, or natural protein-rich materials. In 1957, a soil microorganism belonging to the genus *Micrococcus* (synonym of *Corynebacterium*) was found potent enough to excrete considerable amounts of L-glutamic acid when grown on medium containing glucose and an inorganic ammonium salt. This remarkable discovery led to extensive screening and breeding programs for developing strains and for developing efficient fermentation processes for the production of commercially important amino acids, mainly L-glutamic acid. Consequently, a company now known by the name Ajinomoto produced monosodium glutamate as the first amino acid on an industrial scale.

## PRODUCTION STRAINS

Fermentative production of amino acids got a boost by the discovery of an efficient glutamic acid producer, *Corynebacterium glutamicum* (Figure

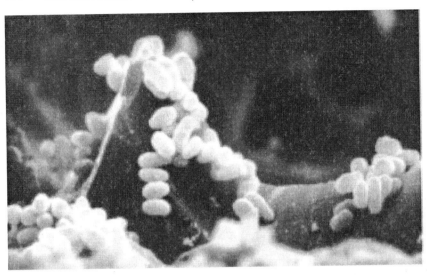

FIGURE III.11. Electron micrograph showing the cells of *Corynebacterium glutamicum*

III.11), originally named *Micrococcus glutamicum* by Kinoshita and colleagues in 1957. Since then, by various screening methods, many different amino acid-producing bacteria have been isolated, including bacteria, yeast, fungi, and actinomycetes. Among them only a limited number of bacterial species were used to obtain production strains for the commercial manufacture of amino acids. This includes the nonpathogenic *Corynebacteria* belonging to the group *Corynebacterium, Brevibacterium,* and the related genera *Arthrobacter* and *Microbacterium.* However, the gunine cytosine (GC) content analysis and DNA-DNA hybridization studies of *Corynebacterium glutamicum, Brevibacterium flavum,* and *Brevibacterium lactofermentum* revealed only minor differences among them, which is not enough to characterize one genus. Hence, it was proposed to consider them one *Corynebacterium glutamicum* species. Together with genera such as *Streptomyces* and *Arthrobacter, C. glutamicum* belongs to the actinomycetes subdivision of Gram-positive bacteria. A major characteristic of these bacteria is that their cell wall contains mycolic acids, which surround the entire cell as a structured layer. In accordance with their best-known representatives, belonging to the families Corynebacteriaceae, Mycobacteriacea, and Nocardiaceae, they are collectively known as CMN bacteria.

## COMMERCIAL NEED FOR AND APPLICATION
## OF AMINO ACIDS

Amino acids are rather simple organic compounds that contain at least one amino group and one carboxylic functional group in their molecular structure. Over the years the demand for individual amino acids has increased dramatically. The amino acids that enter new markets with a growing demand will benefit from the existing experience and the potential that fermentation technology can offer today. Table III.7 presents the current production scale of individual amino acids and the major manufacturing method and area of application.

The food industry looks for flavor enhancers, sweeteners, etc., while the feed industry requires amino acids mainly as feed additives. Most feeds based on crops and oil seeds lack some crucial amino acids, such as L-methionine, L-lysine, and L-threonine, and thus their demand in the feed industry is increasing dramatically. Statistical analysis reveals that in the past two decades the world market for L-lysine increased more than 20-fold. The pharmaceutical industry requires amino acids as infusion compounds, and many of them used for making therapeutic agents. The chemical industry requires amino acids as building blocks for a variety of compounds, including cosmetics, biodegradable surfactants, gelatinizing agents, etc.

TABLE III.7. Current status of amino acid requirement and production

| Amino acid | Major application | Production method | Production scale (tonnes$^{Y-1}$) |
|---|---|---|---|
| L-glutamic acid | Flavor enhancer | Fermentation | 800,000 |
| L-lysine | Feed additive | Fermentation | 350,000 |
| D,L-methionine | Feed additive | Chemical synthesis | 350,000 |
| L-aspartate | Aspartame | Enzymatic synthesis | 10,000 |
| L-phenylalanine | Aspartame | Fermentation | 10,000 |
| L-threonine | Feed additive | Fermentation | 15,000 |
| L-arginine | Pharmaceutical | Fermentation, extraction | 1,000 |
| L-leucine, L-valine | Pharmaceutical Pesticides, pharmaceutical | Fermentation, extraction | 500 500 |
| L-tryptophan L-isoleucine | Pharmaceutical Pharmaceutical | Whole cell process Fermentation | 300 300 |

## *AMINO ACID SECRETION—*
## *PHYSIOLOGY AND METABOLIC CONCEPT*

From a bacterial cell, the secretion of an amino acid occurs as the last step of a sequence of metabolic events as represented schematically in Figure III.12. A suitable substrate is converted within the metabolic network of the cell. From the central metabolic pathways (glycolysis, tricarboxylic acid [TCA] cycle, etc.), the particular biosynthetic pathways to the respective amino acid branch off. The feedback control or the alterations to the expression level of the enzyme involved regulate the complete metabolic network. Various procedures have been developed for effective secretion of amino acids. In some cases the wild-type strain can be used (e.g., L-glutamic acid production by *Corynebacterium glutamicum*). In the case of most other

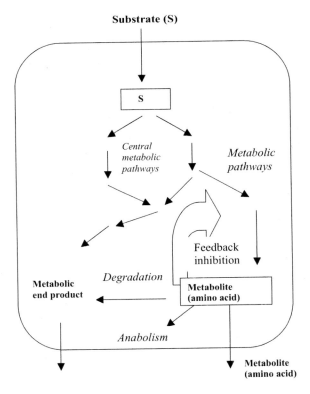

FIGURE III.12. Schematic representation of an amino acid-secreting cell

amino acids secretion is based on alterations in the central and the specific biosynthetic pathways. In the past these changes have been achieved based on random mutagenesis and subsequent selection procedures, such as screening auxotrophic mutants, etc. The availability of genetic engineering tools dramatically changed the whole scenario, and many strains were constructed with significantly increased productivity.

In the case of a mutant, the purposeful alterations made in the specific biosynthetic pathways lead to a high internal steady state of desired amino acid concentration. This can be achieved by several strategies: (1) by enhancing the activity of anabolic enzymes; (2) by altering the regulation pattern, e.g., loss of feedback control; (3) by blocking pathways leading to by-products; and (4) by blocking pathways responsible for product degradation in the cytosol.

### L-Lysine Biosynthesis

L-Lysine is the second amino acid made exclusively with *C. glutamicum* or its subspecies. Almost all genes of *C. glutamicum* required for L-lysine biosynthesis have been cloned. These include kinase *(lysC, asd)*, synthases *(dapA, dapB)*, and dehydrogenases *(dapD, dapE)*, as well as L-lysine exporter and its regulator *(lysE* and *lysG)*. The carbons of L-lysine are derived in the central metabolism from pyruvate and oxaloacetate.

L-Lysine is synthesized via a long pathway, and the first steps of L-lysine biosynthesis are shared with those of L-methionine, L-threonine, and L-isoleucine, the other members of the aspartate family of amino acids (Figure III.13). The first step of the reaction is initiated by the enzyme aspartate kinase. The enzyme is inactive when L-lysine and L-threonine are present together in excess, thus providing a feedback signal.

One other interesting aspect of *C. glutamicum* is its split pathway for L-lysine synthesis (Figure III.13). At the level of piperideine 2,6-dicarboxylate, flux is possible either via the four-step succinyl variant (like in *Escherichia coli*) or the one-step dehydrogenase variant (like in *Bacillus macerans*). The split pathway in *C. glutamicum* is an example of an important principle in microbial physiology. Pathway variants have generally evolved to provide key metabolites under different environmental conditions.

It has been reported that at the start of cultivation the majority of L-lysine is made via the dehydrogenase variant; at the end of the process, at low ammonium concentrations, the newly synthesized L-lysine is almost exclusively made via the succinylase route.

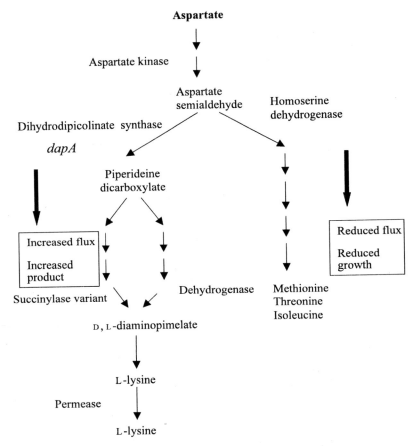

FIGURE III.13. L-Lysine biosynthesis in *C. glutamicum*

One other important step of flux control within lysine biosynthesis is at the level of aspartate semialdehyde distribution. The dihydrodipicolinate synthase activity competes with homoserine dehydrogenase for the aspartate semialdehyde (Figure III.13). Overexpression of the dihydrodipicolinate synthase gene, *dapA,* has shown that with an increasing amount of synthase, a graded flux increase toward L-lysine results. Due to this overexpression of *dapA,* the flux of aspartate semialdehyde into the branch leading to the homoserine is diminished. As a consequence, due to the shortage of homoserine, derived amino acids, the growth of the organism is weakened and it favors L-lysine formation.

## Nitrogen Flux in Amino Acid Formation

For amino acid formation, nitrogen flux is as important as carbon flux. The *amt* gene in *C. glutamicum* encodes the carrier for the uptake of the protonated nitrogen form. Ammonium is then incorporated into L-glutamate and L-glutamine, which provide the nitrogen to almost all cellular amino groups. The key enzymes involved in supplying the amino group for amino acid formation are glutamate dehydrogenase (GDH), glutamine synthatase (GS), and glutamate: oxoglutarate aminotransferase (GOGAT). Dehydrogenase enzyme is essential in the maintenance of high pool concentrations; at low concentrations both GS and GOGAT are increased, showing that a kind of regulation is present to always provide the adequate amount of nitrogen for cellular functions.

## AMINO ACID SECRETION—MECHANISMS AND CONCEPTS

Various mechanisms have been proposed as being responsible for the secretion of different amino acids by bacteria. The major hypotheses are based on simple diffusion (leakage model), inversion of the uptake process induced by changes in chemical potential or regulation, uncoupling due to changes in the membrane structure, or a carrier-mediated process.

Although L-glutamate has been produced for almost four decades, the exact mechanism of its efflux by *C. glutamicum* is not yet understood fully. At the beginning it was suggested that L-glutamate "leaks" through the membrane. Traditionally the efflux of L-glutamate is triggered by biotin limitation, but the possibilities to achieve this condition are many: (1) biotin limitation, (2) addition of detergents such as Tween 40 and Tween 60, (3) addition of penicillin and local anesthetics, and (4) use of auxotrophs such as oleic acid auxotrophs and glycerol auxotrophs. Again, to obtain a massive efflux the cells must be grown for at least one generation in the presence of these components, indicating that cell composition must be altered. Therefore, the membrane status is apparently correlated with efflux. It is already known that during growth under biotin limitation the phospholipid composition of *C. glutamicum* is altered, and this altered cell-wall composition might favor excretion. A recent report showed that as a consequence of genetically modified lipid synthesis, L-glutamate efflux is changed quite dramatically; for instance, overexpression of plsC (acylglycerolacyl transferase) resulted in a detergent-triggered increase of L-glutamate accumulation from 92 to 108 mM, while acp (acyl-carrier protein) overexpression reduced the accumulation to 24 mM. With some of the overexpressed genes, substantial L-glutamate excretion even without detergent addition was observed when the fermentation temperature was elevated. Additional parameters are necessary to result in high L-glutamate efflux: the energetic state of the cell, a low ketoglutarate dehydrogenase activity, the carrier itself, and probably an altered permeability of the mycolic acid layer.

Although it has been shown that the release of some amino acids, e.g., L-glutamate, L-threonine, and L-isoleucine, is at least in part an active process, only recently it has been possible to identify bacterial amino acid exporters, such as LysE and ThrE from *C. glutamicum*, which export basic amino acids and L-threonine, respectively. An exporter related to L-cysteine export has been identified in *E. coli*. Recently the specific L-lysine export carrier has been cloned. It acts as a very good target to improve amino acid excretion and also represents a new translocator structure, which provides a new type of intracellular amino acid control. It is a comparatively small membrane protein (25.4 kDa) and revealed a topology so far unknown for any translocator (Figure III.14). On the basis of hydropathy analysis, six hydrophobic domains were identified, but only five membrane-spanning helices are present. It is assumed that the sixth one may dip into the membrane or be localized on the surface. The amino terminal end of LysE is located in the cytoplasm, while the carboxy terminal end is found in the periplasm. Recent studies based on genome comparison showed at least three distinct families (LysE, YahN, and CadD) of eubacteria which are similar in size and and have similar hydropathy profiles and sequence motifs; together they comprise the LysE superfamily. It is suggested that the members of this superfamily catalyze the export of a variety of biologically important solutes. Thus the exporter serves as a valve that excretes any excess intracellular L-lysine present. A regulator gene, *lysG*, is localized adjacent to LysE and displays all the typical structural features of an autoregulatory transcriptional regulator of the LysR-type family.

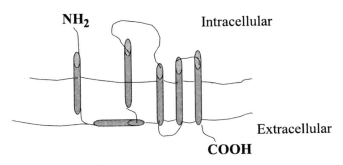

FIGURE III.14. Schematic representation of the topology of the LysE protein encoding the L-lysine exporter of *C. glutamicum*

## OTHER AMINO ACIDS

*Escherichia coli* and *C. glutamicum* mutants can be effectively used for commercial-scale production of L-threonine. The *thrA, thrB,* and *thrC* genes constitute an operon controlled by an attenuation mechanism via L-threonine and L-isoleucine. It is basically a five-step reaction to convert L-aspartate to L-thronine. The operons consists of *thr*A (codes for homoserine dehydrogenase), *thrB* (codes for homoserine kinase), and *thrC* (codes for threonine synthase). Based on this regulation, there are two strategic approaches to construct a producer strain—a stable high-level expression of *thrA, thrB,* and *thrC* and prevention of L-isoleucine formation, since L-threonine is also an intermediate in L-isoleucine biosynthesis. Using an engineered L-thronine producer at the end of fermentation, the maximum yield is about 85 g/l with a conversion yield of about 60 percent based on the carbon source used.

L-Isoleucine is synthesized via a long pathway that is highly structured and regulated. The first steps of its synthesis are shared with those of L-lysine and L-methionine. With high expression of the *homthrB* operon even with wild-type threonine dehydratase, reasonable flux can be obtained and a final L-isoleucine concentration of about 30 g/L with a yield of 22 percent is achieved.

L-Phenylalanine can be produced with *E. coli* or *C. glutamicum.* The pathway for L-phenylalanine synthesis is shared in part with other aromatic amino acids, L-tyrosine and L-tryptophan. There are three DAHP (deoxyarabinoheptulosonate phosphate) synthase enzymes in *E. coli* encoded by *aroF, aroG,* and *aroH.* These enzymes play a key role to control the flux. Production strains have a DAHP activity that is resistant to feedback inhibition and a feedback-resistant chorismate mutase-prephenate dehydratase. In general, the producers are L-tyrosine auxotrophic mutants.

L-Tryptophan is a high-price amino acid. The production process in general involves culturing an *E. coli* mutant overexpressing tryptophan synthase. The pregrown culture is later mixed with L-serine plus indole to convert these substrates into L-tryptophan.

Due to the cost-effectiveness of the process today, L-aspartate is produced exclusively using aspartase rather than depending on fermentation. Fumarate and ammonium serve as substrates for the aspartase.

Both L-cystein and L-methionine require sulfur as an additional element for their synthesis, therefore the first step in engineering *E. coli* was directed toward the provision of L-serine. Strains expressing *serA* (phosphoglycerate dehydrogenase) and *cysE* (acetylserine transferase) alleles were able to excrete nearly 2g/L L-cysteine.

## *CONCLUSIONS*

Amino acid production is an outstanding example of the integration of many different techniques and tools, which include classical strain development, application of recombinant techniques, and intracellular flux analysis. Through the introduction of functional genomics the entire scenario will change dramatically in the future. The availability of the entire sequence of the chromosomes from *C. glutamicum* and *E. coli* opens up tremendous possibilities to compare mutants and to uncover new mutations essential for high overproduction of metabolites. Molecular studies have now identified the L-lysine exporter (LysE) and L-threonine exporter (ThrE) in *C. glutamicum* localized in the inner cytoplasmic bilayer. Export thus represents a new bacterial mechanism for regulating the cellular amino acid balance. The special significance of the cell envelope as a barrier for the production process has been recognized only very recently, and it is a major challenge to discover how these amino acids pass through the various layers of the cell envelope and then to apply these findings for further strain improvement, opening up a wide area to work on.

## SUGGESTED READINGS

Eggeling L, W Pfeffeerle, and H Sham (2001). Amino acids. In *Basic biotechnology*, C Ratledge and B Kristiansan (eds.). London: Cambridge University Press, pp. 281-302.

Kinoshita S, S Udaka, and M Shimone (1957). Studies on the amino acid fermentation. *Journal of General and Applied Microbiology* 3:193-205.

Leuchtenberger H (1996). Amino acids—Technical production and use. In *Products of primary metabolism*, Volume 6, HJ Rehm and G Reed (eds.). Weinheim, Germany: Verlag Chemie Weinheim, pp. 455-502.

Nampoothiri KM and A Pandey (1998). Genetic tuning of coryneform bacteria for the overproduction of amino acids. *Process Biochemistry* 33(2):147-161.

# Antibiotic Production

Javier Barrios-González
Araceli Tomasini
Francisco J. Fernández
Armando Mejía

## INTRODUCTION

Antibiotics are defined as low-molecular-weight organic natural products produced by microorganisms (secondary metabolites), which are active against other microorganisms at low concentration. Their selective action against bacterial and fungal pathogens brought about the antibiotic era, and for 50 years society has benefited from this remarkable property of the so-called "wonder drugs." Its success was so impressive that a small group of antibiotics (which include penicillins, cephalosporins, tetracyclines, and aminoglycosides) have been the only drugs used for chemotherapy against pathogenic microorganisms. In 1996 the antibiotics world market amounted to US$25 billion a year and involved around 300 products. Of the 12,000 antibiotics known in 1995, 55 percent were produced by actinomycetes of the genus *Streptomyces,* 11 percent from other actinomycetes, 12 percent from nonfilamentous bacteria, and 22 percent from filamentous fungi. New antibiotics from microorganisms continue to be discovered at a rate of more than 300 per year.

Antibiotics have mainly medical use and can be classified by their mode of action (e.g., on cell wall or protein synthesis) and activity spectrum. Tetracyclines, the most widely used broad-spectrum antibiotics, are effective against both Gram-positive and Gram-negative bacteria, as well as rickettsias- and psitacosis-causing organisms. The medium-spectrum antibiotics bacitracin, erythromycins, penicillins, and cephalosporins are effective against some Gram-negative and Gram-positive bacteria. Polymyxins are narrow-spectrum antibiotics effective against only a few species of bacteria. On the other hand, antibiotics have found wide nonmedical uses. Some are used in animal husbandry to enhance weight gain of livestock. Others have been used to treat plant diseases such as bacteria-caused infections in tomatoes, potatoes, and fruit trees. Antibiotics are the best known of a group of microbial products known as secondary metabolites (SM).

## SECONDARY METABOLISM

SM are compounds with varied and sophisticated chemical structures, produced by strains of certain microbial species, usually late in the growth cycle. A high percentage of these compounds display diverse biological activity, hence acquiring actual or potential industrial importance. As the structures of these molecules were elucidated, it became evident that these compounds do not play a physiological role during the exponential phase of growth. Moreover, they have been described as secondary metabolites in opposition to primary metabolites such as amino acids, nucleotides, lipids, and carbohydrates that are essential for growth. A characteristic of secondary metabolism is that the metabolites are usually not produced during the phase of rapid growth (trophophase) but are synthesized during a subsequent production stage (idiophase).

Production of SM starts when growth is limited by the exhaustion of one key nutrient: carbon, nitrogen, or phosphate (Figure III.15). In this way, penicillin biosynthesis, by *Penicillium chrysogenum,* starts when glucose is exhausted from the culture medium and the fungus starts consuming lactose, a less readily utilized sugar. Gibberellic acid biosynthesis, by *Gib-*

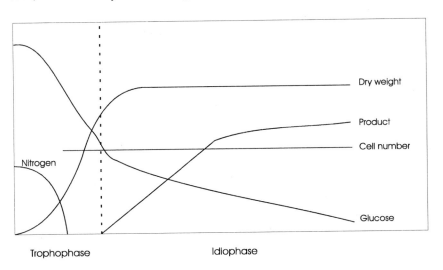

FIGURE III.15. Secondary metabolism and growth

*berella fujikuroi,* starts when the nitrogen source is the depleted nutrient. In a similar way, the depletion of phosphate from the medium is the factor that triggers chlortetracycline biosynthesis by *Streptomyces aureofaciens.*

### Biosynthesis

Microbial SM show an enormous diversity of chemical structures. Their variety can be reduced to a significant order only by analysis of their biosynthetic pathways, which link them to the more uniform network of primary metabolism. It has been shown that SM are formed by pathways that branch off from primary metabolism at a relatively small number of points, which define broad biosynthetic categories or families:

1. Shikimic acid (aromatic amino acids)
2. Amino acids
3. Acetyl-CoA (and related compounds, including Krebs cycle intermediates)
4. Sugars

The metabolites of each family fall into several major classes of structures, which are the basis of further subdivision (see Table III.8).

### Metabolites Derived from the Shikimate Pathway

Microorganisms synthesize a large variety of compounds from intermediates of the shikimate-chorismate pathway, as well as from the products of this route: the aromatic amino acids (phenylalanine, tyrosine, and typtophan). These amino acids are end products of a branched pathway leading to *p*-aminobenzoic acid, a precursor of candicidin. Other examples include chloramphenicol, phenazine antibiotics, and ergot alkaloids.

### Metabolites Derived from Amino Acids

The biosynthetic pathway of important antibiotics such as penicillin, cephamycins, and cephalosporins ($\beta$-lactams) start by the nonribosomal condensation of three amino acids, cysteine, valine, and $\alpha$-aminoadipic acid, to form the tripeptide $\delta$-(L-$\alpha$-aminoadipyl)-L-cysteinyl-D-valine (AVC). This family includes cyclic peptide antibiotics such as gramicidin or the immunosuppressive agent cyclosporine.

TABLE III.8. Secondary metabolites derived from different biosynthetic families

| Family | Example structure subclass | Example compounds | Example activity |
|---|---|---|---|
| Shikimic acid | Pathway intermediates Aromatic amino acid | Candicidin Chloramphenicol Ergot alkaloids | Antifungal Antibacterial Various therapeutic activities |
| Amino acids | β-Lactams Peptidolactones Cyclic peptides Glycopeptides Phosphinopeptide | Penicillins, Cephalosporin Actinomycin D Cyclosporin Vancomycin Bialaphos | Antibacterial Antitumor Immunosuppresive Antibacterial Herbicide |
| Acetyl-CoA Polyketides: | | | |
| Type I modular | Macrolides | Erythromycin, tylosin | Antibacterial Growth promotor |
| | Pentacyclic lactones Ansamycins Polyenes Polyethers | Avermectin, milbemycin Rifamycin, ansatrienins | Insecticidal, antiparasitic Antibacterial Antifungal Growth promotors |
| Type I iterative | Statins | Nystatin, amphotericin B Monensin | Hypocholesterolemic |
| Type II iterative | Tetracyclines Anthracyclines | Lovastatin, pravastatin | Antibacterial Cytotoxic antitumor |
| Terpenes: | Sterolidal Diterpene Triterpene | Oxytetracycline Doxorubicin, aclarubicin | Antitumor, antibacterial Antitumor Antibacterial |
| | | Squalamine Taxol Fusidic acid | |
| Sugars | Aminoglycosides Aminocyclitols | Streptomycin, kanamycin Spectinomycin | Antibacterial Antibacterial |

## *Metabolites Derived from Acetyl-CoA*

This family can be subdivided into polyketides and terpenes.

*Metabolites derived from polyketides.* In polyketide biosynthesis, a molecule of acetate condenses with three or more molecules of malonate to form a polyketomethylene (polyketide) chain which can undergo a variety of further transformations. Because malonate is formed by carboxylation of acetate, these metabolites are often referred to as poly-acetate or acetate-derived. Polyketide synthases (PKS) possess a surprising number of enzyme activities (25 in the case of erythromycin) that are sequentially used during biosynthesis. Depending on their mode of action, PKSs have been described as follows. Type I modular PKSs (each enzyme activity is used only once) include the enzymes of important structure categories such as macrolides and polyene antibiotics. Type I iterative PKSs include the statins antibiotics group. Type II iterative PKSs include tetracyclines and anthracyclines.

There are two distinct phases in polyketide biosynthesis. The first is the assembly of the polyketide chain and its modification, usually by aromatization or reduction, to give a stable product; this phase involves protein-bound intermediates. This product can be the major metabolite or can undergo further transformation(s), i.e., the second phase referred to previously, to give the major metabolite.

*Terpenoid metabolites.* Like the polyketides, the terpenes are derived ultimately from acetate, but instead of the linear condensation characteristic of the polyketides, the terpenes are built up from branched C5 units (the isoprene units) formed from three acetate units. The key intermediate is mevalonate which is converted to isopentenyl pyrophosphate and dimethylallyl pyrophosphate, which condense to form precursors that undergo a variety of cyclization reactions to form mon-, sesqui-, di-, and triterpenes. Fusidic acid and squalamine are examples of these metabolites.

*Metabolites derived from sugars.* Some SM are synthesized from the pool of deoxyribonucleotides and ribonucleotides that microorganisms accumulate during growth. However, the various pentoses and hexoses, which are used mainly in synthesis of the cell wall and storage of polysaccharideas during growth, under limited growth may be diverted to the synthesis of SM like the aminoglycoside antibiotics, such as streptomycin and kanamycin.

## REGULATION

Because secondary biosynthetic routes are related to the primary metabolic pathways and use the same intermediates, regulatory mechanisms, i.e., induction, carbon catabolite regulation, and/or feedback regulation, apparently operate in conjunction with an overall control that is linked to growth rate (Table III.9).

### Induction of Synthesis

In some cases, primary metabolites induce synthases and thus increase production of the final product. These include leucine induction of bacitracin synthetase in *Bacillus licheniformis* and methionine induction of ACV synthetase, cyclase, and expandase in the cephalosporin C pathway of the fungus *Acremonium chrysogenum*.

TABLE III.9. Genetic regulation of some antibiotic biosynthesis

| Mechanism | Antibiotic | Regulatory product |
|---|---|---|
| Catabolic repression by carbon source | Cephalosporin | Glucose, glycerol, maltose |
| | Erythromycin | Glucose, sucrose, glycerol, mannose, 2-deoxiglucose |
| | Kanamycin | Glucose |
| | Penicillin | Glucose, fructose, galactose, sucrose |
| | Tetracycline | Glucose |
| Catabolic repression by nitrogen source | Cephalosporin | Ammonium, L-lysine |
| | Chloramphenicol | Ammonium |
| | Erythromycin | Ammonium |
| | Penicillin | Ammonium, L-lysine |
| | Rifamycin | Ammonium, L-tryptophan, p-aminobenzoate |
| | Tetracycline | Ammonium |
| Feedback regulation (repression or inhibition) | Chloramphenicol | End product |
| | Erythromycin | End product |
| | Kanamycin | End product |
| | Tetracycline | End product |
| Synthases induction | Bacitracin | Leucine |
| | Cephalosporin | Methionine |

An induction effect of endogenous (not primary) metabolites is important in many actinomycete fermentations. A typical example is the induction effect of the A-factor in streptomycin production and morphogenesis in *Streptomyces griseus.*

### Carbon Catabolite Regulation

This mechanism regulates the synthesis of a great number of SM. Catabolite repression is exerted by glucose, on genes from the penicillin (and other β-lactam antibiotics), biosynthetic pathway in *P. chrysogenum.* This is why growth limitation by carbon, i.e., glucose exhaustion, is the factor that triggers antibiotic biosynthesis. Other examples include actinomycin, erythromycin, kanamycin, tetracyclin, neomycin, violacein, mitomycin, and bacitracin.

## Feedback Regulation

Many SM inhibit or repress their own biosynthetic enzymes. Examples include chloramphenicol, kanamycin, erythromycin, and tetracycline. In some cases, primary metabolites, whose pathway is related to the secondary biosynthetic route, can regulate secondary metabolite biosynthesis in this way. This case can be illustrated by L-lysine feedback regulation of penicillin biosynthesis by *P. chrysogenum*. In a similar way, aromatic amino acids inhibit production of candicidin by *S. griseus*.

The genes encoding the biosynthetic enzymes of particular antibiotics are found in a gene cluster that, in actinomycetes, also contains regulatory and resistance genes. Typically there may be more than one specific regulatory gene per cluster. Both activator and repressor genes are known. In *Streptomyces coelicolor*, expression of several such biosynthetic gene clusters also depends on at least 11 globally acting genes, indicating that antibiotic production is also subjected to global, sometimes morphologically coupled, regulation. A protein phosphorylation cascade also seems to be involved (signal transduction). In fungi, structural genes are also clustered, each one under the control of its own promoter. An interesting difference is that, in fungi, regulatory and resistance genes do not seem to be in the biosynthetic cluster.

## PRODUCTION

In industry, improved strains of microorganisms are inoculated into a nutrient medium in flasks and then transferred to a relatively small fermentor. The microbes multiply rapidly, since the environment is controlled to stimulate their growth (exponential or rapid growth phase). This culture is used as the "seed" or "inoculum" and is transferred to a sterilized fermentor tank (typical production vessels range from 30,000 to 200,000 liters), where production phase or idiophase takes place. pH, temperature, and other parameters of the fermenting medium are regulated as per the specific requirements. The different regulatory mechanisms mentioned previously are bypassed by environmental manipulations. Therefore, an inducer such as methionine is added to cephalosporin fermentations, phosphate is restricted in chlortetracycline or candicidin fermentations, and glucose is avoided in penicillin or erythromycin fermentation. After years of empirical development, fermentations of antibiotics regulated by carbon are now conducted with slowly utilized sources of carbon, generally lactose. If glucose is used, it is usually fed at a slow, continuous rate so that metabolites do not accumulate. The use of soybean meal in many industrial fermentations is probably due to its ability to avoid nitrogen metabolite (ammonium) repression of antibiotic biosynthesis.

It is important to note that in some cases a precursor is used which increases and directs production toward the formation of one specific desirable product; this is known as directed biosynthesis. Examples of this include phenylacetic acid in penicillin G fermentation and specific amino acids in the production of actinomycins and tyrocidins.

Finally, it is important to mention that these processes are aerobic, therefore the fermenting medium must be constantly stirred and aerated. Agitation is provided by turbine impellers at a power input of 1 to 4 W/liter. Oxygen uptake rates of a rapidly growing culture can attain 0.4 to 0.8 mmol/liter per minute, so air has to be supplied at flow rates of 0.5 to 1.0 v/v per minute. Exit gas analysis, by infrared for $CO_2$ or by mass spectrometry or gas chromatography for $CO_2$, $O_2$, and $N_2$, can provide metabolic information to regulate feeding rates. Periodic broth sampling is always necessary to determine concentrations of product, phosphate, carbohydrates, etc. Such values can be used to regulate the addition of precursor and other required nutrients. Some natural antibiotic substances are modified chemically to produce semisynthetic antibiotics.

At this point it is interesting to note that research performed in the past ten years indicates that at least some of these compounds could be produced in great amounts, and probably with advantages, by a different culture system: solid-state fermentation (SSF). SM are generally reported to be produced in higher concentrations in solid culture, often in shorter times, requiring less energy, in smaller fermentors, and with easier downstream processing measures. One drawback of this system is the inexperience of engineers in Western nations in the design and scale-up of solid-state fermentors.

## *GENETIC IMPROVEMENT*

Historically, random mutation and selection have been the most successful strategies used for the manipulation and screening of microorganisms to produce higher antibiotic titers. These techniques, although successful, are based on empirical experience and have a moderate probability of success, being labor-intensive methods.

Classical methods have lately been replaced by less empirical, directed-selection (rational selection) techniques such as direct colony selection following overlay bioassay; mutants resistant to toxic precursors or toxic end products; mutants resistant to analogs of intermediary metabolites such as amino acids and carbohydrates (e.g., penicillin mutants resistant to lysine analogs or cephalosporin mutants resistant to methionine analogs); mutants resistant to metallic ions that complex the antibiotic or a biosynthetic intermediary; and use of auxotrophic strains deficient for biosynthetic intermediates, followed by prototrophic reversion.

Industrial strain improvement programs have also used protoplast fusion to combine positive characteristics of different strains, such as good sporulation and high antibiotic production. The clustering of biosynthetic, resistance, and regulatory genes of secondary metabolism in actinomycetes has facilitated the application of genetic engineering techniques for strain improvement in recent years. Such clustering also occurs in bacilli and in fungi. This characteristic allows the transfer of operons or groups of operons from one organism to another by modern genetic engineering methods. In this way, an increase in gene dosage of a limiting enzyme in the pathway or of the whole pathway can be performed in the producing strain. It is important to note that this amplification has been found in penicillin-high-producing industrial strains, obtained by classical (nonrecombinant) methods.

Manipulation of the regulatory genes will be of great importance for industrial strain improvement in the future. Production may be limited by the presence or absence of those genes, rather than by the dosage of structural genes. It is encouraging that disruption of the negatively acting regulatory gene *mmy* of methylomycin biosynthesis increased production 17-fold. On the other hand, the introduction of a single copy of the positively acting gene *actII* raised the synthesis of actinorhodine 35-fold.

## CONCLUSIONS

The most critical reason for the development of new antibiotics, preferably with new structures, is the race to remain one step ahead of antibiotic-resistance development, which is proceeding at an alarming rate. Another important reason is the evolution of previously unknown diseases, such as HIV, Ebola viruses, and Legionnaires' disease; and the existence of bacteria with natural resistance to known antibiotics, such as *Pseudomonas aeruginosa*.

These challenges will be faced with new and powerful tools. The era of antibiotic discovery based on random screening of SM from microbes is being replaced by sophisticated, target-directed, mode-of-action screens, that is, whole cell assay versus enzyme- or receptor-based assays. The application of the new screening procedures brought about the discovery of new antibiotics active against cell walls, such as cephamycins, fosfomycin, and thienamycin. New opportunities for modern chemotherapy include antibiotics with activities against bacterial signal peptidases, inhibitors of β-lactamases, and inhibitors for lipid A biosynthesis. Modern screening procedures to discover new target-directed antibiotics will also trigger the discovery of new SM, such as clavulanic acid, that act as inhibitors of the enzymes responsible for resistance in bacteria. On the other hand, recombinant DNA technology, together with advances in the knowledge of secondary metabolite regulation, will generate a completely new set of strategies and methods for strain improvement in the near future.

Another interesting field will be the development of novel antibiotics, produced by using unconventional compounds as substrates of the biosynthetic enzymes of the microorganism. These enzymes will be modified or mutated to increase their affinity for those unnatural substrates. Generation of new antibiotics can also be performed by the so-called combinatorial biosynthesis. In this case, different activity modules of enzymes such as polyketide synthases can be rearranged by genetic engineering to obtain a microbial strain that synthesizes an antibiotic with novel characteristics.

## SUGGESTED READINGS

Barrios-González J and A Mejía (1996). Production of secondary metabolites by solid-state fermentation. R El-Gewly (ed.), *Biotechnol Annual Rev. 2.* Amsterdam, Netherlands: Elsevier Science B. V., pp. 85-121.

Demain AL (1999). Pharmaceutically active secondary metabolites of microorganisms. *Applied Microbiology and Biotechnology* 52:455-463.

Strohl WR (1997). Industrial antibiotics: Today and the future. In *Biotechnology of antibiotics*, WR Strohl (ed.). New York: Dekker, pp. 1-47.

# Aroma Compound Production

Ali Kademi
Danielle Leblanc
Alain Houde

## INTRODUCTION

Aroma is a mixture of several dozen to several hundred volatile molecules that emanate from plant or animal products. These volatiles (1) have low molecular weights (MW < 400 daltons), (2) have high vapor pressure at room temperature and atmospheric pressure, (3) reach the olfactory organ through the nasal mucus, (4) interact with the receptive membranes of the sensory organ, and (5) have different detection thresholds and chemical structures. The natural aroma of strawberry, for example, is composed of approximately 350 different odorant compounds including alcohols, organic acids, esters, carbonyls, and, to a lesser extent, lactones and furans. The various chemical classes to which aroma compounds may belong are shown in Table III.10.

Aroma compounds in any food are perceived through the nasal and retronasal passages. The nasal passage gathers information about the odor of the food. Once the food is in the mouth, additional information on the taste is gathered through the retronasal passage. These two perceptions are grouped together under the term *flavor,* which includes all the sensations perceived by the tongue, nose, and retronasal passage. Most aroma compounds on the market are chemically synthesized as artificial molecules or "nature identical" (i.e., molecules identical to those found in nature). The major inconvenience of chemical synthesis is the formation of undesirable racemic mixtures. Consumers are also showing an increasingly marked preference for natural compounds in foods, cosmetics, and household cleaning products. This strong consumer demand has stimulated research into so-called natural molecules to replace those synthesized chemically, especially artificial molecules.

TABLE III.10. Common aroma compounds and their notes

| Chemical structure | Example (organoleptic notes) |
|---|---|
| Alcohols | Isoamyl alcohol (fusel oil, whiskey) |
| | 1-Octen-3-ol (mushroom aroma) |
| Carbonyls | 2-Pentanone (Roquefort flavor) |
| (ketones, diketones, and aldehydes) | 2,3-Butanedione (buttery, nutlike) |
| | Benzaldehyde (bitter almond) |
| Carboxylic acids | Oleic acid (olive oil) |
| | Hexanoic acid (coconut oil) |
| Esters | Ethyl butyrate (pineapple) |
| | Ethyl isovalerate (apple on dilution) |
| Lactones | 4-Octalactone (coconut), 4-decalactone (peach) |
| Terpenes | Citronellol (roselike, fresh), menthol (mint) |
| Pyrazines | 2-Methoxy-3-isopropylpyrazine (musty, potatolike) |
| Ethers | *trans*-Anethole (anise) |
| Others | 3-Methyl-2-cyclopenten-2-ol-1-one (caramel-like) |
| | Eugenol (spicy, cloves) |
| | Vanillin (vanilla) |

## PRODUCTION OF AROMA COMPOUNDS

Natural aromas may be obtained through a number of processes, by using (1) extraction from animal or plant materials, (2) distillation (lemon, peppermint, etc.), (3) concentration of fruit extracts or juices, or (4) biotechnological processes including fermentation or biotransformation/bioconversion by plant cells, microorganisms, or enzymes (Figure III.16).

The biotechnological approach for the production of aroma compounds has several advantages:

1. It provides some independence from agriculture, which is highly dependent on climatic variations for supplies of raw materials.
2. It offers the possibility of scaling up processes.
3. Products obtained are labeled "natural" if they have been prepared from natural substrates.
4. Biocatalysts are generally specific and stereoselective, generating optically pure target compounds.

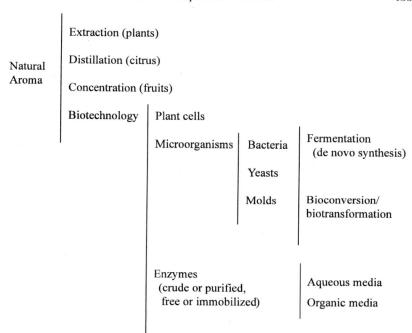

FIGURE III.16. Various processes for the generation of natural aromas

In these processes, isolated enzymes, microorganisms (bacteria, yeasts, or molds), or plant cells can act as biocatalysts. Whole cells are generally used for complex products or compound mixtures, while isolated enzymes can carry out single-step processes.

### *Fermentation or de novo Synthesis*

In the past, the main purpose of using fermentation to process foods with microbial cultures was to extend the product's shelf life (beer, wine, bread, vegetables, etc.). While imparting to the final product a flavor distinct from that of the original food, the microorganisms used play an important role in the development of complex mixtures of aromas through the catabolism of sugars, fats, and proteins. Biotechnology takes advantage of these reactions. Fungi are the major aroma-producing microorganisms, probably due to their secondary metabolism. Culture conditions (medium, pH, temperature, aeration, and fermentation time) play an important role in determining the amount and type of aroma produced. De novo synthesis by microorganisms can often be achieved from relatively inexpensive carbon and nitrogen sources, making the processes very affordable. In general, synthesis of aromas through fermentation generates small amounts of secondary metabolites, because the metabolites produced inhibit the cells or the activity pathway. Incorporation of an aroma-recovery stage becomes necessary to avoid this retroinhibition and therefore may increase productivity. Physiologically optimizing and/or genetically modifying microorganisms can significantly increase production of aroma compounds.

Solid-state fermentation (SSF) involves the growth of microorganisms on water-insoluble substrate in the absence of free water. SSF constitutes an attractive alternative for the production of aroma compounds because solid substrates can be used without pretreatment, the volumetric productivity is high, and compounds are easy to recover. This technique is currently used for cheeses, fermented sausages, and yogurt production.

## Biotransformation/Bioconversion

Unlike fermentation, biotransformation/bioconversion converts specific substrates to target products by using a cell's enzymatic system or directly using crude or purified enzymes. When the reaction occurs in a single step, it is called biotransformation. The term bioconversion is used when the reaction requires several steps. In biotransformation/bioconversion, various reactions, such as oxidation, reduction, hydrolysis, dehydration, formation of new C-C bonds, and several types of breakdowns, may be catalyzed. Biocatalysis is competitive with chemical catalysis in the following reactions: (1) introduction of chirality, (2) functionalization of chemically inert carbons, (3) selective modification of functional group in multifunctional molecules, and (4) resolution of racemic mixtures. Use of whole cells may be an excellent alternative to chemical and enzymatic processes. Many cells have both the redox system necessary for oxidoreduction reactions and the system necessary for cofactor regeneration. Consequently, the use of whole cells avoids problems inherent in the large-scale use of isolated redox enzymes, such as the regeneration of cofactors and the instability of enzymes and cofactors toward oxygen, trace metals, temperature, and organic solvents. On the other hand, use of substrates with low molar concentrations (often on the order of a millimole), low reaction yields, and compound production rates are among the disadvantages of whole-cell processes. Isolated free or immobilized enzymes are used for biotransformation/bioconversion of precursors such as fatty acids or amino acids, which are converted to aroma compounds with higher added value. Aroma compounds can be produced in an aqueous solution or in an organic medium. The organic medium can (1) help to overcome problems of low yields caused by poor substrate solubility in water, (2) shift the balance of the reaction toward product formation, (3) offer the possibility of coupling product formation and recovery into a single process, and (4) in some cases, increase the stability of the enzymes used.

## AROMA COMPOUND BIOSYNTHESIS MECHANISMS

### Formation of Alcohols

Alcohols play a modest and often indirect role as aroma compounds. In wines and spirits, the higher alcohols are quantitatively the largest group of volatile compounds, and their presence is essential to the quality of the aroma. In yeast fermentation, they constitute the major metabolites, with a dominance of ethanol, fusel oil alcohols (propanol, isobutanol, and amyl and isoamyl alcohols), and phenethyl alcohol. Alcohols are also precursors in the preparation of other aroma compounds, including their oxidation to aldehydes or their use in the production of esters through esterification. Alcohols are synthesized by reducing $\alpha$-keto acids which are derived via biosynthesis or alternatively from the breakdown of amino acids. If amino acids are added to the fermentation medium, they undergo deamination, yielding $\alpha$-keto acids, which are decarboxylated to form aldehydes. Then, these aldehydes undergo reduction catalyzed by an alcohol-dehydrogenase, thus producing higher alcohols with one less carbon than the amino acid used as the fermentation substrate.

### Formation of Organic Acids

Short-chain saturated fatty acids are characterized by strongly pungent and unpleasant odors, which are irritating in high concentrations. As the molecular weight increases, these characteristics are increasingly replaced by the rancid, buttery, and cheesy notes, which then become even more fatty and aldehydic. Fatty acids with more than 14 carbon atoms are waxy solids with only slight tallow-like odors. Fatty acids contribute a great deal to aroma compounds and accentuate certain characteristics of the aroma. For example, fatty acids C3 to C6 accentuate fruity notes, while fatty acids C4 and C6 to C10 intensify cheese flavors. In general, branched-chain acids such as isovaleric acid have lower aroma thresholds than the straight-chain acids. Unsaturated acids have distinct flavor nuances. Those with short carbon chains are pungent and acidic, while those with longer chains of the oleic series tend to be spicy, aldehydic, and tallow-like. The presence of a hydroxyl group tends to suppress the odor, while aromatic acids are slightly balsamic, with floral and spicy notes. Di- and tricarboxylic acids are all odorless.

Microbial biogenesis of organic acids may occur by four different processes:

1. The C1 to C5 aliphatic acid series and lactic acid arise essentially as fermentation end products.
2. The classical fatty acid synthesis produces saturated acids with longer carbon chains (C6 to C18), and from these, unsaturated fatty acids are synthesized by the action of an oxygen-dependent desaturase.
3. Iso-acids, such as isovaleric acid and isocaproic acid, seem to be synthesized through the biosynthesis of amino acids via the Strickland reaction.
4. Free fatty acids are also synthesized by the action of lipases/esterases that hydrolyze the ester bonds of the lipids.

## Formation of Esters

Esters are a major group of aroma compounds. Straight-chain and branched aliphatic esters, at very low concentrations varying from 1 to 100 ppm, contribute to the aroma of almost all fruits; for example, ethyl valerate and ethyl isobutyrate have aromatic notes of apple and lemon, respectively. Two biosynthesis pathways may be used to produce esters: (1) alcoholysis of acyl-CoA compounds and (2) direct esterification of an organic acid with an alcohol. During fermentation of beer, the alcohol enzyme acyltransferase in the yeast catalyzes the transfer of the acyl group from an acyl-CoA to an alcohol, leading to the formation of coenzyme A and an ester. In some cases, the addition of precursors such as amino acids or fusel oil to the culture medium stimulates the production of esters. With *Geotrichum fragrans,* amino acids (valine, leucine, and isoleucine) added to the culture medium are deaminated to their corresponding carboxylic acids, which are then transformed into acyl-CoA derivatives. These derivatives are then esterified in presence of alcohols (C2 to C5) added to the culture medium to produce C2 to C5 alkyl esters of C4 and C5 carboxylic acids. Esters can also be synthesized by biotransformation through direct esterification of an organic acid and an alcohol in an aqueous solution or organic medium through the action of isolated lipases and esterases or by using whole microbial cells.

## Formation of Lactones

Lactones are very common in nature and have been isolated from all major food groups including fruits, vegetables, nuts, meats, and dairy products. They are associated with odor impressions such as fruity, coconut-like, buttery, sweet, and nutty. Lactones are generally biosynthesized via the β-oxidation of saturated or unsaturated hydroxy fatty acids or their lipid precursors. The peach note, γ-decalactone, is synthesized from ricinoleic acid by *Yarrowia lipolytica*. The process involves a bioconversion of castor oil by the yeast. The oil is obtained by pressing seeds of *Ricinus communis* and is composed of 80 percent triglyceride of 12-hydroxy-9-octadecenoic acid, also known as ricinoleic acid. The yeast hydrolyzes the castor oil and the liberated fatty acid is metabolized via β-oxidation, leading to the formation of 4-hydroxydecanoic acid. This acid is then spontaneously lactonized into γ-decalactone in the culture medium by heating under acidic pH conditions. The position and stereochemical orientation of the hydroxyl group in the molecule of the natural precursor determine the type of lactone that will be synthesized.

## Formation of Ketones

The aromatic note of ketones is often found in cheeses, from which many saturated and unsaturated cyclic, aromatic, and aliphatic ketones have been isolated. For instance, 2-heptanone has a spicy aromatic note. Methyl ketones are biosynthesized by β-oxidation of fatty acids through the addition of an acyl group, leading to β-keto acids, which undergo decarboxylation, producing a methyl ketone with one carbon less than the original fatty acid. Short- or long-chain fatty acids can be metabolized to produce a variety of methyl ketones.

# APPLICATIONS OF AROMA COMPOUNDS

## Agri-Food Industry

Aromas play an important part in the composition of foods and beverages. They can be synthesized by fermentation or biotransformation using microorganisms or enzymes (Table III.11).

## Cheese Making

Cheese production uses several complex biochemical processes involving microorganisms such as bacteria, molds, and yeasts. A group of micro-

TABLE III.11. Biocatalysts and some of their applications for aroma production

| Food | Source | Description |
| --- | --- | --- |
| Cheese | Enzymes | Neutrase/palatase, Peptidase/protease |
| | Bacteria | *Lactococci, Lactobacilli, Propionibacteria* |
| | Yeasts | *Brevibacterium linens* |
| | Molds | *Penicillium camemberti, P. roqueforti* |
| Yogurt | Bacteria | *Lactobacillus bulgaricus, Streptococcus thermophilus* |
| Bread | Yeasts | *Saccharomyces cerevisiae, Candida* sp. |
| Meat | Enzymes | Protease |
| | Bacteria | *Enterobacteria, Lactobacilli, Pediococcus pentosaceus, Staphylococcus carnosus* |
| | Molds | *Penicillium nalgiovense* |
| Beer | Yeasts | *Saccharomyces cerevisiae* |
| Wine | Bacteria | *Leuconostoc oenos, Lactobacilli, Pediococci* |
| | Yeasts | *Saccharomyces cerevisiae* |
| Vegetable | Bacteria | *Lactobacilli* |
| | Yeasts | *Pichia, Hansenula, Saccharomyces* |

organisms starts the process by producing lactic acid and by helping the cheese ripening with enzymes involved in proteolysis (breakdown of proteins into peptides). Peptides are then broken down into amino acids, the main precursors of cheese flavor. In this first group, bacteria, mainly *Lactococcus, Lactobacillus, Streptococcus, Leuconostoc,* and *Enterococcus,* may occur naturally in milk or be added to it. Another group of microorganisms, composed mainly of a mixture of bacteria, yeasts, and molds (secondary flora), contributes significantly to ripening of cheese and brings specific flavors to various cheeses.

*Brewing*

Brewing draws on an extensive knowledge of microbiology and biochemistry. Once the raw materials have been selected, prepared, and processed, inoculation with yeasts triggers the main fermentation (alcoholic fermentation), in which a large amount of alcohol is produced. In addition, a precise and typical mixture of carefully balanced flavors characterizes the product. The main aroma compounds are synthesized at this stage. The next stage, secondary fermentation, or aging, results in only minor changes. In traditional brewing, this stage may last few weeks to several months.

## Vanillin

The production of natural vanillin is considered to be a biotechnology application offering a very promising market. Vanillin accounts for approximately 2 percent of the *Vanilla planifolia* bean from which it is extracted. Vanillin may be produced by enzymatic synthesis, microbiologically, or by plant cell culture. In enzymatic synthesis, several precursors of the metabolic pathway may be transformed into vanillin using different enzyme systems, such as (1) transformation of stilbene isorhapontin by oxidation, (2) transformation of eugenol generating ferulic acid or coniferaldehyde as intermediates, or (3) transformation of lignin. These substrates are cheap and readily available, but yields are still low.

## L-Menthol

L-Menthol is one of the most important terpene alcohols and the only one of the eight stereoisomers that combines a mint flavor and a refreshing sensation. It can be obtained by crystallization of peppermint oil from the plant, generating a mixture of isomers. Esterification of the D,L-menthol mixture with acids yields menthyl esters. Resolving the racemic mixture constitutes an important step in the process. One approach is based on the fact that stereospecific microbial lipases and/or esterases will hydrolyze D,L-menthyl esters to L-menthol, which will then be crystallized. Furthermore, another process involving a *Rhodotorula minuta* esterase/lipase immobilized in a polyurethane resin resolves this racemic mixture by producing L-menthol with an optical purity close to 100 percent.

## Fragrance Industry

The fragrance industry accounts for a significant part of the aroma market. It is not limited to perfumes but also involves uses in derived products (soaps, cosmetics, shampoos, cleaners). Norpatchoulenol, an ingredient used in perfumery, is present in trace amounts in essential oil of patchouli but constitutes one of the major odorant compounds in that oil. Patchoulol, which is the dominant constituent of the essential oil (30 to 45 percent), can be hydroxylated by various fungi and then converted chemically into norpatchoulenol. Another compound is Ambrox, a major constituent of ambergris. It is produced naturally by sperm whales and has traditionally been used in perfume making. The decline of the whale population is causing a supply problem for aroma specialists, but the yeast *Hyphozyma roseoniger* and some strains of *Cryptococcus* can oxidize the sclareol extracted from clary sage into the intermediate diol for further chemical transformation into Ambrox.

## CONCLUSIONS

Aromas play a very important role in a number of industries. With the increasing consumer demand for natural additives in food and cosmetics, biotechnological production of aromas constitutes an alternative source of supply and may offer many advantages such as low production cost, continuous availability, and stereospecifically pure products. With new pathways that might be explored and the contribution of genetic engineering to increase production yields, aroma biotechnology is a field that should expand in the near future.

## SUGGESTED READINGS

Berger RG (ed.) (1995). *Aroma biotechnology.* Jena: Springer-Verlag.
Cheetham PSJ (1993). The use of biotransformations for the production of flavor and fragrances. *TIBTECH* 11:478-488.
Christen PA and A López-Munguía (1994). Enzymes and food flavor—A review. *Food Biotechnology* 8:167-190.
Welsh FW, WD Murray, and RE Williams (1989). Flavours and fragrances chemicals. *Critical Reviews in Biotechnology* 9:105-169.

# Bioconversion of Agroindustrial Residues for Bioprocesses

## Cassava Industry Residues

Carlos Ricardo Soccol
Ashok Pandey

### *INTRODUCTION*

#### Nature and Origin of Cassava

The *Manihot* genus consists of more than 200 species, among which *Manihot esculenta* Crantz is the most important for food and industrial applications. Cassava is known under several appellations, notably tapioca in countries of Asia, mandioca, aipim, castelinha, and macaxeira in Brazil, yuca in Spanish-speaking countries, and manioc in the French-speaking countries of Africa.

Cassava was believed to have originated in Venezuela around 2700 B.C. However, in a significant research report published in May 1999, biologists at the University of Washington reported that cassava originated from the extreme south of the Amazon River in Brazil. They used a sophisticated DNA sequencing technique that traced variation in a single gene *(G3pdh)* found in cultivated and wild cassava. Cassava was introduced to Africa by the Portuguese during the sixteenth century and to Asia in the eighteenth century.

A cassava plant consists of aerial and underground parts. The aerial part can reach 2 to 4 m in height with a trunk and branches. The underground part consists of two types of roots: those responsible for the feeding of the plant and those for axial disposition surrounding the trunk. The latter are called tubers and represent the edible part of the plant. Every plant can possess 5 to 20 tubers that can reach 20 to 80 cm in length and 5 to 10 cm in diameter. The clean weight of each tuber could vary between about 100 grams to 5 kilograms. Tubers of cassava are rich in starch (80 percent dry matter) but low in proteins (1.2 percent dry matter).

Cassava occupies the sixth position in world food cultures and is a staple for more than 700 million people in the world. It has the remarkable capacity to adapt to various agroecological conditions. It is also considered a low-risk crop. In view of its drought-resistant nature and non-requirement of any specific growth conditions, much attention has been paid in the past 15 to 20 years to increasing its production all over the world, which has been well achieved. World production of cassava has steadily increased from about 75 million tons in 1961-1965 to 153 million tons in 1991. In 1994, the world production reached approximately 167 million tons, but fell slightly in 1998 to 162 million. Africa is the largest producer, with about 53 percent of the world production, followed by Asia with about 29 percent and Latin America with about 18 percent. Although cassava is cultivated in some 88 countries, only five countries account for 67 percent of its production. These are Nigeria (approximately 31 million tons), Brazil (23 million tons), Thailand (19 million tons), Zaire (18 million tons), and Indonesia (16 million tons).

About 60 percent of the world production of cassava is destined for human consumption. It is consumed in its natural form cooked in water, as flour, or in fermented forms such as gari, fufu, etc. The animal feed industry absorbs about 33 percent of the world production of cassava, and the remaining 7 percent is used in industries such as textiles, food, and fermentation. With the advent of biotechnological approaches, the focus has shifted to widening the application of cassava and its starch for new applications with the aim of added value.

### Industrial Processing of Cassava Roots

The industrial processing of cassava root is oriented toward flour production and extraction of starch. Most processing units are generally small or medium sized with varying capacities of production. Figure III.17 shows the general process of extraction of flour/starch from the tubers, which results in several by-products such as bagasse, peels, unusable roots, etc. Two types of wastes are generated: solid and liquid. Solid wastes include peels and bagasse. Processing of 250 to 300 tons of cassava tubers results in about 1.6 tons of solid peels and about 280 tons of bagasse with high moisture content (85 percent). Liquid wastes include wastewater (about 2,655 m$^3$) with about 1 percent solids. Solid wastes are generally discarded in the environment as landfill.

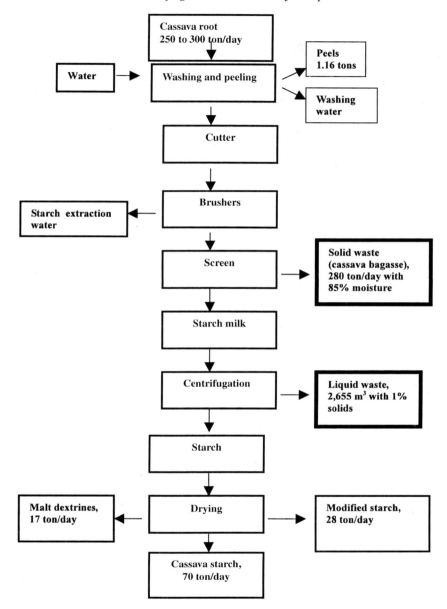

FIGURE III.17. Industrial processing of cassava for starch and other products

### Cassava Bagasse

Cassava bagasse (CB) is a fibrous residue containing 40 to 70 percent starch on dry matter basis. In spite of the absence of cyanide in CB, its utilization in food or feed has not been considered attractive because of its low protein content. Compared to other agroindustrial residues, cassava bagasse can be thought of as a rich energizing reserve in carbohydrates.

Table III.12 shows the composition of cassava bagasse. These analyses were conducted on bagasse samples obtained from different processing units at different times in the state of Paraná, Brazil. The composition shows variation probably because most processing is done under poorly controlled technological conditions. In addition, the composition may also differ due to the use of different crop varieties. Starch, however, is the main carbohydrate component in all the varieties.

Because of its low ash content, cassava bagasse could offer numerous advantages in comparison to other crop residues such as rice straw and wheat straw, which have 17.5 percent and 11 percent ash content, respectively, for usage in bioconversion processes using microbial cultures. In comparison to other agricultural residues, cassava bagasse can be considered to be a rich solar energy reservoir due to its (cassava's) easy regeneration capacity. When compared to sugarcane bagasse, it offers advantages because it does not require any pretreatment and can be easily attacked by microorganisms.

## MICROBIAL STRAINS CULTIVATED ON CASSAVA BAGASSE

Microorganisms that utilize starch as the substrate for growth and activity have generally been preferred for bioconversion processes utilizing cassava bagasse because of its high starch content. Some yeasts and fungi have been used for cultivation on cassava bagasse, and filamentous fungi have been most widely employed. Table III.13 shows different microorganisms cultivated on cassava bagasse and hydrolyzed cassava bagasse for various purposes.

TABLE III.12. Physicochemical composition of cassava bagasse

| Component | g/100 g dry weight |
|---|---|
| Moisture | 5.02-11.20 |
| Protein | 0.32-1.61 |
| Lipids | 0.53-1.06 |
| Fibers | 21.10-50.55 |
| Ash | 0.66-1.50 |
| Carbohydrates | 40.50-63.85 |

TABLE III.13. Bioprocesses involving cassava bagasse

| Microorganism | Process | Application |
|---|---|---|
| *Aspergillus niger* | SSF | Citric acid |
| *Candida lipolytica* | SmF | Citric acid |
| *Ceratocystis fimbriata* | SSF | Aroma compounds |
| *Kluyveromyces marxianus* | SSF | Aroma compounds |
| *Lentinus edodes* | SSF | Mushroom |
| *Pleurotus sajor-caju* | SSF | Mushroom |
| *Rhizopus* sp. | SSF | Biotransformation |
| *R. arrhizus* | SmF | Fumaric acid |
| *R. ciricians* | SmF | Fumaric acid |
| *R. delemar* | SmF | Fumaric acid |
| *R. formosa* | SmF | Fumaric acid |
| *R. oligosporus* | SmF | Fumaric acid |
| *R. oryzae* | SmF | Fumaric acid |
| *R. oryzae* | SSF | Aroma compounds |
| *Monascus* sp. | SSF | Pigments |
| *Xanthomonas campestri* | SmF | Xanthan gum |

SSF: solid-state fermentation; SmF: submerged fermentation

## BIOPROCESSES INVOLVING CASSAVA BAGASSE

### Protein Enrichment of Cassava Bagasse

Protein enrichment of cassava bagasse has generally been carried out using filamentous fungi. Under laboratory conditions a four- to fivefold increase in the protein contents has been achieved using the optimized conditions of initial substrate moisture and pH about 70 percent and 5.7 to 6.4, respectively, C:N ratio 4.7 to 14.0, inoculation rate $10^5$ spores/g of dry cassava bagasse, and 28 to 32°C as incubation temperature. A strain of *Rhizopus oryzae* was reported to utilize nongelatinized cassava bagasse. During the scale-up, a tray type fermentor demonstrated better performance in comparison to a column fermentor. The utilization of perforated bottom steel trays permitted better heat transfer and also better growth of the fungi on cassava bagasse.

Some studies have been performed on the effect of thickness of layer of cassava bagasse in the tray fermentor. The temperature increase during the fermentation is a function of the thickness of the substrate layer. The increase in the temperature is directly proportional to the increase in the thickness of the layer. For a thickness of 8 cm, the temperature of the product could be in the order of 44°C between 18 and 20 h of culture, while with 6 and 4 cm layers the temperature could be 42.5 and 37.5°C, respectively. In these studies, higher protein contents were achieved with lower thickness of the substrate bed. However, reasonable protein contents could be achieved with a 6 to 8 cm thick bed substrate where the higher conversion rates are obtainable (based on consumed starch).

### Glucoamylase Production from Cassava Bagasse by Solid-State Fermentation

Studies have shown that cassava bagasse served as substrate in solid-state fermentation (SSF) for the production of glucoamylase enzyme by the strains of *Rhizopus* sp. *Rhizopus oryzae* MUCL 28627 presented the most important specific activity after fermentation of crude bagasse. Higher specific activity values (>10 Kat/kg) were obtained after 72 hours of fermentation at 32°C. No pretreatment of bagasse was required.

### Mushroom Production

Cassava bagasse, used alone or mixed with other substrates such as sugarcane bagasse, can be used as a substrate for the production of mushrooms, e.g., *Pleurotus*. Production is dependent on several factors such as temperature of fermentation, initial pH of the substrate, inoculation concentration, etc. Best results were achieved in SSF with a mixture of cassava bagasse (80 percent) and sugarcane bagasse (20 percent). With this mixture, the production of *Pleurotus* (fresh mushrooms) was 300 g/kg of dry substrate. C:N ratio also plays a crucial role in the production of *Pleurotus*. Addition of natural nitrogen-rich materials such as soybean cake has been found to be beneficial. When added at 20 percent to cassava bagasse, mushroom production increased from 300 g to 690 g/kg of dry substrate. A C:N ratio of 12 to 14 is generally regarded as most suitable for *Pleurotus* cultivation on lignocellulosic materials.

Cassava bagasse has also been used for cultivating another mushroom, *Lentinula edodes* (shiitake). The best results for its production were achieved by using a mixture containing cassava bagasse (80 percent) and sugarcane bagasse (20 percent). This mixture permitted a yield of 729 g of fresh mushrooms per kg of dry substrate. Because conventional production of shiitake on trunks of oaks takes five to six months, its cultivation on cassava bagasse could have good commercial implications, since it takes only about 60 days for fruiting body formation.

## Production of Organic Acids

There are reports on the production of fumaric acid ($C_4H_4O_4$), which is a dicarboxylic acid and has a wide range of applications, using cassava bagasse (hydrolysate) in submerged fermentation by fungal strains belonging to *Rhizopus* sp. Fumaric acid possesses a double bond and two carboxylic groups and is an excellent intermediate in chemical synthesis involving esterification reactions. It is also used as an acidulant in the food industry, in beverages, and in the pharmaceutical industry due to its nontoxic and nonhygroscopic properties. Bioprocess optimization was achieved by applying factorial design experiments on different media compositions using cassava bagasse hydrolysate. A laboratory process has been described using a strain of *Rhizopus formosa,* yielding 21.28 g fumaric acid per liter in a media containing cassava bagasse hydrolysate as the sole carbon source, $KNO_3$ as nitrogen source (C:N ratio of 168), 20 g/l of $CaCO_3$, 10 μg/l of biotin, 0.04 g/l of $ZnSO_4 \cdot 7H_2O$, 0.25 g/l of $MgSO_4 \cdot 7H2O$, 0.15 g/l of $KH_2PO_4$, and 15 ml/l of methanol.

Another important organic acid that has been produced from cassava bagasse is citric acid ($C_6H_8O_6$, 2-hydroxyl-1,2,3-propane tricarboxylic acid). Citric acid is used mainly in the food industry (60 percent) for its pleasant taste and elevated solubility in water. Citric acid production from cassava bagasse has involved the SSF technique using mostly fungal strains of *Aspergillus* sp. In comparison to other agroindustrial residues such as sugarcane bagasse, wheat bran, rice bran, sugarcane press mud, coffee husk, etc., cassava bagasse has been found superior as a carbon source in laboratory processes using *Aspergillus niger*. Yields such as 13.6 to 27.0 g citric acid per 100 g dry substrate were obtained, which corresponded to 41.8 to 70.0 percent conversion (based on sugars consumed). Maximum yield, however, has been as high as 88 g citric acid/kg dry cassava bagasse.

## Aroma Compound Production

Flavor and aroma (including fragrance) compound synthesis by biotechnological process currently plays an increasing role in the food, feed, cosmetic, chemical, and pharmaceutical industries. This is mainly due to an increasing preference by consumers for natural food additives and other compounds of biological origin. Attempts are being made to produce such compounds by fermentation of simple nutrients such as sugar and amino acids. SSF using agroindustrial residues offers good opportunities in this regard. A wide range of aroma compounds were obtained in a process involving cassava bagasse as a substrate by *Ceratocystis fimbriata,* which included one acid, six alcohols, one aldehyde, two ketones, and five esters, resulting in a strong fruity aroma. *Kluyveromyces marxianus* can also be used for the production of fruity aroma by SSF using cassava bagasse. In general, an acidic pH and high C:N ratio in the substrate have been found useful for aroma production.

### Hydrolysis of Cassava Bagasse

One alternative approach for utilizing cassava bagasse has been to subject it to hydrolysis using acid or enzymes and then to use hydrolysate for cultivation of microorganisms for the production of various products. One important technoeconomic consideration is the amount of the reducing sugar recovered and the operational costs. As mentioned previously, cassava bagasse has been used for the production of fumaric acid. Studies have been performed to optimize the hydrolysis in lab conditions and subsequently scaled-up in which a cylindrical reactor (1,500 L) with flat top and bottom was used with 150 kg of cassava bagasse and 1,350 kg of water to calculate the energy consumption, the heat necessary to heat the material, and the heat necessary to keep the reactor temperature at the required level. The costs with chemicals were also considered. The reaction time appeared to be a very important factor for the process. The yield of the acidic hydrolysis was 62.35 g of reducing sugar from 100 g of cassava bagasse (having 66 percent starch). It represented 94.5 percent of reducing sugar recovery. The yield of the enzymatic hydrolysis was 77.1 g of reducing sugar from 120 g of cassava bagasse (having the same starch content). It represented 97.3 percent of reducing sugar recovery. Concerning the time, a batch of acid hydrolysis required 10 minutes, plus the time to heat and cool the reactor, while a batch of the enzymatic hydrolysis needed 25 hours and 20 minutes, plus the time to heat and to cool the reactor. Concerning the costs, for acidic and enzymatic hydrolysis of 150 kg of cassava bagasse US$34.27 and 2471 were spent, respectively.

### Xanthan Gum Production with Cassava Bagasse Hydrolysate

Xanthan gum has great industrial potential. Attempts are being made to develop bioprocesses with technoeconomical feasibility for its production from various sources. Cassava bagasse hydrolysate offers this possibility. In a laboratory process, xanthan gum production was achieved that utilized cassava bagasse hydrolysate consisting of 20 g/l glucose. The yield was about 14 g/l after 96 hours of fermentation at 28°C. Rheological analyses and data on absorption in infrared spectra of the xanthan gum produced were similar to the data of the analyses accomplished with the commercial xanthan gum.

## *Natural Pigment Production Using Cassava Bagasse*

Recently there have been increased effort toward the production of pigments from microbial sources. Several agroindustrial residues including cassava bagasse have been used as the substrate. For example, different strains of *Monascus* sp. were tested to produce natural pigments in cassava bagasse by solid-state fermentation. One of the strains, *Monascus* LPB showed good capacity to grow in cassava bagasse supplemented with defatted soybean flour. The concentration of red pigment produced in cassava bagasse was similar to that produced in the conventional process utilizing rice as the substrate.

## CONCLUSIONS

Vast quantities of cassava bagasse are available in tropical countries and do not find any appropriate application at present. Rather, the disposal of cassava bagasse causes pollution concerns. Apparently not much work has been done to utilize this residue globally. However, a dedicated effort by the Laboratory of Process Biotechnology, Federal University of Paraná, Brazil, and others at a few locations around the world has shown that cassava bagasse could be an attractive substrate for bioprocesses and could be used in an economical way for varied applications. For example, it could be used for the production of enzymes, organic acids, aroma compounds, edible mushrooms, pigments, xanthan gum, and foods and feed. Cassava bagasse hydrolysate, which is rich in glucose, could be used for microbial processes for the production of value-added products. Attempts are also ongoing to use cassava bagasse as substrate to cultivate bacteria that possess probiotic properties.

## SUGGESTED READINGS

Pandey A and CR Soccol (1998). Bioconversion of biomass: A case study of lignocellulosic bioconversion in solid-state fermentation. *Brazilian Archives of Biology and Technology* 41(4):379-391.

Pandey A and CR Soccol (2000). Economic utilisation of crop residues for value addition: A futuristic approach. *Journal of Scientific and Industrial Research* 59:12-22.

Pandey A, CR Soccol, and DA Mitchell (2000). New developments in solid-state fermentation: Bioprocesses and products. *Processes Biochemistry* 35:1153-1169.

Pandey A, CR Soccol, P Nigam, VT Soccol, L Vandenberghe, and R Mohan (2000). Biotechnology potential of agro-industrial residues: II. Cassava bagasse. *Bioresource Technology* 74(1):81-87.

Soccol CR (1996). Biotechnology products from cassava root by solid-state fermentation. *Journal of Scientific and Industrial Research* 55(5):358-364.

Soccol CR and N Krieger (1998). Brazilian experiments for the valorisation of agro-industrial wastes by solid-state fermentation. In *Advances in biotechnology*, A Pandey (ed.). New Delhi: Educational Publishers, pp. 25-40.

# Coffee Industry Residues

Carlos Ricardo Soccol
Ashok Pandey

## INTRODUCTION

Coffee (*Coffea* sp.) is one of the most important agricultural commodities in the world. Arabica and Robusta are the two principal varieties cultivated for commercial production. Several hundred million consumers drink more than 1.5 billions of cups of coffee every day, and about 20 million people annually use about 100 million 60 kg bags produced in some 70 tropical countries. After petroleum, coffee is the second most valuable product on the world market, and it has a prime position in the world market of agricultural products along with sugarcane, wheat, and cotton. Constituting 4 percent of world trade of food products, it represents on the international market about 10 billion dollars per year. Because coffee is the most consumed nonalcoholic drink in developed countries, imports of coffee are directed toward more industrialized countries. The largest importer of coffee in the world is the United States (18 million 60 kg bags), followed by Germany, France, and Japan. The five largest producers of coffee are Brazil, Colombia, Indonesia, Mexico, and the Ivory Coast, which account for about 60 percent of world production.

## INDUSTRIAL PROCESSING OF COFFEE CHERRIES

Coffee cherries collected from gardens are processed either by the humid method or the dry method to isolate coffee grains (Figure III.18).

### The Humid Method

Cherries are first washed with water to remove dirt and other refuse and then are subjected to depulping, which separates the pulp from the grains. Subsequently they undergo fermentation at 18 to 25°C for 24 to 36 h and then are washed again with a strong water current to remove remainders of the pulp. Finally, the grains are dried either in the sun on cement floors or in driers and then packed in 60 kg bags. This technique is generally applied to the Arabica variety and consumes large quantities of water.

453

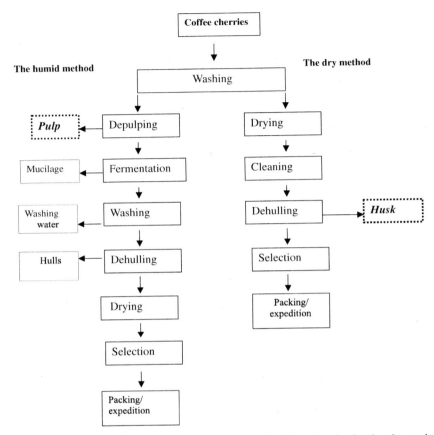

FIGURE III.18. Different stages of the treatment of coffee cherries by the dry and humid methods

## *The Dry Method*

In the dry method, after picking from gardens, cherries are immediately dried in the sun by spreading them in thin layers (about 30 kg/m$^2$), moving them frequently, and putting them under cover during the night and in the rain. It is sometimes difficult to dry the cherries adequately (approximately 12 percent or less moisture content) by simple sun drying. In such cases artificial drying is done using static, rotary, or vertical types of driers.

During processing of the cherries, major residues generated include coffee pulp (in the humid method) and coffee husk (in the dry method). Coffee pulp and husk contain toxic components such as caffeine, polyphenols, and tannins, and hence do not find suitable application. However, these are rich in organic nature.

## PHYSICOCHEMICAL COMPOSITION
## OF COFFEE PULP AND HUSK

Table III.14 shows the composition of coffee pulp and husk. Although the nature of the compounds present in the both of these are largely similar, there is some difference between the components and their concentrations. These differences could be attributed to different processing mode and efficiency, crop variety, and cultivation conditions such as soil type, etc.

Caffeine, one of nature's most powerful and addictive stimulants, is the principal substance causing the mild stimulating effect of coffee. It is also present in coffee pulp and husk at about 1.3 percent concentration on dry weight basis. Tannins are generally thought to be an antinutritional factor and prevent coffee pulp from being used at greater than 10 percent in animal feed. Information on coffee pulp tannins is sometimes contradictory, and such data as are available have sometimes been difficult to interpret because nonspecific analytical methods have been used. Depending upon the type of cultivars, the tannin contents may also differ. For example, coffee pulp from yellow-fruited cultivars could be richer in condensed tannins (proanthocyanidins) than pulp from the associated red-fruited cultivars.

## APPLICATIONS OF COFFEE PULP AND HUSK

Traditionally, coffee pulp and husk have found only limited applications as fertilizers, livestock feed, compost, etc. These applications utilize only a

TABLE III.14. Composition of coffee pulp and husk

| Components | Coffee pulp (% dry wt basis) | Coffee husk (% dry wt basis) |
|---|---|---|
| Carbohydrates | 44-50 | 57.8 |
| Proteins | 10-12 | 9.2 |
| Fibers | 18-21 | – |
| Fat | 2.5 | 2 |
| Caffeine | 1.2-1.3 | 1.3 |
| Tannins | 1.8-8.56 | 4.5 |
| Polyphenols | 1 | – |
| Pectin | – | 12.4 |

fraction of the available quantity and are not technically very efficient. Recent attempts have focused on their application as a substrate in bioprocesses because they contain fermentable sugars. Attempts have also been made to detoxify them for improved application as feed and to use the detoxified material as an efficient substrate for producing several value-added products such as enzymes, organic acids, flavor and aroma compounds, mushrooms, etc.

## Biological Detoxification of Coffee Husk and Pulp

Fungal strains such as *Rhizopus arrhizus, Phanerochaete chrysosporium, Penicillium curtosus, Pleurotus ostreatus, Lentinula edodes,* and *Flammulina velutipes* have the capacity to degrade caffeine and tannins present in coffee pulp and husk. Among these, *Rhizopus arrizhus* and *Aspergillus* sp. have been termed as the most suitable, which could degrade 87 to 92 percent of caffeine and 65 percent of tannins present in coffee husk, respectively Degradation of caffeine and tannins improves the feed value of coffee pulp and husk. Edible mushrooms such as *Pleurotus ostreatus, Lentinula edodes,* and *Flammulina velutipes* can also be cultivated on coffee pulp and husk and degrade 10 to 60 percent of caffeine and 12 to 80 percent of tannins.

## Production of Microbial Aroma

A novel approach to value addition of coffee husk has been to use it as a substrate for the production of aroma compounds for food industry applications using yeast and fungi. There has been a remarkable shift in the consumer's preference for naturally produced food and flavor compounds (in comparison to synthetic ones) for human use globally. Thus, production of aroma compounds through fermentative means has a promising future. The yeast *Pachysolen tannophilus* and the fungi *Ceratocystis fimbriata* were used in solid-state fermentation for synthesizing aroma compounds. These cultures produced a strong pineapple aroma. Along with ethanol, which could be the major compound produced, aldehyde and esters such as ethyl acetate, isobutyl acetate, ethyl-3-hexanoate, and isoamyl acetate may also be produced. Supplementation with nutrients such as amino acids could change the flavor. For example, when leucine was added to the medium, a strong banana odor was produced.

## Production of Enzymes, Citric Acid, and Gibberellic Acid

One of the earliest approaches to the application of coffee pulp and husk has been for the production of enzymes such pectinases, tannase, caffeinase, cellulases, protease, β-amylase, β-glucoamylase, and lipase using fungal strains and anaerobic bacteria. Citric acid has been produced using coffee husk by a strain of *Aspergillus niger,* and yields were higher than wheat bran, rice bran, and deoiled rice bran. Yields on the basis of amount of starch consumed have been almost similar for sugarcane press mud and coffee husk.

Coffee husk can also be used as a carbon source for the production of bioactive secondary metabolites such as gibberellic acid ($GA_3$). Fungal cultures such as *Gibberella fujikuroi* have commonly been used. Pretreatment of coffee husk with alkali solution could be useful in removing the phenolic compounds present in it and thereby increase the yields of gibberellic acid. Another important factor in this regard is the C:N of the substrate, which has been generally reported between 20 and 100. In the case of coffee husk, however, a lower C:N (between 13 and 15) has been recommended. Interestingly, mixed-substrate SSF, such as mixing of coffee husk with cassava bagasse, has been termed more suitable than single-substrate SSF, which under optimized conditions resulted as high as about 890 mg $GA_3$ per kilogram dry weight fermented matter.

### Composting and Biogas Production

Coffee pulp can be used as raw material for preparing compost comprising macro- and microfauna such as Acarida, Coleoptera, Collembola, Diptera, *Eisenia, Oligochaeta, Perionyx,* Thysanoptera, etc. Open pile systems or newer methods could de adopted. Vermicomposting, which takes advantage of biological and physiological capabilities of the growing macrofauna in solid residue, could be also a useful method to effectively use these residues.

Coffee pulp and husk can also be used for biogas production in anaerobic digestion. It has been found that from one ton of coffee pulp, about 131 $m^3$ biogas could be produced by anaerobic digestion, which would be equivalent to 100 liters of petrol in fuel value. Thus, composting (or vermicomposting) and anaerobic digestion could be considered useful ways to utilize these residues effectively.

### Production of Mushrooms

As mentioned previously, several mushrooms can be cultivated on coffee pulp and husk. In addition to coffee pulp and husk, coffee plant leaves and spent coffee grounds can also be used for this purpose. These substrates can be used individually or in combination. Cultivation of *Pleurotus ostreatus* on three different substrates, coffee husk, spent coffee grounds, and in a mixture of spent coffee grounds + coffee leaves (60:40, w/w), showed high biological efficiency (96.5, 90.4, and 76.7 percent, respectively, after 60 days of culture). Although *Lentinus edodes* can grow in coffee husk, it generally cannot produce the fruiting body. Pretreatment of coffee husk with boiling water and then using the husk, however, could be effective. The treatment of the coffee husk with the boiling water removes the toxic components present in it that inhibit the formation of the fruiting body. After such a treatment, the first flashes of *L. edodes* took place after 60 days and the biological efficiency was 85.8 percent. This mushroom easily grew on spent coffee grounds and gave the first flash after 56 days of culture with a biological efficiency of 88.7 percent.

*Flammulina velutipes* has also been cultivated on coffee husk. It took a relatively shorter time to grow and produce the first flash (25 days), although the biological efficiency was also relatively less (55.8 percent). However, when spent coffee grounds were used, biological efficiency improved to 78.3 percent in 21 days.

### *Hydrolysis of Coffee Husk*

One way to use coffee pulp and husk through biotechnological means involves the hydrolysis of these residues and use of the hydrolysate for different purposes. Hydrolysis could be performed using diluted acids such as diluted sulfuric acid or steam, which results in the formation of xylose, arabinose, fructose, glucose, sucrose, and maltose. Arabinose concentration is generally maximum, followed by glucose. Efficiency of hydrolysis could be around 60 to 70 percent for total and reducing sugars. Steam treatment (under pressure) has also been found to produce hydrolysate containing about 45 to 50 percent reducing sugars.

## CONCLUSIONS

From these discussions, it can be concluded that coffee pulp and husk can be effectively used as substrates for bioprocesses. Processes such as cultivation of edible mushrooms on treated or untreated coffee husk have great potential for commercial exploitation. Several other products, such as industrial enzymes, food-grade aroma compounds, etc., can be produced in SSF. Removal of antiphysiological and antinutritional factors, namely, caffeine and tannins, from these residues enhances their applicability as cattle feed. Adoption of new methods of composting and vermicomposting with these residues as raw material could also be an attractive alternative.

Hydrolysis of coffee husk using diluted acids or steam could be a cost-effective method. The hydrolysate can be used as a substrate for the production of various microbial products. Thus, application of coffee pulp and husk as a substrate for cultivating microorganisms provides a new raw material for bioprocesses and simultaneously resolves the problem of safe disposal of these residues from the coffee processing industries.

## SUGGESTED READINGS

Brand D, A Pandey, S Roussos, and CR Soccol (2000). Biological detoxification of coffee husk by filamentous fungi using a solid-state fermentation system. *Enzyme and Microbial Technology* 26(1-2):127-133.

Pandey A, CR Soccol, P Nigam, R Mohan, and S Roussos (2000). Biotechnological potential of coffee pulp and coffee husk for bioprocess. *Biochemical Engineering Journal* 6(2):153-162.

Sera T, CR Soccol, A Pandey, and S Roussos (eds.) (2000). *Coffee biotechnology and quality*. Dordrecht, The Netherlands: Kluwer Academic Publishers.

# Palm Oil Industry Residues

Poonsuk Prasertsan
S. Prasertsan

## INTRODUCTION

Oil palm is the highest oil-yielding crop. It is grown in many tropical countries in Asia and Africa. Palm oil wastes are mainly lignocellulosic material, which can be converted into valuable products. At present, palm oil residues are left unused, although many research works have indicated the potential of these wastes.

## RESIDUES FROM THE PALM OIL INDUSTRY

Oil palm trees (*Elaeis guineensis* Jacq.), a long-life rotation crop (25 to 30 years), give the highest oil yield per area, 3.27 tons of oil per hectare per year, which is six times higher than sunflower. Approximately 20 tons of fresh fruit bunches (FFB) are harvested per hectare per year. Oil yield is about 15 to 20 percent by weight of FFB. Southeast Asia, predominantly Malaysia, Indonesia, and Thailand, produces about 82 percent of the world production. Biomass yielded from the replantation of oil palm trees is 190.4 $m^3$/ha or 75 ton/ha. Oil palm wood can be a good material for the furniture industry because of its distinctive appearance from ordinary wood. However, sawing of oil palm wood is not easy because of the abrasive nature of the wood. Drying of the wood is also difficult because its density varies enormously within the trunk, which causes dimensional instability. Furthermore, oil palm wood is not suitable for power plant firing because its high potassium content causes ash meltdown.

Palm oil could be extracted by either standard process (wet process) or dry process. For standard process, steam and water are employed to inactivate the lipase activity of palm fruits and to extract the oil, respectively. The products are crude palm oil and palm kernel oil. The wastes include empty fruit bunches (EFB), palm press fiber (PPF), palm kernel cake (PKC), palm kernel shell (PKS), sludge cake or decanter cake, and palm oil mill effluent (POME). Based on the percentage of FFB, the expected wastes are 20 to 28 percent EFB, 11 to 12 percent PPF, and 5 to 8 percent PKS. POME is generated at approximately 0.6 to 1.0 ton per ton of FFB. In the dry process, dry heat is used for inactivation of lipase, and the whole palm fruit is fed to a screw press. The product is mixed crude palm oil and kernel oil, and the only waste generated is palm cake, without any wastewater.

## VALUABLE PRODUCTS FROM PALM OIL WASTES

### Energy

Energy could be a valuable product from palm oil mill solid wastes. PPF is used as boiler fuel in all palm oil mills due to its surplus. PKS use is more limited because it produces black smoke, leading to air pollution problems. The heating value of PKS is 17.4 MJ/kg. Many mills have installed cogeneration power plants (which produce heat and electricity) for their own consumption. Excess electricity can be sold to the grid.

The new scenario is to maximize the utilization of wastes by replacing the combustion of solid wastes with the biogas from POME as an energy source. This would allow solid wastes to be used for other products. Most mills use anaerobic pond systems for treatment of POME because of their low capital and operating cost. However, the ponding system requires a large area, and malodor consequently irritates nearby communities. This leads to the advantage of using a closed digester for methane production. In Malaysia, thermophilic anaerobic contact digestion of POME has been studied. Biogas yield of 0.9 to 1.5 $m^3$/kg of total solids (TS) utilized is achieved with loading of 3 to 5 kg TS/$m^3$ per day. One cubic meter of biogas is equivalent to 0.7 liter of fuel oil, and processing a ton of FFB produces 1 $m^3$ POME, which produces 28.3 $m^3$ biogas. Thus, heat of 784 MJ is expected from biogas per ton of FFB processed. Processing one ton of FFB requires 0.73 ton of steam at 3 bars (1,897 MJ of process heat) and 20 to 25 kWh of electricity. Assuming that the heat-to-electricity conversion efficiency is 25 percent, the heat required for 25 kWh electricity generation is 360 MJ. Biogas is therefore sufficient for electricity generation and partly sufficient for steam production. The energy deficit of 2,500 MJ for steam generation (assuming boiler efficiency of 65 percent) is obtainable from the solid wastes.

Apart from boiler and steam turbine technology, biogas can be used to produce electricity through an internal combustion engine or, in a more advanced technique, a gas turbine. The gas is first scrubbed to reduce $H_2S$ to less than 1,000 ppm, using iron and wood shavings. This is necessary to prevent corrosion in the gas engine. It is estimated that for a mill in Malaysia discharging a capacity of 576 $m^3$ of POME per day, the cost for producing

1 m$^3$ of biogas and 1 kWh electricity are US$0.05 and US$0.03, respectively. Digested POME can be used as fertilizer, which is claimed to increase plantation productivity by 15 percent.

Another form of energy is producer gas from the gasification of solid biomass. Producer gas is a mixture of gases, and the combustible components are CO, H$_2$, CH$_4$, and C$_x$H$_x$. The gas heating value is approximately 6 to 7 MJ/m$^3$. There are several types and sizes of gasifiers for application; the updraft gasifier is suitable only for process heat generation, while the downdraft gasifier can be used to run internal combustion engines for shaft power production.

### Activated Carbon

Because PKS contains 20.3 percent fixed carbon, it is suitable for making charcoal and activated carbon. PKS is pyrolyzed and physically or chemically activated to become activated carbon. After carbonization at 500°C for 30 minutes, charcoal yield of 31.6 percent was obtained with fixed carbon of 73.6 percent. Activation by steam at 900°C for 2 h produces activated carbon with an iodine value of 964 mg/g and specific pore area of 792.2 m$^2$/g. Chemical activation by zinc chloride at 700°C for 1 h yielded a better product, with an iodine value of 1,037 mg/g and specific pore area of 1,141 m$^2$/g. Palm shell charcoal activating at 900°C using CO$_2$ as the activating agent was studied. In general, as the activation time increases, both the micropore and the surface area are increased. Its surface area could be higher than 1,000 m$^2$/g for 3 h activation.

### Hardboard, Particleboard, Pulp, and Paper

Oil palm fiber and its inherent properties, namely, physical, morphological, mechanical, and chemical, have been well established. In general, the fiber properties of oil palm have a close resemblance to those of tropical hardwood. Much research has been conducted in the development of oil palm materials into useful products both in solid and reconstituted forms. Sawn timber, veneer and plywood, furniture production, particleboard, medium-density fiberboard, hardboard, chemically modified particleboard, cement-bonded particleboard, pulp and paper, chemical feed stock, animal feed, cellulose gel, and wood polymer composite have been produced and their properties evaluated. However, due to the inherent properties of the oil palm materials and fiber, such as very high initial moisture content and high dimensional instability, it is generally believed that the greatest potential for utilization lies in the composite and reconstituted forms.

The simplest method of EFB utilization is the physical separation of fibrous material from the empty bunches. EFB fiber is coarser, longer, and stronger than that of PPF. By adding a binding agent, such as rubber latex, EFB fiber is used for cushion-filling material.

Rather than emplying a wet process that needs a binding agent and generates wastewater, hardboard could be produced by a dry process. The binderless board is achieved using steam-exploded fibers of oil palm biomass (the cut-down trunk for replantation) which is rich in hemicellulose. The palm biomass residue is soaked in high steam pressure (28 bars) for five minutes and instantaneously released to atmospheric pressure. Pulp yield from the steam explosion is 70 percent. Mats of defibrated fiber are formed and hot pressed at 150°C for 10 minutes. Experiments revealed that the steam-exploded fiber is suitable for hardboard making to meet the JIS A5905-1994 standard. The main bonding strength of the board is believed to be due to a lignin-furfural linkage.

Oil palm fiber can be pulped mechanically or chemically. Mechanical pulping apparently uses less energy consumption compared to corresponding wood production, while the overall properties of paper made from oil palm trunk fiber are superior to those of bagasse and some tropical and temperate hardwood species such as eucalyptus and aspen.

### Feed

Palm oil mill wastes are a good source for feed supplements. PPF could be used as ruminant feed at 10 to 20 percent of the diet, and its quality could be improved by adding 5 to 6 percent ammonium hydroxide or urea and fermenting for two to three weeks. PKC has a very high protein content (19 percent) and is a good feed, as 20 to 40 percent could be added for broiler use and 10 to 50 percent for swine. Dried decanter cake as well as palm cake are used as feed supplements. POME, either dried or concentrated, could be supplemented to feed for cattle and goat.

### Composting/Fertilizer

The optimum C:N ratio for composting is in the range of 25 to 30:1. Solid palm oil mill wastes are rich in carbon but low in nitrogen sources. The deficiency of nitrogen can be solved by adding nitrogen-rich seafood processing wastes or other nitrogen sources. EFB is used for composting to obtain better nutrient balance for mushroom cultivation or efficient microbial activity. Higher biodegradation rate and shorter incubation period could be achieved using commercial composite microorganisms or animal wastes such as goat dung, cow dung, or chicken manure. The decrease of EFB volume after the ripeness of the compost would be beneficial for transportation and handling. The compost and residue from mushroom production are stable humus suitable for crop production.

Decanter cake mixed with boiler ash is a good source of fertilizer. EFB ash contains high potassium content, which can be a mineral source for fertilizer. POME is usually irrigated to oil palm plantation after treating in two to three anaerobic ponds. Dried POME (6.5 percent moisture content) mixed with other ingredients is sold as fertilizer or feed under the trade name Super Grow.

### Enzymes

Lignocellulosic enzymes are complex in nature due to the heterogeneous component of the substrate. Solid wastes from palm oil mills consist of three major components: cellulose (25 to 50 percent), hemicellulose (20 to 35 percent), and lignin (18 to 35 percent). They can be used as substrates for production of cellulases, hemicellulases, and ligninases from various microorganisms. Pretreatment is usually required prior to the fermentation stage. Steam-explosion pretreatment on palm cake and palm fiber results in higher contents of the water-extractable hemicellulose fraction and methanol-extractable lignin. Heating and alkali treatment of ground palm cake, however, give no further improvement in enzyme production from *Aspergillus niger* ATCC 6275. The fungus produces higher xylanase activity when grown on palm cake than on palm fiber in solid-substrate fermentation. The crude enzyme is applied to treat POME for separation of oil (99 percent) and suspended solids (71 percent). In addition, culture filtrate of the isolate Cf-27 is able to release about 8 percent or more of the trapped oil from PPF, giving an increase in total oil extraction of about 0.3 percent.

### Biopolymers

POME is suitable as a culture medium for biopolymer production due to its high carbon to nitrogen ratio. Volatile fatty acids or organic acids from the anaerobic treatment of POME can be converted to polyhydroxyalkanoate (PHA) by *Rhodobacter sphaeroides* (IFO 12203), giving the maximum yield of 0.5 g/g organic acid consumed and 67 percent PHA content in the cells. The intracellular PHB possesses thermoplastic and biodegradable properties. Two thermotolerant fungal isolates, ST4 and ST29, cultivated in POME at 45°C could produce extracellular polymers that are able to harvest oil and suspended solids from the POME.

## Antibiotics

POME is a cheap medium suitable for antibiotic production. It is first filtered to remove suspended solids, then ultrafiltered to reduce the ash content to a desirable level. Pretreated POME supplemented with $(NH_4)_2SO_4$ to obtain the C:N ratio of 20:1 is used for cultivation of *Penicillium chrysogenum*. The carbohydrate content of the medium is 35 g/l, which gave a biomass yield of 16 g/l, and penicillin produced is 88 percent of the best value reported elsewhere.

## CONCLUSIONS

Many valuable products can be obtained from the leftover wastes in palm oil mills. The processes involve many disciplines ranging from mechanical engineering to biotechnology. Although research shows that technically it is possible to do so, industrial-scale production seems not to be fully established yet. Therefore, the increasing demand for green products could provide opportunity for this industry in the future.

## SUGGESTED READINGS

Laemsak N and M Okuma (2000). Development of boards made from oil palm frond. II: Properties of binderless boards from steam-exploded fibers of oil palm frond. *Journal of Wood Science* 46:322-326.

Prasertsan P and S Prasertsan (1996). Biomass residues from palm oil mills in Thailand: An overview on quantity and potential usage. *Biomass and Bioenergy* 11(5):387-395.

# Seafood Industry Residues

Poonsuk Prasertsan
S. Prasertsan

## INTRODUCTION

Seafood is a large industry in terms of worldwide production scale. Residues from the industry are nutrient rich and often pollute the environment if proper treatment is not in place. On the other hand, if proper technology is employed, wastes can be converted into valuable products. This chapter reviews the potential of seafood wastes as a bioresource for valuable products.

## RESIDUES FROM THE SEAFOOD INDUSTRY

Seafood industries are very diversified in raw material types and species, as well as their processes. Type and quantity of residues generated therefore depend on type of raw materials and methods used during the processes. In general, seafood-processing residues account for approximately three-quarters of the total weight of the catch. Fish solid wastes (residues), consisting of head, tail, frame, and skin, are in the amount of 28 to 30 percent with 5 to 7 percent of viscera, while crustacean wastes are in the range of 40 to 80 percent. Liquid wastes include blood, thawing solution, and precooking water.

Seafood residues are very perishable due to their high protein content and neutral pH, therefore they are potentially contributory to environmental pollution. Considering the fact that seafood wastes are enormous in quantity, it is worthwhile to convert these wastes into utilizable products. Such an approach will, no doubt, result in avoidance of environmental pollution as well as monetary gain.

## VALUABLE PRODUCTS FROM SEAFOOD-PROCESSING RESIDUES

Seafood-processing residues serve as excellent raw material sources for production of numerous valuable products. These include fish meal, fish silage, protein hydrolysate, fish extract, fish sauce, single-cell proteins, enzymes, fish oil and omega-3 fatty acids, fish gelatin, chitinous material, carotenoid pigment and flavorant, as well as other products.

## Fish Meal

Fish meal is probably the most common value-added product from sea-food-processing waste. Its importance in animal feed is enormous and is increasing. It is the preferred protein source for many farmed fish and shrimp species and is valued for its amino acid balance, vitamin content, palatability, and unidentified growth factors. The process involves the removal of water and oil from solid wastes using filter press or centrifugation, resulting in liquid waste (or stickwater), and subsequently the solid residues are dried in a dryer. Fish meal has 6 to 12 percent moisture content and is composed of 50 to 70 percent protein, 5 to 15 percent fat, <1 percent fiber, and 8 to 33 percent ash, with essential amino acids and vitamins.

## Fish Silage

Fish silage is the product from fish wastes preserved by addition of acid or by lactic fermentation. Molasses or cassava may be added as a carbohydrate source, i.e., for preparation of shrimp head silage. Control of the degree of proteolysis and lipid oxidation is required to produce silages of high nutritive value. *Lactobacillus plantarum* is mostly used, and the presence of *Saccharomyces* sp. will improve the odor and increase the amount of reducing sugar, as well as being the source of probiotics to increase disease resistance. Fish neural-tissue silage contains 5.5 to 46.5 percent lipids (by dry weight) with $n$-3 highly unsaturated fatty acids, especially docosahexaenoic acid (DHA) (22:6 $n$-3). Its DHA:EPA (eicosapentaenoic acid) ratios range from 3.5 to 5.4. The codried product of the lactic fermented silage and the sulfuric acid silage from salmon viscera contains 9 to 11 percent nitrogen and is deficient in methionine.

Fish silage can be used as feed, enrichers for rotifer *(Brachionus plicatilis)* and Artemia *(Artemia nauplii)* for feeding marine fish larvae before weaning, and liquid fertilizer. Fertilizer, prepared by the addition of 3.5 percent formic acid and 20 percent molasses and fermented for 20 days, must be neutralized and diluted to 1:50 or 1:100 before applying.

## Protein Hydrolysate

Fish wastes or by-catch fish are the bioresource for fish protein hydrolysate (FPH) production. FPH is made by enzymatic hydrolysis of a protein-rich source yielding small peptides and free amino acids. The traditional method is that the acid is added to lower the pH to 3 to 4 and the fish endogenous enzymes, active and stable at low pH, such as pepsins, quickly hydrolyze most of the protein. The hydrolysate from fish viscera (an enzyme-rich raw material) contains about 12 percent peptides and amino acids and a small amount of lipids. In this case, addition of other enzyme sources neither accelerates the autolysis nor improves the hydrolysate. For low-protease-activity raw materials, commercial microbial enzymes are commonly added. Enzymatic process gives FPH with higher nutritional values since essential amino acids are not destroyed. Nevertheless, overhydrolysis by enzymes will give peptides with a bitter taste.

Protein hydrolysate has a wide range of applications as food, medical food, feed, and culture media. By controlling the degree of hydrolysis, FPH with acceptable functional properties for human consumption is obtained. The functional properties, on the other hand, depend on the size of the molecular weights of the hydrolyzed protein. Cod frame protein hydrolysate with molecular weights of 10 kDa and 30 kDa has shown excellent emulsion properties and whippability. The 10 kDa hydrolysate has high antioxidative activity, while the 3 kDa hydrolysate has excellent angiotensin I converting enzyme (ACE) inhibitory activity, preventing high blood pressure. In addition, FPH appears to be useful in treatment of rare diseases such as pancreatitis, irritable bowel syndrome, Crohn's disease, ulcerative colitis, fistulas, severe trauma, and food allergies. Unique peptides are speculated to exist with important physiologic functions, such as stimulation of growth factors and blood-flow regulation. In addition, FPH is used as a milk replacer for young animals, such as calves and piglets, and as nitrogen sources for microbial growth media. Fish peptones are produced commercially in Norway and Japan.

### Fish Extract

Precooking water, fish stickwater, and fish soluble are used as raw materials for fish extract production. Fish extract is produced by heating raw materials at 85 to 90°C for 6 h, followed by cooling, centrifugation, and digestion (using commercial protease at 50°C, pH 7 to 8 for 1 h). Subsequently, the enzymes are inactivated at 90°C before removal of solids by filter press, and the product is concentrated to reduce the moisture content to 43 percent before desalting and packaging. The product contains 60 percent protein, a dark-brown color, good flavor, and no fishy smell. In Thailand, tuna precooking water, which accounts for 20 percent of tuna weight and contains 5 percent protein, is used for fish extract production.

### Fish Sauce

Fish sauce is the aqueous soluble phase obtained after fermentation and autolysis of the fish raw material for several months at very high salt concentrations. Fish sauce is rich in essential amino acids such as lysine and methionine, which are not present in cereal. Fish cannery wastes including viscera and the juice extracted from the solid wastes prior to the drying of these wastes to fish meal can be used as raw materials for the production of fish sauce with the addition of *koji* of *Aspergillus oryzae* as a source of proteolytic enzyme. Good-quality fish sauce is obtained within three months as compared to 12 months from the traditional process.

### Enzymes

Out of 300 commercially available enzyme preparations, only 15 have been prepared from marine resources, and most of these are used as biochemical research reagents. Fish viscera contain a wide variety of proteolytic enzymes, of which trypsin, chymotrypsin, and pepsin are the most important ones. Pepsin is found in the stomach, while trypsin is present in pyloric caeca. Trypsin is widely used in medical treatment, leather-tanning processes, meat tenderization, and wine and beer refining. Cold-temperature enzymes from gastrointestinal tracts of fish may serve as processing aids in the food industry. Proteinase extracted from tuna pyloric caeca is applied for production of cod frame protein hydrolysate. Prawn waste, on the other hand, is used for chitinase production by solid-state fermentation of the marine fungus *Beauveria bassiana* (BTMF S10).

The enzymes from the viscera of yellowfin tuna *(Thunnus albacares)* exhibit higher protease activities (72.17 Units/ml) and lipase activities (1.26 U/ml) than those of skipjack tuna *(Katsuwonus pelamis)* and longtail tuna *(Thunnus tonggol)*. Among the individual viscera organs, spleen has been found to be the best source for protease (53.38 U/ml), while pancreas gives the highest lipase activity (0.72 U/ml). The enzymes have an optimum pH in the range of 9.5 to 10.0, while the optimum temperature of protease and lipase are at 50°C and 60°C, respectively. For enzymes from fish *(Epinephelus tauvina* F.) pyloric caeca, the optimum protease activity is at pH 8 and 45°C.

### Fish Oil and Omega-3 Fatty Acids

Fish oils are produced from the whole body or guts of many fish species. The major component is triacylglycerol, rich in omega-3 polyunsaturated fatty acids (PUFA) such as EPA and DHA. Omega-3 fatty acids in marine lipid from fish liver (also rich in vitamin A and D) or by-products from fish meal production can be used for pharmaceutical and food applications. Crude tuna oil (0.1 percent of the fish weight) obtained from the centrifugation process contains 29.5 to 36.5 percent PUFA consisting of 4.4 to 6.7 percent EPA and 22.5 to 26.9 percent DHA. Crude tuna oil is purified by removal of the impurities using water and phosphoric acid, neutralization by sodium hydroxide, decolorization by 3 percent decolorizing agent under 10 mm Hg pressure at 100°C for 15 min, and deodorization at 1.5 to 3 mm Hg at 170°C. The DHA content of the crude tuna oil is half of that contained in DHA-rich (50 to 65 percent) fish oils, commercially available using enzymatic modification and chemical esterification of acyl groups. EPA-rich product (more than 92 percent EPA ethyl ester) from sardine oil is commercially available in Japan as a pharmaceutical for arteriosclerosis and hyperlipidemia.

### Fish Gelatin

Fish skins are rich in collagen that can be recovered and converted into valuable products such as gelatin. Fish gelatin preparation is as follows: the fish skins are initially washed to remove surface slime, cut into small pieces, and treated with proteases to remove noncollagenous protein material. The deproteinized material is demineralized and then centrifuged at a low temperature to separate the fat layer. Gelatin is extracted from the degreased material by heating with protease in citric acid solution. The gelatin liquor obtained is clarified by filtration through cheesecloth and concentrated by rotary evaporation under vacuum. The concentrated gelatin liquor is chilled to thicken, air dried, and then powdered by grinding. Fish gelatin has relatively higher concentrations of serine, threonine, methionine, and total essential amino acids than calf gelatin or mammalian gelatin. Highly purified fish gelatin is used in special purposes such as precision printing.

### Chitinous Materials

Chitin, chitosan, and chitosan derivatives are biopolymers of great economic importance. Chitin content from shrimp, crab, squid, and krill are in the range of 11 to 49 percent. Chitin is a homopolymer of $N$-acetyl-D-glucosamine (NAG), which is known to have anti-inflammatory properties. Chitin is insoluble in aqueous solution and organic solvents. Production of chitin from crustacean wastes is obtained after deproteinization and demineralization using alkali and acid, respectively. Recovery of chitin can also be achieved by lactic acid fermentation using *Lactobacillus paracasei* strain A3 treated on scampi *(Nephrops norvegicus)* waste. Chitosan, a polycationic biopolymer, is obtained by the *N*-deacetylation of chitin using concentrated alkali at elevated temperatures or enzyme chitin deacetylases (EC 3.5.1.41). The enzyme can also be used for preparation of chitosan oligomers.

Acid-free, water-soluble chitosan has been developed using an immobilized chitinolytic enzyme complex from *Streptomyces kurssanovii*. The products are a 22 to 24 kDa chitosan of low solubility in water and a 2 to 9 kDa acid-free, water-soluble chitosan. In addition, partially hydrolyzed chitosan and oligosaccharides are produced from chitosan using an immobilized enzyme chitosanase (694 U/g protein) from *Bacillus pumilus* BN-262 and an ultrafiltration membrane reactor.

Chitin, chitosan, and chitosan derivatives are applied in food, agriculture, processing, and additives, as well as in water treatment, biomedical applications (including wound dressing and artificial skin), and personal care products. Chitin and chitosan possess hypocholesterolemic activity and antihypertensive action. Their oligomers possess additional functional properties, such as antitumor activity, immuno-enhancing effects, and antimicrobial activity, and are soluble in neutral aqueous solutions. Chitosan derivatives, *O*-carboxymethylchitin and *O*-hydroxypropylchitosan, are used in cosmetics and as a structural component of liposomes. *N,O*-carboxymethylchitosan and its lactate, acetate, and pyrrolidine carboxylate salts are used to control lipid oxidation in meats.

### Carotenoid Pigments and Flavorant

Crustacean wastes are rich sources for pigments and flavor compounds. Carotenoid pigments can be extracted into nonpolar solvents such as edible oils at 50 to 80°C. The maximum extraction was achieved at 60°C at an oil to crustacean waste ratio of 2:1 (v/w). The carotenoid content in shrimp and crab wastes varies from 119.6 to 147.7 µg/g, and the main components are astaxanthin (3.95 and 21.16 percent, respectively) and its monoester (19.72 and 5.11 percent, respectively) as well as diester (74.29 and 56.57 percent, respectively). Carotenoid and carotenoprotein extracts, prepared from shellfish processing wastes, are used in aquaculture feed formulations intended for pigmentation of salmonids.

Flavor compounds in fish and shellfish can be divided into two major groups: nitrogenous and nonnitrogenous compounds. The nitrogenous compounds include free amino acids, low-molecular-weight peptides, nucleotides, and organic bases. The nonnitrogenous compounds consist of organic acids, sugars, and inorganic constituents. Nitrogenous flavoring compounds from shrimp heads are extracted using 0.25 percent bromelain, pH 6, at 50°C for 5 h with sodium chloride as the binder. The total amino acid content in shrimp flavor extracted with enzyme is about 2.5-fold higher than that extracted with water. Free amino acids such as arginine, alanine, glutamic acid, serine, and glycine are among the major contributors to the distinctive sensory features of crustacea. Membrane process by electrodialysis is a more effective method for recovery of flavor compounds than diafiltration.

Among 80 volatile components in blue crab *(Callinectes sapidus)* processing by-product, trimethylamine, carbon disulfide, dimethyltrisulfide, two alkanes (C15 and C17), geranylacetone, and 1-dodecanol are the highest. Flavorants, recovered from cooking water or shellfish processing wastes, could be blended into aquatic feed to enhance the feed uptake of some fish. Protein hydrolysate from fish and shrimp wastes possess high flavoring amino acids and therefore are used as flavoring agents in food products such as surimi, cereal products, or feed supplements for fish and shrimp.

### *Culture Media*

Fish-processing wastes are good culture media for production of single-cell proteins. Tuna precooking water is a good source for growth of the photosynthetic bacteria *Rhodocyclus gelatinosus* R7. The highest biomass of 12.27 g/l is achieved by repeated-batch cultivation under anaerobic-light (3 lux) condition. The cell contains 56 percent protein, 2.21 mg carotenoid, and 22.52 mg bacteriochlorophyll/g dry cell weight, as well as vitamin $B_{12}$. Besides *R. gelatinosus* R7, *Bacillus subtilis, Candida tropicalis* F-129, and *C. utilis* IFO 0396 could also grow well in tuna precooking water.

Effluent from frozen-seafood-processing plants can be used as culture medium for growth of *Chlorella* sp. T9. Maximum biomass (5.4 g/l) is achieved by supplementation with 85 mg/l $NaNO_3$ and 2 percent $CO_2$ feeding into the effluent at the light intensity of 5200 lux. Feeding of $CO_2$ not only increased the biomass yield but also decreased the cultivation time by nearly half (from 18 to 10 days).

### *Other Products*

Antimicrobial agents can be produced from marine resources. Protamine is a basic peptide containing over 80 percent arginine and is found in the testicles of more than 50 fish species. Its unique properties include thermostability and the ability to prevent the growth of *Bacillus* spores. Hence, it is being used as an antibacterial agent in food processing and food preservation. Production of protamine and salmine, and curpeine was from salmon and sardine, respectively.

The antifreeze proteins from blood plasma of cold-water fish are important both for production of transgenic fish and for extending the shelf life of human organs intended for transplant purposes. Collagen from cod swim bladder is used as a clarifier in the brewing of beer and wine.

## CONCLUSIONS

Seafood-processing residues are nutrient-rich bioresources in both quantity and quality. Many valuable products could be derived from these wastes. However, making them commercially viable needs more research and development as well as evaluations of their marketing potential. Such attempts are increasingly being recognized in food-exporting industrial countries.

## SUGGESTED READINGS

Gildberg A (1993). Enzymatic processing of marine raw material. *Process Biochemistry* 28:1-15.

Hall GM and NH Ahmad (1992). Functional properties of fish protein hydrolysate. In *Fish processing technology,* GM Hall (ed.). London: Blackie Academic and Professional, pp. 249-270.

Shahidi F (1994). Seafood processing by-products. In *Seafoods: Chemistry, processing technology and quality,* F Shahidi and JR Botta (eds.). London: Blackie Academic and Professional, pp. 320-330.

# Biodiesel Production and Application

Edward Crabbe
Ayaaki Ishizaki

## INTRODUCTION

Over the past two centuries the world's economic growth has relied heavily on fossil-derived liquid fuel for energy generation and transportation. These sources are nonrenewable, and at the present rate of consumption known crude oil reserves could be depleted by the end of the twenty-first century. However, there is an increasing demand for liquid fuels for transportation, for energy generation stemming from rapidly increasing populations and industrialization in many developing economies, and to power new technologies. Liquid fuels are a necessity for agricultural production, which largely depends on diesel fuel. Emissions from the combustion of these fuels, such as carbon dioxide ($CO_2$), carbon monoxide (CO), nitrogen oxides ($NO_x$), and sulfur-containing residues, are the principal cause of global warming and public health diseases. As a result, many countries have passed legislation to arrest their adverse environmental consequences. Therefore, there is an ongoing effort to develop alternative sources of liquid fuel to ensure that new technologies are available to keep pace with society's need for new renewable power alternatives for the future. Key requirements are that the alternative source(s) must be abundant, readily available, and renewable, and emissions from combustion of any derivative liquid fuels must reduce the incidence of related public health diseases and protect the environment.

Biodiesel refers to liquid fuels made from renewable biomass, such as vegetable oils or animal fats, and an alcohol, such as methanol or ethanol. Technically, it is the transesterified product (alkyl esters) of a triglyceride (or a fatty acid) and an alcohol, usually methanol or ethanol. They are therefore fatty acid alkyl esters. When the product is intended for use as liquid fuel it is referred to as biodiesel. In a general sense, it refers to any diesel fuel substitute derived from natural renewable biomass.

Biodiesel production has received a lot of attention because of the economic, environmental, and health benefits that it could offer. It is considered a renewable fuel because it is biodegradable: the carbon dioxide emitted when the oil is combusted as liquid fuel forms part of the life cycle of the carbon of vegetable crops and can be sequestered into plants and recycled, facilitating a near net zero increase in carbon dioxide emission. Most biodiesels marketed are cleaner-burning fuels and can help reduce greenhouse gas emissions, global warming, air pollution, and related public health risks. These include reduction in particulate matter (PM), carbon monoxide (CO), hydrocarbons (HC), sulfur oxides ($SO_x$), nitrogen oxides ($NO_x$), and air toxins. They can be used alone or as a blend with petroleum diesel, extending limited supplies of fossil fuels. For countries with agriculture-based economies, it can reduce a country's dependence on petroleum imports and boost its domestic economy.

## SOURCES OF RAW MATERIALS

Biodiesel can be produced from any naturally occurring renewable oil. Any abundant source of cheap fatty acid or oil can serve as raw materials. Sources include crude and refined vegetable oils, used or recycled vegetable oil and animal fat or tallow, oil extracted from algae and other oilseeds, and soap stock. Oilseed crops are the largest group of exploitable renewable biomass resource for biodiesel production. There are more than 350 oilbearing crops identified, among which only sunflower, safflower, soybean, rapeseed, cottonseed, peanut, and palm oils are considered as potential alternative fuels for diesel engines. Unlike fossil fuel, however, different regions of the world have their own vegetable oil resource that is being or can be used for commercial biodiesel production. For example, rapeseed biodiesel dominates the market in Europe, soybean is used predominately in the United States, while safflower is the oil source in Turkey. In Malaysia, biodiesel production from crude palm oil is being developed. Vegetable oils have long been considered as alternative or emergency fuels for diesel engines because they have heat contents approximately 90 percent of that of #2 diesel fuel, the transportation fuel. The problem associated with using unesterified oils is that their high viscosities, about ten times that of #2 diesel fuel, affect engine performance and limit their use in modern direct-injection-type diesel engines. Used cooking oil recovered from homes can be another possible source. Discharge of used cooking oil from homes into drains without treatment is now strictly restricted by regulations.

## METHODS OF MANUFACTURE
## AND FACTORS AFFECTING PRODUCTION

Biodiesel can be produced by a variety of esterification technologies. The oil and fats are filtered and preprocessed to remove water and contaminants. It is then chemically or enzymatically reacted with a simple short-chain primary alcohol, usually methanol or ethanol. Glycerol is produced as a by-product. Methanol is the most widely used alcohol for biodiesel production because it is easy to process and is relatively inexpensive. Therefore, most biodiesel is produced as methylated fatty acids (MFA) or fatty acid methyl esters (FAME). There are four basic routes to ester production from oils and fats:

1. Base-catalyzed transesterification of the oil with alcohol
2. Direct acid-catalyzed esterification of the oil with alcohol
3. Conversion of the oil to fatty acids, and then to alkyl esters with acid catalysis
4. Using biocatalysts, such as a lipase, to accomplish the transesterification process

The majority of the biodiesel produced today is done using base-catalyzed transesterification (with sodium or potassium hydroxide as catalyst) because it is the most economical in terms of operating conditions for processing (low temperature [150°F] and pressure [20 psi]); high rate of reaction; high conversion (98 percent) with minimal side reactions and reaction time; and direct conversion to methyl ester with no intermediate steps. By this method, the three most important parameters affecting triglyceride transesterification (biodiesel synthesis) are the molar ratio of the methanol to the triglyceride, the nature and the amount of catalyst, and the reaction temperature. Stoichiometrically, complete transesterification should occur at a molar ratio of 3:1 (methanol to triglyceride) yielding 3 moles of ester and 1 mole of glycerol. At this stoichiometry however, the reaction rate is slow and rarely proceeds to completion, necessitating the use of excess methanol. Although alkali-catalyzed transesterification proceeds faster than acid catalysis, the type of oil used determines the mode of chemical catalysis. Alkali-catalyzed reactions are one-step reactions and proceed faster when the acid value is low (i.e., in refined oils), whereas acid catalysis favors vegetable oils with high acid value (i.e., in crude oils). A high free fatty acid concentration also deactivates alkali catalysts, and the addition of excess amount of alkali as compensation gives rise to the formation of emulsion, which increases viscosity and leads to the formation of gels and to problems associated with glycerol separation and loss in ester yield.

## PROPERTIES OF BIODIESEL
## VERSUS PETROLEUM DIESEL

Table III.15 compares the fuel properties of acid-catalyzed production of crude palm oil methyl ester (CPOME) to #2 diesel fuel. This biodiesel has physical properties very similar to conventional diesel, but the emission properties are better for biodiesel than for conventional diesel. The greatest differences are in the sulfur, nitrogen, cetane number (CN), and distillation range, which were all higher in CPOME biodiesel. The higher sulfur and nitrogen content, attributed to sulfates and nitrogenous compounds in the broth and the acid used as catalyst, are readily eliminated by repeated wash-

TABLE III.15. Fuel properties of CPOME and CPOME+ABE[a] mix and #2 diesel fuel

| Property | #2 Diesel (JIS K2280) | CPOME only | CPOME +ABE |
|---|---|---|---|
| Density (g/cm$^3$), 15°C | 0.805-0.895 | 0.8587 | 0.8548 |
| Cetane number | 32.5-56.5 | 49 | 52 |
| Flash point (°C) | 52 | 27 | 26 |
| Elemental composition (w%) | | | |
| Carbon | 85 | 74.3 | 74.16 |
| Hydrogen | 16 | 13.0 | 12.4 |
| Oxygen | 0.22[b] | 12.7 | 13.0 |
| Sulfur | 0.05[b] | 6 | 1.0 |
| Nitrogen | 0.01[b] | 3 | 1.0 |
| Distillation range | | | |
| IBP (°C) | – | 63 | 54 |
| 10% | 171-259 | 71 | 69 |
| 50% | 212-308 | 335 | 339 |
| 90% | 251-363 | 360 | 360 |
| FBP (°C) | – | 610 | 597 |

[a]From batch extractive ABE fermentation using 40 g/l glucose in tryptone yeast extract acetate medium. CPOME contained 5.74 g/l butanol extracted from the broth during cultivation.
[b]Specifications are quoted from equivalent ASTM.

ing with deionized water. The CN is a prime indicator of diesel fuel quality and is related to the ignition delay time of a fuel in the combustion chamber. The higher CN of CPOME translates into a shorter ignition delay time or reduced cold starts. It also indicates that there would be good control of the fuel combustion which would enhance engine performance while reducing the level of contaminants in exhaust gases. Moreover, storage and transportation are facilitated because the boiling points of the 50 and 90 percent fractions are higher than that of #2 diesel fuel.

Biodiesel operates in combustion-ignition engines just like petroleum diesel. Blends of up to 20 percent biodiesel (mixed with petroleum diesel fuels) can be used in nearly all diesel equipment and are compatible with most storage and distribution equipment. These low-level blends (20 percent and less) do not require any engine modifications and can provide the same payload capacity and range as diesel. Higher blends, even pure biodiesel (100 percent biodiesel), can be used in many engines built since 1994 with little or no modification. Using biodiesel in a conventional diesel engine substantially reduces emissions of unburned hydrocarbons, carbon monoxide, sulfates, polycyclic aromatic hydrocarbons, nitrated polycyclic aromatic hydrocarbons, and particulate matter. These reductions increase as the amount of biodiesel blended into diesel fuel increases. The best reductions are seen with 100 percent biodiesel. The use of biodiesel decreases the solid carbon fraction of particulate matter (since the oxygen in biodiesel enables more complete combustion to $CO_2$) and reduces the sulfate fraction (biodiesel contains less than 24 ppm sulfur), while the soluble, or hydrocarbon, fraction stays the same or increases. Therefore, biodiesel works well with new technologies such as catalysts (which reduce the soluble fraction of diesel particulate but not the solid carbon fraction), particulate traps, and exhaust gas recirculation.

## POTENTIAL TECHNOLOGY DEVELOPMENT: BIODIESEL AS A SOLVENT EXTRACTANT FOR IN SITU BIODIESOHOL PRODUCTION

In addition to their fuel properties, FAMEs of vegetable oil origin are known to extract butanol, an excellent fuel extender, which efficiently blends with petroleum diesel to form diesohol. Butanol is preferred to ethanol in diesohol formulation because it has a lower vapor pressure and mixes with petroleum diesel at all temperatures. Diesohol production can also be achieved using FAME of vegetable oil origin as a butanol extractant in acetone-butanol-ethanol (ABE) fermentation because the composite product (FAME-butanol mix) would have fuel properties comparable to diesohol obtained by blending petroleum diesel and commercial butanol. In this regard, different ABE fermentation systems (batch, fed-batch, or continuous systems) can be integrated with in situ solvent extraction to produce biodiesohols.

In situ extractive ABE fermentation removes butanol, the end product, from culture broth to extractant, vegetable oil methylester, resulting in lower product concentration in the culture broth. Oleyl alcohol is better extractant for butanol since it has a high partition coefficient for butanol, but unfortunately it is poisonous to the microorganism.

As butanol extractant for in situ ABE fermentation culture, both CPOME (produced from crude palm oil) and UCOME (used cooking oil methyl esters from used cooking oil from Japanese restaurants) biodiesel are nonmetabolizable and biocompatible with *Clostridium saccharoperbutylacetonicum* N1-4 (ATCC 13564). They also remain thermally and chemically stable even after sterilization at high temperature (121°C) and pressure and when employed as an extractant in in situ batch fermentation. Both CPOME and UCOME biodiesel selectively extract about 40 to 50 percent of the total butanol produced in the broth and thus enhance its production and the overall productivity of the bioprocess system (Table III.16). This concept of employing MFAs as extractants appears attractive because these extractants could be used directly as liquid fuels (that is, as biodiesel) in agricultural machineries and transit buses, thereby eliminating the recovery step from solvent extraction.

Another possible application is in waste management to reduce environmental pollution from food and agro-based industrial effluent streams. In conventional ABE fermentation, the carbon source was mashed starch and molasses. Today, these agricultural products are too expensive to use in butanol fermentation. Many agroindustrial effluents contain mixed carbohydrate substrates that can be exploited to produce butanol by many clostridial strains to reduce its biological oxygen demand and fuel consumption

TABLE III.16. Total ABE fermentation products from batch culture

| Fermentation system | Product (g/l) | | | | |
|---|---|---|---|---|---|
| | Butanol | Acetone | Ethanol | Acetic acid | Butyric acid |
| Nonextractive | 15.9 | 4.09 | 1.23 | 1.83 | 0.11 |
| Extractive | | | | | |
| Oleyl alcohol | 19.2 | 7.81 | 0.83 | 1.82 | 0.11 |
| CPOME | 20.9 | 8.01 | 0.86 | 1.84 | 0.10 |

*Note:* Cultivation time 80 h; glucose 40 g/l

for incineration. Home refuse, garbage, and food residues discharged from homes, restaurants, and hotels are possible raw materials for ABE fermentation. Waste from the food industry, distilleries, and agroindustry, such as the palm oil industry, the rubber industry, and sago starch mills, are confirmed as good mediums. The butanol produced can be then extracted with biodiesel to produce biodiesohol.

## SUGGESTED READINGS

Crabbe E, CN Hipolito, G Kobayashi, K Sonomoto, and A Ishizaki (2001). Biodiesel production from crude palm oil and evaluation of butanol extraction and fuel properties. *Process Biochemistry* 37:65-71.

Ishizaki A, S Michiwaki, E Crabbe, G Kobayashi, K Sonomoto, and S Yoshino (1999). Extractive aceton-butanol-ethanol fermentation using methylated crude palm oil as extractant in batch culture of *Clostridium saccharoperbutylacetonicum* N1-4 (ATCC 13564). *Journal of Bioscience Bioengineering* 87(3):352-356.

Petersen CL (1986). Vegetable oil as a diesel fuel: Status and research priorities. *Trans ASAE* 29:1413-1421.

Schwab AW, MO Bagby, and B Freedman (1987). Preparation and properties of diesel fuels from vegetable oils. *Fuel* 66:1372-1378.

Sheehan J, V Camobreco, J Duffield, M Gabroski, and H Shapouri (1998). *An overview of biodiesel and petroleum diesel life cycles.* A joint study sponsored by U.S Departments of Agriculture and Energy. Golden CO: National Renewable Energy Laboratory.

# Biofertilizers: Production, Application, and Quality Control

Anil Kumar Tripathi

## INTRODUCTION

All living organisms need nitrogen and phosphorus, which are the basic building blocks of cells. Although a huge amount of nitrogen is present in the air and phosphorus is available as insoluble phosphates in the soil, plants often fail to obtain enough of either to grow vigorously. Microorganisms possessing the potential to increase plant and crop growth through increased availability of nutrients via biological nitrogen fixation (BNF), phosphate solubilization, and/or growth-promoting hormonal substances are considered to be potential biofertilizers. Their importance lies in their ability to supplement or mobilize soil nutrients with minimal use of nonrenewable resources and as components of integrated plant nutrient systems. Application of biofertilizers improves physicochemical and biological characteristics of soil, provides macro- and micronutrients to plants, restores biological activity in soils, improves development of roots, increases retention of soil water, raises pH of soils, and augments the absorption of nutrients. Thus, farmers can reduce the input of chemical fertilizers because biofertilizers improve nutrient utilization efficiency of crops.

The introduction of beneficial microorganisms into soil or rhizosphere is known as inoculation. Bioinoculants refer to products containing microorganisms for application as biopesticides, biofertilizers, phytostimulators, or soil bioremediation agents. Preparations of biofertilizers are used for the inoculation of soils that need to be restored in their fertility or are so stressed that the populations of native biofertilizer microorganisms declines after every drought year. Inoculation of agricultural fields with biofertilizers, therefore, has special significance, as it is a cost-effective, eco-friendly, and renewable source of plant nutrients suitable for sustainable agricultural pro-

483

duction systems. The prospects of improving agriculture by inoculation with biofertilizers are of great importance for less intensive, low-input agricultural systems existing in many developing countries. Agricultural fields that are deficient in a nutrient and are devoid of native populations of microorganisms capable of supplying the deficient nutrients are the appropriate locations for using biofertilizers for inoculation. Biofertilizers are useful for dry land and irrigated agriculture, and are available for a wide variety of crops such as cereals, legumes, millets, oilseeds, spices, vegetables, fruits, and plantation crops. Some of the important biofertilizer microorganisms that make nitrogen and phosphorus available to plants are as follows:

> Nitrogen-fixing bacteria: *Rhizobium, Azorhizobium, Bradyrhizobium, Azospirillum, Klebsiella, Azotobacter, Burkholderia, Acetobacter diazotrophicus, Frankia,* blue-green algae, *Azolla.*
> Phosphate-solubilizing microorganisms: Fungi such as *Penicillium, Aspergillus,* and *Trichoderma;* vesicular arbuscular mycorrhizal (VAM) fungi, including *Glomus, Gigaspora, Acaulospora, Sclerocystis,* etc.; and bacteria belonging to *Bacillus, Flavobacterium,* and *Pseudomonas.*

Many of these microorganisms also promote plant growth via phytohormone production, which causes morphological and physiological changes in plant roots, resulting in enhanced water and mineral uptake by plants. Some of them also benefit their host plants by inhibiting infection and proliferation of pathogens via antibiosis, production and secretion of siderophores, and induction of systemic disease resistance.

Biofertilizer inoculation technology includes selection of appropriate bacterial strains, large-scale production of their biomass, development of formulations (liquid, powder, or granules), and their application methods in the field (Figure III.19). Reliable commercial use of bioinoculants on a large scale depends on formulations that are simple, economical, unaffected by long storage, and easy to transport and apply. It also depends on application technology that facilitates timely, easy, and precise delivery in the field. The study of a formulation process is generally undertaken when the choice of an efficient strain has already been made. However, the optimization of formulation is largely independent of the strain, since strains within one genus or species share many cultural properties. A process developed for one strain of a genus may also be generally applicable to the other strains of the same genus, requiring only a few adaptations or modifications.

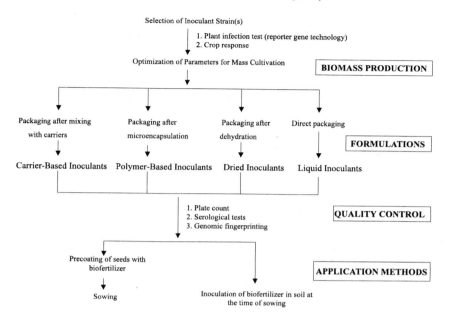

FIGURE III.19. Schematic representation of the components of biofertilizer inoculant technology

## BIOMASS PRODUCTION

Large-scale commercial use of inoculants requires considerable biomass. Except for *Azolla* and blue-green algae, most other bacterial biofertilizers can be produced by large-scale liquid fermentation. Optimization of the fermentation process is required for the production of desired quality bacterial biomass. The first step for batch fermentation in a fermentor is the optimization of medium and culture conditions. The composition of the medium, particularly the sources of carbon and nitrogen, plays a very crucial role in biomass production. For economic reasons, however, an industrial medium is often much simpler than that used in the laboratory. To maximize yields and productivity of the inoculum, optimal levels of dissolved oxygen required by each type of bacteria should be maintained in the fermentor. The fed-batch culture, in which nutrients are added in the medium during the culture, can help in reaching the desired physiological state as well as increasing biomass productivity. The fermentor culture must be stopped at a precise time corresponding to the most adequate physiological state of the cells to give the highest number of viable cells once the product is formulated. Physiological status of the cell affects the survival of the inoculant in the carrier and on the seed, colonization of the rhizosphere, and the extent of plant response.

Most laboratories utilize logarithmic or late logarithmic phase cultures, whereas others prefer a stationary phase in order to obtain cysts or flocs, which have a survival advantage. In *Azospirillum* and *Azotobacter,* resistance to high temperature, starvation, and desiccation are achieved by encystation in which vegetative cells undergo morphological and biochemical changes to form resting cysts, preparing them for long-term survival on the shelf and in the soil. There is a direct correlation between accumulation of poly-$\beta$-hydroxybutyrate (PHB) granules and extent of cyst formation. Knowledge of culture conditions to initiate a metabolic shift toward PHB production is useful in producing PHB-rich inocula; for example, *n*-butanol, hydroxybutyrate, or mineral deficiencies are known to induce encystation in *Azotobacter. Azospirillum* differentiates into cysts when grown in culture media containing fructose and nitrate as carbon and nitrogen sources. The formation of the capsule and production of extracellular polysaccharides are the prerequisites for the development of a mature cyst.

In liquid culture, cysts produce copious amounts of adhesive capsular polysaccharides resulting in aggregates of cysts called "flocs," a process known as flocculation or aggregation. Bacterial aggregation is of great interest in the production of bacterial inoculants because the flocs or aggregates can be produced on a large scale and separated easily from the growth medium. The capacity of *Azospirillum, Azotobacter, Klebsiella,* and *Rhizobium* to aggregate and flocculate is related to the formation of cellulose fibrils and helps in dispersal, survival in soil, and attachment to plant roots.

## FORMULATIONS

Maintaining high viable populations of the inoculant strain in the biofertilizer under adverse environmental conditions during the prolonged period from manufacture to inoculation is the most important constraint. Bacteria can be applied to the seed or to the soil directly, but their numbers usually decline rapidly. A good-quality carrier, which supports the viability and proliferation of the inoculum during storage, is therefore a prerequisite for good-quality biofertilizer preparation. The characteristics of the formulations used to deliver bacterial inoculants can strongly influence their behavior in the soil or rhizosphere. Humus-based formulations are preferred because they show reasonable shelf life and good field performance. However, more economical formulations based on sugarcane industry by-products, such as press mud and bagasse, are also being tried.

A high-quality formulation and application must maintain and deliver, in a convenient and economical fashion, a high population of the inoculated bacteria. It should be made of raw materials that are nontoxic, biodegradable, chemically and physically uniform, and of consistent quality. It should have high water-holding capacity, permit easy adjustment of pH and addition of nutrients, and be easily mixable in the factory as well as on the farm. It should be compatible with as many bacterial species/strains as possible, have prolonged shelf life, and be easy to use and apply with standard agrotechnical machinery.

### Carrier-Based Products

Most of the classical inoculants are based on carriers, mainly peat or vermiculite, which are abundant and cheap. Their quality varies according to their origin. They are neutralized and sterilized before mixing with the desired inoculant strain to achieve $10^8$ to $10^9$ viable cells per gram. Bacterial inoculants can also be multiplied directly in the vermiculite by supplementing nutrients. Therefore, in carrier-based formulations, bacteria remain metabolically active for a considerable period. Due to the ease of their production, the cost of peat-based inoculants is relatively low. The main drawbacks include release of toxic compounds upon heat sterilization and sensitivity to pesticides coated on the seeds and to temperature variations during storage, which result in reduced shelf life of the inoculant.

### Polymer-Based Products

Although peat formulations are economical as carriers, new trends in formulations using biopolymers such as alginate or xanthan gum offer several advantages over peat. The preparations of macro- or microbeads encapsulating sufficient number of bacteria in alginate provide protection against environmental stresses. They are nontoxic and biodegradable and facilitate slow release of bacteria into the soil. They offer consistent batch quality and a better-defined environment for inoculant bacteria. They can be manipulated easily according to the needs of specific bacteria and can be stored dried at ambient temperatures for prolonged periods. These inoculants can also be amended with nutrients to improve the short-term survival of bacteria upon inoculation. The fine powder of the microbeads, which can be prepared by several simple techniques, is used for coating the seeds before they are sold to farmers. In comparison to peat-based inoculants, polymer-based inoculants are rather expensive and require more biotechnical handling by the industry.

## Dried Inoculants

The main limitation of peat-based or polymer-based inoculants is the survival of microorganisms during storage. Drying or dehydration is recognized as a key step in inoculant preparation because it can affect inoculant survival and increase the lag time before the expression of a beneficial effect. A metabolically inactive state of dehydrated bacteria ensures longer shelf life, better stress tolerance, and better compatibility with pesticides and avoidance of contamination. Differences in the extent and process of dehydration and additives (carriers, protectants, etc.) affect the survival of inoculants differentially. Population estimates are higher with dried products when an initial slow rehydration is utilized to minimize rehydration upshock before continuing the dilution. Although water activity controls survival during storage, the survival just after dehydration depends on culture medium, physiological stage of the cells at the time of their harvest, process of encapsulation, use of protective agents, and the rate of drying.

## Liquid Inoculants

Liquid formulations of cyst-based liquid inoculants facilitate packaging and convenient delivery of the inoculants to seeds or seedlings. They are commercially distributed in liquid form and have been shown to benefit a wide variety of crops without using any carrier material. They are claimed to have longer shelf life than the carrier-based ones. Farmers in both mechanized and more traditional farming systems seem to prefer the convenience that liquid formulations offer. The cysts of *Azotobacter* in liquid formulations have been shown to survive and retain nitrogen-fixing ability for over two years.

## Mixed Inoculants

Some biofertilizer strains of bacteria show unpredictable behavior under field conditions, limiting their utility on a commercial scale. The new trend of microbial inoculant preparations consists of consortia of bacterial inoculants (biofertilizers, phytostimulators, and biocontrol agents) and beneficial fungi (e.g., VAM fungi). In order to improve the performance of inoculants, application of synergistic combinations or consortia of beneficial bacteria including phytohormone producers, nitrogen fixers, phosphate solubilizers, biological control agents, lignocellulose degraders, etc., are mixed in a single carrier. Although such combinations may bring about multiple benefits to the plant, optimization of appropriate media, growth conditions, and carriers accommodating all members of the consortium are required.

## APPLICATION METHODS

The method used to inoculate plants is extremely important. It must match common agricultural practices and must allow the delivery of the right number of cells at the right place with standard equipment. The choice of application method is linked to the formulation process. Inoculants can be applied either directly on the seed or in the furrows, in a liquid or a solid formulation. The simplest inoculation method is by application of bacteria in liquid suspension either directly to the soil or to the seeds. However, some inoculants such as *Azospirillum* survive poorly in the soil in the absence of a carrier.

### Inoculation on Seeds

Inoculum may be applied to the seeds just before sowing in the field or before their storage and packaging. When applying just before sowing, seeds are mixed with the inoculants, with or without the addition of water and some sticker to improve adhesion. This method is relatively cheap and is used mostly with peat-based inoculants, but the process of moistening and mixing reduces viability of bacteria and adversely affects germination of seeds. In clay-based preinoculant, cultures are mixed with the clays, dried, and ground into a fine powder. Seed processors are then used to apply the dried product to the seed while mixing to provide a uniform application.

Seed companies use formulations that can maintain a high bacterial population on seeds before their sale. Seeds can be coated with a homogeneous suspension/film of dehydrated bacteria and stored before distributing them as "quality seeds." The practice of applying the inoculant to the seeds up to several months before sowing is known as preinoculation. A dormant state of bacteria supports their survival on seeds during several months of storage. Seeds can also be sprayed with liquid adhesives or polymers, to which pesticides, biological control agents, and other plant beneficial bacteria may be added. Materials commonly used in film coating include methyl cellulose, dextran, vegetable or paraffin oil, and polysaccharides, especially alginates.

Seed pelleting is a kind of preinoculation in which peat inoculant is applied as a slurry utilizing a sticker and the inoculated seeds are covered with finely ground calcium carbonate. Addition of slurry or stickers improves the seed adhesion, but it requires additional time and labor to the already labor-intensive inoculation process. Therefore, liquid inoculants, packageable in plastic bags, have been developed, which can be applied to the seeds in either a batch treatment or continuous application system with the aid of an applicator kit. A uniform moist coating of the seeds is achieved before the inoculant quickly dries.

### Inoculation of Soil

Inoculants can also be applied in the field at the time of sowing so as to place the inoculant directly in the furrows in the vicinity of the seeds. Application of nonsterile peat granule containing bacteria by a granular applicator is able to place the soil inoculant in the furrow with the seeds. The liquid in-furrow inoculants are diluted with water and delivered into the soil with the help of liquid delivery equipment, mounted on a tractor or planted. This kind of device is able to place the inoculant in the furrow on top of the seed before the furrow is closed.

In microgranulate application the product is delivered in the furrow with the help of a specific granular applicator, which is also used for the delivery of insecticide microgranules. This method ensures the presence of viable bacteria in the vicinity of the seeds. The microgranulate is a chemically inert carrier such as marble powder, sand, clay, or calcium carbonate, which is either premixed or mixed by the farmer with the inoculum. The process can be used with all kinds of inoculants after optimizing the compatibility between the carrier and the inoculum.

## INOCULANT QUALITY CONTROL

Market success of agricultural inputs depends on the confidence of the farmers in the quality and performance of the product. However, in many countries, biofertilizer inoculants are highly variable in quality due to lack of mandatory quality control. Quality of the inoculants is determined by the proper identification of the effective inoculant strain, their numbers in the biofertilizer formulation (e.g., $>5 \times 10^8$/g of peat), and the ability of the formulation to promote survival of the inoculant after application to seed or soil.

Techniques that rapidly identify bacterial strains, even at the genus or species level, are used for controlling the quality of inoculant products entering the market. Identification methods using media that select for individual species are also useful. Serological methods, enzyme reactions specific to a genus or species, and methods that combine antibody or enzyme reactions with vital strains have been proposed as suitable quality-assurance methods for industry and regulators.

The most reliable control of any *Rhizobium* inoculant is the plant infection test, which is quite laborious and takes at least three weeks to perform. Another type of control, often used in tandem with the plant test, is plate counting, which is rapid but does not distinguish between different *Rhizobium* strains unless they differ by some marker such as resistance to an antibiotic. This is a drawback when the inoculant contains several strains or is mixed with unsterilized peat carrier. A more advanced method for identifying target strains is by using monoclonal antibodies raised against individual inoculant strains, but this technique also suffers from the possibility of change in the antigen due to a change in the conditions of growth or storage, leading to a loss or variation of the specificity of the antibody. The production of specific antibodies may also involve some difficulties and can take two months to produce a new monoclonal antibody.

The application of DNA-based techniques has been demonstrated for the quality control of peat-based *Rhizobium* inoculants, which takes advantage of the intrinsic genomic characters for the identification of the strains without any need for using mutants, genetically engineered bacteria, or specific antibodies. The DNA-DNA hybridization and polymerase chain reaction (PCR) amplification of signature amplicons appear to be rapid tools for identifying the inoculant strain, even if they cannot completely substitute for plant infection tests. Both of these techniques are capable of detecting $10^2$ to $10^3$ cells per gram of soil sample. Considering that the commercial inoculants should have bacterial densities of $5 \times 10^8$/g of peat, PCR is sensitive enough to be used for inoculant quality control.

The competitive ability of an inoculant is a major factor in determining the success of rhizobial inoculation. Many soils contain high numbers of indigenous rhizobia, which are often poor in nitrogen-fixation ability but highly competitive, as they are well adapted to the local conditions. Therefore, effectiveness of the inoculant strain vis-à-vis native rhizobia in terms of nodule occupancy needs to be evaluated before recommending any rhizobial strain for inoculation in a specific soil in a specific location. Reporter genes such as the β-glucuronidase gene *(uidA)* or the thermostable β-glucosidase gene *(celB)* allow detection of rhizobial strains in nodules when they are still attached to the root system. Use of differentially marked strains with *gusA* and *celB* has facilitated comparison of the competitive effectiveness between the two strains in terms of nodule occupancy. Such analyses are extremely simple and fast and permit high data throughput. Because this technique does not require sophisticated equipment, an easy-to-use *gus* gene-marking kit has been developed which helps in determining nodule occupancy by allowing rapid screening of competitive ability of inoculant strains. Because the marked strain can be detected directly on the plant, picking up nodules and preparing bacterial isolates are not required.

The response to inoculant is inextricably linked to the numbers of viable bacteria applied to seeds. Although the number of viable bacterial cells declines during the storage of the biofertilizer formulation, the real constraint to the performance of inoculant formulation is not shelf life but survival after inoculation. Adaptation to the needs of individual or highly localized situations is essential for the successful adoption of this technology. Research is needed to develop formulations that increase the survival of rhizobia on seed and in soil following inoculation. Superior formulations are likely to result from exploiting the additive effects of physical protectants, physiological conditioning to promote tolerance to rapid changes in water potential, inactivating toxic substances diffusing from seed, and genetic improvement for better survival.

## CONCLUSIONS

In spite of several advantages and substantial potential of improving crop productivity by inoculating plant growth-promoting bacteria, biofertilizer technology has not become popular due to low quality of inoculants which perform inconsistently in farmers' fields. Improving quality-control methods and enforcing quality standards are required to improve the acceptability of biofertilizers among farmers. Bacterial strains to be recommended for use as biofertilizer for a specific crop should be tested rigorously for their ability to survive, multiply, and colonize the plant roots and to improve crop productivity in the field. Due emphasis should also be given to optimizing their large-scale production so as to obtain a physiological state of the bacteria that is best suited for their long-term survival on the shelf and in the field. Research is also needed to develop superior formulations that increase their survival on the seed and in the soil. Success of biofertilizers in the farmers' fields can be realized only if research and development sections of commercial companies pay due attention to the specificity of bacterial strains to crops and soils and ensure survival and optimum colonization of host crops by the potential bacterial strains.

## SUGGESTED READINGS

Bashan Y (1998). Inoculants of plant growth-promoting bacteria for use in agriculture. *Biotechnology Advances* 16:729-770.

Fages J (1994). *Azospirillum* inoculants and field experiments. In *Azospirillum/ plant associations,* Y Okon (ed.). Boca Raton: CRC Press, pp. 77-86.

Mulongoy K, S Gianinazzi, PA Roger, and Y Dommergues (1992). Biofertilizers: Agronomic and environmental impacts and economics. In *Biotechnology: Economic and social aspects,* EJ DaSilva, C Ratledge, and A Sasson (eds.). Cambridge, UK: Cambridge University Press, pp. 55-69.

Okon Y, GV Bloemberg, and BJJ Lugtenberg (1998). Biotechnology of biofertilization and phytostimulation. In *Agricultural biotechnology,* A Altman (ed.). New York: Marcel Dekker, pp. 327-349.

Sessitsch A, G Hardoarson, WM De Vos, and KJ Wilson (1998). Use of marker genes in competition studies of *Rhizobium. Plant and Soil* 204:35-45.

Smith RS (1995). Inoculant formulations and applications to meet changing needs. In *Nitrogen fixation: Fundamentals and applications,* IA Tikhonowich, NA Provorov, VI Romanov, and WE Newton (eds.). Dordrecht: Kluwer Academic Publishers, pp. 653-657.

# Biopulping

Juan Carlos Villar
Luis Jiménez Alcaide

## INTRODUCTION

The processes by which cellulose pulp for paper manufacturing are produced are of the chemical or mechanical types, or a combination thereof. The purpose of these technologies is to remove fibers from the raw materials. In chemical processes, wood chips are cooked with suitable chemical reagents to dissolve the lignin that binds cellulose fibers together. On the other hand, mechanical processes remove fibers under the shearing action of various types of grinders and disk refiners. The most widely used chemical process is the *kraft* or sulfate process, which provides strong, dark pulp that is difficult to bleach. Chemical processes exhibit low yields (typically close to 50 percent), which entails using about two tons of wood per ton of pulp. Mechanical processes provide light-colored pulp that is not always bleached; because they use little or no chemical reagent, wood components are not dissolved and yields are high (close to 90 percent) as a result (only 1.1 ton of chips is required to obtain one ton of mechanical pulp).

Pulp quality varies widely. Kraft pulp is strong. It is used for purposes in which strength is the essential requirement or to strengthen weaker pulp. Mechanical pulp is weak but possesses excellent features for making printing paper. Bleaching also differs among pulp types. Chemical pulp such as kraft pulp is bleached by dissolving residual lignin. This is usually accomplished by using chlorinated compounds that produce highly toxic, scarcely biodegradable chlorolignins. On the other hand, mechanical pulp is not bleached with chlorinated reagents, which would decrease pulp yield and opacity; rather, they are treated with hydrogen peroxide or sodium hydrosulfite to alter chromophores in the lignin without removing it from the pulp.

One of the most salient features of kraft pulping is that the reagents are recovered. As a result, only a small amount of reagents needs be added in each cycle to offset any losses. Also, cooking by-products, dissolved as

*495*

black liquors, are burned during the reagent recovery step, thereby removing potential pollutants and obtaining energy from the process (Figure III.20). It is, therefore, unnecessary to reduce reagent consumption in kraft pulping, so efforts toward improvement have so far focused on increasing the bleaching efficiency and avoiding the use of chlorinated compounds as much as possible.

With mechanical pulp, the situation is rather different; in fact, the defibrating and refining steps use large amounts of energy, which severely hinders implementation of this technology in countries where energy is expensive. In any case, energy consumption in this process can be reduced by impregnating the raw materials with chemical reagents prior to defibrating. The reagents soften lignin and increase the mechanical strength of the pulp (Figure III.21). However, these improvements are partly offset by a decreased pulp yield, which can easily drop to 80 percent, and the consequent loss of opacity in the paper and increase in chemical oxygen demand (COD) and biochemical oxygen demand (BOD) in the wastewater. In short, modifications of the mechanical pulping processes are aimed at reducing both the polluting power of the effluent and the consumption of energy.

Environmentally, chemical and mechanical pulping pose different problems. While the main problem with chemical pulping lies in the bleaching step, that of mechanical pulping arises from the need to reduce the amount of energy used in the defibrating step and the subsequent refining step while improving yields and minimizing the organic load in the wastewater.

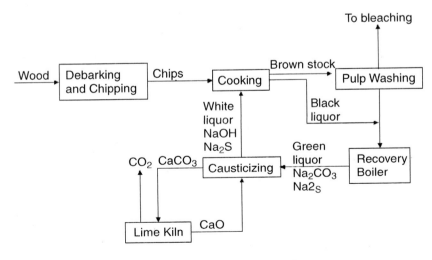

FIGURE III.20. Flowchart for the kraft process

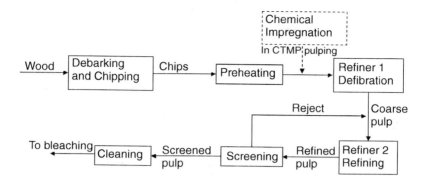

FIGURE III.21. Flowchart for the thermomechanical process

Fungal treatments of lignocellulosic materials (wood, pulp, annual plants) have received substantial attention over the past two decades as effective, nonpolluting solutions to problems arising from the bleaching of kraft pulp, the efficient use of energy in the production of mechanical pulp, and the need to reduce pitch in kraft pulp or recycle old paper. The use of ligninolytic fungi or their enzymes in the bleaching of kraft pulp and in mechanical pulping are typical examples of *biobleaching* and *biopulping*, respectively. There is no precise definition for either term because both have been applied to various procedures. Thus, biopulping has been used not only to process wood with ligninolytic fungi with a view to obtain kraft or mechanical pulp, but also to treat pulp in order to improve its response to refining. The term could also be applied to the treatment of these materials with enzyme broths produced by the fungi, which affect the degradation of wood components.

One possible definition for biopulping is the production of pulp by using a procedure that includes a biological treatment. Biopulping replaces chemical reagents or mechanical energy with the action of microorganisms capable of degrading lignin, thereby resulting in a more environmentally friendly pulping process.

Fungi are known to be the principal agents for natural rotting wood. Although different fungal species can attack wood in different manners, three clear-cut types of wood decay have been identified: soft, brown, and white rotting. Soft rotting is caused mainly by ascomycetes and deuteromycetes; it occurs under high-moisture conditions and is characterized by the formation of cylindrical cavities in the secondary walls of fibers. The name comes from the softening effect produced on wood surfaces. Fungi degrade cellulose and hemicellulose by attacking the surface of fibers and penetrating them once they have destroyed the outermost layer—a difference from the other two types of rotting.

Brown-rot fungi are mostly basidiomycetes that degrade cellulose and hemicellulose while leaving lignin untouched; as a result, the wood acquires a brown color (after which this type of rotting has been named). Fungal hyphae occupy fiber lumen, from which they can penetrate adjacent fibers via pits or perforations caused by their own action. The attack therefore takes place from the secondary wall to the primary wall of each fiber and is especially frequent in conifers.

White rotting affects all major components of wood, namely, cellulose, hemicellulose, and lignin. Attacked wood becomes increasingly brittle as rotting develops. This type of rotting is the most interesting in regard to biopulping, particularly with specially selective fungi capable of degrading lignin while leaving polysaccharide chains as intact as possible. The presence of moisture is essential for the growth and metabolism of the fungal species involved in wood decay. While soft-rot fungi are the only ones present under high-moisture conditions, the others also require some moisture to grow; in fact, wood containing less than 20 percent moisture cannot be attacked by fungi. However, some species, such as *Serpula lacrymans* and *Meruliporia incrassata,* can grow even in the absence of moisture, which they extract from the wood itself.

The Forest Products Laboratory (FPL) (Madison, Wisconsin), Swedish Pulp and Paper Institute (STFI) (Stockholm), and Pulp and Paper Research Institute of Canada (Paprican) (Pointe Claire, Quebec) pioneered the search for biological solutions to the problems of the paper industry. *Phanerochaete chrysosporium,* a white-rot fungus, was the most widely studied in the early research; lignin peroxidase, one of the enzymes involved in lignin degradation, was first isolated by FPL in 1983. This fungus was also studied by STFI researchers with a view to obtaining mutants with no cellulolytic activity in order to achieve the selective degradation of lignin. On the other hand, the researchers at Paprican, who focused on pulp bleaching, chose the fungus *Trametes versicolor* for this purpose.

## LIGNIN-DEGRADING ENZYMES

Lignin peroxidase (LiP), manganese peroxidase (MnP), and laccase (Lac) are the enzymes playing the most crucial roles in lignin degradation. LiP is a nonspecific oxidant that catalyzes the oxidation of phenols. It oxidizes the benzene ring of lignin, the oxidized form then undergoing cleavage of C-C bonds, opening of the aromatic ring, demethylation, or quinone formation. MnP is similar to LiP in its action; however, it is a milder oxidant and acts on phenol groups only. It has the additional advantage that the oxidizing agent coming into contact with lignin is oxidized manganese, which allows it to reach areas that are inaccessible to enzymes. Laccases are phenol oxidase enzymes that use molecular oxygen as a substrate and oxidize it to water. To this end, the enzyme captures four electrons in a sequential manner from a wide variety of phenol compounds, or even nonphenol ones if appropriate intermediate substances are present.

For lignin to be degraded by peroxidases, the medium must contain hydrogen peroxide, which is produced by the enzymes glyoxal oxidase, glucose oxidase, and aryl-alcohol oxidase. It is believed that the degradation of lignin involves several enzymes and that some reductive enzymes such as cellobiose dehydrogenase and cellobiose quinone oxidoreductase play crucial roles as they help stabilize the radicals formed by the oxidative enzymes, thereby preventing lignin from repolymerizing.

The size of an enzyme is one factor governing the efficiency of its attack on wood. It has been assumed that the attack takes place only at fiber lumen—the sole areas accessible by enzymes. One other possible mechanism of action involves the cooperation of the enzyme with some mediator (a low-molecular-weight compound that would reach and oxidize the lignin not directly accessible by the enzyme). Mediators can result from fungal metabolism or be external agents. Especially prominent among the former are veratryl alcohol and oxalate, malate, and fumarate ions.

Tannins and polyphenols in tree bark are thought to possess antifungal properties. Occasionally, however, fungi have been found to grow on barks; also, the outcome of biopulping is more favorable when the fungus is brought into contact with the tree bark or some component thereof.

## USE OF BIOPULPING FOR THE PRODUCTION OF CHEMICAL PULP

From the previous discussion, it might seem that fungal treatments are of interest only for obtaining mechanical pulp and that such advantages of chemical pulping as chemical savings would be lost because recovering chemicals during the black liquor burning and recycling step poses no special problem. Replacing chemical delignification processes with the action of white-rot fungi is not easy either because lignin degradation is always accompanied to a greater or lesser extent by cellulose and hemicellulose degradation; thus, a strong attack on cellulose will leave exceedingly damaged fibers and detract from the mechanical strength of the resulting pulp. This is reflected in poor values for paper quality parameters such as the tensile or tear index.

Circumventing the previous shortcomings entails careful selection of fungal strains. *Phanerochaete chrysosporium* and *Ceriporiopsis subvermispora* strains were used to treat hardwood (*Betula papyrifera* and *Populus tremuloides*) and softwood *(Pinus taeda)* species. Only with the hardwood species and *Ceriporiopsis subvermispora* could most of the lignin (50 to 80 percent) be removed without excessive degradation of cellulose; by contrast, only 42 percent of the lignin in *Pinus taeda* could be removed, and with increased losses of polysaccharides. It should be noted that even in the most favorable cases, the incubation time was 12 weeks, which was too long for the treatment to be attractive.

However, one can reasonably expect selective degradation of lignin within a fairly short time to ensure that wood fibers are left virtually intact. In this situation, fungal treatments would extract only a small fraction of lignin but would render the wood more accessible to the action of the cooking reagents. In other words, fungi would favor mass transfer within the wood chips, thereby increasing the cooking efficiency and reducing the cooking time and also, possibly, the proportion of uncooked materials. The net outcome would be increased production to an extent that would by itself justify using the biological pretreatment. This assumption was confirmed by using cellulolytic and hemicellulolytic enzymes on pine wood chips. The result was increased diffusion within the chips, both in the longitudinal and tangential directions. This effect resulted in the breakage of pit membranes. The results obtained by cooking fungal-treated wood chips confirmed the previous assumptions. Thus, the pretreatment shortened the time needed to reach a given degree of delignification or, in other words, with equal cooking times, the amount of residual lignin in the pulp and reagent consumption were both smaller with fungal-treated chips.

Table III.17 summarizes some features of using biopulping to obtain kraft pulp. Among the potential disadvantages are a slightly decreased yield but also a decreased kappa number; as a result, yield differences between fungal pretreated and untreated pulp with a similar kappa number are insubstantial. One additional problem arises from the viscosity of the pulp, an indirect measure of the integrity of cellulose chains, which is usually affected by the fungal action. The search for highly selective ligninolytic fungal species on biopulping may eventually provide an effective solution to this shortcoming.

TABLE III.17. Features of biopulping as applied to the production of kraft pulp

| Strains: | *Phanerochaete chrysosporium, Coriolus versicolor, Ceriporiopsis subvermispora* |
|---|---|
| Kappa reduction | 3-5 |
| Pulp yield reduction | 2-4 percent |
| Cooking time reduction | 15-30 percent |
| Viscosity reduction | 4-30 percent |

## *USE OF BIOPULPING FOR THE PRODUCTION OF MECHANICAL PULP*

As stated earlier, chemical and mechanical pulping pose different environmental problems, and using alternative processes makes more sense in the case of mechanical pulp. Treating wood with ligninolytic fungi with a view to obtaining mechanical pulp results in substantial savings of defibrating energy, which could save up to 30 percent of energy with respect to the process using untreated wood. The exact savings, however, depends on the degree of refining of the pulp and increases with decreased refining.

One other way of using biopulping to obtain mechanical pulp is to start from unrefined mechanical pulp rather than from chips of the raw material in order to save energy in the subsequent refining step. The main difference from the direct use of the fungus on chips is an increased exposed surface area with unrefined pulp, which can accelerate the fungal attack. Some experiments conducted to examine the effect found no significant differences between the fungal attack on chips and unrefined pulp. The treatment of unrefined pulp with ligninolytic fungi substantially reduced the amount of energy required in the subsequent refining relative to untreated pulp. The magnitude of the energy savings was found to depend on the starting species: it amounted to 66 percent with some hardwood species but only to 33 to 36 percent with softwood species. In addition, the mechanical strength of the refined pulp was improved, the effect increasing with increasing duration of the fungal treatment. The most marked effect of the type of wood used was on the tear index: with pulp from hardwoods, the fungal treatment improved the tear index; with pulp from conifers, the index remained virtually unaltered or even decreased slightly as a result of the treatment.

The inclusion of a chemical step involving impregnation of the raw material in a mechanical pulping process results in improved pulp quality and in decreased yield and intensity to an extent that depends on the strength of the treatment. Similarly, the use of a biological pretreatment improves the properties of the final pulp but also at the expense of decreased yield and opacity. The differences increase with increasing duration of the treatment. This co-incidence between the two types of treatment is unsurprising as ligninolytic fungi depolymerize lignin and, as a rule, increase its degree of oxidation; these effects are identical to those caused by chemical impregnation re-agents such as hydrogen peroxide or sodium sulfite.

Table III.18 summarizes the features of biopulping as applied to the production of mechanical pulp. The greatest disadvantage encountered so far is the decreased brightness of the pulp. This appears to be the result of the fungi producing colored substances that detract from the final brightness. The effect, however, is usually small (2 to 5 percent ISO [International Organization for Standardization] brightness) and rarely poses a serious problem as, following bleaching with hydrogen peroxide, the brightness of biologically treated pulp can even exceed that of untreated pulp.

The enzymes produced by ligninolytic fungi have also been used as such with a view to improving the characteristics of mechanical pulp. Experiments with lignin peroxidase as applied to thermomechanical pulp from conifer wood provided results similar to those obtained by using the fungus directly on wood chips. The pulp tensile strength was slightly increased and the tear index slightly decreased. Again, the biological treatment, involving the enzyme rather than the fungus in this case, resulted in decreased brightness relative to untreated pulp, but the subsequent bleaching restored it to levels virtually identical to those in the latter.

In a case study, similar results were found in experiments with hardwoods treated with a concentrated broth of MnP. The tensile strength of the resulting pulp was 10 percent higher and the tear index 15 percent lower. The enzyme treatment decreased pulp brightness, but the effect depended on the consistency of the pulp. Thus, with a consistency of 10 percent, the brightness of fungal-treated pulp surpassed that of untreated pulp. An energy-savings of 25 percent was achieved in refining enzyme-treated pulp; also, fiber shortening as a result of refining was less marked than in untreated

TABLE III.18. Features of biopulping as applied to the production of mechanical pulp

| Strains: | Phanerochaete chrysosporium, Coriolus versicolor, Ceriporiopsis subvermispora |
|---|---|
| Energy savings | 25-66 percent |
| Physical mechanical properties | |
| Tensile index | +10 percent to +60 percent |
| Tear index | −10 percent to +150 percent |
| Brightness reduction | −10 percent to −2 percent |

pulp. The results were ascribed to increased fiberization in the pulp. The enzyme removed the material between cellulose microfibrils, thereby releasing cellulose fibers and increasing fiberization, which in turn increased the ability of fibers to bind to one another. In addition to the microscopic observations, which exposed this effect, the results revealed an increased tensile and burst index, as well as an increased density of the paper obtained from the pulp, all of which are consistent with the previous explanation.

## CONCLUSIONS

The current prospects for biopulping are quite promising. The laboratory results obtained so far have shown major advantages in the use of fungi or their enzymes for the production of both chemical and mechanical pulp. Biopulping has been successfully applied not only to wood but also to annual plants such as kenaf or sisal. The use of biopulping to obtain chemical pulp seemingly reduces the amount of residual lignin present in the pulp and shortens the cooking time. By using selective strains to degrade lignin, cellulose integrity can be preserved and pulp of a high viscosity obtained.

Early attempts at producing mechanical pulp by biopulping on a large scale have met with success. Thus, FPL has succeeded in treating up to 50 tons of chips with the fungus *Ceriporiopsis subvermispora*. The results have confirmed that fungal-treated wood uses less energy and yields mechanical pulp of improved quality. The biological impregnation system for chips is about to be made commercially available.

## SUGGESTED READINGS

Eriksson KE and L Vallander (1982). Properties of pulp from thermomechanical pulping of chips pretreated with fungi. *Svenk Papperstidning* 85:R33-R38.

Jacobs-Young CJ, RA Venditti, and TW Joyce (1998). Effect of enzymatic pretreatment on the diffusion of sodium hydroxide in wood. *Tappi Journal* 81(1):260-266.

Leonowicz A, A Matuszewska, J Luterek, D Ziegenhagen, M Wojtás-Wasilewska, NS Cho, M Hofrichter, and J Rogalski (1999). Biodegradation of lignin by white-rot fungi. *Fungal Genetics and Biology* 27:175-185.

Morita S, Y Yakazi, and GC Johnson (2001). Mycelium growth promotion by water extractives from the inner bark of radiata pine (*Pinus radiata* D. Don). *Holzforschung* 55:155-158.

Sigoillot JC, M Petit-Conil, I Herpoël, JP Joseleau, K Ruel, B Kurrek, C de Choudens, and M Asther (2001). Energy saving with fungal enzymatic treatment of industrial poplar alkaline peroxide pulps. *Enzyme and Microbial Technology* 29:160-165.

# Biosurfactant Production and Application

Yiannis Kourkoutas
Ibrahim M. Banat

## INTRODUCTION

Concern about environmental protection has increased recently from a global viewpoint. Accordingly, chemical products working in harmony with the environment are highly sought after. Under these circumstances, natural products are advantageous as substitutes for synthetic chemicals. Surfactants are amphiphilic molecules that partition preferentially at the interface between fluid phases and alter the conditions prevailing at interfaces. The presence of both a hydrophilic and a lipophilic moiety is recognized within the surfactant molecule of definite molecule structure, which gives the typical properties of a surfactant.

Recently, surface-active compounds produced by microorganisms have attracted attention from the standpoint of being ecologically adaptable and biologically safe. These are new kinds of surfactants having particular chemical structures and effective functional performance. These new surfactants have been named biosurfactants, via microbial surfactants and emulsifiers. Microbial biosurfactants are a structurally diverse group of surface-active molecules, including a wide variety of chemical structures, such as glycolipids, lipopeptides, polysaccharide-protein complexes, phospholipids, fatty acids, and neutral lipids. They consist of distinctive hydrophilic and hydrophobic moieties. The former can be either ionic or nonionic and consist of mono-, di-, or polysaccharides, carboxylic acids, amino acids, or peptides, while the latter are usually saturated, unsaturated, or hydroxylated fatty acids.

Organisms that produce surfactants include many of the yeasts, bacteria, and filamentous fungi, although the majority of microbial emulsifiers have been reported in bacteria. Bacteria are strictly correlated with surfaces and concentrated at interfaces, and production of surface-active agents, together with a large surface-to-volume ratio, is vitally important in terms of competition with other microorganisms.

The term biosurfactant is used loosely in that it also includes emulsifying and dispersing agents. They have advantages over chemical surfactants, such as lower toxicity, higher biodegradability, higher selectivity, and specific activity at extreme temperatures, pH, and salinity. Almost all surfactants currently in use are chemically derived from petroleum. However, interest in microbial surfactants has been steadily increasing due to their diverse properties and structures and their potential applications: environmental protection, crude oil recovery, health care and food processing industries, use in agriculture as a fungicide, and the ability to be synthesized from renewable feedstocks through fermentation.

## CLASSIFICATION

Biosurfactants are categorized mainly by their chemical composition and their microbial origin. The major classes of biosurfactants include glycolipids, lipopeptides and lipoproteins, phospholipids and fatty acids, polymeric biosurfactants, and particulate biosurfactants.

### Glycolipids

Glycolipids are the best-known biosurfactants. They consist of carbohydrates (mono-, di-, tri-, and tetrasaccharides including glucose, mannose, galactose, glucuronic acid, rhamnose, and galactose sulfate) combined with long-chain aliphatic or hydroxyaliphatic acids, usually similar in composition to the phospholipids of the microorganism that produced them. The following are the three best-known glycolipids:

1. Rhamnolipids: The best-studied glycolipids are those consisting of one or two molecules of rhamnose linked to one or two molecules of β-hydroxydecanoic acid. The best-known microorganisms that produce them are members of the genus *Pseudomonas*. Rhamnolipids are able to lower surface tension in *n*-hexadecane-water solutions and emulsify different hydrocarbons.
2. Trehalolipids: They consist of the disaccharide trehalose linked to mycolic acids (long-chain, α-branched-β-hydroxy fatty acids). They are produced by many species of *Mycobacterium, Nocardia, Corynebacteria,* and *Brevibacteria*. Size, structure, number of carbon atoms, and degree of unsaturation of the mycolic acid depend on the microorganism.

3. Sophorolipids: They consist of the disaccharide sophorose, which consists of two β-1,2-linked glucose units, linked to a long-chain hydroxy fatty acid. They are produced by different strains of the yeast *Torulopsis (T. apicola, T. bombicola, T. petrophilum)*.

## Lipopeptides and Lipoproteins

A large number of lipopeptides and lipoproteins possess remarkable surface-active properties. The best known are gramicidin S produced by *Bacillus brevis*, the lipopeptide antibiotic polymixin produced by *Bacillus polymyxa*, surfactin (subtilisin) produced by *Bacillus subtilis*, lichenysin-A produced by *Bacillus Licheniformis*, and antibiotic TA produced by *Myxococcus xanthus*.

## Phospholipids and Fatty Acids

Phospholipids and fatty acids are components of microbial membranes. Many bacteria and yeasts produce large quantities of phospholipids and fatty acid surfactants when grown on alkane substrates. Microorganisms producing phospholipid and fatty acid biosurfactants are species of *Aspergillus, Acinetobacter, Arthrobacter, Pseudomonas aeruginosa*, and *Thiobacillus thiooxidans*.

## Polymeric Biosurfactants

Polymeric biosurfactants are usually polymeric heterosaccharide-containing proteins. The best-studied are emulsan produced by *Acinetobacter calcoaceticus*, liposan produced by *Candida lipolytica*, and mannoprotein produced by *Saccharomyces cerevisiae*.

## Particulate Biosurfactants

Extracellular vesicles from *Acinetobacter* species form a microemulsion. They consist of proteins, phospholipids, and lipopolysaccharides and appear to play a role in the uptake of alkanes. Many microbial cells have a strong affinity for hydrocarbon-water and air-water interfaces and act as surfactants themselves. Their surfactant activity is attributed to several cell-surface components. They are usually hydrocarbon-degrading and pathogenic bacteria (e.g., some species of *Cyanobacteria*).

## ROLE AND PRODUCTION MECHANISMS

### Physiological Role

The physiological role of biosurfactants is not yet clear. Although most of them are considered to be secondary metabolites, some may play an essential role. From a physiological point of view, production of such large compounds by cells would be a waste of energy and resources if they had no function. Their function is most likely related to their amphipathic properties which may be necessary for their survival either through facilitating nutrient transport or as biocides.

The production of biosurfactants can enhance the emulsification and solubilization of hydrocarbon compounds, facilitating the growth of cells on hydrocarbon substrates. It has been demonstrated that the growth of *Pseudomonas aeruginosa* on *n*-alkane could be accelerated by adding small amounts of rhamnolipid into the nutrient solution. However, there has been speculation about their involvement in emulsifying water-insoluble substrates.

Some biosurfactants, mainly lipopeptides and lipoproteins, seem to act as biocides. Their biocidic activities may have a connection with their amphipathic properties. Most of the antiobiotic biosurfactants (e.g., surfactin produced by *B. subtilis*) function to solubilize major constituents of the cell membranes. By producing biosurfactants, which act as cell antiadhesives in a hostile environment, the cells may have a better chance of surviving.

### Biosynthesis

The biosynthesis of biosurfactants is generally complex and not well characterized. The diverse structures of biosurfactants involve various biosynthetic pathways. Biosurfactants consist of a hydrophobic and a hydrophilic moiety. The hydrophobic moiety is either a long-chain fatty acid, a hydroxy fatty acid, or a $\alpha$-alkyl-$\beta$-hydroxy fatty acid, while the hydrophilic moiety can be a carbohydrate, carboxylic acid, phosphate, amino acid, cyclic peptide, or alcohol. Therefore, hydrocarbon and carbohydrate metabolic pathways are involved in the biosynthesis of biosurfactants.

The following four possibilities exist for the synthesis of the two different moieties of biosurfactants:

1. Both hydrophilic and hydrophobic moiety are synthesized de novo.
2. The hydrophilic moiety is synthesized de novo while hydrophobic moiety synthesis is substrate dependent.

3. The hydrophobic moiety is synthesized de novo and the synthesis of the hydrophobic moiety is induced by the substrate.
4. Both hydrophilic and hydrophobic moiety synthesis are substrate dependent.

## *Fermentation*

As with all microbial fermentations, biosurfactant production technology aims to achieve high productivities and yields, high concentrations of the desired final product, and minimum other undesired metabolic by-products. The processes used for biosurfactant production are similar to those used for other secondary metabolites. Many production systems, such as fed-batch, continuous culture, stirred-tank reactor (STR), solid-state fermentation, and even immobilized biocatalysts, have been proposed for the production of biosurfactants. However, all of these techniques have low production rates and yields. The main reasons for such low production yields are mass-transfer limitation, feedback inhibition, and competition between cell growth and biosurfactant production.

At present, most of the effort is focused on the improvement of economics and efficiency of the processes. The high production costs combined with the general lack of public acceptance of microbial-based technologies for biosurfactant production and the purification steps usually required during product preparation for use by the cosmetic, food, and pharmaceutical industries are the main drawbacks that reduce biosurfactant competitiveness with chemically produced surfactants. Table III.19 shows the sources and properties of some important biosurfactants.

## *Kinetics of Production Through Fermentation*

The kinetic parameters can be grouped into the four following types:

1. *Growth-associated production:* In this case, biosurfactant production is related to cell growth and substrate utilization. Examples of this type are the production of rhamnolipids by *Pseudomonas* sp., glycoprotein by *Pseudomonas fluorescens,* and biodispersan by *Bacillus* sp.
2. *Production under growth-limiting conditions:* In this case, biosurfactant production is stimulated under limitation of one or more nutrients. A characteristic example of this type is the production of biosurfactants by *Pseudomonas* sp. under nitrogen and iron limitation.
3. *Production by resting or immobilized cells:* In this case, biosurfactant production is enhanced in nongrowing cells. Examples of this type are

the production of sophorolipids by *Torulopsis bombicola* and *Candida apicola* and the production of cellobiolipid by *Ustilago maydis*. Biosurfactant production by resting cells is very important for the product recovery process, as cell growth and product formation can be separated.

4. *Production by addition of precursors:* In many cases, the addition of biosurfactant precursors results in an increase in their production. For example, addition of lipophilic compounds in the culture medium increased biosurfactant production by *Torulopsis magnoliae, T. bombicola,* and *T. apicola.*

### Product Recovery

The recovery of the product is responsible for a large portion (up to 60 percent) of the production cost. The optimal conditions for biosurfactant recovery depend on fermentation conditions, physicochemical properties of the product (ionic charge, water solubility), and location (intracellular, extracellular, or cell bound).

The most widely used recovery techniques are solvent extractions using different solvents or combination of solvents such as butanol, ethyl acetate, pentane, hexane, acetic acid, ether chloroform-methanol, and dichloromethane-methanol. Examples of biosurfactant recovery using solvent extraction techniques include rhamnolipids produced by *Pseudomonas* sp., trehalose lipids produced by *Mycobacterium* sp. and *Arthrobacter paraffineus,* trehalose corynomycolates and tetraesters produced by *Rhodococcus erythropolis,* cellobiolipids produced by *Ustilago* sp., and liposan produced by *C. lipolytica.*

Other techniques that have been proposed for biosurfactant isolation are acid precipitation at low temperature (used for recovery of glycolipids from *P. aeruginosa* and *Ustilago zeae*), acidification followed by extraction in chloroform-methanol mixture (used for recovery of rhamnolipids from *P. aeruginosa* and *C. lipolytica*), acetone precipitation (used for biosurfactant recovery from *Pseudomanas* sp., *Endomycopsis lipolytica, Candida tropicalis,* and *Debaryomyces polymorphus*), and ammonium sulfate precipitation (used for recovery of emulsan and biodispersan from *Acinetobacter calcoaceticus*).

Investigations of continuous removal (harvesting) of biosurfactants from the fermentation supernatant results in a severalfold increase in production yields due to the elimination of product inhibition. The techniques that can be used for continuous biosurfactant recovery include foam fractionation, adsorption on activated carbons or hydrophobic adsorbents (e.g., adsorption

TABLE III.19. Source and properties of some important microbial surfactants

| Biosurfactant | Organisms | Surface tension (mN/m) | Critical micelle concentration (CMC) | Interfacial tension (mN/m) |
|---|---|---|---|---|
| Glycolipids | | | | |
|   Rhamnolipids | *P. aeruginosa* | 29 | | 0.25 |
| | *Pseudomonas* sp. | 25-30 | 0.1-10 | 1 |
|   Trehalolipids | *R. erythropolis* | 32-36 | 4 | 14-17 |
| | *Nocardia erythropolis* | 30 | 20 | 3.5 |
| | *Mycobacterium* sp. | 38 | 0.3 | 15 |
|   Sophorolipids | *T. bombicola* | 33 | | 1.8 |
| | *T. apicola* | 30 | | 0.9 |
| | *T. petrophilum* | | | |
|   Cellobiolipids | *U. zeae, U. maydis* | | | |
| Lipopeptides and lipoproteins | | | | |
|   Peptide-lipid | *B. licheniformis* | 27 | 12-20 | 0.1-0.3 |
|   Serrwettin | *Serratia marcescens* | 28-33 | | |
|   Viscosin | *P. fluorescens* | 26.5 | 150 | |
|   Surfactin | *B. subtilis* | 27-32 | 23-160 | 1 |
|   Subtilisin | *B. subtilis* | | | |
|   Gramicidins | *B. brevis* | | | |
|   Polymyxins | *B. polymyxa* | | | |
| Fatty acids, neutral lipids, and phospolipids | | | | |
|   Fatty acids | *C. lepus* | 30 | 150 | 2 |
|   Neutral lipids | *N. erythropolis* | 32 | | 3 |
|   Phospolipids | *T. thiooxidans* | | | |
| Polymeric surfactants | | | | |
|   Emulsan | *A. calcoaceticus* | | | |
|   Biodispersan | *A. calcoaceticus* | | | |
|   Mannan-lipid-protein | *C. tropicalis* | | | |
|   Liposan | *C. lipolytica* | | | |
|   Carbohydrate-protein-lipid | *P. fluorescens* | 27 | 10 | |
| | *D. polymorphus* | | | |
|   Protein PA | *P. aeruginosa* | | | |
| Particulate biosurfactants | | | | |
|   Vesicles and fimbriae | *A. calcoaceticus* | | | |
|   Whole cells | Variety of bacteria | | | |

on Amberlite followed by purification and freeze-drying), and adsorption chromatography on ion-exhange resins.

## FACTORS AFFECTING BIOSURFACTANT PRODUCTION

The type, quality, and quantity of the produced biosurfactant mainly depend on carbon and nitrogen source, salt concentration, and environmental factors and growth conditions such as pH, temperature, dilution rate (in continuous processes), agitation, and oxygen availability.

### Carbon Source

The source of carbon often has a critical effect on the biosurfactant structure and production yield. The effect of hydrocarbons (as insoluble water substrates) and other water-soluble carbon sources present in the media during biosurfactant production varies. Biosurfactant production is usually induced by hydrocarbons, while water-soluble carbon sources repress their biosynthesis. Different biosurfactants were produced by *A. paraffineus* when grown on different carbon sources. Water-soluble carbon sources such as glycerol, glucose, mannitol, and ethanol resulted in an inferior product compared to water-immiscible substrates such as *n*-alkanes and olive oil during rhamnolipid production by *Pseudomonas* sp. Although the composition of biosurfactants produced by *Pseudomonas* sp. was affected by the carbon source, the chain length of the substrate had no effect on the chain length of fatty acid moieties in glycolipids. On the other hand, the carbon number of alkanes resulted in a qualitative variation during biosurfactant production by *Acinetobacter* sp.

### Nitrogen Source

Ammonium and nitrate salts, urea, and amino acids are usually used as nitrogen sources. Lichenysin-A production from *B. licheniformis* was enhanced by addition of L-glutamic acid and L-asparagine. Addition of aspartic and glutamic acid, asparagine, and glycine to the culture medium resulted in an increase in biosurfactant production by *A. paraffineus*. In many cases, biosurfactant production is stimulated under nitrogen-limiting conditions. For example, nitrogen limitation caused an overproduction of biosurfactant in *P. aeruginosa, C. tropicalis,* and *Nocardia* sp.

## Environmental Factors and Growth Conditions

The pH of the growth medium, level of oxygen, agitation, and temperature may play important roles in biosurfactant production: biosurfactant production by *Pseudomonas, Ustilago maydis,* and *Torulopsis bombicola* was affected by pH, and biosurfactant production by *Arthrobacter paraffineus, Rhodococcus erythropolis,* and *Pseudomonas* sp. was affected by temperature.

Salt concentration and the presence of some compounds such as ethambutol, penicillin, chloramphenicol, and EDTA (ethylene diaminete traacetic acid) may also affect biosurfactant production. Surfactin production by *Bacillus subtilis* was increased when iron or manganese salts were added in the medium.

## APPLICATIONS OF BIOSURFACTANTS

For a number of years, enhanced oil recovery, applications related to oil spill bioremedation/dispersion, both inland and at sea, and removal/mobilization of oil sludge from storage tanks were considered to be the most important growth areas of biosurfactants. One well-known example was the *Exxon Valdez* oil spill. In this case, biosurfactants were used to emulsify hydrocarbon-water mixtures, so as to enhance the degradation of hydrocarbons in the environment. Biosurfactants are also used in food and agriculture. In the food industry, they are used as food emulsifiers, antioxidant agents, and antiadhesives, while in agriculture they are used for solubilizing hydrophobic compounds from contaminated soils, for decontaminating soils from pesticides, in metal-contaminated soil remediation, and in plant pathogen elimination.

Another large market for biosurfactants is emulsion polymerization for paints, paper, and industrial coatings. It is also important to understand that biosurfactants might find applications for therapeutic purposes. Rhamnolipids, lipopeptides, and mannosylerythritol lipids have been shown to have antimicrobial activities, while some other biosurfactants are being investigated for their biological activities in leukemia, inhibition of HIV virus, and inhibition of adhesion of pathogenic enteric bacteria. The lipopeptide biosurfactant viscosin, for example, has a powerful antibiotic activity against mycobacteria and bronchitis virus of chickens, as well as being active against influenza A virus of mice.

Biosurfactants have found a niche in the personal care market because of their lower moisturizing properties and skin compatibility. In oral hygiene products, they are helpful in dental plaque removal. Sophorolipids have found commercial utility in the cosmetic industry and as a skin moisturizer. Other possible applications of biosurfactants are in mining and manufacturing processes as an agent for solubilizing and dispersing inorganic minerals.

## CONCLUSIONS

Because of the high hazard for human health of synthetic surfactants and increasing consumer demand for natural products, microbial surfactants have become increasingly important. High availability and production of microorganisms, which are able to produce biosurfactants by simple biotechnological methods, allow large quantities of biosurfactants to be obtained from microbes. In addition, biosurfactants possess many advantages over synthetic surfactants. The chemical diversity of biosurfactants offers a wider selection of surface-active agents with properties closely tailored to specific applications.

However, the production cost of biosurfactants is much higher than that of chemical surfactants. Much effort has been made for process optimization at the engineering and biological levels. Cheap raw materials and industrial effluents such as olive oil mill effluent, potato-processing industrial and chicken fat residues, agroindustrial by-products, and wastewater pressate from fuel-grade peat processing are promising substrates for low-cost biosurfactant production. There have also been attempts to improve yields by genetic manipulation. For example, the *lac* plasmid from *Escherichia coli* has been inserted to *P. aeruginosa* cells, and biosurfactant production is feasible using whey as a substrate.

It is evident that the expected breakthrough in biosurfactant commercialization will arrive when their production costs become comparable to or more cost effective than those of chemical surfactants. Biosurfactants will gain a significant share of the market when improved knowledge and ability to manipulate the metabolism of the producer strain may permit their growth on cheaper substrates, or when the improvement of process technology will facilitate complete product recovery.

## SUGGESTED READINGS

Banat IM, RS Makkar, and SS Cameotra (2000). Potential commercial applications of microbial surfactants. *Applied Microbiology and Biotechnology* 53:495-508.
Desai JD and IM Banat (1997). Microbial production of surfactants and their commercial potential. *Microbiology and Molecular Biology Reviews* 61(1):47-64.
Fiechter A (1992). Biosurfactants: Moving towards industrial application. *Tibtech* 10:208-217.

Karanth NGK, PG Deo, and NK Veenanadig (1999). Microbial production of biosurfactants and their importance. *Current Science* 77(1):116-126.

Lin SC (1996). Biosurfactants: Recent advances. *Journal of Chemistry, Technology and Biotechnology* 66:109-120.

# Microbial Enzymes: Production and Applications

## L-Glutaminase

### Abdulhameed Sabu

#### INTRODUCTION

L-Glutaminase (L-glutamine amidohydrolase—EC 3.5.1.2) is a potent antileukemic drug and has found application as a flavor-enhancing agent in the food industry. It deamidates L-glutamine and plays a major role in the cellular nitrogen metabolism of both prokaryotes and eukaryotes. L-glutaminase is useful in the food industry because it increases the glutamic acid content of fermented foods, thereby imparting a unique flavor. Because glutaminase is the key enzyme responsible for glutamine metabolism at many different levels, it plays a regulatory role in gene expression as well. In addition to its role as a flavor enhancer in fermented foods, the ability of this enzyme to bring about degradation of glutamine positions it as a possible candidate for enzyme therapy, which may soon replace or combine with L-asparaginase in the treatment of acute lymphocytic leukemia.

#### SOURCES OF L-GLUTAMINASE

Glutaminase activity is widely distributed in plants, animal tissues, and microorganisms including bacteria, yeast, and fungi. Although L-glutaminase synthesis has been reported from many bacterial genera, members of the Enterobacteriaceae family have been best characterized. Among these, *Escherichia coli* glutaminases have been studied in much detail. Some examples of bacterial strains producing L-glutaminase include *E. coli, Pseudomonas* sp., *Pseudomonas aeruginosa, Pseudomonas aureofaciens, Pseudomonas aurantiaca,* and *Pseudomonas fluorescens, Acinetobacter* sp., *Bacillus* sp., *Proteus morganii, Proteus vulgaris, Xanthomonas juglandis, Erwinia carotovora, Ewinia aroideae, Serratia marcescens,*

*Enterobacter cloacae, Klebsiella aerogenes,* and *Aerobacter aerogenes.* Among yeast, species of *Hansenula, Rhodotorula, Candida scottii, Cryptococcus albidus, Cryptococcus laurentii, Candida utilis, C. nodaensis, Torulopsis candida, Zygosaccharomyces rouxii, Tilachlidium humicola, Verticillum malthoasei,* etc., and among fungi *Aspergillus sojae* and *Aspergillus oryzae* have been reported to produce glutaminase. *Escherichia coli* is the only other organism used for industrial applications. Thus, seemingly enormous scope exists for the search for potential strains that could produce L-glutaminase in high yields and with novel properties under economically viable bioprocesses.

## PRODUCTION OF L-GLUTAMINASE

Different methods of fermentation technology can be applied for the production of L-glutaminase. Although commercial production of glutaminase is carried out using the submerged fermentation (SmF) technique and the majority of the reports on microbial glutaminase production also deal with SmF, the solid-state fermentation (SSF) technique using natural and inert solid materials has gained attention. The technique of whole-cell immobilization has also been applied for the production of microbial glutaminase. Table III.20 gives a brief account of the various methods used for glutaminase production. Glucose and L-glutamine have been the most favored substrates for L-glutaminase production under SmF.

## STRUCTURE OF L-GLUTAMINASE

The structure and chemical nature of microbial glutaminase differs from species to species. The structure of the glutaminase domain of glucosamine g-phosphate synthase reveals that the protein fold has structural homology to other members of the superfamily of N-terminal nucleophile (Ntn) hydrolases, being a sandwich of antiparallel beta sheets surrounded by two layers of helices. The structural homology between the glutaminase domain of GLMS (glucosamine-6-phosphate synthetase) and that of PRPP (phosphoribosylpyrophosphate) amidotransferase indicates that they may have diverged from a common ancestor. Cys1 is the catalytic nucleophile in GLMS, and the nucleophilic character of its thiol group appears to be increased through general base activation by its own alpha-amino group. Cys1 can adopt two conformations, one active and one inactive. Glutamine binding locks the residue in a predetermined conformation. It has been proposed that when a nitrogen acceptor was present, Cys1 was kept in the active con-

TABLE III.20. Sources and methods for glutaminase production

| Microorganism | Substrate | Technology |
|---|---|---|
| *Aspergillus oryzae* AJ ii 7281 | Wheat bran | SSF |
| *Aspergillus oryzae* CNCM I 1881 | Proteinacious materials | SmF |
| *Aspergillus awamori* ATCC 14335 | Glucose | SmF |
| *Beauveria bassiana* BTMF S10 | Glucose and glutamine in polystyrene | SSF |
| *Beauveria bassiana* BTMF S 10 | L-Glutamine and methionine | SmF |
| *Cryptococcus albidus* ATCC 20293 | Glutamine | Immobilization |
| *Cryptococcus nodaensis* G 60 | Lactose | SmF |
| *Pseudomonas aurantiaca* | L-Glutamine | SmF |
| *Pseudomonas fluorescens* ACMR 347 and 43 | L-Glutamine | SmF |
| *Pseudomonas nitroreducens* IFO 12694 | Glucose | SmF |
| *Pseudomonas nitroreducens* IFO 12694 | Glucose | Immobilization |
| *Vibrio cholerae* ACMR 347 | L-Glutamine | SmF |
| *Vibrio costicola* ACMR 267 | L-Glutamine | SmF |
| *Vibrio costicola* ACMR 267 | L-Glutamine, glucose, wheat bran, rice husk, sawdust, copra cake, groundnut cake | SSF |
| *Zygosaccharomyces rouxii* | Sesamum oil cake and groundnut oil cake | SSF |

formation, explaining the phenomenon of substrate-induced activation of the enzyme, and that Arg26 was central in this coupling.

The amino acid sequence and a 2 Å resolution crystallographic structure of *Pseudomonas* 7A glutaminase-asparaginase (PGA), which belongs to the family of tetrameric bacterial amidohydrolases and deamidates glutamine and asparagines, has a high degree of similarity to the sequences of other members of the family. PGA has the same fold as other bacterial amido-hydrolases, with the exception of the position of a 20-residue loop that forms part of the active site. In the PGA structure the active site loop is observed clearly in only one monomer, in an open position, with a conformation different from that observed for other amidohydrolases. In the other three monomers the loop is disordered and cannot be traced, because of the direct consequence of a very low occupancy of products of the enzymatic reaction bound in the active sites of PGA in these crystals. The active sites are composed of a rigid part and the flexible loop. The rigid part consists of the residues directly involved in the catalytic reaction as well as residues that assist in orienting the substrate. The flexible loops actively participate in the transport of substrate and product molecules through the amido-hydrolase active sites and participate in orienting the substrate molecules properly in relation to the catalytic residues.

## PROPERTIES

Properties of any enzyme determine its suitability and efficiency for application in bioprocesses. There has been wide variation in the properties of glutaminases obtained from different sources. These are generally active at an alkaline pH. While optimal activities of glutaminase A and B of *P. aeruginosa* were at alkaline pH of 7.5 to 9.0 and 8.5, respectively, glutaminase from *Pseudomonas* sp. was reported to be active over a broad range of pH (5 to 9) with an optimum near pH 7.0. An intracellular glutaminase from *Cryptococcus albidus* preferred an optimal pH of 5.5 to 8.5.

The temperature stability of glutaminases shows wide variation. Glutaminase from *Pseudomonas* sp. showed maximum activity at 37°C and was not stable at high temperatures, whereas the enzyme from *Clostridium welchii* retained activity at 60°C. Glutaminase from *Cryptococcus albidus* retained 77 percent of its activity at 70°C even after 30 minutes of incubation. Glutaminase I and II from *Micrococcus luteus* had temperature optima of 50°C, and the presence of NaCl (10 percent) increased the thermostability.

Sodium chloride influences the activity of glutaminase from both fungi and bacteria of terrestrial origin. Glutaminase from *E. coli, Pseudomonas fluorescens, Cryptococcus albidus,* and *Aspergillus sojae* showed only 65, 75, 65, and 6 percent, respectively of their original activity in presence of 18 percent NaCl. Similar results were obtained with glutaminase from *Candida utilis, Torulopsis candida,* and *A. oryzae.* Salt-tolerant glutaminase have been observed in *C. albidus* and *Bacillus subtilis.* Use of salt-tolerant glutaminase from marine bacteria could provide an interesting alternative in the soy sauce fermentation industry.

Glutaminases also differed in their affinity toward L-glutamine. While the enzyme from *Acinetobacter* sp. recorded a Km of $5.8\pm1.5 \times 10^{-6}$ M, those from *C. welchii* had a Km of $10^{-3}$ M. The enzyme from *Achromobacteraceae* had a Km of $4.8\pm1.4 \times 10^{-6}$ M. The average Km values for glutaminase-asparaginase from *Pseudomonas* sp. 7A was $4.6\pm0.4 \times 10^{-6}$ M, whereas, that from *Pseudomonas acidovorans* had $2.2 \times 10^{-5}$ M. The isoelectric point of glutaminase varied for different organisms. It was 5.5 for *Clostridium welchii;* 5.4 for *E. coli;* 8.43 for *Acinetobacter glutamina-*

*sificans;* 5.8 for *Pseudomonas;* 7.6 for another species of *Pseudomonas;* and 3.94 to 4.09 for *Cryptococcus albidus* and *Pseudomonas acidovorans.*

Various substances and heavy metals inhibited glutaminase activity. Cetavlon, while accelerating glutaminase of *Clostridium welchii, E. coli,* and *Proteus morganii* in crude extracts and intact cells, inhibited the purified enzyme. Glutaminase of *E. coli* was found to be sensitive to heavy metals, and *Acinetobacter* glutaminase-asparaginase was inactivated by glutamine analog 6-diazo 5-oxo L-norleucine, even at very low concentration, while being unaffected by EDTA (ethylene diaminete traacetic acid), $NH_3$, L-glutamate, or L-aspartate. In the case of fungi, both intra- and extracellular glutaminase from *Aspergillus oryzae* were inhibited by Hg, Cr, and Fe but were not affected by sulphydroxyl reagents. EDTA and $Na_2SO_4$ strongly inhibited the *Micrococcus luteus* glutaminase I, while glutaminase II was inhibited by EDTA, $HgCl_2$, $Na_2SO_4$, $CuCl_2$, and $FeCl_3$.

There has been wide variation in the molecular weight of glutaminases from different sources, which could generally be between 120 and 147 kDa, although higher (e.g., *P. acidovorans* had molecular weight of approximately 156 kDa) or lower (e.g., flutaminase B from *E. coli* had molecular weight of 90 kDa) could also be found.

## *GLUTAMINASE GENE*

Due to the increased demand for glutaminase with better characteristics, good potential exists for recombinant DNA technology for isolation and manipulation of the glutaminase gene. The glutaminase gene from both bacteria and fungi have been isolated and transferred to other hosts using suitable vectors. Recombinant organisms thus obtained expressed many better characteristics such as improved yield and tolerance to pH, salt, temperature, etc.

The complete nucleotide sequence of the glutaminase-encoding gene from the *koji* mold *Aspergillus oryzae* was elucidated. N-terminal and internal amino acid sequences were determined. A 700 base pair (bp) fragment was amplified by polymerase chain reaction (PCR) using oligonucleotide primers designed from partial amino acid sequences and was used as a homologous probe for screening an *A. oryzae* genomic DNA library. Reverse transcription (RT)-PCR showed that the gene contained seven short introns. Sequence analysis revealed an open reading frame that encodes a protein of 690 amino-acid residues with a predicted molecular mass of 76 kDa. The *A. oryzae* glutaminase gene was expressed in *A. nidulans* to confirm the presence of a functional gene.

The structural *glsA* gene of *Rhizobium etli* glutaminase A was amplified by PCR and cloned in the expression vector pTrcHis. After purification the enzyme protein showed the same kinetic properties as native glutaminase A. The physicochemical and biochemical properties of native and recombinant glutaminase were also identical. These results suggest that *R. etli* glutaminase A is composed of four identical subunits.

In order to make organisms with the ability to produce salt-tolerant and resistant glutaminase, many researchers have attempted to create recombinant organisms by expressing the glutaminase gene in other organisms using appropriate plasmid vectors. The gene encoding for salt-tolerant glutaminase I from marine *Micrococcus luteus* K-3 was cloned in *Escherichia coli* JM109 using plasmid pUC18 and plasmid pUC19. Clones were screened by hybridization with degenerate oligonucleotide probes designed using the known N-terminal protein sequence of glutaminase I from K-3. A 2.4 kb Hind III DNA fragment from a 8 kb primary cloned DNA fragment was subcloned and sequenced. The DNA fragment had an open reading frame of 1,368 nucleotides encoding 456 amino acids. Attempts have also been made to enhance the enzyme production capacity of bacteria and fungi by mutagenesis. Protoplast fusion among the species of *A. sojae* has also been employed to improve glutaminase production.

## APPLICATIONS OF L-GLUTAMINASE

### Food Sector

The ever-increasing consumption of soy and soy products all over the world shows the significance of L-glutaminase in the food industry Glutaminases are widely used in the production of soy sauce and enzymatically hydrolyzed protein. L-Glutaminase enhances the flavor of fermented foods by increasing their glutamic acid content and thereby imparting a palatable taste. Glutaminase from some bacteria and fungi are approved by the Food and Drug Administration (FDA) in the "generally regarded as safe" (GRAS) category and widely used in China, Japan, Korea, and other Asian countries where fermented foods such as soy sauce are a valuable commodity. The use of L-glutaminase as a flavor-enhancing agent in Chinese dishes has replaced the use of monosodium glutamate (MSG), which is an allergen for some persons.

Most of the basic flavor components of fermented condiments are amino acids produced by enzymatic degradation of protein contained in raw materials. In order to ensure a palatable taste, about one half of the nitrogenous compounds present must be free amino acids and over 10 percent should be free glutamic acid. The unique flavor of fermented soy sauce or shoyu is mainly due to glutamic acid. Activity of L-glutaminase, which is responsible for the synthesis of glutamic acid, makes it an important additive during enzymatic digestion of shoyu koji. It has been observed that the glutamic acid content of shoyu increases on addition of glutaminase. Attempts to increase the glutamate content of soy sauce using salt-tolerant and heat-stable glutaminase have drawn large attention.

### Medical Sector

L-Glutaminase is used in the treatment of cancer (lung carcinoma, mamma carcinoma, colon carcinoma, etc.). Cancerous cells compete for nitrogen compounds which induces in the host a negative nitrogen balance and a characteristic weight loss and in the tumor reciprocal nitrogen increase. Glutamine is the most abundant free amino acid in the human body, which is essential for the growth of normal and neoplastic cells and for the culture of many cell types. Cancer has been described as a nitrogen trap, and the presence of a tumor produces great changes in host glutamine metabolism in such a way that host nitrogen metabolism is accommodated to the tumor-enhanced requirements of glutamine. To be used, glutamine must be transported into tumor mitochondria. Thus, an overview of the role of glutamine in cancer requires a discussion of not only host and tumor glutamine metabolism but also its circulation and transport. Because glutamine depletion has adverse effects for the host, the effect of glutamine supplementation in the tumor-bearing state should also be studied.

Tumor inhibition is mediated by inhibition of both nucleic acid and protein synthesis of tumor cells. Because specific inhibition of tumor cell glutamine uptake could be one of the possible ways to check the growth, use of glutaminase enzyme as a drug gains importance in this respect.

The in vivo antiretroviral activity of glutaminase has potential applications in the medical field. The murine leukemia virus requires glutamine for replication, and glutaminase-mediated depletion of glutamine in animals results in potent inhibition of retrovirus replication, thereby increasing the median survival time of the animals. In 1993, a patent was registered for a *Pseudomonas* sp. recombinant glutaminase that could be economically produced and active against HIV virus. Another patent was registered in 1994 for a recombinant glutaminase derived from *Pseudomonas* 7A. This enzyme was active against HIV virus replication, and the inventors proposed a new method for tumor gene therapy by transfecting tumor infiltrating lymphocytes with plasmid and administration to the patient. Studies on clinical and biochemical aspects of microbial glutaminase toxicity in rabbit and rhesus monkey have showed that treatment with chemically modified glutaminases was lethal to rabbits and rhesus monkeys, and lesions were produced in kidney, liver, and intestine, while treatment with unmodified glutaminase induced similar changes in rabbits but not in rhesus monkeys.

### In Biosensors

Another important application of L-glutaminase is in biosensors for monitoring the glutamine levels in mammalian and hybridoma cell cultures without the need for a separate measurement for glutamic acid. Determination of glutamine in mammalian cell cultures is usually done by high performance liquid chromatography (HPLC), but the technique is time-consuming and expensive and requires specialized operators; thus, it is not optimally suited for online monitoring. Optical methods such as near-infrared (IR) spectroscopy and chemiluminescence have also been recently described. These methods have high sensitivity, but matrix interferences in the case of near-IR and background fluorescence in the case of chemiluminescence can degrade the selectivity of the measurements.

Online simultaneous monitoring of ammonia and glutamine in a hollow fiber reactor using flow injection analysis is possible using a glutaminase biosensor. Glutamine was determined by a difference method in which ammonia was measured before and after passage through a module containing immobilized glutaminase. Use of tetrathiafulvalene (TTF)-mediated amperometric enzyme electrodes was reported for the determination of glutamine and glutamic acid in mammalian cell cultures. An integrated thin-film biosensor was developed for the simultaneous measurement of L-glutamine and L-glutamic acid in a micro-flow cell using glutaminase from *Pseudomonas boreopolis*. Immobilized L-glutaminase and L-glutamate oxidase enzyme-based biosensors have been used for the determination of L-glutamate and L-glutamine by flow injection analysis and chemiluminiscence detection.

### CONCLUSIONS

Because the sources for L-glutaminases are limited, the search for potential microbial strains and technologies that can be used for the production of glutaminase in high titres with novel properties for their applications in various fields is being pursued all over the world. However, the large-scale application of glutaminase in cancer chemotherapy is still under experimental conditions and there is a need for advanced research on enzyme therapy against cancer.

## SUGGESTED READINGS

Abell CW and JR Uren (1981). Enzymes. In *Antitumor compounds of natural origin: Chemistry and biochemistry,* A Aszalos, (ed.). Boca Raton, FL: CRC Press, pp. 123-153.

Davidson L, DR Brear, P Wingrad, J Hawkins, and BG Kitto (1977). Purification and properties of an L-glutaminase-L-asparaginase from *Pseudomonas acidovorans. Journal of Bacteriology* 129:1379-1386.

Sabu A, M Chandrasekaran, and A Pandey (2000). Biopotential of microbial glutaminases. *Chemistry Today* 11/12:21-25.

# Inulinases

Pushpa R. Kulkarni
Rekha S. Singhal

## INTRODUCTION

Among the enzymes that hydrolyze polymers into interesting monomers, inulinases have attracted much attention in recent years. Inulin is the primary substrate for inulinases. A polymer of plant origin, inulin serves as a reserve carbohydrate in Compositae and Gramineae. Inulin and its analogs are polyfructans, consisting of linear β-2,1-linked polyfructose chains displaying a terminal glucose unit. The average chain length varies as a function of the plant and the season. Inulin is present in large amounts in Jerusalem artichoke (*Helianthus tuberosus* L.), chicory (*Cichorium intybus* L.), dandelion (*Taraxacum officinale* Weber), dahlia (*Dahlia pinnata* Cav.), burdock *(Articum),* scorzonera (*Scorzonera hispanica* L.), cardoon (*Cynara cardunculus* L.), costus *(Saussurea lappa),* Agave americana, and rye grass.

As early as 1900, the yeast *Saccharomyces marxianus* was known to utilize inulin. By 1924 and 1933, respectively, *Aspergillus niger* and *Kluyveromyces fragilis* were identified to grow at the expense of inulin. Until then, a single enzyme from yeast, a β-fructofuranosidase capable of hydrolyzing sucrose, inulin, raffinose, stachyose, and gentianose, was known, and no separate existence of inulinase was considered. In 1943 it was established that even purified invertase from yeast strains displayed varying inulinase activity, and it had a pH and temperature optima very different from that of invertase from the same preparation.

## INULINASES: ACTION AND TYPES

Most inulinases are in fact β-fructofuranosidase and split off fructose moieties from the nonreducing end of the inulin molecule or from certain sugars displaying a fructose unity at the terminal β-2-1 position. These enzymes can be designated as 2-1-β-D-fructan fructanohydrolases (EC 3.2.1.7), whereas invertases that specifically hydrolyze sucrose into glucose and fructose can be classified as β-D-fructofuranoside fructohydrolases (EC 3.2.1.26). Inulinases with β-fructosidase activity are found in plants and microorganisms. Although tubers from Jerusalem artichoke, chicory, dandelion, and dahlia do not display any invertase activity, many purified microbial inulinases are known to possess invertase activity. Though inulinases were first isolated from plants, it is very difficult to obtain these inulinases in sufficient quantities. As a result, microbial inulinases produced by growing microbes in an inulin-based growth medium are receiving much attention all over the world. Important species of yeast, filamentous fungi, and bacteria producing inulinases are summarized in Table III.21.

Inulinases are both endoacting and exoacting on inulin. Exoacting inulinases produce monosaccharides as the main end product, and oligosaccharides are produced in low amounts. The endoacting inulinases produce oligosaccharides as the main end product and monosaccharides in minor amounts. Inulinases from *Penicillium* sp. were purified into three exoacting types: P I, P II, and P III, with molecular weight of 80,000, 63,000, and 66,000, respectively. *Aspergillus niger* sp. 12 inulinase has also been fractionated into P I (exo), P II, and P III (endo), with molecular weights of 59,000, 54,000, and 59,000, respectively. Inulinases from *Aspergillus ficcum* have now been characterized into inulinase exo II, III, IV, and V and inulinase endo I, II, and III with molecular weights of 75,000, 76,000, 74,000, 74,000, 74,000, 64,000, 64,000, and 64,000, respectively. *Fusarium oxysporum* produces exoacting inulinases (mycelial as well as extracellular) with molecular weight of 300,000.

Inulinases are also both extra- and intracellular. Table III.22 lists microorganisms producing both of these types of enzymes. Some organisms also show a mixed form. In *Candida kefyr*, a cationic surfactant such as alkyldimethylbenzyl ammonium chloride is used to release intracellular enzyme during stationary growth of the cells. Rhizosphere soil samples and decomposing Compositae plant materials are common sources of inulinase-producing microorganisms. For screening, inulin is used as the sole source of carbon. A screening medium containing inulin 2 percent, $K_2HPO_4$ 0.1 percent, $MgSO_4 \cdot 7H_2O$ 0.05 percent, $NaNO_2$ 0.15 percent, $(NH_4)_2HPO_4$ 0.2 percent, KCl 0.05 percent, $FeSO_4 \cdot 7H_2O$ 0.01 percent, and pH 6.0 is popu-

TABLE III.21. Important species of inulinase-producing microorganisms

| Fungi | Yeast | Bacteria |
|---|---|---|
| *Aspergillus* sp. | *Kluyveromyces* sp. | *Arthrobacter* sp. |
| *Aspergillus niger* sp. | *Candida* sp. | *Bacillus* sp. |
| *Penicillium* sp. | *Debaryomyces* sp. | *Achromobacter* sp. |
| *Cladosporium* sp. | *Saccharomyces* sp | *Cladosporium* sp. |
| *Fusarium* sp. | *Schizosaccharomyces* sp. | *Clostridium* sp. |
| *Sporotrichum* sp. | *Pichia* sp. | *Staphylococcus* sp. |
| | *Hansenula* sp. | |

TABLE III.22. Location of inulinases in some microorganisms

| Intracellular | Extracellular |
| --- | --- |
| *Kluyveromyces fragilis**  | *Sterigmatocystis nigra* |
| *Candida kefyr**  | *Aspergillus* sp. 1 |
| *Debaryomyces phaffii* | *Aspergillus niger* 12 |
| *Aspergillus niger* | *Aspergillus ficuum* |
| *Kluyveromyces* ATCC 12424 | *Fusarium oxysporum** |
| *Clostridium acetobutylicum* ABKn8 | *Arthrobacter ureafaciens* |
| *Clostridium thermosuccinogenes* | *Penicillium* |
| *Candida salmanticensis* | *Kluyveromyces marxianus* CBS 6556 |

*Both extracellular and intracellular

larly used. Growth in this medium or clear zones of solubilized inulin in the agar layer confirms presence of inulinase producers.

## MICROBIAL PRODUCTION OF INULINASES

Although inulin is the most commonly used substrate for production of inulinase, a variety of substrates (carbon and energy sources) have been used in different microorganisms. These include pure substances, naturally occurring inulin-rich materials, and mixed substrates. Among pure substances, inulin and sucrose have been the preferred carbon sources. In general, if a microbial strain shows only inulinase activity, inulin serves as the best substrate. If the organism also produces invertase, sucrose is a better substrate. In the case of *K. fragilis, Candida kefyr,* and *Penicillium* sp., the highest yields of inulinase have been obtained with inulin followed by raffinose, fructose, and sorbitol, and very low yields resulted from use of sucrose, galactose, glucose, and mannitol. Inulinase production in *Aspergillus niger* van Teighem is inducible and subject to catabolic repression. Isolation of a constitutive mutant of *K. fragilis* has provided genetic evidence for the inducible nature of inulinase in the wild type, while in the case of *Kluyveromyces marxianus,* the production has been proved to be partially constitutive. In the case of *Aspergillus niger,* the highest yields of inulinase were produced with maltose rather than with inulin, suggesting that the enzyme production is constitutive. *Bacillus subtilis* and *Panaeolus papilionaceus* also produce inulinase constitutively. Derivatives of natural dahlia inulin such as caprylated inulin and cholesteryl inulin have been successfully proved to be inulinase-producing substrates for *K. marxianus.* Fructan- and fructosan-containing media have proved to be supportive of growth as well as inulinase production in *Fusarium oxysporum*. Roots and tubers of several Compositae and Graminae appear to be good sources of inulin. Dahlia, chicory, Jerusalem artichoke, and costus roots have widely been used for this purpose. A Japanese patent describes the use of a mixture of roots of Jerusalem artichoke and chicory in slurry or powder form with maltose as a carbon source to make the process of inulin production cheaper.

Complex nitrogen sources such as yeast extract, peptone, corn steep liquor, and urea, and inorganic nitrogen sources such as $(NH_4)_2SO_4$, $(NH_4)_2HPO_4$, $(NH_4)H_2PO_4$, $NH_4Cl$, $NaNO_3$, and $KNO_3$ have been widely used in inulinase-producing media. *Kluyveromyces fragilis* grew best with a high yield of inulinase in medium containing casamino acids as a nitrogen source. With *C. kefyr*, the highest inulinase levels were observed upon addition of 0.35 percent yeast extract and 0.2 percent urea to a medium containing 5 percent lactose and 2 percent inulin. Peptone and corn steep liquor stimulated, while urea and yeast extract had less influence on inulinase production in *Penicillium* sp. 1. Among inorganic nitrogen sources, $(NH_4)H_2PO_4$ and $(NH_4)_2HPO_4$ gave the highest yield, while $KNO_3$ and $NaNO_3$ were reasonably productive. This is also true in case of the *Aspergillus niger* 12 strain. Yeast extract stimulated the highest enzyme production in LC B41 bacterial thermophilic strain, while corn steep liquor resulted in good enzyme production in *A. niger* and *Penicillium* sp.

Inulinase production is also influenced by factors such as presence of metal ions, pH of the medium, aeration, and temperature of fermentation. Although many details are not available, the positive influence of KCl (0.01 M), $MgSO_4$ (0.01 M), and $FeSO_4$ (0.001 M) has been observed in *Penicillium* sp. 1 and *A. niger* 12 when added to a medium containing 1 percent inulin, 1 percent corn steep liquor, and 1 percent $(NH_4)H_2PO_4$ at pH 5.0. The highest extracellular inulinase production occurs at pH 7.5 in *Debaryomyces castellii*, *Arthrobacter ureafaciens*, and LCB4, while in *Penicillium* sp. 1 it is at pH 5.0. *Kluyveromyces fragilis* produced comparable cell and enzyme yield in a broad pH range of 3.5 to 6.0. Although a variation in dissolved oxygen tension from 2.5 to 40 percent saturation did not have any influence on inulinase production in *K. fragilis,* culturing without aeration displayed poor growth and low inulinase levels. Shaker conditions have been found necessary for inulinase production in *Penicillium* sp. 1, *K. marxianus,* and *A. niger* van Teighem.

Optimum temperature for production of inulinase for *C. kefyr, K. fragilis,* and *Penicillium* sp. 1 are 27 to 30°C, 30 to 34°C, and 30 to 33°C, respectively. Thermophilic bacterial strains require 50°C for the purpose.

Several media are known for production of inulinase. A typical fermentation medium for *A. niger* 12 inulinase contains inulin 3 percent, corn steep liquor 2 percent, $(NH_4)H_2PO_4$ 1.2 percent, KCl 0.07 percent, $MgSO_4 \cdot 7H_2O$ 0.05 percent, $FeSO_4 \cdot 7H_2O$ 0.001 percent, and pH 4.5. In a medium containing inulin 2 percent, $(NH_4)H_2PO_4$, $NaNO_3$, $(NH_4)_2SO_4$, urea, and corn steep liquor each at 1 percent, and trace element solution ($FeSO_4 \cdot 7H_2O$ 0.1 g, $MnCl_2 \cdot 4H_2O$ 0.1 g, $ZnSO_4 \cdot 7H_2O$ 0.1 g per 100 ml) 1.5 ml percent, *A. niger* van Teighem produced 160 U/ml inulinase at pH 5.4 in 72 h, while its UV mutant produced 377 U/ml. Several strains of *Aspergillus* species, namely, *A. fischeri* and *A. nidulans,* produce as high as 1,000 to 12,000 U/l of extracellular enzyme after nine days of growth. While *A. niger* 42 yields 4,200 U/g dry cell weight, Novo Nordisk Industries have developed a commercial preparation of inulinase from *A. ficuum* useful in hydrolysis of inulin to fructose.

*Kluyveromyces marxianus* CBS 6656 produces extracellular inulinase in high cell density fed-batch cultures giving yields as high as 300,000 U/l. *Kluyveromyces fragilis* ATCC and *Candida pseudotropicalis* produce inulinase in liquid medium at 1,000 and 25,000 U/g dry cell. One of the advantages of using bacterial strains for inulinase production is the thermophilic nature of the strains. Thermophilic strains belonging to *Bacillus* species such as *B. circulans* and *B. subtilis* 430 A yield inulinase at 72 to 282 U/l. Newer strains of *Clostridium thermosuccinogenes* produce cell-bound inulinase. *Clostridium acetobutylicum* $ABK_n8$ produces enzyme with specific activity of 3.03 U/mg protein. Reports on isolation of *Staphylococcus* species and *Pseudomonas* sp. capable of producing inulinase have appeared in recent years for the first time. Production of inulinase using *Streptomyces* sp. in a medium containing inulin 1 percent, $(NH_4)_2HPO_4$ 0.4 percent, $(NH_4)H_2PO_4$ 0.8 percent, KCl 0.05 percent, $MgSO_4 \cdot 7H_2O$ 0.05 percent, $FeSO_4 \cdot 7H_2O$ 0.001 percent in a jar fermentor for 96 h has been described recently.

Although all commercial production, as well as reported work on microbial inulinases, deals with submerged fermentation (batch, fed-batch, continuous mode) as the preferred technique for fermentation, there have been attempts to use solid-state fermentation (SSF) for this purpose. Inulinase production in SSF using *K. marxianus* ATCC 52466 is reported. Wheat bran, coconut oil cake, and corn flour have been tried individually and in combination. Under optimum conditions, extracellular inulinase levels reached peak in 72 h, giving 122 U/dry fermented substrate.

Generally inulinases from fungal strains show a pH optima between 4.5 to 7.0, the yeast strains 4.4 to 6.5, and the bacterial strains 4.8 to 7.0. Fungal and bacterial inulinases show temperature optima in the mesophilic as well as thermophilic range, while yeast show optima in the mesophilic range.

All the reported values of inhibition or activation of inulinase with metal ions are with 0.001 M solution of metal ions. Thus $Fe^{+3}$ has been shown to inhibit *Aspergillus* inulinase up to 80 percent and *F. oxysporum* between 55 to 77 percent. $Cu^{+2}$ inhibits to varying levels in different organisms. In *Penicillium* sp. 1, inhibition is 10 to 60 percent, in *Aspergillus* sp. 15 to 20 percent, and in *F. oxysporum* 88 to 89 percent. $Hg^{+2}$ inhibits inulinase activity in *Aspergillus* sp. totally and up to 55 to 65 percent in *F. oxysporum*. In *Penicillium* sp., *Aspergillus niger* 12, $Mn^{+2}$ enhanced the inulinase activity.

## PURIFICATION OF INULINASES

Conventional methods of centrifugation, ultrafiltration, or salt/solvent precipitation followed by column chromatography have been used for purification of extracellular inulinases. For intracellular inulinases, a step for cell wall destruction is added before using the conventional procedures. Inulinases from *F. oxysporum* were purified by column chromatography in Sephadex G 100 with yields of 65 to 75 percent. For the enzyme from *Penicillium* sp., ammonium sulfate precipitation, ion exchange chromatography on diethylaminoethyl (DEAE) Sepharose and DEAE Sephacel, ultrafiltration, and gel filtration on Sephadex G 100 have been used. A crude inulinase preparation from *Aspergillus* sp. was dialyzed for 48 h and the lyophilized powder loaded onto a carbozymethyl (CM) Sepharose column for purification. Chromatography on DEAE cellulofine A 500 column further separation on a Q-Sepharose HP column is used for enzyme from *A. niger*. Ethanol precipitation and chromatography on Sephadex G 200 DEAE cellulose and CM cellulose purified enzyme from *K. fragilis*.

## APPLICATIONS OF INULINASES

Production of fructose syrup from inulin or inulin-rich materials is the major application area for inulinases. Fructose formation from inulin in this manner is a single-step reaction. This offers advantages compared to the conventional enzymic method converting starch to fructose via three enzymes, namely, $\alpha$-amylase, glucoamylase, and glucose isomerase. Processes have been developed for continuous production of fructose syrups from inulin using immobilized inulinase from *A. niger* and *A. ficuum* in packed-bed column reactors. Jerusalem artichoke and agave pulp have been used as sources of inulin successfully.

Continuous ethanol production from Jerusalem artichoke tubers using free as well as immobilized cells of *K. marxianus* UCD (FST) 55 to 82 strains has been achieved. *Kluveromyces* sp. has been used to produce ethanol by fermentation of Jerusalem artichoke juices. Acetone and butanol are efficiently manufactured with inulin from Jerusalem artichoke with *Clostridium acetobutylicum* under anaerobic conditions. Using inulin, single-cell proteins have been produced with *K. marxianus*. Inulinases also find application for production of inulooligosaccharides that have microphage-activating properties and lipid-removing activity. A fully enzymatic method for the determination of inulin in serum or plasma without deproteinization is described.

## SUGGESTED READINGS

Pandey A, CR Soccol, P Selvakumar, VT Soccol, N Kriegeri, and JD Fontana (1999). Recent developments in microbial inulinases: Production, properties and applications. *Applied Biochemistry and Biotechnology* 81(1):35-52.

Poorna V and PR Kulkarni (1995a). *Saussurea lappa* as a new source of inulin for fermentative production of inulinase in a laboratory stirred fermenter. *Bioresource Technology* 52:181-184.

Poorna V and PR Kulkarni (1995b). A study of inulinase production by *A. niger* van Teighem using fractional factorial design. *Bioresource Technology* 54:315-320.

Selvakumar P and A Pandey (1999). Solid state fermentation for synthesis of inulinase by *Staphylococcus* and *Kluyveromyces*. *Process Biochemistry* 34(8): 851-855.

Vandamme EJ and DG Derycke (1984). Microbial inulinases: Fermentation process, properties and applications. *Advances in Applied Microbiology* 29:139-176.

# Laccase

Jerzy Rogalski
Andrzej Leonowicz

## INTRODUCTION

Laccase (benzendiol: oxygen oxidoreductase, EC 1.10.3.2), an enzyme belonging to the group of copper-containing proteins, was first described in 1883 by Yoshida, who studied the material used to create Oriental lacquer finishing. The lacquer, used for a wide variety of purposes throughout East Asia, is commonly prepared from the sap of trees from the *Rhus* or *Melanorrhoea* genera.

### Laccase Structure

Initially, plant laccases involved in the lignin formation process are capable of oxidizing coupling monolignols to dimers and trimers, which can next be oxidized by peroxidase to higher ligomers and lignin structures. Biochemically, laccase is a glycosylated monomer or homodimer protein generally having fewer saccharide compounds (10 to 25 percent) in fungi and bacteria than in the plant enzymes. The carbohydrate compound contains monosaccharides such as hexoamines, glucose, mannose, galactose, fucose, and arabinose. Copper atoms found in laccase are classified into three types. Type 1, a blue copper site, has one copper ion, characteristic absorption features (~600 nm), and a small parallel hyperfine coupling (~40 to 90 × $10^{-4}$/cm) in the electron paramagnetic resonance (EPR) spectrum. Type 2, a mononuclear copper center, has regular spectral features (~150 to 200 × $10^{-4}$/cm) and no intense feature in the visible spectrum region. In type 3, a binuclear copper site, coppers are antiferromagnetically coupled through a bridging ligand which makes them EPR silent. This type of copper is a binary complex with absorption at 330 nm disappearing on the reduction of the active site. Type 2 and type 3 coppers form a trinuclear site within 3.8X, in which binding dioxygen and four-electron reduction to water occur. Copper of the first type can be acted upon by solvents, including water, and removed from the enzyme molecule by various complexes. Copper of the second type is easy to eliminate, which can frequently be done during purification procedures. On the other hand, type 2 copper can be reconstructed both in aerobic and anaerobic conditions.

The study of laccase derivatives showed that type 2 copper is bound to three nitrogen atoms. A water molecule is the fourth copper ligand. Type 2 copper has proven to play an important role in structural nonspecific stabilization of anionic binding in the copper 3 active site. It has also been found that type 1 copper centers that lack a liganding methionine, which is true for all fungal laccases, are relatively unstable.

In the 1990s, a novel combination of prosthetic groups was proposed for the laccase of *Phlebia radiata*. This particular laccase was shown to have about two atoms of copper per molecule; the claim is that these work in concert with a pyrroloquinoline quinone (PQQ) factor. Later it was demonstrated that the laccases isolated from solid-state fungal cultures were yellow-brown and did not have typical blue oxidase spectra, showing simultaneously atypical EPR spectra. The comparison of N-terminal amino sequences of the *Phlebia radiata, Panus tigrinus, Coriolus versicolor,* and *Phlebia tremellosus* laccases showed high homology between blue and yellow-brown laccase forms. The yellow enzyme seems to have an altered oxidation state of copper in the active center, which is probably caused by the integration of aromatic lignin-degradation products. Interestingly, evidence has been provided that yellow laccases are capable of oxidizing nonphenolic lignin models (-O-4) and veratryl alcohol directly in the presence of $O_2$ but in the absence of any diffusible mediator. Other enzymes containing copper, e.g., polyphenol oxidase (PPO), are a small group of enzymes widely distributed in all types of cells from bacteria to mammals. The most abundant PPO in animals is tyrosinase (monophenol monooxigenase, EC 1.18.14.1). This enzyme is involved in the control of melanin formation, catalyzing hydroxylation and subsequent oxidation of L-tyrosine to L-dopaquinone. A multipotential PPO showing all the activities of tyrosinase and laccase was found only in *Marinomonas mediterranea.* Ceruloplasmin is the only protein present in the serum of animals that has homology to laccases. Its function could be connected with the ferroxidase activity as well as other activities, such as preventing oxidation of serum catecholamines and copper transport. Laccase activities have been mainly detected in fungi and in the *Azospirillum lipoferum,* Aquificales, and Protobacteria bacteria, which opens the possibility that the enzyme is not restricted only to Eucaryotes.

### Fungal Laccase: Properties and Application

Fungal laccase has been detected and purified from many species of Basidiomycetes, Ascomycetes, and Deuteromycetes. The highest amounts of laccase are produced by wood-decaying Basidiomycete white-rot fungi. The fungal enzyme catalyzes the removal of an electron and a proton from phenolic hydroxyl or aromatic amino groups to form free phenoxy radicals and amino radicals, respectively. Having all four copper atoms in the 2+ oxidation state in the active site (i.e., blue oxidase), laccase not only oxidizes phenolic and methoxyphenolic acids but also decarboxylates them and attacks their methoxyl groups through demethylation or demethoxylation. These reactions may represent an important step in the initial transformation of the lignin polymer. It has also been reported that the enzyme is involved in the transformation and detoxification of reactive lignin degradation products. Laccase reacts with polyphenols and other lignin-derived aromatic compounds, which in turn can be both polymerized and depolymerized; the latter can also act as low-molecular-weight mediators.

Laccase and similar polyphenol oxidases can be used as native or immobilized biocatalyts in aqueous and organic solvents in several biotechnological processes. For example, laccase can be used as a bleaching agent in the pulp and paper industry; as a stabilizer during must and wine processing; or as a dechlorinating agent. Also, its broad specificity with respect to hydrogen donors creates interesting opportunities in the detoxification of organopollutants in soils or in the removal of phenolic and other aromatic compounds from natural and industrial wastewaters. The oxidation of phenolics generates phenoxy radicals and quinoid intermediates, which are subsequently transformed into dimers and insoluble polymers. After sedimentation such polymers may be easily removed from water. Organopollutants in soil can be oxidized to less toxic polymers by laccase immobilized in certain soil fractions. Following subsequent transformations, these emergent polymers may be incorporated in the soil humus. Laccase is also involved in various physiological processes of economic and ecological relevance. It is engaged in the development of fungal fruit bodies, pigmentation of fungal spores, pathogenicity of molds, sexual differentiation, and rhizomorph formation.

## ACTIVITY ON LIGNOCELLULOSE CONSTITUENTS

Enzymatic activities are responsible for the biodegradation of lignocellulose constituents: cellulose, hemicelluloses, and lignin. The conversion of cellulose and hemicelluloses into simple sugars has been studied for a long time. A large number of microorganisms (bacteria, fungi, protozoans) make use of a whole string of hydrolases, which are capable of producing large quantities of mono- and disaccharides from all polysaccharide components in lignocellulose. The degradation, however, is affected by the occurrence of polysaccharides in a complex with lignin, because the latter forms a barrier against the microbial attack by hydrolytic enzymes. The lignin barrier also complicates cellulose production in the pulp and paper industry. For these ecological, economic, and other reasons, research into the biotransformation of lignin has been carried out for decades. The wood tissue is penetrated by wood-rotting basidiomycete fungi, which first come into contact with easily assimilable carbohydrate constituents of the lignocellulosic complex. The white-rot group of these fungi, equipped with a versatile machinery of enzymes cooperating with certain secondary fungi metabolites, is capable of attacking the lignin barrier efficiently. These fungi use a multienzyme system comprising laccase, other wood-attacking oxidases, hydrolases, and so-called feedback-type enzymes to transform and degrade all structural elements of the lignocellulosic complex (polysaccharides and lignin; see Figure III.22).

The currently known enzymes of white-rot fungi involved in wood degradation can be divided into three groups. The first group of enzymes can attack wood constituents or their primary degradation products directly; this group includes laccase, different peroxidases, protocatechuate-3,4 dioxygenase, etc., as well as cellulase and hemicellulase complexes. The second group of enzymes, comprising, among others, aryl alcohol oxidase and glyoxal oxidase, cooperates with the first group by providing $H_2O_2$ for peroxidases, but these enzymes do not attack wood components directly. The third enzyme group represented by glucose oxidase and cellobiose: quinone oxidoreductase (cellobiose dehydrogenase) includes feedback-type enzymes which play a key role in joining metabolic chains during the biotransformation of high-molecular-mass wood constituents. All these enzymes, including laccase, can act separately or in cooperation.

### Low-Molecular-Mass Mediators

According to several publications, the molecular size of wood-attacking enzymes does not permit penetration of the undegraded plant cell wall. However, certain studies contain evidence that some of these enzymes (e.g., laccase) are capable of bleaching hardwood pulp by depolymerizing and solubilizing lignin in the presence of so-called mediator compounds. Therefore, in recent years research has been focused on such potential low-molecular-mass mediators of internal or external origin that possess sufficiently high redox potentials (>900 mV) to attack lignin and which can migrate from enzymes into the tight lignocellulose complex. 3-Hydroxyanthranilic acid (3-HAA), the first natural mediator of laccase, supporting ligninolysis in *Pycnoporus cinnabarinus,* a white-rot fungus which does not produce man-

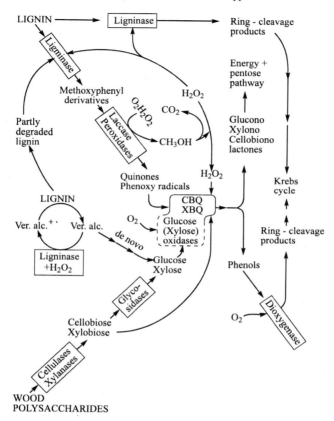

FIGURE III.22. Hypothetical scheme for degradation of lignin, cellulose, and xylan in wood. (*Source:* Adapted from Eriksson et al., 1990, and Leonowicz et al., 2001.)

ganese and lignin peroxidase, was described by Eggert in 1996. The laccase/3-HAA system mediates the oxidation of nonphenolic lignin model dimers, while laccase alone cannot act on these compounds. Consequently, it has been suggested that many low-molecular-mass compounds permeate wood cell walls and initiate decay. Examples of such substances include veratryl alcohol, oxalate, 3-hydroxyanthranilic acid, and Gt-chelators. These are produced as a result of fungal metabolism, and their secretion enables fungi to colonize and degrade the wood cell-wall structure more effectively than other organisms. Veratryl alcohol synthesis was first observed in *Phanerochaete chrysosporium;* oxalate and other organic acids were found in culture liquids of a number of wood-rotting fungi (e.g., *Armillaria mellea, Fomes annosus, Pleurotus ostreatus*) by Takao in 1965. Later their secretion was also demonstrated for solid-state fungal cultures. 3-Hydroxyanthranilic acid was isolated and identified from *Pycnoporus cinnabarinus*. A special phenolate derivative, the so-called Gt-chelator (molecular mass <1 kDa), has been isolated from the *Gloeophyllum trabeum* brown-rot fungus. Dimeric ethers possessing phenolic groups are either oxidized or cleaved by the laccase/3-HAA system. Apart from the production of veratric acid and guaiacol, the laccase/3-HAA activity on nonphenolic dimers also results in a six-electron oxidation of 3-HAA. This leads to the formation of a phenoxazinone ring containing a compound from 3-HAA, i.e., cinnabarinic acid (CA), which is a common secondary metabolite of *Pycnoporus cinnabarinus*. However, Temp and Eggert have demonstrated that in the presence of a suitable cellulose-derived electron donor, cellulose dehydrogenase (CDH) can regenerate the fungal mediator 3-HAA from cinnabarinic acid.

### Pulp Delignification

Mediators have also been used in the paper industry. The first attempt at using laccase-mediator couples for delignification in the pulp industry was the development of the Lignozym process, which was described in detail in Call's and Mucke's review in 1997. According to Bourbonnais, the delignification of kraft pulp by laccase can be supported by a number of external synthetic, low-molecular-mass dyes or other aromatic hydrogen donors. ABTS [2,2'azinobis-(3-ethylbenzenthiazoline-6-sulfonic acid)] was the first mediator shown to be effective in the delignification of kraft pulp and lignin transformation by laccase. According to Sealey, the reaction mechanism mediated by ABTS appears to proceed as follows: Oxygen activates laccase, and the mediator is oxidized by the enzyme. The oxidized mediator diffuses into pulp and oxidizes lignin, disrupting it into smaller fragments which are easily removed from the pulp by means of alkaline extraction. Additionally, superoxide dismutase (SOD) inhibits polymerization of soluble lignin by laccase and accelerates the delignification process. In 1999, Majcherczyk demonstrated the oxidation of aromatic alcohols (used as nonphenolic lignin models) by the *Trametes versicolor* laccase in the presence of ABTS. Cation radical and dication formation were proposed to be involved in this laccase mediator system.

Apart from ABTS, 1-hydroxybenzotriazole (HBT) was recently introduced as an effective laccase mediator in pulp processing. An R-NO (organic azides) radical is an active form of this mediator; it is also selective in lignin oxidation. The laccase-HBT couple can be responsible for up to 50 percent of pulp delignification. HBT is as effective in the bleaching processes as ABTS. The HBT discovery introduced a new class of mediators with N-OH as the functional group, which is oxidized to a reactive radical. Other mediators of this type described by the Bourbonnais group, such as 4-hydroxy-3-nitroso-1-naphtalenesulfonic acid (HNNS), 1-nitroso-2-naphthol-3,6-disulfonic acid (NNDS), and Remazol brilliant blue (RBB), have also been shown to promote delignification. However, they are not as efficient as HBT and ABTS.

It is necessary to mention at this point that there are differences among laccases produced by various fungi, both in the delignification degree and the recovery of residual enzyme activities. It seems that such differentiation may be a result of the varied status of copper in the activity center of particular laccases as well as different redox potentials.

Pulp delignification supports the sequential xylanase- and laccase-mediator system treatments followed by the alkaline peroxide treatment. The final pulp brightness and the reduction of viscosity after the xylanase treatment followed by two "traditional" alkaline peroxide stages were higher than those for laccase/HBT alone followed by two peroxide stages. This procedure has yielded the greatest brightness of pulp in all biochemical or traditional techniques applied so far. Nevertheless, in the case of laccase-containing systems, the darkening effect of the enzyme should be taken into consideration. It is worth mentioning that laccase alone, working in pulp under high oxygen pressure (5 Atm), resulted in pulp brightness comparable to that of the laccase-mediator systems without increased oxygen pressure. Such an experiment was conducted eight years ago, when both ABTS and other laccase mediators were not known or had just been discovered. Remazol brilliant blue R (RBBR) and carminic acid (CA) were also used as laccase mediators for bleaching pulp black liquor (kraft effluent). In the experiment conducted by Leonowicz and colleagues in 1993, CA used as a mediator caused considerably greater brightness of black liquor resultant from pulp chlorination than RBBR did. On the other hand, inducible forms of laccase of *Kuehneromyces mutabilis* and *Pleurotus ostreatus* decolorized both RBBR and CA, which can be interpreted as ligninolytic activity of the enzyme-degrading dyes. Some authors reported previously that decolorization of several polymeric dyes by basidiomycete fungi usually occurs under the conditions that favor lignin degradation, thus pointing to the interrelations of dye decolorization and ligninolysis.

In conclusion, ligninolytic enzymes, particularly laccase, frequently act by cooperating with low-molecular-weight compounds serving as redox mediators. The ideal mediator should form a high redox potential oxidation product in a highly reversible reaction.

## Feedback Interdependence

As far as the biotransformation of lignocellulose is concerned, it has been unequivocally stated that lignin degradation is accelerated in the presence of cellulose or its oligomers. The idea of a feedback-type interdependence of delignification and cellulose degradation was postulated by Westermark and Eriksson as early as 1974. They postulated that the processes of depolymerization of cellulose and lignin are interrelated in certain points and even accelerate each other. In the proposed complex system, laccase, lignin peroxidase (LiP), manganese-dependent peroxidase (MnP), and various hydrolases are secreted by fungal hyphae close to the hyphae environment, where they cooperate with one another as well as with mediating factors. Yielded chelators and mediating radicals are exported further to the wood tissue where they work as enzyme "messengers" in ligninocellulose degradation. Accordingly, it has been proposed that this feedback-type enzyme system is involved in ligninocellulose transformation with a meaningful participation of various ligninolytic enzymes.

The process of transformation of lignocellulose complex by fungal enzymes and mediators works probably as follows. Laccase oxidizes lignin-derived radicals to quinones. These can serve as the oxygen source for glucose oxidase and aryl alcohol oxidase, producing $H_2O_2$ and preventing polymerization; $H_2O_2$ formed serves as the cosubstrate for ligninolytic peroxidases (Figure III.22). The cellobiose quinone oxidoreductase/cellobiose dehydrogenase (CDH/CBQ) system requires the presence of dioxygen and hydrogen peroxide for functioning; dioxygen is supplied from the air, but external hydrogen peroxide (required at least by lignin peroxidase) is produced only in small amounts by CDH and CBQ, as suggested by the literature. Superoxide ($O_2^-$), probably yielded from quinone cycling by generating $H_2O_2$ through the oxidation of $Mn^{2+}$, is the crucial radical in $H_2O_2$ production. Simultaneously, highly reactive $Mn^{3+}$ is formed, which is known from manganese peroxidase to be an efficient lignin-attacking agent. $H_2O_2$ produced here accelerates both the production of $Mn^{3+}$ from $Mn^{2+}$ by manganese peroxidase and the oxidation of lignin and derived fragments. However, because $H_2O_2$ production by this system, which is crucial for the process, is not sufficient for all $H_2O_2$-consuming reactions, it was necessary to look for other natural systems generating enough $H_2O_2$ for the biodeterioration of the ligninocellulose complex. A number of possibilities have been considered. First, the possible involvement of certain enzymes was proven, e.g., of glyoxal oxidase, veratryl alcohol oxidase, manganese peroxidase, or glucose oxidase. Several of these enzymes can function both intracellularly and extracellularly. Other enzymes generating hydrogen peroxide, such as pyranose-2-oxidase (mentioned previously), methanol oxidase, and fatty-acyl-CoA oxidoreductase, act intracellularly only. Because wood transformation is an exclusively extracellular process, these enzymes should not be taken into consideration.

The enzymes listed in the first group are relatively stable and resistant to the conditions outside cells. Among them, only glucose oxidase can join both lignin and carbohydrate metabolic chains. This means that glucose oxidase possesses two possible functions for the acceleration of lignocellulose degradation: it produces $H_2O_2$ by glucose oxidation (required for lignin peroxidases), and it reduces quinoids and phenoxy radicals originating from the action of laccase during lignin oxidation (Figure III.22).

The other group of enzymes also reducing quinones and producing $H_2O_2$ (e.g., aryl/veratryl alcohol oxidases) has been taken into consideration, albeit to a lesser extent because their $H_2O_2$ does not result from the oxidation of glucose, which is a key metabolite in carbohydrate transformation. Consequently, it seems that only glucose oxidase cooperates with the cellulolytic system by using glucose as the substrate generated by hydrolytic enzymes from cellulose. The enzyme is produced by all white-rot fungi tested, including *Phanerochaete chrysosporium,* which also secrete laccase and/or peroxidases and show strong ligninolytic ability. The *Phanerochaete chrysosporium* mutant that was deprived of glucose oxidase by mutagenesis was not able to decompose lignin at all.

## CONCLUSIONS

In summary, laccase and other oxidases appear to be helpful in lignocellulose transformation both in nature and in paper and dye industries. Glucose oxidase is probably a feedback-type enzyme accelerating these processes. When oxygen is indispensable in the second stage of the glucose oxidase-glucose reaction, it can be supplied by radicals or quinones generated when phenolic or methoxyphenolic compounds are exposed to laccase. When excess quinones produced by laccase inhibit the enzyme, glucose oxidase counteracts the poisonous level of quinones in the medium and enables laccase and other enzymes to continue functioning.

## SUGGESTED READINGS

Alexandre G and IB Zhulin (2000). Laccases are widespread in bacteria. *TIBTECH* 18:41-42.
Call HP and I Mucke (1997). History, overview and application of mediated lignolytic systems, especially laccase-mediator-system (Lignozyme process). *Journal of Biotechnology* 53:163-202.

Eriksson, K-E, RA Blanchette, and P Ander (1990). *Microbial and enzymatic degradation of wood and wood components.* Berlin: Springer-Verlag.

Leonowicz A, N-S Cho, J Luterek, A Wilkolazka, M Wojtaś-Wasilwska, A Matuszewska, M Hofrichter, D Wesenberg, and J Rogalski (2001). Fungal laccase: Properties and activity on lignin. *Journal of Basic Microbiology* 41:185-227.

Leonowicz A, Y Matsumo, R Fuji, and A Ishizu (1993). Production of laccase with various properties and its application to pulp and paper industry. *Proceedings of 6th Paper and Pulp Symposium.* JSPPT Research Press, pp. 62-65.

Thurston CF (1994). The structure and function of fungal laccases. *Microbiology* 140:19-26.

Westermark U and K-E Eriksson (1974). Cellobiose: quinone oxidoreductase, a new wood-degrading enzyme from white-rot fungi. *Acta Chem Scand* B28: 209-214.

Woonsup S and K-Y Sung (1999). Laccases and their catalytic activities. In *Proceedings of the International Conference on New Horizons of Bioscience in the Forest Products Field,* April 21-22, 1999. Chengju, Korea: Chungbuk National University, pp. 101-111.

Yaropolov AI, OV Skorobogatko, SS Vartanov, and SD Varfolomeyev (1994). Laccase—Properties, catalytic mechanism and applicability. *Applied Biochemistry and Biotechnology* 49:257-279.

# Lignin Peroxidase

Carlos G. Dosoretz
Gary Ward
Yitzhak Hadar

## INTRODUCTION

White-rot fungi are obligate aerobes, deriving their energy and nutrient requirements from the biological combustion of wood and associated materials, using molecular oxygen ($O_2$) as the terminal electron acceptor. Lignin, which is one of the most abundant and widely distributed polymers in the biosphere, is the limiting factor in the biodegradation of cellulose and hemicellulose from wood, due to its recalcitrant chemical structure. The main mechanism of lignin degradation by these fungi involves one-electron oxidation reactions catalyzed by extracellular phenol oxidases (laccases) and peroxidases.

Lignin degrading-peroxidases are heme-containing enzymes, which require hydrogen peroxide ($H_2O_2$) as an electron acceptor to oxidize lignin and lignin-related compounds. They are monomeric, with molecular weights and isoelectric points ranging from 35 to 47 kDa and 2.8 to 5.4, respectively. Three types of lignin-degrading peroxidases have been reported in white-rot fungi: lignin peroxidase (LiP), manganese-dependent peroxidase (MnP), and, more recently, versatile peroxidase (VP). Laccases are multicopper phenol oxidases. Rather than $H_2O_2$, these enzymes utilize $O_2$ as the electron acceptor, reducing it by four electrons to $H_2O$. Laccases have a molecular weight of 50 to 300 kDa and acidic isoelectric points. In most white-rot fungi species, peroxidases and laccases are expressed as several isozymes. Both types of enzyme are glycosylated, which may increase their stability.

The ligninolytic system of white-rot fungi also includes extracellular $H_2O_2$-generating enzymes, essential for peroxidase activity. To date, a number of oxidase enzymes have been reported to be involved in the production of $H_2O_2$, including glyoxal oxidase, glucose 1-oxidase, methanol oxidase, and aryl-alcohol oxidase. LiP is perhaps the most unusual of the ligninolytic enzymes, and this chapter will focus on its production, mode of action, and potential applications.

## *LiP PROPERTIES AND PRODUCTION*

LiP from *Phanerochaete chrysosporium*, the most extensively studied white-rot fungus, possesses a higher redox potential and lower pH optimum than any other isolated peroxidase or oxidase (Table III.23). Like other peroxidases, LiP is capable of oxidizing phenols through the generation of phenoxy radicals. However, due to its exceptionally high redox potential and low pH optimum, it is able to directly oxidize nonphenolic aromatics typically not oxidized by other peroxidases, including the nonphenolic phenylpropanoid units of lignin. Stable cation-centered radicals formed during the oxidation of nonphenolic aromatic nuclei may serve as redox mediators for LiP-catalyzed oxidations, effectively extending the substrate range. The ability to form relatively stable cation radicals therefore enables LiP to oxidize a broader range of substrates than other peroxidases. Reactions catalyzed by LiP include benzyl alcohol oxidations, side-chain cleavages, ring-opening reactions, dimethoxlations, and oxidative dechlorinations. The ability of LiP to attack such a variety of linkages suggests it plays a key role in lignin degradation.

### *Catalytic Cycle*

The catalytic cycle of LiP is similar to that of other peroxidases (Figure III.23). Reaction of native ferric LiP with $H_2O_2$ yields the two-electron-oxidized intermediate, compound I (Cpd I), with a ferryl iron and a porphyrin cation radical. One-electron reduction of Cpd I with a reducing substrate yields the one-electron-oxidized ferryl intermediate, compound II (Cpd II). Finally, a one-electron reduction step by a second substrate molecule returns the enzyme to its native ferric state.

In the absence of suitable reducing substrate, or for that matter in the presence of excess $H_2O_2$ concentrations, Cpd II is further oxidized to com-

TABLE III.23. Oxidative properties of some key oxidases and peroxidases

| Enzyme | Redox potential, $E_o$ (mV)* | pH optimum |
|---|---|---|
| Plant laccase | +434 | 7.5 |
| Fungal laccase | +785 | 5.5 |
| Horseradish peroxidase (HRP) | +920 | 6.0 |
| Fungal LiP | +1100 | 2.5 |

*Source:* Adapted from Call and Mucke, 1997.
*$E_o$ is the potential versus normal hydrogen electrode.

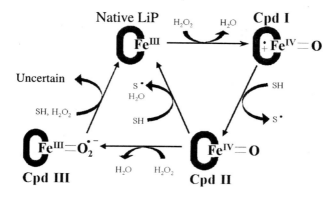

FIGURE III.23. Catalytic cycle of LiP. Cpd I, Cpd II, and Cpd III are compounds I, II, and III, respectively; SH is a reducing substrate; S· denotes an aryl radical.

pound III (Cpd III), a species with limited catalytic activity. LiP is different from other peroxidases in that it exhibits an unusually high reactivity between Cpd II and $H_2O_2$. Because Cpd III is inactivated in the presence of excess $H_2O_2$, if it is not rapidly converted to the native state, the enzyme has a "suicidal" tendency. Cpd III has been shown to readily return to the native ferric state in the presence of $H_2O_2$ and veratryl alcohol (VA). Ligninolytic cultures of *P. chrysosporium* normally produce VA, one of the proposed physiological roles of which is to convert Cpd III to the native state, thereby protecting LiP from $H_2O_2$-dependent inactivation. This is of particular significance, since during oxidation of certain chemicals such as phenols, Cpd III has been shown to accumulate, indicating that they are either poor substrates for Cpd II or they lack the ability to convert Cpd III to the native state. $H_2O_2$-dependent inactivation during LiP-catalyzed oxidation of ferulic acid (FA) was attributed to the high turnover rate ($k_{cat}$ = 41.7 s), which effectively amplified the reaction between Cpd II and $H_2O_2$, forming Cpd III. FA (or its phenoxy radical) was capable of converting Cpd III to the native state, albeit ineffectively, and the enzyme therefore underwent inactivation.

VA has also been shown to act as a charge-transfer mediator in LiP-catalyzed reactions. During the catalytic cycle of LiP, VA is oxidized to VA cation radical (VA+), which in the presence of suitable reducing substrate is reduced back to VA and ready for another LiP-catalyzed charge-transfer reaction as depicted in Figure III.24.

Low-molecular-weight redox mediators such as VA are believed to be essential for degradation of lignin, since the enzymes appear to be too large for the penetration of the cell wall or the middle lamella. The mediation mecha-

Primary substrate        Secondary substrate

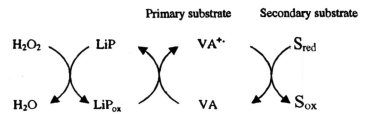

FIGURE III.24. Proposed mechanism of the veratryl alcohol-mediated oxidation of reducing substrates by LiP. (*Source:* Modified from Harvey and Thurston, in *Fungi in Bioremediation,* 2001.)

nism is believed to account for how the enzyme can oxidize substrates that it cannot directly gain access to due to size exclusion, as well as substrates that are incompatible with the active site of the enzyme. Nonphenolic aromatic compounds other than VA, such as 3,4-dimethoxycinnamic acid, 1,2-dimethoxybenzene, and 2-chloro-1,4-dimethoxybenzene, have also been shown to be capable of mediating oxidation of phenols. The mediation phenomenon appears to be driven by the difference in the oxidation potential (OP) and site-binding affinity of the mediators (possessing higher OP values and higher affinity) and the target phenolic substrates (possessing lower OP values and lower affinity).

### *Substrate Interaction Sites*

The ability of LiP to oxidize a broad range of substrates suggests that it may possess multiple binding sites. The presence of a substrate interaction site in plant peroxidases at the δ-meso carbon of the "exposed heme edge" is well established. However, the substrate access channel and heme edge of LiP is relatively inaccessible, which prompted the suggestion that the classical heme-edge site may not be the only substrate interaction site present in this enzyme. Site-directed mutagenesis has indicated that VA and probably other hydrophobic substrates are oxidized at the surface of the enzyme, with Trp 171 being implicated in catalysis by long-range electron-transfer routes. Two mutants lacking Trp 171 lost all activity toward VA yet retained substantial activity toward two dye substrates. Hydrophobic amino acid residues are located in the vicinity of Trp 171, forming a large hydrophobic surface region supporting hydrophobic interaction with lignin and other aromatic substrates. After a charge neutralization mutation in the classical heme edge of the enzyme, in which Glu 146 was substituted by Gly, LiP showed substantial activity with respect to VA and a marked (2.4 pH units) increase in

$pK_a$ for the oxidation of a negatively charged difluoro azo dye. This indicates that hydrophilic substrates are most probably oxidized at the classical heme edge of the enzyme.

Further evidence for the presence of more than one binding site has emerged from quantum structure/activity relationship (QSAR) studies. A linear relationship (semilogarithmic plot) was observed between the Michaelis-Menten constant $(K_m)$ and OP values for phenols and anilines, indicating that substrates with lower OP values have more affinity for LiP. In contrast, no correlations were observed between OP and $K_m$ values of nonphenolic dimethoxy aromatic substrates. The differential behavior observed between nonphenolic dimethoxy aromatics and phenols and anilines with respect to the QSAR may be indicative of the fact that the modes and sites of oxidation differ for both.

### Production of Wild-Type LiP

The production of ligninolytic enzymes and lignin degradation generally occurs at the onset of the secondary growth phase of white-rot fungi, when utilizable nutrients are depleted and primary fungal growth ceases. Carbon, nitrogen, and manganese are all critical nutritional variables in the production of ligninolytic enzymes by white-rot fungi. The level of $O_2$ in liquid culture has been reported to have a strong stimulating effect on the production of ligninolytic enzymes in several fungi. Liquid cultures of *P. chrysosporium* need to be concomitantly starved and exposed to a pure $O_2$ atmosphere to trigger LiP expression. Nutrient or carbon starvation is signaled by a rise in intracellular cyclic adenosine monophosphate (cAMP) concentrations. However, starving cultures without excess $O_2$ is not enough for triggering LiP synthesis, indicating that both effects need to be simultaneous. Increasing $O_2$ availability leads to an increase in the titer of LiP even when atmospheric air is supplied and balanced (nonlimiting) medium is employed. Such a high $O_2$ concentration presumably leads to increased production of reactive oxygen species (ROS) relative to that during normal metabolism, subjecting the fungus to an ROS-rich environment. A major loss in the organization of cellular ultrastructure of hyphal cells, the presence of numerous chlamydospores, and cells with impaired mitochondrial function indicate accumulation of ROS during LiP synthesis in cultures of *P. chrysosporium* grown under a pure $O_2$ atmosphere. Similar levels of LiP activity were obtained in oxygenated cultures of *P. chrysosporium* and in manganese-deficient cultures under atmospheric air. In the latter, no manganese-containing superoxide dismutase (MnSOD) activity was detected, suggesting that both cultures were saturated by the ROS. All of these findings would suggest that ROS are required to trigger LiP expression.

A multiplicity of LiP isozymes has been noted in different strains of *P. chrysosporium,* as well as in other white-rot fungi. LiP of *P. chrysosporium* has been reported to be produced in several isoforms designated as isozymes H1, H2, H6, H8, and H10, which differ slightly in their physical characteristics, substrate specificity, and stability. As part of the process leading to their secretion, LiP isozymes are proteolytically cleaved and glycosylated. In addition, the LiP isozymes H2, H6, H8, and H10 have been reported to be phosphorylated, via a mannose-6-phosphate moiety, contained in an asparagine-linked oligosaccharide. Extensive dephosphorylation of LiP-isozymes H2, H6, and H8 was noticed in nonimmersed liquid cultures of *P. chrysosporium* grown with excess nitrogen, forming the dephosphorylated isoforms H1, Ha, and Hb, respectively.

Many attempts have been made to achieve the highest possible yield of ligninolytic enzymes from *P. chrysosporium* in static, submerged, or immobilized cultures. Various inert materials have been tested for immobilizing *P. chrysosporium,* such as inclusion in gel beads; in polyurethane and porous plastic material; and on plastic disks, silicone tubes, nylon web, sintered glass, and porous ceramic carrier. Noninert materials such as corncob have also been studied.

Optimization of the culture parameters for maximal production of LiP in batch or semicontinuous operations has been widely reported. Shear forces have been reported to decrease LiP titer, and therefore, in most cases low shear configurations or devices have been employed. The most commonly used bioreactors are completely mixed ones with or without mechanical agitation, such as continuously stirred tank reactors, airlift reactors, or bubble columns. Attached-growth bioreactors such as up flow-fixed bed, rotating disk, and silicone membrane and hollow fiber reactors have also been evaluated. All configurations provide a peak of activity that decreases after several hours. The amount of enzyme obtained is also strongly dependent on the $O_2$ supply, i.e., pure $O_2$ gas or atmospheric air. In most cases, nutrient limitation enhances production efficiency since excessive fungal growth increases resistance to $O_2$ transfer rate and decreases LiP titer. The efficiency of LiP production by *P. chrysosporium* under different conditions, summarized from numerous works performed in the past fifteen to twenty years, ranges from 1 to 5 U/l per h in suspended growth system to 10 to 60 in attached growth system.

### Production of Recombinant LiP

The expression of recombinant fungal peroxidases in different hosts has been extensively studied in the past decade. Expression of LiP H8 in

*Escherichia coli* resulted in production of the inactive apoproteins in inclusion bodies, and the active enzyme was recovered after controlled refolding in vitro, albeit at low yields. LiP H2 has also been expressed in *E. coli,* and after refolding, the active recombinant enzyme had spectral characteristics and kinetic properties identical to that of native enzyme isolated from *P. chrysosporium.* However, the thermal stability of recombinant LiP H2 and LiP H8, which were expressed without glycosylation in *E. coli,* was lower than those of corresponding native peroxidases isolated from *P. chrysosporium,* indicating that glycosylation plays a crucial role in protein stability.

The baculovirus expression system has been employed in insects for producing active LiP H8 and LiP H2. However, this system suffers from low yields, and enzymes with only partial activity (60 percent for H8 and 77 percent for H2) were obtained. Because the procedure also has high production costs, it is not suitable for use on a large scale. The development of a homologous expression system for LiP H8 in *P. chrysosporium* has been reported. The constitutively expressed *P. chrysosporium* glyceraldehyde phosphate dehydrogenase *(gpd)* promoter was used to drive the expression of the recombinant genes, using nutrient-rich media in which the endogenous genes are not expressed. Despite the use of the strong promoter, production levels of the recombinant proteins remained at the same low level as normally produced by the endogenous genes under starvation conditions.

The reports on the expression of fungal peroxidases in filamentous fungi indicate that their overproduction is difficult to accomplish. The expression of the LiP gene of *Phlebia radiata* in *Trichoderma reesei,* although resulting in detectable mRNA levels, failed to produce any extracellular LiP. Also, significant *lip* transcript but weak extracellular activity was found upon expression of a LiP H8 cDNA clone in a Tunisian *Aspergillus niger* strain. More success was obtained in the expression of the *P. chrysosporium* MnP *(mnp1)* gene in *Aspergillus oryzae;* active protein was produced in the culture medium, but the levels were similar to those of the parental host. Expression of LiP H8 and MnP H4 from *P. chrysosporium* in a protease-deficient *A. niger* strain resulted in secretion of recombinant MnP into the culture medium as an active protein which showed specific activity and a spectrum profile similar to those of the native enzyme. Recombinant MnP production could be increased up to 100 mg/liter upon hemoglobin supplementation of the culture medium. On the contrary, although LiP was secreted into the extracellular medium, the protein was not active, presumably due to incorrect processing of the secreted enzyme. Expression of the *lipA* and *mnp1* genes fused to the *A. niger* glucoamylase gene did not result in improved production yields.

# MAIN APPLICATIONS OF LIGNINOLYTIC ENZYMES

Ligninolytic enzymes, like other peroxidases and oxidases, have been considered for many useful applications. Some of the most studied applications are listed as follows.

## Biopulping

One of the most obvious applications of white-rot fungi and their oxidative enzymes is biobleaching and biopulping in the pulp and paper industry to replace environmentally unfriendly chemicals (e.g., chlorine), to save on mechanical pulping energy costs, and to improve the quality of pulp and the properties of paper. The ligninolytic enzymes of white-rot fungi selectively remove or alter lignin and allow cellulose fibers to be obtained. Recent data suggest that biopulping has the potential to be an environmentally and economically feasible alternative to current pulping methods.

## Decolorization of Dyes in Textile Industry Wastewater

One of the most-studied applications of ligninolytic enzymes is in the treatment of dyes and dyestuffs, which find use in a wide range of industries but are of primary importance to textile manufacturing. Over 100,000 commercial dyes are available to textile industries which consume vast quantities of water and chemicals during processing, ultimately producing dye containing effluent which consists of complex, synthetic, and often recalcitrant compounds. Dyes are designed to be resistant to light, water, and oxidizing agents and are therefore difficult to degrade once released into aquatic systems. Many azo dyes, constituting the largest dye group, are decomposed into potential carcinogenic amines under anaerobic conditions after discharge into the environment. The ability of LiP, MnP, VP, and laccase to degrade and decolorize a wide range of synthetic dyes has been demonstrated and warrants their potential use in treating textile wastewater.

## Polymerization of Toxic Aromatic Compounds

The polymerization of aromatic compounds in the presence of peroxidases and oxidases has been the focus of much attention due to its potential use for the decontamination of wastewater. The main target contaminants of such a process would be phenols and anilines, which both polymerize readily upon oxidation. Phenols are a major class of pollutants found in various industrial wastewaters, e.g., petroleum refinery, resin manufacture, flame retardant, and coal processing. They are oxidized to generate phenoxyl radicals, which couple to form oligomeric and polymeric products. The polymeric products formed have limited water solubility and tend to precipitate quite readily. The increase in molecular weight and precipitation of the products is thought to be accompanied by a detoxification effect and presents a possible alternative for the treatment of industrial wastewater when conventional methods are ineffective.

## SUGGESTED REFERENCES

Call, HP and I Mucke (1997). History, overview and applications of mediated lignolytic systems, especially laccase-mediator-systems [Lignozym(R)-process]. *Journal of Biotechnology* 53(2-3):163-202.

Dunford, HB (1999). *Heme peroxidases.* New York: John Wiley and Sons, Inc.

Gadd, GM (2001). *Fungi in bioremediation.* Cambridge, UK: British Mycological Society, Cambridge University Press.

Harvey PJ and CF Thurston (2001). The biochemistry of ligninolytic fungi. In *Fungi in Bioremediation,* GM Gadd (ed.). Cambridge, UK: Cambridge University Press, pp. 27-52.

Kirk, TK and D Cullen (1998). Enzymology and molecular genetics of wood degradation by white-rot fungi. In *Environmentally friendly technologies for the pulp and paper industry,* AR Young and M Akhtar (eds.). New York: John Wiley and Sons, Inc., pp. 273-307.

Martinez, AT (2002). Molecular biology and structure-function of lignin degrading heme peroxidases. *Enzyme and Microbial Technology* 30:425-444.

Reddy, CA and TM D'Souza (1994). Physiology and molecular biology of the lignin peroxidases of *Phanerochaete chrysosporium. FEMS Microbiology Reviews* 13(2-3):137-152.

Tien, M and TK Kirk (1988). Lignin peroxidase of *Phanerochaete chrysosporium. Methods in Enzymology* 161:238-249.

# Lipases

Ali Kademi
Danielle Leblanc
Alain Houde

## INTRODUCTION

Lipases (triacylglycerol acylhydrolase, EC 3.1.1.3) are part of the family of hydrolases that act on carboxylic ester bonds. Their physiological role is to hydrolyze triglycerides to diglycerides, monoglycerides, fatty acids, and glycerol. These enzymes are found widely throughout the animal and plant kingdom, as well as in molds and bacteria. Another enzyme, esterase, can also hydrolyze carboxylic esters. However, esterase activity and lipase activity differ fundamentally in their ability or inability to be activated by an interface. Esterase activity increases as a function of substrate concentration according to Michaelis-Menten kinetics, and the maximum reaction rate is achieved before the solution is saturated by substrate. Formation of a substrate/water emulsion has no effect on the rate of reaction. On the contrary, lipases show almost no activity on a given substrate as long as it is in a monomeric state. However, once the substrate solubility limit is exceeded, activity increases significantly with the same substrate in an emulsified state. Lipase activity therefore depends on the presence of an interface, a phenomenon known as interfacial activation. A number of years elapsed before the molecular bases of interfacial catalysis were established.

Resolution by X-ray diffraction of the three-dimensional structure of the lipase from the fungus *Rhizomucor miehei,* revealed the presence of an amphiphilic α-helical structure on the surface of the protein, which was called the lid, covering the active site. The hydrophobic side of the helix is turned toward the inside of the active site, which is therefore inaccessible to the substrate molecules. However, when a lipase is bound to a lipid interface, a conformational rearrangement takes place causing the lid to move away, whereby the lipase active site becomes fully accessible. As a result, the hydrophobic side of the lid becomes exposed to the lipid phase, enhancing hydrophobic interactions between the enzyme and the lipid surface.

Other three-dimensional lipase structures have subsequently been described and the presence of a lid corroborated, but the number and position of the α-helices involved in the composition of the lid differ among lipases. However, some lipases do not show activation in the presence of emulsified substrates; instead, their activity continuously increases, indicating these enzymes are able to degrade both emulsion and monomeric substrates, whereas true esterases degrade only monomeric substrates. For this reason, a lipase can be defined not only according to its interfacial activation behavior, but also by its capability to hydrolyze emulsions of long-chain acylglycerides.

## KINETIC MODEL OF LIPOLYSIS

Lipase kinetics at an interface cannot be described by the classical Michaelis-Menten model, which applies only in the case of homogeneous catalysis, i.e., in which the enzyme and substrate are soluble. Therefore, a simple model has been proposed to describe lipase activity at an interface. This model consists of two successive equilibria. The first one describes the physical adsorption of the enzyme at the interface, and the second describes the formation of the E*S complex involving the adsorbed lipase (E*) and a lipid molecule present at the interface. The latter equilibrium is equivalent to the Michaelis-Menten equilibrium for the enzyme-substrate complex. Once the E*S complex is formed, the catalytic steps take place, ending with the release of the products and the regeneration of the enzyme. This model takes into account the basic fact that the concentration of substrate in the vicinity of the lipase adsorbed at the interface is not the volumetric concentration established in the environment, but rather the concentration at the surface (expressed in moles per unit of surface area). In this model, the regenerated lipase remains adsorbed at the interface and is liberated only after several catalytic cycles.

## REACTION MECHANISM

The reaction mechanism for lipases is common to all members of the "serine hydrolase" family. The active site of these enzymes is formed by a catalytic triad consisting of the amino acids serine, histidine, and aspartic (or glutamic) acid. The various steps involved in this mechanism were established using α-chymotrypsin as a model, which hydrolyzes the peptide bonds of soluble proteins. The initial step consists of the formation of an enzyme-substrate complex in which the region of the molecule that will be hydrolyzed is stabilized in the catalytic cavity by several hydrogen bonds (Figure III.25). The reaction is then initiated by the nucleophilic attack by the

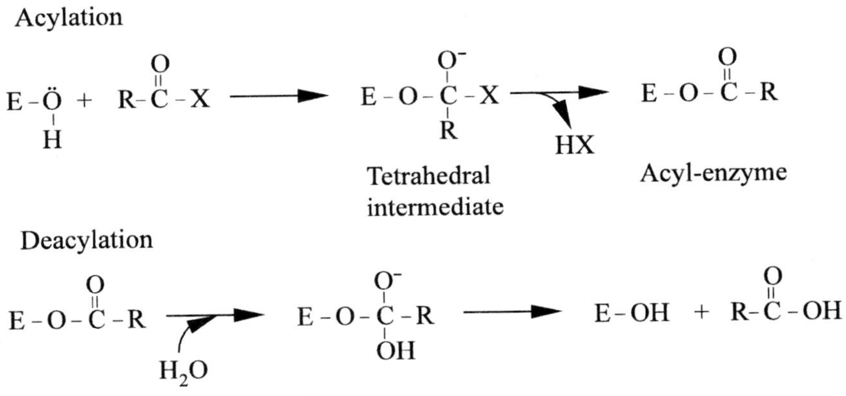

Acylation

$$E-\overset{|}{\underset{H}{\ddot{O}}} + R-\overset{O}{\overset{\|}{C}}-X \longrightarrow E-O-\overset{O^-}{\underset{R}{\overset{|}{C}}}-X \rightarrow E-O-\overset{O}{\overset{\|}{C}}-R$$

Tetrahedral          HX          Acyl-enzyme
intermediate

Deacylation

$$E-O-\overset{O}{\overset{\|}{C}}-R \rightarrow E-O-\overset{O^-}{\underset{OH}{\overset{|}{C}}}-R \longrightarrow E-OH + R-\overset{O}{\overset{\|}{C}}-OH$$

$H_2O$

FIGURE III.25. Reaction mechanism of serine hydrolyses

hydroxyl group of the serine on the carbonyl carbon atom of the ester bond, resulting in the formation of a covalent tetrahedral intermediate. Stabilization of this transition state is reinforced by two hydrogen bonds on the negatively charged oxygen (or oxyanion) carried by the substrate. A proton is then transferred from the serine side-chain to the group that is then liberated as the first product (alcohol) of the reaction. The covalent complex involving the enzyme and the remaining substrate is called the acyl-enzyme covalent complex. The acylation, i.e., formation of the acyl-enzyme, is then followed by deacylation reactions which lead to the release of a second product (fatty acid) and the regeneration of the native enzyme. The deacylation involves an analogous process to the acylation. A water molecule acts as the nucleophile and attacks the carbonyl group of the acyl-enzyme. A second tetrahedral intermediate is formed and then cleaved to release the enzyme-product complex, which is later separated by simple dissociation. The carboxylic acid and histidine residues of the triad become involved in a charge-relay system, making the hydroxyl group of the serine a strong nucleophile and therefore a highly reactive catalyst. Both serine and carboxylic acid residues are linked to the histidine by hydrogen bonds.

## *PRODUCTION OF MICROBIAL LIPASES*

Lipids are insoluble in water and must be hydrolyzed in the extracellular environment to more polar compounds, which are then readily absorbed by cells as nutrients. As a result, microbial lipases are usually extracellular. A very broad variety of culture conditions that stimulate or suppress the production of microbial lipases are described in the literature, and there is no overall procedure for improved enzyme production. A mineral culture medium can be used with an organic nitrogen source such as urea, or an inorganic nitrogen source such as ammonium sulfate. Also, a rich medium containing peptone, tryptone, or yeast extract can be used. Although the presence of lipids in the culture medium is essential to the production of lipases, the type of lipid used may vary widely. Often olive oil or long-chain fatty acid triglycerides are used as carbon sources and as a means of inducing the production of microbial lipases. In certain cases, they have an inhibiting effect on the production instead. Other vegetable oils, including palm, sesame, coconut, and sunflower oil, are less costly than olive oil and also have a positive effect on enzyme production. Finally, using gum arabic to emulsify a culture medium containing oil can enhance enzyme production by improving the availability of the substrate. The same effect is observed with Tween 80, Triton X-100, bile salts, and glycerol.

Various sugars, including fructose, maltose, and glucose, can have a stimulating effect on enzymatic production. However, in certain cases, glucose causes catabolic repression on enzyme production. Aeration has a highly variable effect on the production of lipases. Certain microorganisms produce great amounts of lipases when the culture medium is gently aerated, while significant aeration is required for other microorganisms. Oxygen concentration is often used as a criterion for determining whether a fermentation is oxygen dependent or oxygen independent. However, it is the oxygen transfer rate that appears to be critical to the production of lipases.

Various operational strategies are used in the production of microbial lipases: submerged fermentation (SmF) in batch, in fed-batch, or in continuous culture. In the past ten years, considerable interest in the use of solid-state fermentation (SSF) for the production of microbial lipases has appeared. In this process, agroindustrial wastes (wheat bran, rice bran, etc.) are mixed with oils and used as solid substrates for the production of lipases. In most cases, the oleaginous plant residues (e.g., olive oil cake, coconut oil cake, palm oil cake) remaining after oil extraction contain a significant amount of fat and are used directly as solid substrates. Lipase yields in the SSF process often exceed those obtained in SmF systems, and SSF is therefore an excellent option for the industrial production of microbial enzymes. Moreover, the residues used are inexpensive, and the enzymes are recovered in concentrated form at the end of fermentation, thereby reducing the cost of effluent treatment.

## INDUSTRIAL APPLICATIONS OF LIPASES

The industrial use of enzymes in food processing began thousands years ago with bread making, alcohol, and cheese production. An understanding of the catalytic cycles of various enzymes has led to their wide use in a range of biotechnological applications.

### Enzymes As Biocatalysts

Once the mechanisms governing enzymatic catalysis were understood, the advantages of using enzymes as biocatalysts in chemical processes became obvious. Enzyme-catalyzed reactions proceed $10^8$ to $10^{10}$ times faster than equivalent nonenzymatic reactions. As a result, although certain enzymes are still costly, the overall efficiency of enzymatic processes may surpass that of conventional processes. Moreover, the fact that, once immobilized, enzymes can be reused also helps lower costs. Enzymes act at mild conditions of pH (5 to 8) and temperature (between 20°C and 40°C), an advantage that significantly reduces the risk of secondary reactions such as decomposition, isomerization, racemization, and rearrangement. Finally, unlike heavy metals, biocatalysts are biodegradable. Enzymes exhibit great specificity in terms of the type of reaction they catalyze but are also capable of accepting a broad range of substrates, including nonnatural ones. Almost all organic reactions have equivalent enzymatic processes.

Other advantages, such as regioselectivity and enantioselectivity, confirm the supremacy of enzymes. Because of their regioselectivity, the complex three-dimensional structure of enzymes enables them to distinguish among functional chemical groups located in different regions of the same substrate molecule. In the case of lipases, such regioselectivity leads to the preferential hydrolysis of ester bonds in outer positions (1,3-specificity) or in an intermediate position (2-specificity) in the structure of triglycerides. However, 2-specificity is rarely observed.

Almost all enzymes are synthesized from L-amino acids and are therefore chiral catalysts. As a result, any type of chirality present in a substrate molecule is recognized once the enzyme-substrate complex is formed. This means that a prochiral substrate (potential to become chiral under the action of an enzyme) may be transformed into an optically pure product, and two enantiomers of a racemic mixture may react at different rates, leading to a kinetic resolution.

Of all known enzymes, lipases have attracted the most scientific attention. Because they are hydrolases, lipases do not require a cofactor during catalysis. Also, in addition to their natural function of hydrolyzing carboxylic ester bonds, lipases catalyze the esterification reaction that leads to an ester synthesis from a fatty acid and an alcohol in a nonaqueous environment (Figure III.26). A third type of catalyzed reaction involves the transfer of an acyl group between two esters (interesterification), between an ester and an acid (acidolysis), between an ester and an alcohol (alcoholysis), or between an ester and an amine (aminolysis).

Lipases can therefore synthesize an entire range of interesting molecules, and lipase has become the enzyme of choice for organic chemists, biotechnologists, microbiologists, and enzymologists. Potential applications for lipases exist in the pharmaceutical, leather, detergent, oil, and agri-food industries. The main biotechnological applications of lipases are summarized in Table III.24.

## Applications of Lipases

### Lipases in the Pharmaceutical Industry

The enantioselectivity of lipases has contributed much to the renewal of interest in these enzymes. Their main application in the pharmaceutical industry involves the use of lipases in the resolution of racemic mixtures, an area in which chemical catalysis encounters enormous constraints in terms of the completion of certain multistep reactions.

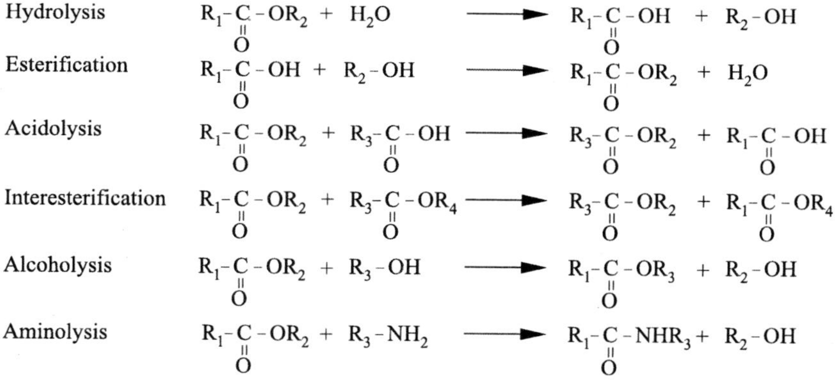

Hydrolysis

$$R_1\text{-}\underset{O}{C}\text{-}OR_2 + H_2O \longrightarrow R_1\text{-}\underset{O}{C}\text{-}OH + R_2\text{-}OH$$

Esterification

$$R_1\text{-}\underset{O}{C}\text{-}OH + R_2\text{-}OH \longrightarrow R_1\text{-}\underset{O}{C}\text{-}OR_2 + H_2O$$

Acidolysis

$$R_1\text{-}\underset{O}{C}\text{-}OR_2 + R_3\text{-}\underset{O}{C}\text{-}OH \longrightarrow R_3\text{-}\underset{O}{C}\text{-}OR_2 + R_1\text{-}\underset{O}{C}\text{-}OH$$

Interesterification

$$R_1\text{-}\underset{O}{C}\text{-}OR_2 + R_3\text{-}\underset{O}{C}\text{-}OR_4 \longrightarrow R_3\text{-}\underset{O}{C}\text{-}OR_2 + R_1\text{-}\underset{O}{C}\text{-}OR_4$$

Alcoholysis

$$R_1\text{-}\underset{O}{C}\text{-}OR_2 + R_3\text{-}OH \longrightarrow R_1\text{-}\underset{O}{C}\text{-}OR_3 + R_2\text{-}OH$$

Aminolysis

$$R_1\text{-}\underset{O}{C}\text{-}OR_2 + R_3\text{-}NH_2 \longrightarrow R_1\text{-}\underset{O}{C}\text{-}NHR_3 + R_2\text{-}OH$$

FIGURE III.26. Various reactions catalyzed by lipases

TABLE III.24. Important areas of industrial application of microbial lipases

| Industry | Application | Product |
|---|---|---|
| Dairy | Hydrolysis of milk fat | Flavoring agents for dairy products |
| Oil processing | Hydrolysis of oils and fats<br>Reagents for lipid analysis | Fatty acids, diglycerides, and monoglycerides |
| Leather | Removal of subcutaneous fat | Leather products |
| Cosmetics and perfume | Esterification | Surfactants and aroma |
| Detergents | Removal of oil stains | Detergents for laundry and household uses |
| Medical and fine chemistry | Blood triglyceride assay | Diagnostic kits |
| | Resolution of racemic mixtures | Chiral intermediates for drug production |
| | Esterification | Esters |

Optically pure enantiomers are increasingly used in the production of pharmaceuticals and in agrochemistry because they are more active and their side effects are milder than those of racemic mixtures. Moreover, biological activity is often associated with a single enantiomer, and the undesired enantiomer is considered to be an impurity.

*Resolution of racemic carboxylic acids.* Ibuprofen, 2-(4-isobutylphenyl) propionic acid, is an important member of the family of nonsteroidal anti-inflammatory drugs. Ibuprofen is a racemic carboxylic acid and one of the most studied racemates. It contains both the S-(+) and R-(−) enantiomers, but the S-(+) enantiomer is primarily responsible for its anti-inflammatory activity. The resolution of the mixture is achieved by a lipase-catalyzed esterification reaction. The ibuprofen is esterified with a methanol- or *n*-butanol alcohol in organic media. Due to the enantioselectivity of the lipase used, only the S-(+) ibuprofen enantiomer is esterified to form the S-ester. Following a complete separation between the S-ester formed and the remaining R-(−)-ibuprofen, the S-ester is chemically hydrolyzed to obtain the S-(+) ibuprofen enantiomer. Optically pure ibuprofen can also be obtained through a lipase catalyzed enantioselective hydrolysis of its chemically synthesized ester.

*Resolution of racemic alcohols and amines.* Whereas in hydrolysis the nucleophile is water, in a transesterification reaction it is replaced by other nucleophiles such as alcohols. In the case of racemic alcohols, use of lipases may allow only one enantiomer to be acylated, thereby leading to enantioselective transformations. Acyl-group donors may be vinyl esters, anhydrides, or diketenes. The reaction is irreversible, and the separation of the remaining alcohol and the newly formed ester is simple to achieve. This principle is now routinely used in many reactions by the German company BASF to produce optically pure alcohols. Amines may also be used as nucleophiles, and racemic amines are resolved using ethylmethoxyacetate as an acyl-group donor, a process that has also been used by BASF since 1993. Its products, the R-amide and the S-amine, can be recovered and separated by distillation and have high chemical and optical purities. This process is applicable to a broad spectrum of amines, which are of considerable interest as auxiliaries for the synthesis of bioactive ingredients.

*Resolution of racemic esters.* Naproxen, 2-(6-methoxy-2-naphthyl) propionic acid, is a nonsteroidal anti-inflammatory belonging to the family of 2-aryl propionic acid derivatives. This ester is widely used as a drug for human connective tissue diseases such as arthritis. The S-form of naproxen is 28 times more physiologically active than the R-form. For this reason, only the S-form is used as a drug for humans. The S-form can be produced by hydrolysis of the racemic ester in an aqueous-organic biphase system or by esterification of the corresponding racemic fatty acid with an alcohol (trimethylsilyl methanol).

## Lipases in the Detergent Industry

The use of lipases in washing preparations remains the only significant industrial application of enzymes. Initially, the fine-chemical industry used ground porcine or bovine pancreas, rich in lipases, as detergent additives. In 1988, following screening programs backed by genetic engineering techniques, the Novo Nordisk company introduced the first commercial recombinant lipase developed for the detergent industry: Lipolase, a *Humicola* lipase expressed in *Aspergillus oryzae*. Lipolase is effective in alkaline conditions (up to a pH of 12) and active over a broad range of temperatures. Lipolase can remove fat stains caused by such sources as lipstick, butter, cooking oil, sauces, etc. Lipolase is now added to a significant number of major brands of washing preparations throughout the world. The company later launched two other variants of Lipolase: Lipolase Ultra and LipoPrime. Lipolase Ultra is more effective than Lipolase at low wash temperatures, while LipoPrime gives, after one wash cycle, the same effect as with Lipolase after three washes in certain types of detergent.

## Lipases in the Dairy Industry

Lipases are routinely used in the dairy industry to intensify the flavor of cheeses, to accelerate cheese maturation, and to carry out lipolysis of butter and cream. Milk fat contains a variety of lipids, over 98 percent of which are triglycerides. Other lipids include mono- and diglycerides, phospholipids (lecithin), fatty acids (in small quantities), and sterols (cholesterol). In cheese processes, triglycerides are hydrolyzed to liberate fatty acids. Short-chain fatty acids (C4 and C6) develop a sharp taste, while the release of fatty acids consisting of medium-length carbon chains (C12 and C14) impart a soapy taste to the product. Every type of cheese has a distinctive fatty-acid profile. Fatty acids can also undergo simple chemical reactions leading to the synthesis of other flavor compounds such as acetoacetate, β-keto acids, methyl ketones, flavor esters, and lactones. Hydrolysis of fats in cheese can be achieved by commercial lipases added in powder form or by the natural lipases present in unpasteurized milk. In certain varieties of cheese, fat degradation can be achieved by lipases produced by molds such as *Penicillium roqueforti, P. camemberti,* or by certain lactic acid bacteria.

## CONCLUSIONS

Lipases have important industrial applications in several sectors. However, factors such as their high production cost mean that they are still used only on a limited basis. Nevertheless, because of recent advances in molecular biology, it should soon be possible to obtain lipases that are not only more effective and more specific but also less expensive.

## SUGGESTED READINGS

Harboe MK (1994). Use of lipases in cheese making. *Bulletin of the International Dairy Federation* 294:11-16.

Jaeger KE, S Ransac, BW Dijkstra, C Colson, M Van Heuvel, and O Misset (1994). Bacterial lipases. *FEMS Microbiology Review* 15:29-63.

Saxena RK, PK Ghosh, R Gupta, WS Davidson, S Bradoo, and R Gulati (1999). Microbial lipases: Potential biocatalysts for the future industry. *Current Science* 77:101-115.

Schmid A, JS Dordick, B Hauer, A Kiener, M Wubbolts, and B Witholt (2001). Industrial biocatalysis today and tomorrow. *Nature* 409:258-268.

# Pectinases

Cristóbal Noe Aguilar
Juan Carlos Contreras-Esquivel
Ernesto Favela-Torres

## *INTRODUCTION*

Pectinases are a group of hydrolytic enzymes, called pectolytic enzymes, that play an important role in food processing industries and alcoholic beverage industries. They are employed as processing aids in textiles, pulp and paper, animal feeding, detergents, and in the treatment of wastewaters. Pectinases also find application as analytic tools in phytochemistry, in particular to elucidate the structure of the cellular wall of vegetables. Pectolytic enzymes degrade pectin and reduce the viscosity of solutions so that they can be handled easily. In 1995, the industrial value of sales of pectinases was around $75 million, covering 10 percent of global industrial enzymes, and this figure is expected to increase drastically, to almost $2 billion by 2005.

Pectinases are a complex system of proteins, which include hydrolases, lyases, and oxidases, that play important roles in the degradation or modification of pectic substance, their natural substrate that occurs as structural polysaccharide in the middle lamella and primary cell wall of young plant cells. These enzymes are found in higher plants and are also produced by filamentous fungi, bacteria, and some yeast and insects. In general, pectinases are extracellular metabolites, but they could be intracellular as well, being responsible for the metabolism of degradation products generated by the action of extracellular pectinases. A great deal of work has been done about the enzymes involved in the biosynthesis of pectin. These enzymes include the transferases, which eject bindings among monomeric units and substitute the final product. Study of pectinases is closely related to the advancement and improvement of analytic methods used to elucidate complex structures of carbohydrates.

## SUBSTRATES OF PECTINASES

Natural substrates of pectinases are the pectic polysaccharides, localized mainly in the matrix of cell walls of higher plants, where they control the porosity and passive diffusion of several solutes and participate in the regulation of elongation and abscission processes. Their chemical structure is the backbone of galacturonic acid residues linked by $\alpha(1\text{-}4)$ linkages. The side chains of the pectin consist of L-rhamnose, L-arabinose, L-galactose, and L-xylose. Several compounds are identified in a pectin chain: homogalacturonans (HG), rhamnogalacturonans (RG), xylogalacturonans (XG), and apiogalacturonans (AG). Carboxyl groups of galacturonic acid are partially esterified by methyl groups and partially or completely neutralized by sodium, potassium, or ammonium ions. Study of pectic polysaccharides has importance in plant physiology, phytopathology (defense mechanisms), food sciences (in connection with textural changes during ripening and fruit and vegetable processing), nutrition (role of pectin as a dietetic fiber), and pharmaceutical and industrial technology (by their use as an antidiarrheic, as tablet and biodegradable films, and as a copolymer of polyurethane). Historically, pectic polysaccharides have been considered to be those acid compounds in plant tissues that can be extracted with hot water, acid or ammonium oxalate, and other binding chemicals. Based on the type of modifications of the backbone chain, pectic polysaccharides are classified into protopectin (parent pectic substance that upon restricted hydrolysis yields pectin or pectinic acid), pectic acid (galacturonans that contain negligible amounts of methoxyl groups and precursors of pectates), pectinic acid (galacturonans with various amounts of methoxyl groups and precursors of pectinates), and pectin (generic name of the mixture of widely differing compositions containing pectic acid as the major component).

## CLASSIFICATION OF PECTINASES

Until recently, pectinases were described solely as those enzymes that acted on HG chains. Recently, however, several enzymes that act on RG chains have been discovered. Pectinases can be divided into depolymerizing and deesterfying enzymes following some criteria such as rupture type of glucoside linkages, reaction mechanisms (exo- or endo-types), and esterification degree. Table III.25 shows a general classification of pectinases according to the International Commission of Enzymes.

On the other hand, deesterifying enzymes are classified according to type of ester group (methyl, acetyl, or feruloyl ester). Other pectinases are the oxidases (i.e., galacturonic acid oxidase) and those responsible for the

TABLE III.25. Modern classification of pectin-degrading enzymes

| Enzyme (common name) | | EC Code | Glicosyl-hydrolase family | Main products or action mode |
|---|---|---|---|---|
| Hydrolases | | | | |
| Esterases | pectin methylesterase | 3.1.1.11 | 8 | low methoxyl HG + methanol |
| | pectin acetylesterase | 3.1.1.6 | | HG deacetylated + acetic acid |
| | rhamnogalacturonan acetylesterase | | 12 | RG deacetylated + acetic acid |
| | feruloyl esterase | | | RG + ferulic acid |
| Glycosydases | endo-polygalacturonase | 3.2.1.15 | | oligogalacturonates + galacturonic acid |
| | exo-polygalacturonase | 3.2.1.67 | | galacturonic acid, digalacturonate |
| | rhamnogalacturonan hydrolase | | | random hydrolysis of linkages between galacturonic acid and rhamnose on RG |
| | rhamnogalacturonan-galacturonic hydrolase | | | release end-galacturonic acid linked to rhamnose on RG (exo-hydrolysis) |
| | rhamnogalacturonan ramnohydrolase | | | release end-rhamnose linked to galacturonic acid on RG (exo-hydrolysis) |
| | xylogalacturonan hydrolase | | | release xylose from XG |
| | endo-galactanase | | 53 | random hydrolysis of galactans |
| | α-galactosidase | 3.2.1.22 | 27, 36 | remove residues of galactose |
| | β-galactosidase | 3.2.1.23 | 35 | remove residues of galactose |
| | endo-arabinase | | | random hydrolysis of arabans |
| | α-L-arabinofuranosidase | | 51, 54 | remove residues of arabinose |
| Lyases | | | | |
| | pectin lyase | 4.2.2.10 | | unsaturated methyl-oligo-galacturonates |
| | pectate lyase | 4.2.2.2 | | unsaturated oligogalacturonates |
| | rhamnogalacturonan lyase | | | random hydrolysis of RG |
| Oxidases | | | | |
| | galacturonic oxidase | | | oxidation of galacturonic acid |

metabolism of degradation products of pectin. Such classification refers to the mode of action of pectinases on water-soluble substrates. Some authors have described an additional class of pectinases, taking into account their action on water-insoluble substrates; they are called protopectinases (PPases), which are defined as enzymes degrading protopectin, giving as products water-soluble pectins of high molecular weight. However, after characterization of several PPases, it was determined that their action mechanism was similar to that described for hydrolytic and transeliminative pectinases, specific to HG and RG regions. Moreover, it was demonstrated that the gene codifying PPase from *Trichosporum penicillatum* showed a consistent homology with classical polygalacturonases. Hence, PPases should not be considered an additional group of the pectic enzyme classification. An important step in glycosylase classification has been their division into 28 families considering their similarities in sequence. Figure III.27 shows a scheme of reaction involved during the action of homogalacturonan-degrading enzymes on pectin.

## *ACTION OF PECTINASES*

Polygalacturonases (PGases) act on HG and can be divided in three groups: endo-PGases, exo-PGases type I, and exo-PGases type II. The first group hydrolyzes $\alpha$-(1-4)-glycosydic bonds on polysaccharide chains releasing oligomers of galacturonic acid. The second group [galacturonan $\alpha$-(1-4)-galacturonosidase] hydrolyzes residues of D-galacturonic acid from nonreducing ends, and the third group (exo-Poly-$\alpha$-galacturonosidase) releases digalacturonate from nonreducing ends of polygalacturonic acid.

Lyases degrade HG or RG through a transeliminative mechanism, introducing a double bond between C4 and C5 in the nonreducing ends generated during the reaction. HG lyases are of two types, those acting on pectins with a low esterification degree (pectate lyases), and those with a high esterification degree (pectin lyases). Exo-pectate-lyases and oligogalacturonate lyases require $Ca^{++}$ during their action on reducing ends of pectin. Enzymes involved in the hydrolysis of branches of pectins and hemicellulose are generally called accessory enzymes (Figure III.28). These include (1) $\alpha$-L-arabinofuranosidases and arabinoxylan arabonifuranhydrolases that act on pectins and hemicellulose, (2) endo-arabinases that hydrolyze araban bonds, (3) $\alpha$- and $\beta$-galactosidases that act on galactans, (4) endo- and exo-galactanases, which remove the branches of arabinogalactans, and (5) feruloyl, and *p*-coumaryl esterases that release feruloyl and coumaryl residues. Due to their property to act on xylan and pectin and other polysaccharides, such as lignin and cellulose, these enzymes have an important role in the structural integrity of cell walls. They also enhance the degradative action of those enzymes, which attach to the structural base of the cell wall, generating finally the group of products that microorganisms need to transport and metabolize.

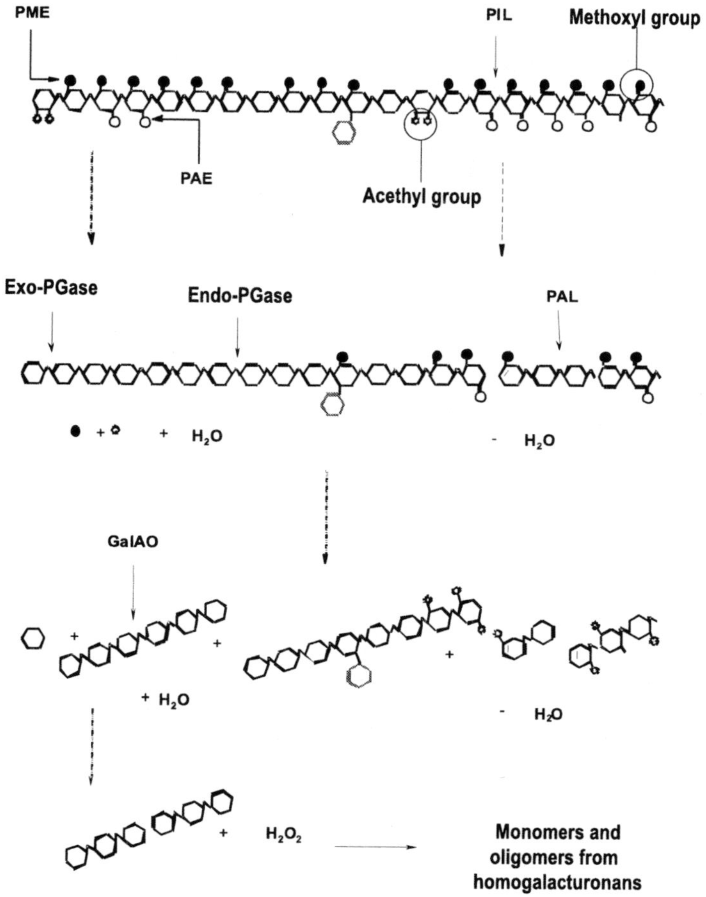

FIGURE III.27. Homogalacturonan-degrading enzymes. PME = pectin-methyl-esterase; PAE = pectin-acetylesterase; PIL = pectin-lyase; PGase = polygalac-turonase; PAL = pectate-lyase; Xgase = xylogalacturonase; GalAO = galacturonic-oxidase.

## PRODUCTION OF PECTINASES

Pectinases can be obtained from different sources such as higher plants (especially fruits and leaves), microorganisms, and insects. The main source for industrial production is *Aspergillus niger,* which produces different pectic enzymes in response to culture conditions. Molecular biology techniques

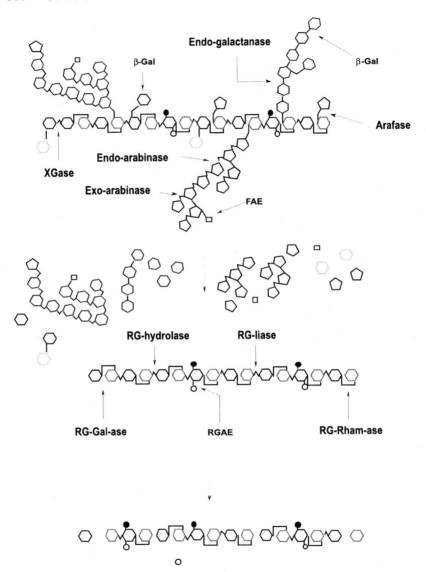

FIGURE III.28. Rhamnogalacturonan-degrading enzymes. Arafase = arabino-furanosidase; XG = xylogalacturonase; β-Gal = β-galactosidase; RGAE = RG-acetylesterase; RG-Gal-ase = RG-galacturona-hydrolase; RG-Rham-ase = RG-rhamnose-hydrolase.

are used to clone the corresponding genes, and the expression of these enzymes can take place in equivalent concentrations to mg/l or g/l of enzymatic protein. Simultaneously, the production process with recombinant strains allows for obtaining a pure product. Thus, according to industrial demand, better mixtures of enzymes can be formulated and tailor-made. This strategy is used in the food industry.

## *APPLICATIONS OF PECTINASES*

Pectinases have been applied in the food and beverage industry for more than 60 years. Depending on the fruit source and final product, pectinases may be added to increase yield, lower viscosity, increase clarity, and facilitate filtration and concentration. The most traditional application of pectinases is in the clarification of juices. In some cases, the juice obtained from apples or grapes is cloudy due to the presence of fragments of cellular walls and complexes formed by surrounded, positively loaded proteins of a pectin layer with a negative load. At present, pectinases are used as processing aids in the manufacture of apple, grape, cranberry, pear, blueberry, black currant, stone fruit, and tropical fruit juices. The repulsion of these complexes among them favors their suspension. The addition of a mixture of PGase and PE or pectin lyase alone produces the degradation of the external layer of pectin, promoting the electrostatic interaction of the complexes, their precipitation, and the increased clarification of the juice. In some cases, the loss of turbidity of the juice is undesirable, such as in citric juices. When the fruits are squeezed, the endogenous PE de-esterify pectin and promote their interaction with the present $Ca^{++}$ in the juice, giving place to the precipitation of the calcium pectate and the rising autoclarification. The partial degradation of the pectin by means of the selective use of a PGase or pectin lyase generates products of low molecular weight nonprecipitable with calcium, and this way avoids autoclarification.

Other applications of pectinases are pulp enzyming, maceration, and liquefaction. In pulp enzyming, the pectinases are added to the pressed mass of fruits, generally those that contain large amounts of pectin (e.g., strawberries, cherries, currants, raspberries, and even apples and grapes), where pectinases degrade the pectin, causing the jellification of the pulp and facilitating the filtration process. This enzymatic treatment has also been applied to increase yield in the production of olive, palm, and coconut oils. Another process of great interest is maceration, in which the objective is to degrade restrictively the middle lamella of cell walls of the plant tissue to produce relatively intact free cells. This process was originally developed to obtain viscous and cloudy drinks with pulp, called nectars. Some of the fruits used for these products include pears, peaches, damasks, papaya, passion fruit, and guava. In the same way, maceration is employed to obtain purees from vegetables such as carrots, potatoes, tomatoes, and others, with high contents of solids, pigments, and vitamins that are used in baby and geriatric foods and food preserves. The enzymes used for the maceration of the vegetable fabrics are PGases, pectin, or pectate-lyases.

Through the combined action of pectinases and cellulases it is possible to achieve the complete degradation of the cell wall, thus increasing liberation of the cellular juice. This process is applied for the production of juices of fruits difficult to filter such as mango, banana, or guava. However, use of pure cellulases in the elaboration of foods is not accepted by regulatory agencies.

## CONCLUSIONS

Although the importance of some aspects for the microbial production of pectinases, such as the influence of kind and amount of carbon sources, inducers, optimum media, pH, temperature, and airflow are well known, it is necessary to study the optimization in different reactors supported with extensive work on reactor kinetics to analyze the whole production process. With respect to applications of pectinases, it is important to note that these enzymes are used more and more each year in several sectors; however, their potential uses have not been fully applied. It is necessary to evaluate the action mode of these substances on the pectin chains to develop their new uses and products.

## SUGGESTED READINGS

Contreras-Esquivel JC, RA Hours, CN Aguilar, ML Reyes-Vega, and J Romero (1997). Microbial and enzymatic extraction: A review. *Archivos Latinoamericanos de Nutrición* 47:208-216.

Kashyap DR, PK Vohra, S Chopra, and R Tewari (2001). Application of pectinases in the commercial sector: A review. *Bioresource Technology* 77:215-227.

Naidu GSN and T Panda (1998). Production of pectolytic enzymes—A review. *Bioprocessing Engineering* 19:355-361.

Prade RA, D Zhan, P Ayoubi, and AJ Mort (1999). Pectins, pectinases and plant-microbe interactions. *Biotechnology and Genetic Engineering Reviews* 16:361-391.

# Phytases

Chundakkadu Krishna
Ashok Pandey
Ambat Mohandas

## *INTRODUCTION*

Phosphorus, an essential mineral salt for animal growth and development, comes from either the feedstuffs or inorganic feed phosphates added to animal diets. Although the total phosphorus content of feedstuffs should be sufficient for the required phosphorus supplement, up to 80 percent of the total phosphorus present in most feedstuffs of plant origin exists in the form of phytic acid phosphorus (hexaphosphate of myoinositol). Monogastric animals, such as swine and poultry, lack sufficient amounts of intrinsic phytases necessary to hydrolyze phytic acid complexes. Phytic acid has antinutritive properties and forms insoluble complexes with protein and multivalent cations such as $Zn^{2+}$, $Ca^{2+}$, and $Fe^{3+}$, thus reducing their bioavailability. Phytic acid is also known to inhibit a number of nutritionally important enzymes in vivo. These nutritional impediments regarding phytic acid result in the release of undigested phytate P in the feces and urine.

Phosphorus in the environment accelerates the eutrophication of fresh waters and has been identified as the main problem in surface-water quality, resulting in restricted water use for fisheries, recreation, industry, and drinking. In Europe, stringent environmental legislation controls the amount of phosphorus that can be released into the environment, and the United States is also beginning to face similar regulations. Recent reports suggest that due to the economic and environmental significance of the problem, any method that can improve phosphorus digestibility in feedstuffs or reduce the amount of phytate in plants would be beneficial.

Phytic acid can be hydrolyzed chemically or enzymatically with phytase—an osphomonoesterase—to inorganic orthophosphate, lower esters of myoinositol, and free inositol, thereby making phosphorus available for bioabsorption. The phytases (myoinositol hexakisphosphate 3- and 6-phosphohydrolases; EC 3.1.3.8 and 3.1.3.26), enzymes in the subfamily of the histidine acid phosphatases, convert phytic acid (myoinositol 1,2,3,4,5,6-hexakis dihydrogen phosphate) to inositol and phosphoric acid (Figure III.29), making phosphorus available for bioabsorption. Phytases can be de-

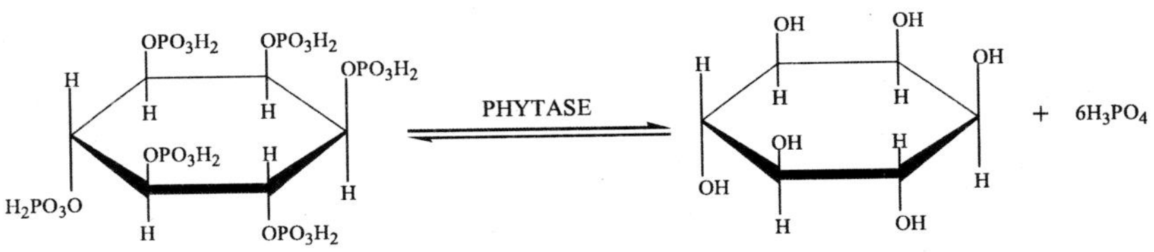

FIGURE III.29. Structure showing the enzymatic hydrolysis of phytic acid to inositol and phosphoric acid by phytase

rived from a number of sources, including plants, animals, and microorganisms. Recent research has also shown that microbial sources are more promising and more economical for the production of phytase on a commercial scale.

Supplementation of microbial phytase to animal diets alters the phytic acid complexes and also increases the bioavailability of proteins and essential minerals, thereby providing growth performance equivalent to or better than those with phosphate supplementation, and also reduces the amount of phosphorus in the animal manure to approximately 30 percent. If phytase were added to the diets of all monogastric animals reared in the United States, the value of the phosphorus released would be $1.68 \times 10^8$ per year, and it would reduce environmental loading of P by $8.23 \times 10^7$ kg. The Food and Drug Administration (FDA) has approved a GRAS (generally recognized as safe) petition for use of phytase in food, and phytase has been marketed as a feed additive in the United States since 1996.

Feed enzymes such as protease, xylanase, phytase, amylase, cellulase, lipase, and β-glucanase are the newest segment of the multi-billion dollar animal nutrition market, which is fast growing. At present, only 6 percent of manufactured animal feeds contain enzymes, whereas vitamins constitute 80 to 90 percent, which is considered to be the largest animal nutrition category. Several major animal nutrition companies, such as Novo Nordisk, Cenzone, Alltech, Gist- Brocades, Finnfeeds International, BASF, Roche, etc., are getting involved in this area very actively, and various products under different trade/brand names are already available on the market.

## SOURCES OF MICROBIAL PHYTASES

Phytases are present in plants, animal tissues, and microorganisms. Recent research has shown that microbial sources are more promising for the production of phytases on a commercial level. Table III.26 cites several examples of microorganisms as the source of microbial phytases.

Several strains of bacteria (wild or genetically modified), such as *Lactobacillus amylovorus, Escherichia coli, Bacillus subtilis, Bacillus amyloliquefaciens,* and *Klebsiella* sp., have been employed for phytase synthesis. However, bacterial phytase synthesis yields are low and the pH optimum is neutral to alkaline, which hinders their use as feed additives as well as the commercial exploitation.

The yeast cultures *Schwanniomyces castellii, Schwanniomyces occidentalis, Hansenula polymorpha, Arxula adeninivorans,* and *Rhodotorula gracilis* are reported to produce phytase in submerged fermentation (SmF) systems. Phytase production was influenced by pH, dilution rate, phytic acid content, nature of carbon source, etc.

Table III.26 cites several examples of fungal cultures used for phytase production. Although several strains of bacteria, yeasts, and fungi have been used for production under different conditions, two strains of *Aspergillus*

TABLE III.26. Sources of microbial phytases

| Bacteria | Yeasts | Fungi |
|---|---|---|
| *Bacillus* sp. | *Arxula adeninivorans* | *Aspergillus* sp. |
| *B. amyloliquefaciens* | *Hansenula polymorpha* | *A. carbonarius* |
| *B. subtilis* | *Rhodotorula gracilis* | *A. carneus* |
| *Enterobacter* sp. | *Schwanniomyces castellii* | *A. ficuum* |
| *Escherichia coli* | *S. occidentalis* | *A. flavipes* |
| *Klebsiella* sp. | | *A. fumigatus* |
| *K. aerogenes* | | *A. niger* |
| *K. oxytoca* | | *A. oryzae* |
| *K. terrígena* | | *A. terreus* |
| *Lactobacillus amylovorus* | | *Emericella nidulans* |
| *Megasphaera elsdenii** | | *Lentinus edodes* |
| *Mitsuokella multiacidus** | | *Myceliophthora thermophila* |
| *Selenomonas ruminantium** | | *Penicillium* sp. |
| *Treponema* sp.* | | *Peniophora lycii* |
| | | *Talaromyces thermophilus* |
| | | *Thermomyces lanuginosus* |
| | | *Trichoderma reesei* |

*Anaerobic bacteria

sp., *A. niger* and *A. ficuum,* have most commonly been investigated and employed for the commercial production of phytases in submerged fermentation or solid-state fermentation (SSF) systems.

## PRODUCTION OF MICROBIAL PHYTASES

### Screening and Assay Procedures

Many investigators aiming at isolation of different groups of bacteria, fungi, and yeast having extracellular phytase activity have carried out several screening programs. A simple and rapid method described for determining microbial phytase activity consists of determining the inorganic orthophosphate released on hydrolysis of sodium phytate at pH 5.5. In another method, differential agar media were used, and the disappearance of precipitated calcium or sodium phytate was considered to be an indication of enzyme activity. Bacterial phytase activity is determined from the enzymatic hydrolysis of sodium phytate under controlled conditions and measuring the amount of orthophosphate released.

### Production Techniques

Phytases can be produced by several microorganisms including bacteria, yeasts, and fungi (Table III.26). During the past five decades, the use of filamentous fungi for the production of industrial enzymes has rapidly increased, and phytases are no exception to this. Submerged fermentation has largely been employed as the enzyme-production technology. However, the high cost of the enzyme was cited as the limiting factor in using the enzyme in animal diets. In recent years, solid-state fermentation has gained much interest for the production of primary and secondary metabolites. The potential of SSF for the development of bioprocess such as bioremediation and biodegradation of hazardous compounds, biological detoxification of agroindustrial residues, bioconversion of crops and crop residues for nutritional enrichment, biopulping, and production of value-added products such as bioactive secondary metabolites including antibiotics, alkaloids, plant growth factors, etc., enzymes, organic acids, biopesticides, etc., has been well documented.

Microbial phytases are produced commercially by SmF and SSF systems. SSF involves the growth of microorganisms on moist solid substrates in the absence of free liquid. SSF is a promising technology for commercial phytase production, because it can use unrefined agroindustrial waste products as substrate, in general uses a less expensive process, requires lower capital investment and operational costs, and results in a higher volumetric productivity over submerged fermentation. The entire fermented product can be dried, ground, and sold as animal feed, resulting in less waste and less downstream processing.

Types of strain, culture conditions, nature of substrates, and availability of nutrients are the important critical factors affecting the yield, so care should be taken in choosing the appropriate technology. For example, a filamentous fungus in SmF is exposed to hydrodynamic forces, but in SSF the surface of the solid particles acts as the matrix for the culture. Microbial growth in such systems depends upon the availability of nutrients and the geometric configuration of the matrix. Filamentous fungi are the most important group of microorganisms for SSF cultivation due to their physiological capabilities and hyphal mode of growth. Inoculum quality and quantity, age of the colony, media composition, nature of substrate, and duration of fermentation were found to be important factors influencing enzyme production. Phytase production was strongly growth associated and less time consuming in SSF when inoculated with younger liquid cultures.

## MOLECULAR BIOLOGY AND GENE EXPRESSION

In the past decade, there has been much advancement in molecular biology and gene expression of phytases, starting with the cloning of phytases of the fungi *Emericella nidulans* and *Talaromyces thermophilus*. Phytases encoded by the *E. nidulans* sequence consisted of 463 amino acids, and that of *T. thermophilus* 466 amino acids with a M-r of 51785 and 51450, respectively. Both predicted amino acid sequences exhibited high identity, 48 to 67 percent, to known phytases. The unavailability of naturally occurring phytases of the required thermostability for application in animal feed has prompted investigators to construct consensus phytases using primary protein sequence comparisons. A consensus enzyme based on 13 fungal phytase sequences had normal catalytic properties but showed an unexpected 15 to 22°C increase in unfolding temperature compared to each of its parents. To gain more understanding of the molecular basis of increased heat resistance, the crystal structure of consensus phytase was determined and compared with that of *A. niger* phytase which unfolded at a much lower temperature. It was concluded that for fungal phytase apparently an unexpected direct link exists between protein sequence conservation and protein stability.

The expression of *A. niger* phytase gene, *phyA*, in *Saccharomyces cerevisiae* was studied to determine the effects of glycosylation on the activity of phytase and its thermostability. A 1.4 kb DNA fragment containing the coding region of the *phyA* gene was inserted into the expression vector pYES2 and was expressed in *S. cerevisiae* as an active extracellular phytase. The signal peptide and the medium composition affected the yield of extracellular phytase activity. The expressed phytase had two pH optima at 2.0 to 2.5 and 5.0 to 5.5, temperature optima between 55 and 60°C, and a molecular size of approximately 120 kDa. Deglycosylation of the phytase resulted in losses of 9 percent of its activity and 40 percent of its thermostability. The *phyA* gene for the *A. niger* phytase with optima at pH 5.5 and 2.2 was expressed in *E. coli* under the control of the T7lac promoter.

In another study, the expression of the phytase gene, *phyA*, from *A. niger* in *Pichia pastoris* was investigated. The gene was inserted into an expression vector pPICZ alpha A with a signal peptide alpha-factor, under the control of AOX1 promoter. The resultant plasmid was transformed into two *P. pastoris* strains, the methanol utilization slow strain KM71 and the wild-type X33. Both strains produced high levels of active phytase that were largely secreted into the medium. The result of SDS-PAGE (sodium dodecyl sulfate-polyacrylamide gel electrophoresis) of the phytase expressed by *P. pastoris* showed that the modified *phyA2* had been overexpressed and secreted. The phytase concentration in *P. pastoris* with modified *phyA2* had a 3,000-fold increase over that of original *A. niger* 963, and was 37 times higher than that of recombinant *P. pastoris* with nonmodified *phyA2*.

Molecular characterization and expression of a phytase gene from the thermophilic fungus *Thermomyces lanuginosus* involved the cloning of the *phyA* gene encoding an extracellular phytase. The *phyA* gene encoded a primary translation product, PhyA, of 475 amino acids (aa), which included a putative signal peptide (23 aa) and a propeptide (10 aa). The deduced amino acid sequence of PhyA showed limited sequence identity with *A. niger* phytase. The *PhyA* gene was inserted into an expression vector under transcriptional control of the *Fusarium oxysporum* trypsin gene promoter and used to transform a *Fusarium venenatum* recipient strain. The secreted recombinant phytase protein was enzymatically active in the pH range of 3.0 to 7.5. The *Thermomyces* phytase retained activity at 75°C and showed superior catalytic efficiency to any known fungal phytase at 65°C as optimum temperature.

In an efficient expression system developed in *B. subtilis* for the large-scale expression of phytase, the phytase gene with a native promoter derived from *B. amyloliquefaciens* was cloned in the *Bacillus* expression vector pJH27 under a strong BJ27 promoter and its expression was optimized. A gene-encoding phytase was also cloned from *Bacillus* sp. DS11 in *E. coli*. The *phy* cloned was encoded by a 2.2-kb fragment. This gene comprised 1,152 nucleotides and encoded a polypeptide of 353 amino acids with a deduced molecular mass of 41,808 Da. The phytase content was 20 percent of total soluble proteins in *E. coli*. However, the DNA sequence of *E. coli* phytase (AppA) was reported as early as 1990.

## PURIFICATION AND PROPERTIES

Similar to any other enzyme, microbial phytases have also been purified using conventional methods of salt or solvent precipitation under cold and then subjected to various chromatographic techniques such as ion-exchange chromatography, gel filtration, chromatofocusing, etc., and purification as high as 400-fold has been achieved. Their molecular weight has been generally between 36 to 120 kDa, with monomeric protein nature of the native enzyme. However, a phytase from *Schwanniomyces castellii,* had a very high molecular weight (490 kDa), and one from *Klebsiella aerogenes* had low molecular weight (10 to 13 kDa). Phytases have been active mostly in acidic pH, with optimum activity around 4.5 to 5.5. Some bacterial phytases have been reported to be most active at pH near to neutrality. For example, *Enterobacter* sp. phytase was active at pH 6.0 to 8.0, with optimum value between 7.0 and 7.5. Most of the phytases show their temperature optima at 50 to 60°C. However, phytase from *S. castellii* had an uncommon preference for high temperature, with optimum activity at 77°C.

A phytase was purified from *B. subtilis* strain VTT E-68013 and its gene *(phyC)* was cloned. The different homology sequence indicated that phyC was not a member of the phytase subfamily of histidine acid phosphatases but a novel enzyme having phytase activity. The metal ion requirement of a *B. subtilis* phytase showed that removal of metal ions from the enzyme by ethylene diamine tetraacetic acid (EDTA) resulted in complete inactivation, but active conformation was partially restored in the presence of calcium.

Thermostability is an important and useful criterion for industrial application of phytase. The enzyme from *Aspergillus fumigatus* was found to be heat-stable with great potential. Attempts were made to determine if a high level of functional expression of the *A. fumigatus* phytase gene could be produced in *Pichia pastoris,* and how the recombinant phytase reacted to different substrates, heating conditions, and proteases. Results have shown that *P. pastoris* was a potential host to express high levels of *A. fumigatus* phytase. Other studies have also demonstrated that some heat-stable phytases are able to withstand temperatures up to 100°C over a period of 20 min, with a loss of only 10 percent of the initial enzymatic activity.

Studies have been carried out to determine the primary and crystal structure of phytase through chemical sequencing and by a two-wavelength anomalous diffraction method using strong anomalous scattering of tungsten. The structure was found to closely resemble the overall fold of other histidine acid phosphatases, despite a lack of sequence similarity. Without using a conventional precipitant crystals of *E. coli* phytase were also obtained through bulk crystallization. A self-rotation function showed a clear twofold noncrystallographic symmetry relating two molecules of *E. coli* phytase in the asymmetric unit. The X-ray crystallographic analysis of a phytase from *B. amyloliquefaciens* strain using the hanging drop vapor-diffusion method showed that the amino acid sequence did not show any homology to those of other known phytases or phosphatases, with the exception of a phytase from *B. subtilis*. The enzyme exhibited a strong calcium-ion-dependent thermal stability. A new folding architecture of a six-bladed propeller for phosphatase activity revealed by the 2.1 Angstrom crystal structures of a novel, thermostable phytase determined in both the partially and fully $Ca^{2+}$-loaded states has also been reported. Binding of two calcium ions to high-affinity calcium binding sites resulted in a dramatic increase in thermostability by joining loop segments remote in the amino acid sequence.

## CONCLUSIONS

The increasing economic pressure currently being put on animal producers demands more efficient utilization of low-grade feedstuff. In addition, consumer awareness and new legislation require that any increase in animal production cannot be achieved through growth-promoting drugs or other chemical substances. Improved nutritional quality in animal feeds, improved feed yield rations, and reduced environmental costs associated with the disposal of animal wastes are the three major factors associated with the quality of animal feeds, and it is at this juncture that the major role of phytases become relevant. Microbial phytases offer technoeconomical feasibility for their production and application.

## SUGGESTED READINGS

Gowthaman MK, C Krishna, and M Moo-Young (2001). Fungal solid-state fermentation—An overview. In *Applied mycology and biotechnology*, Volume I, *Agriculture and food production,* GG Khachatourians and DK Arora (eds.). Dordrech, the Netherlands: Elsevier Science, pp. 305-352.
Krishna C and SE Nokes (2001). Predicting vegetative inoculum performance to maximize phytase production in solid-state fermentation using response surface methodology. *Journal of Industrial Microbiology and Biotechnology* 26(3):161-170.

Pandey A, CR Soccol, JAR Leon, and P Nigam (2001). *Solid-state fermentation in biotechnology.* New Delhi, India: Asiatech Publishers Inc.

Pandey A, CR Soccol, and DA Mitchell (2000). New developments in solid-state fermentation. I. Bioprocesses and products. *Process Biochemistry* 35:1153-1169.

Pandey A, G Szakacs, CR Soccol, JAR Leon, and VT Soccol (2001). Production, purification and properties of microbial phytases. *Bioresource Technology* 77(3):203-214.

Wodzinski RJ and AHJ Ullah (1996). Phytase. *Advances in Applied Microbiology* 42:263-302.

# Proteases

Rintu Banerjee

## INTRODUCTION

Proteases are a highly complex group of enzymes that vary enormously in their physicochemical and catalytic properties. Since the past few decades proteases have been regarded as degradative enzymes having substrate specificity in action. As the most important industrial enzyme, proteases account for nearly 60 percent of total enzyme sales, of which two-thirds are from microbial origin. Proteases are either extracellular or intracellular depending on the nature of the microorganisms. Extracellular proteases mainly degrade different types of exogenous proteins and have an active role in sporulation, spore germination, and formation of peptides and amino acids. Intracellular proteases take part in different types of modulation of substrate proteins, thus modifying it suitably for its proper function.

Many bacteria and fungi produce extracellular proteases in the early and late log phases, respectively, which may be due to the deficiency of nutrients during their growth and metabolic activities. Production in the stationary phase is thought to be due to the control of transcription level. In some bacteria, production of proteases is constitutive. Although there are numerous reports available on the synthesis of proteases, very little is known about the mechanism controlling their production. Among bacteria, *Bacillus* sp. and *Pseudomonas* sp. are the well-studied organisms, whereas among fungi *Aspergillus* sp., *Neurospora crassa,* and a few basidiomycetes have been studied thoroughly.

## CLASSIFICATION OF PROTEASES

Based on their nature of attack, the International Union of Biochemists classified proteases into two major groups: peptidase and proteinase based. Peptidases have been further classified according to the following three major criteria:

1. The reaction catalyzed
2. The chemical nature of the catalytic site
3. The evolutionary relationship as revealed by the structure

On the basis of the reaction catalyzed, proteases have been classified into four classes by the International Union of Biochemistry and Molecular Biology: serine proteases, cysteine proteases, aspartic proteases, and metallo proteases. This indicates that the different types of proteases have different types of catalytic activities.

### Serine Proteases

There are two distinct types of serine proteases. They belong to either the chymotrypsin family, a mammalian enzyme such as chymotrypsin, trypsin, or elastase, or the substilisin family, which includes bacterial enzymes such as subtilisin. While characterizing the enzyme and determining the three-dimensional structure, some differences were observed in the two families, but they have the same active site geometry, and catalytic reaction proceeds via the same mechanism. Serine proteases exhibit different substrate specificities, which are related to amino acid substitutions in the various enzyme subsites interacting with the substrate residues. According to their side chain, a specifically against oxidized insulin $\beta$-chain, serine proteases can be divided in to four subgroups.

### Cysteine Proteases

The cysteine protease family includes plant proteases such as papain, actinidin, or bromelain, several mammalian lysosomal proteases, as well as several parasitic proteases. Papain is the archetype and the best-studied member of the family. Recent elucidation of the X-ray structure has revealed a novel type of fold for cysteine proteases. Like the serine proteases, catalysis proceeds through the formation of a covalent intermediate and involves a cysteine and a histidine residue. The attacking nucleophile is the thiolate-imidazolium ion pair in both steps, and then a water molecule is not required.

### Aspartic Proteases

Most aspartic proteases belong to the pepsin family. The pepsin family includes digestive enzymes, such as pepsin and chymosin as well as lysosomal cathepsins D, processing enzymes, such as rennin, and certain fungal proteases. A second family comprises viral proteinases such as the protease from the AIDS virus (HIV), also called retropepsin. Crystallographic studies have shown that these enzymes are bilobed molecules with the active site located between two homologous lobes. These two aspartyl residues are in close geometric proximity in the active molecule, and one aspartate is ionized, whereas the second one is unionized at the optimum pH range of 2 to 3. Retropepsins are monomeric, i.e., carry only one catalytic aspartate, and dimerization is required to form an active enzyme.

### Metallo Proteases

Metallo proteases are one of the older classes of proteases and are found in bacteria, fungi, and higher organisms. They differ widely in their sequences and their structures, but the great majority of enzymes contain a zinc atom, which is catalytically active. In some cases, zinc may be replaced by another metal such as cobalt or nickel without loss of the activity. Bacterial thermolysin has been well characterized, and its crystallographic structure indicates that zinc is bound by two histidines and one glutamic acid.

## PRODUCTION OF PROTEASES

Conventionally, commercial production of proteases has been carried out using submerged fermentation (SmF). However, solid-state fermentation (SSF) has been deemed to hold tremendous potential in the production of enzymes. It has numerous advantages over SmF because of its high volumetric productivity, relatively higher concentration of products, less effluent generation, and simple reactor system. Recently, there have been increased attempts to produce different types of proteases, such as acid, alkaline, and neutral proteases through the SSF technique. Different substrates have been used for the production of these enzymes, including wheat flour, sunflower flour, coffee husk, soybean meal, wheat bran, wheat husk, polyeurethane foam, wheat bran and bean cake mixture, rice bran, soybean, sweet potato residues, and aspen wood, as well as by using various microorganisms such as *Pseudomonas* sp., *Aspergillus oryzae, Aspergillus niger, Aspergillus flavus, Rhizopus oligosporus,* and *Neurospora sitophila.* Among all the agricultural residues used for different types of proteolytic enzyme production, wheat bran holds the key role. The basic raw material not only provides the necessary nutrients for proper growth of the organisms but also provides necessary support for the filamentous fungi to anchor. Major parameters that govern the production of microbial protease synthesis are selection of suitable substrate, particle size, moisture content, and $a_w$ of the substrate, relative humidity, temperature, initial pH, period of cultivation, rate of oxygen consumption, and release of carbon-dioxide generation. A commercial process for the production of alkaline serine protease was developed in SSF using *Rhizopus oryzae* at the Indian Institute of Technology (ITT) at Kharagpur.

## APPLICATION OF PROTEASES

### Detergents

Proteases were the first enzyme to be used in detergent formulations, but powdered enzyme detergents received unfavorable publicity because some workers handling the enzyme, prepared as a finely ground powder, developed an allergic reaction. This led to the discovery of the new formulation of the product in which the enzyme was supposed to be present in the encapsulated form. The pH of the laundry detergent is generally 9.0 to 10.5, and temperature can be as high as 95°C. In most of the formulations, there are some oxidizing, chelating, and surface-active agents, which sometimes denature the enzyme. The ideal detergent enzyme can be defined as that enzyme which remains stable to the conditions mentioned previously. Alkaline saline protease from *Rhizopus oryzae* developed at IIT fulfilled all these (active at pH 3.0 to 11). The most efficient application of proteases in detergents is in the presoaking process. Proteolytic enzymes are also used in dry cleaning. Proteinaceous material becomes degraded by the action of proteases to smaller molecules, which subsequently are removed by other solvents during washing.

### Cheese Manufacture

Rennet is a partially purified enzyme extract consisting of the major milk coagulating enzymes in the extract rennin and bovine pepsin. Both of these enzymes play a vital role during cheese ripening. The variety of cheese produced depends on the type of milk. Most cheese is manufactured from cow milk, but goat, sheep, or buffalo milk are also used in the manufacture of different varieties of cheese. Some other enzymes also actively participate during this process, e.g., lipase, which plays a significant role in the development of flavors of certain cheese varieties. Multiple-enzyme systems are useful in modifying the natural cheese, which occurs during traditional cheese ripening. Various enzyme-modified cheeses are available and are called processed cheese spreads and cheese dips. The enzymes either enhance the intensity of flavor without increasing the solid or maintain the cheese flavor when its solid contents are reduced.

### Soy Sauce Production

Soy sauce is prepared by incubating soybeans, wheat, and salt with a mixture of mold, yeast, and bacteria. During fermentation, proteins, carbohydrates, and other constituents present in soybean are hydrolyzed to peptides, amino acids, sugars, and other low-molecular-weight compounds by the enzymes. Addition of salts prevents the development of toxins from the microorganism. Defatted soybean flakes are used for soy sauce production. The beans are moistened and steamed under pressure, mixed with coarsely crushed wheat kernel, and finally inoculated with the starter culture, as this is a fungal fermentation. Different species of *Rhizopus* are used for enzyme production. The neutral and alkaline proteases play a significant role in the digestion of soybean protein during soy sauce processing. Tofu (bean curd), sufu (bean cake), miso (bean paste), and shoyu are the traditional foods prepared from soybeans.

### Clinical and Medical Applications

Proteolytic enzymes are used as digestive aids and closers of serious wounds. Because enzymes are proteins, digestive enzymes are suitably coated to protect the enzyme during passage through the stomach, where the acidic environment could cause protein denaturation. Injection of some foreign proteases into humans reduces tissue inflammation. The highly purified crystallized form of enzyme minimizes the immune response. The natural defense of live cells against protease attack is usually inactivated in dead cells. This convenient difference allows application of solution of proteases to virulent or oozing wounds. Selective liquification of dead tissue and cells is achieved, which facilitates wound drainage and thereby decreases the time needed for healing.

### Baking Industry

Proteolytic action on the gluten component is vital for the quality of the bread product. Partial hydrolysis of gluten reduces the dough viscosity and improves the grain and texture of baked bread. Because cereals usually have a low protease level, supplementation with fungus *(Aspergillus oryzae)* protease is routine. Thermostable proteases are used only in biscuit and pizza dough, in which the higher cooking temperature rapidly inactivates the enzyme and prevents overt proteolysis and stickiness.

### Brewing Industry

The brewing industry is a major user of proteases. In the production of brewing wort, *Bacillus subtilis* protease are used to solublize protein from barley adjuncts, thereby releasing peptides and amino acids which can fulfill the requirement of the nitrogen supply. The proteolytic enzymes are used in chill proofing, a treatment designed to prevent the formation of precipitates during cold storage. In beer, hazes are formed due to the presence of proteinaceous substances which also precipitate the polyphenols and oligosaccharides. Hydrolysis of the protein component prevents aggregation of the insoluble complex.

### Photography Industry

The photography industry uses large quantities of silver in the light-sensitive emulsion that it produces. When such film is processed, to recover the expensive silver, the procedure involves separating the silver containing the gelatin from the film base. The aqueous solution that results contains both gelatin and silver, but the presence of protein hinders the separation of silver. Addition of proteolytic enzymes at a temperature of 50°C and pH 8.0 rapidly degrades the gelatin and allows the silver particles to separate out.

## CONCLUSIONS

Industrially important enzyme proteases play a very important role in performing different intracellular as well as extracellular activities. Proteases hydrolyze the proteinaceous substances and thereby selectively and specifically modify the protein molecule. Proteases can be produced from different sources, including plant, animal, and microbial. Today, plenty of reports are available on the production and properties of different industrial enzymes. For economic production of protease microbes can be the best choice. The basic properties of enzymes for these applications are that the enzyme should withstand high temperatures along with a wide pH stability. Proteases find major applications in detergent, tannery, and photographic industries, although they are also used in several food processing industries such as bakery, brewery, cheese, soy sauce, and meat industries. Currently, scientists are also applying proteolytic enzymes in therapeutic and pharmaceutical industries, mainly for health care products such as digestive enzymes and HIV treatment. For such applications, absolute purity of the product is required, which can be done by either conventional or non-conventional purification techniques. Proteases have a huge demand in genetically modified product preparation, as well. At present, application of microbial proteases is used in the modification of certain products such as chocolate, cocoa, beer, and wine, in addition to their applications in fruit juice preparation. Thus, with enhanced development of greater numbers of products, the applications for proteolytic enzymes are likely to be increased in the near future.

## SUGGESTED READINGS

Banerjee R and BC Bhattacharyya (1992). Extra-celluar alkaline protease of newly isolated *Rhizopus oryzae. Biotechnology Letters* 14:301-304.

Holzer H and H Tschesche (eds.) (1972). *Biological functions of proteinases.* Berlin: Springer-Verlag.

Kalisz HM (1988). Microbial proteinase. In *Advances in biochemical engineering/biotechnology,* A. Fiechter (ed.). Volume 36, *Enzyme studies.* Berlin: Springer-Verlag, pp. 1-66.

Stroud RM, M Krieger, RE Koeppe, AA Kossiakoff, and JL Chambers (1975). In *Protease in biological control,* Volume 2, E Reich, DB Rifkin, E Shaw (eds.). Cold Spring Harbor Lab, p. 13.

# Therapeutic Enzymes

## J. S. Pai

### INTRODUCTION

Enzymes are protein molecules with or without other moieties attached to them, which catalyze various reactions in living cells. Worldwide sales of industrial enzymes were projected at $1.6 billion for 2003, but by 2008, enzymes will consitute sales of $3 billion per year, an annual growth rate of 6.5 percent. About 45 percent of enzyme use is in foods, 34 percent in detergents, 11 percent in textiles, 2.8 percent in leather, and 1.2 percent in pulp and paper.

Many enzymes are being used in the health care industry, and their application is increasing both in value and in quantity. Some enzymes, such as penicillin acylase, are used for preparing health care products, whereas others, such as asparaginase, are used directly in treatment of disorders such as cancer, inflammation, and digestive disorders.

Enzyme therapy began in the 1920s, when plant enzymes were used to prevent and cure digestive disorders. Protease, amylase, lipase, and cellulase were used in these treatments. Cellulase was particularly helpful because the human body does not produce it. Animal enzymes were also used, especially pancreatic enzymes which are used today as digestive enzymes. Enzyme supplements are often prescribed for patients suffering from disorders affecting digestive process, such as cystic fibrosis and celiac disease.

Modern biotechnology has enabled production of microbial enzymes, which are cost effective, of uniform activity and properties, of high purity, and available in ample supply. Availability and cost of animal and plant enzymes were uncertain and depended on many factors, such as geographical location, climatic conditions, etc. Microbial enzymes are now produced in fermentors, thus many of these factors were eliminated. With the advent of genetic engineering, it was possible to produce even plant and animal enzymes using microorganisms. This eliminated certain problems such as adverse reactions and incompatibility. These changes have made microbial enzymes extremely lucrative and commercially attractive, and there is likely to be a big surge in the growth in number as well as quantity of these enzymes produced in the near future.

Some diseases being treated with therapeutic enzymes are acute inflammation, back pain, cancer, celiac disease, colitis, cystic fibrosis, food allergies, gastric duodenal ulcer, gout, premenstrual syndrome (PMS), and stress. Some enzymes are also used in the preparation of pharmaceutical products such as antibiotics including semisynthetic penicillins and cephalosporins, steroids, and chiral products. Some examples of microbial enzymes that are already being produced commercially include streptokinase, penicillin acylase, serratiopeptidase, asparaginase, and hyaluronidase. Many more may be added to the list in years to come. Some of these enzymes are discussed in this chapter with respect to their action, production, and applications.

## SPECIFIC THERAPEUTIC ENZYMES

### Penicillin Acylase

Penicillin acylase catalyzes the hydrolysis of penicillin to yield 6 amino penicillanic acid (6-APA). The product 6-APA can then be reacylated using appropriate side chains to obtain various semisynthetic penicillins such as ampicillin and amoxycillin. The production of 6-APA is estimated to be about 7,000 tons/year, and this is produced by several companies such as Rohm Pharma, Gist-Brocades, Boehringer Mannheim, Novo Nordisk, Toyo Jozo, and Beecham, mostly to prepare 6-APA.

Penicillin acylase is produced by many bacteria (*Escherichia coli, Proteus rettgeri, Alcaligenes faecalis, Bacillus megaterium,* and species of *Pseudomonas* and *Micrococcus*), fungi (*Penicillium, Aspergillus, Cephalosporium,* and *Fusarium*), and actinomycetes *(Streptomyces lavendulae).* Depending on the substrate specificity, it has been classified as penicillin G acylase and penicillin V acylase. The enzyme is produced intracellularly, as is the case in most organisms. *Bacillus megaterium* and *S. lavendulae* are different because they produce it extracellularly.

Penicillin acylase from most microorganisms is composed of two dissimilar subunits held together by hydrophobic interactions, an α-subunit with molecular weight between 20,500 and 24,500 and a β-subunit ranging between 60,000 and 66,000 Da. The active holoenzyme is formed by combination of α and β subunits. The α subunit is involved in the binding of the side chain moiety of the penicillin molecule and determines the substrate specificity, whereas the β subunit is involved in catalysis. The enzyme from *B. megaterium* was found to be much larger (120,000).

Enzyme production by microorganisms is controlled by several regulatory mechanisms, which are affected by fermentation conditions. Enzyme production is induced by phenyl acetic acid and repressed by glucose, fructose, maltose, and lactose. Mild temperature conditions of 25 to 30°C and neutral pH favor enzyme production. While *E. coli* prefers low aeration rates, *B. megaterium* requires much higher aeration rates of up to 2 vvm. Several *E. coli* strains have been mutated as well as genetically modified, including penicillin acylase genes from other organisms into them. This has enabled the commercial strain to produce several times more enzymes than the wild strain.

Various protocols have been adopted for purification of enzymes from different microorganisms. Extracellular enzymes from *B. megaterium* do not require cell disintegration, which is cumbersome and expensive. Enzymes from *E. coli* are normally precipitated by using ammonium sulfate and then purified further using chromatography. The large volume with *B. megaterium* enzyme necessitates concentration using either ultrafiltration or adsorption. Thereafter, chromatography is used to further purify the enzymes. Purity of several hundred fold is reported, with large variation in recovery of enzyme from 3 to 63 percent. Two-phase partitioning between aqueous phases has been applied with a recovery rate of 93 percent. Purified enzyme has been stabilized by polyols such as polyethylene glycol (PEG) and sucrose.

### Serratiopeptidase

Serratiopeptidase is an enzyme produced by bacteria belonging to *Serratia*. The purified enzyme is used as an effective anti-inflammatory agent. Clinically it is used alone or with other drugs in the treatment of inflammation in bronchitis, asthma, dentistry, obstetrics, gynecology, and healing of wounds after surgery. It acts rapidly on localized inflammation. Besides its anti-inflammatory action, it has some antiedemic and fibrinolytic activity as well.

*Serratia* sp. belong to the Gram-negative Enterobacteriaceae family. They are known to produce different enzymes including asparaginase, chitinase, lipase, streptokinase, and β-lactamase, but the most prominent is the extracellular protease called serratiopeptidase, produced primarily by *Serratia marcescens,* which has been isolated from soil, gut of silkworm, cow's milk, boll weevil, and ulcer patients by different researchers.

Typical strains of *Serratia* sp. secrete one to four proteases into the medium. The majority of the protease belongs to the metallo protease class. The others include thiol protease, serine protease, and serralysin protease. Media components have an effect on the production of enzymes during fermentation. Because the enzyme is inducible, presence of proteins and peptides has a favorable effect. However, easily metabolized substrates such as carbohydrates and especially sugars will exert catabolite repression, resulting in low amounts of the enzyme, although the growth of the microorganism will be quite rapid. Media consisting of proteinaceous substances such as casein, whey, gelatin, soy, or their hydrolyzed products have been used as the major or only source of carbon. Calcium seems to stabilize the enzyme, and its accumulation is quite substantial in its presence. Calcium chloride with potassium phosphate as buffering salt gives high yields of the enzyme around neutral pH. Temperature of around 25°C in a medium composed of soybean meal with a trace of tryptone gives high yields of the enzyme.

Serratiopeptidase is an extracellular enzyme. It is liberated into the medium after biosynthesis, and no active enzyme remains bound to the cell. Its formation increases in the logarithmic growth phase, and its concentration is highest at the onset of the stationary phase. As the enzyme is extracellular, the concentration is low in the medium, so the first step in the recovery is the removal of water. There are two methods of concentration: membrane filtration and precipitation by ammonium sulfate. Much of the early work utilized the second method but some have also used ethanol or acetone for precipitation. More recently, availability of ultrafiltration membranes made it a cost effective means of removal of water with less damage to the activity. The enzyme has a molecular weight of between 50,000 and 60,000 Da, so the selection of the molecular weight cut-off for the membrane is very critical.

Most of the purification strategies involved chromatography using Sepharose, diethyl amino ethyl (DEAE)-cellulose, Sephadex, and other materials, giving a final purification of up to 450-fold with enzyme recovery of 15 to 52 percent. *Serratia marcescens* also produces a pigment, prodigiosin, along with the peptidase. This pigment is red in color, and although it may have activity against some pathogenic protozoa and fungi, due to its possible toxicity it is removed during purification. It has similar favorable and unfavorable conditions of formation with the enzyme and normally occurs when enzyme is produced. The pigment can be removed by using ammonium sulfate precipitation.

This protease is available in highly purified form for medical applications as well as enzymatic studies. Properties have been studied with respect to kinetics, as well as effects of various parameters on its activity. Other studies report intestinal absorption and medical action from the point of view of application. It is stable between pH 5 and 7, with an optimum around 9, and is stable at temperatures up to 40°C. Using the radioimmunoassay (RIA) method, it was shown that the enzyme was absorbed to a significant level within one hour after administration in rats. Activity of the enzyme in sputum liquefaction and inhibition of inflammation has been evaluated using animals. It is commonly used for its anti-inflammatory and antiedema action, as well as to promote the lysis and discharge of sputum and pus. More recently, it has also been used in drug delivery, especially transfer of antibiotics in infected tissues.

## Asparaginase

L-Asparaginase catalyzes the hydrolysis of L-asparagine to L-aspartic acid and ammonia. Lymphoma cells lack the ability to synthesize the essential nutrient L-asparagine produced by the normal cells. Asparagine synthetase, which is needed by the cells to prepare their own L-asparagine, is lacking in tumor cells and depends on the supply of this nutrient from outside. Administering L-asparaginase derived from bacteria in the blood of leukemic patients lowers its concentration and leukemic cells are starved and destroyed.

Asparaginase occurs in a wide range of prokaryotic and eukaryotic organisms. Despite the wide distribution, only a few organisms produce asparaginase having properties for treatment of acute lymphoblastic leukemia. Clinically useful sources are *Erwinia carotovora, Escherichia coli, Serratia marcescens,* and *Proteus vulgaris.* Production and purification of asparaginase from *E. coli* has been most extensively studied. However, preparation from *Erwinia* sp. was found to be less toxic. *Erwinia carotovora* asparaginase is ten times more effective than the *E. coli* enzyme. There is higher L-glutaminase activity in the enzyme preparation from *Erwinia* sp., which may partially account for its higher effectiveness. There is greater availability of *Erwinia* enzyme in the cells, and it has a lower $K_m$ value. Some of the other microorganisms that produce asparaginase with antitumor activity are *S. marcescens, Vibrio succinogenes, Citrobacter freundii,* and *Azotobacter vinelandii,* while enzymes from *Fusarium tricinctum, Bacillus coagulans,* and *Acinetobacter calcoaceticus* show no activity. Molecular weight of the enzyme has been reported to be mostly between 128,000 and 150,000 Da, but a few species have shown lower molecular weight of around 85,000. The pH optima of all the enzymes lies in the alkaline region between 7.5 and 8.5.

Asparaginase production is affected by a variety of cultural conditions such as C and N sources, activators, temperature, and pH during growth of the microorganism. The enzyme is produced only in the logarithmic phase, reaching a maximum in the middle of the stationary phase. Lactose is a good carbon source for enzyme production. Organic acids and amides such as fumarate, malate, citrate, aspartate, and asparagine produce good growth and enzyme synthesis. Glucose and sucrose support good growth but exert catabolite repression, giving very low enzyme units. Asparagine acts as an inducer, and when its concentration is 0.1 to 0.3 percent, enzyme activity increases up to sevenfold. Corn steep liquor, when used as a nitrogen source, gives very high enzyme production, but purification becomes cumbersome. Tryptone and yeast extract are thus the preferred nitrogen sources and give equally good production. Asparaginase yield is very high if the pH of the medium is kept near neutral. Various buffers such as $CaCO_3$ and phosphate are useful in maintaining the pH during fermentation.

Asparaginase are used with a very high degree of purification in medicines. Large-scale purification was done using harvested cells, which were dried with acetone after washing. The acetone powder was extracted with borate buffer of pH 9.5. After centrifuging and filtration to remove cell debris, various combinations of adsorption, ion-exchange, and gel permeation chromatography were carried out. One combination used DEAE-cellulose, Sephadex G100, hydroxyapatite, and Sepharose CL-6B to give a recovery of 60 percent and purity of 30-fold. Another scheme of ammonium sulfate fractionation, gel filtration with Seralose 6B, and SP Sephadex C50 cation exchanger gave 43 percent recovery and a purification of 92-fold.

Although asparaginase does not possess the myelotoxic effects associated with most antitumor agents, it has a wide range of toxic effects on other organs, including the liver, pancreas, kidneys, blood-clotting systems, and brain. These changes are usually reversible, but to reduce the toxicity due to the enzyme, its substrate analogs such as *S*-carbamoyl cysteine, which closely resembles asparagine, enhance the effectiveness of the enzyme. Some of the side effects of the treatment are nausea and vomiting, confusion, decreased appetite, allergic reactions, bone marrow depression, soreness of the mouth and throat, and mood changes. The toxic effects are seen less with asparaginase from *Erwinia* than from other sources.

## CONCLUSIONS

Many more enzymes with applications in the health care industry are expected to be produced using microorganisms in the future because of the obvious advantages. In addition, biotechnology has enabled insertion of genes from one species into another. This has already been carried out with penicillin acylase, wherein one microbial gene has been introduced into another, resulting in substantial increase in productivity. Because the advances in genetic engineering have facilitated transfer of genes from animals or plants into microorganisms, one can make bacteria produce human enzyme or protein, as in the case of production of human insulin. Such developments may decrease the problems of reactions and toxic effects. The industry will see many new applications of microbial enzymes in the near future.

## SUGGESTED READINGS

Christie RB (1980). The medical uses of proteolytic enzymes. In *Topics in enzyme and fermentation biotechnology,* Volume 4, A Wiseman (ed.). Chichester, England: Ellis Horwood Ltd., pp 54-64.

Gallagher MP, RD Marshall, and R Wilson (1989). Asparaginase as drug for treatment of acute lymphoblastic leukemia. In *Essays in biochemistry,* RD Marshall and KP Tipton (eds.). New York: Academic Press, pp. 1-40.

Kalisz HM (1988). Microbial proteinases. *Advances in Biochemical Engineering/ Biotechnology* 36:3-65.

Rao MB, AM Tanksale, MS Ghatge, and VV Deshpande (1998). Molecular and biotechnological aspects of microbial proteases. *Microbiology and Molecular Biology Reviews* 62(3):597-635.

Senthilvel SG and JS Pai (1996). Purification of penicillin acylase of *Bacillus megaterium. Biotechnology Techniques* 10(8):611-614.

# Xylanases: Production

## Ufuk Bakir

### *INTRODUCTION*

All plant cell walls are mainly composed of three polymers, cellulose, hemicellulose, and lignin, in varying quantities depending on the plant source, growth stage, and development. The most abundant of these cell-wall components is cellulose, which is a homogeneous polysaccharide composed of β-(1,4)-linked D-glucose units. Hemicellulose, on the other hand, is not a single homogeneous polymer like cellulose but contains different heterogeneous polymers such as xylan, mannan, and galactan. The third type of polymer, lignin, is a complex polyphenolic compound which cross-links to hemicelluloses and, together with them, fills the space between the cellulose fibrils which are formed by cellulose polymer interactions.

Being the major hemicellulose in most plants and the second most abundant polymer in nature, xylan accounts for roughly one-third of the renewable biomass available on earth. The xylan percentages of hardwoods, softwoods, and annual plants are in the ranges of 15 to 35, 7 to 10, and up to 30 percent on dry weight basis, respectively. The backbone of xylan is composed of β-D-xylose units linked by 1,4-glycosidic bonds. However, xylans having no other residues than the homogeneous backbone are rarely present in nature and are isolated from very few plants, including esparto grass, tobacco stalks, and guar seed husks. Xylans, in general, contain different chemical groups, the most common of which are arabinosyl, acetyl, and glucuronosyl residues. To illustrate, hardwoods contain $O$-acetyl-4-$O$-methylglucuronoxylan and softwoods contain arabino-4-$O$-methylglucuronoxylans.

The complete hydrolysis of xylan can be achieved by synergistic action of a series of hydrolytic enzymes due to the heterogeneity of the polymer (Figure III.30). However the major enzyme is 1,4-β-D-endoxylanase (1,4-β-D-xylan xylohydrolase; EC 3.2.1.8) that cleaves the internal β-1,4 glycosidic linkages, producing substituted or nonsubstituted xylooligosaccharides. The other main chain-cleaving enzyme is β-D-xylosidase (β-D-xyloside xylohydrolase; EC 3.2.1.37), which hydrolyzes these short xylooligosaccharides from the nonreducing ends to produce D-xylose. Meanwhile,

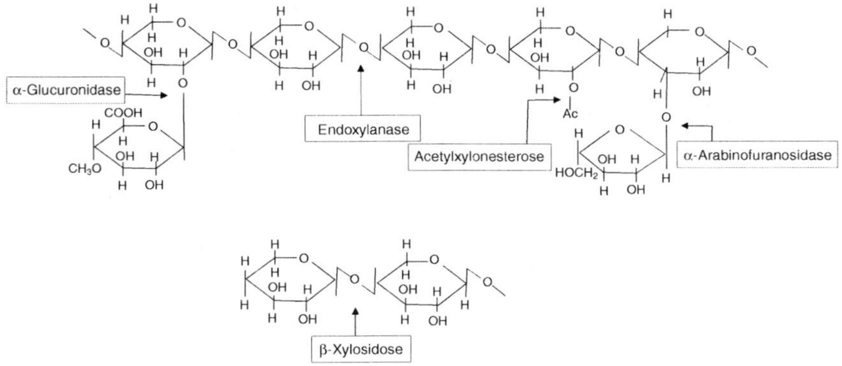

FIGURE III.30. A hypothetical xylan molecule and the xylanases involved in xylan degradation

debranching enzymes cleave the substituent groups from the main chain not only to liberate the substituent groups but also to facilitate backbone hydrolysis against the blocking effect of substituents. The main debranching enzymes and their functions are as follows: α-L-arabinofuranosidase (EC 3.2.1.55) liberates arabinose residues; α-D-glucuronidase (EC 3.2.1.131) cleaves D-glucuronic acid and 4-*O*-methyl-D-glucuronic acid residues; acetyl xylan esterase (EC 3.1.1.72), ferulic acid esterase (EC 3.1.1.73), and *p*-coumaric acid esterase (EC 3.1.1.-) remove acetic acid, ferulic acid, and *p*-coumaric acid residues from the main chain, respectively.

The conversion of xylan together with other renewable lignocellulosics into valuable products has attracted considerable attention as an alternative chemical and nutritional feedstock and energy source. Although nonenzymatic hydrolysis methods are also available, enzymatic hydrolysis is usually preferred, owing to many well-known advantages of enzymatic conversions. Several important industrial applications, including paper and pulp, textile, food, and feed industries, in addition to biomass biodegradation, boosted the research on microbial xylanase production, especially during the last two decades of the twentieth century.

Xylanases are widespread in nature and are produced by many prokaryotic and eukaryotic cells, including bacteria, fungi, archaea, algae, protozoa, gastropods, arthropods, and seeds of terrestrial plants. However, microbial sources have gained great popularity for the economical production of xylanases for many different industrial applications. Owing to this popularity, numerous studies have been conducted on

- microbial screening of sites where hemicellulose degradation occurs, including the gastrointestinal tract of ruminants and extreme environments such as volcanic springs and cold polar regions, in order to find more potent microbial strains producing xylanases with desired characteristics;
- mutation and genetic engineering for strain improvement to obtain hyperproducing mutants with desirable characteristics;
- fermentor design and fermentation optimization to increase xylanase production; and
- isolation and purification not only to find economical and practical methods for large-scale purification but also to characterize the xylanases.

## XYLANASE PRODUCTION

Microbial xylanase production can be performed by submerged (SmF) or solid-state fermentation (SSF). In SmF, substrates are either dissolved or suspended in an aqueous medium, then mixed by airflow or an agitator so that fermentation takes place in a homogeneous environment which can be firmly controlled. SSF, on the other hand, is performed on moist natural substrates in the absence of free-flowing water in a nonhomogeneous environment. Although SSF is a simpler and more economical process, especially preferred to produce product in smaller volumes, SmF should be the option whenever firm control of fermentation conditions is vitally important. SSF, on the other hand, is more suitable for filamentous fungi due to their low moisture requirement for growth. In general, xylanase production per unit volume gives higher results in SSF, but enzyme yield per unit substrate weight is higher in SmF. Commercial xylanase productions by SmF are reported from *Aspergillus niger, Trichoderma reesei, Trichoderma longibrachiatum,* and *Humicola insolens,* and by using SSF from *Aspergillus niger, Trichoderma reesei,* and *Trichoderma koningii.*

### Factors Affecting Xylanase Yield

#### Microorganism Selection

The major parameter affecting xylanase yield in a microbial fermentation process is the choice of microorganism among many different kinds of filamentous fungi, yeasts, and bacteria, including actinomycetes and archaea (Table III.27). The main criteria in the selection of a microorganism are its xylanolytic nature and productivity. Microorganisms may produce all of the

TABLE III.27. Common xylanase-producing microorganisms

| Fungi | Bacteria | Yeast |
|---|---|---|
| Filamentous fungi | *Aeromonas caviae* | *Aureobasidium* |
| *Aeromonas* sp. | *Bacillus* sp. | *pullulans* |
| *Aspergillus* sp. | *B. acidocaldarius* | *Pichia stipitis* |
| *A. awamori* | *B. circulans* | *Trichosporon* |
| *A. fumigatus* | *B. pumilus* | *cutaneum* |
| *A. kawachii* | *B. stearothermophilus* | |
| *A. nidulans* | *B. subtilis* | |
| *A. niger* | *Cellulomonas fimi* | |
| *A. oryzae* | *Clostridium* sp. | |
| *Chaetomium globosum* | *C. acetobutylicum* | |
| *Humicola insolens* | *C. stercorarium* | |
| *Neurospora crassa* | *Micrococcus* sp. | |
| *Penicillium* sp. | *Staphylococcus* sp. | |
| *P. chrysogenum* | *Thermoanaerobacterium* sp. | |
| *P. purpurogenum* | *Thermotoga* sp. | |
| *Rhizoctonia solani* | *T. maritima* | |
| *Rhizomucor pusillus* | *T. thermarum* | |
| *Rhizopus oryzae* | Actinomycete | |
| *Schizophyllum commune* | *Streptomyces* sp. | |
| *Trichoderma* sp. | *S. thermoviolaceus* | |
| *T. harzianum* | Archaea | |
| *T. koningii* | *Thermococcus zilligii* | |
| *T. longibrachiatum* | *Pyrodictium abyssi* | |
| *T. reesei* | | |
| *Thermomyces lanuginosus* | | |

main and debranching xylanases or only some of them, depending on their nature and fermentation conditions. Therefore, the type of xylanase activities needed and their properties for the application should be identified first and then a suitable microorganism selected accordingly. Great care should be given to the comparison of xylanase activities cited in literature, since the activity levels deviate highly depending on the methods used, substrate type, and the reaction conditions. For example, Nelson-Somogyi and dinitrosalicylic acid (DNS) methods that are used to measure reducing sugar concentrations, on which xylanase activity calculations are based, yield eight- to tenfold different xylanase activities. In general, filamentous fungi produce comparatively larger amounts of xylanases than yeast and bacteria. Some of the maximum xylanase activities given in literature are about 1,000 to 4,000

IU/ml for *Trichoderma reesei* and *Schizophyllum commune,* 400 IU/ml for *Bacillus circulans* in submerged culture, and about 20,000 IU/g for *Trichoderma reseei, Thermomyces lanuginosus,* and *Schizophyllum commune* in solid-state culture.

Microorganisms produce enzymes extracellularly, intracellularly, or, less frequently, both forms simultaneously. Extracellular enzymes are usually preferred to intracellular ones in large-scale production to facilitate downstream processing operations. Nevertheless, xylanases are, in most cases, secreted to the medium due to the large molecular weight of their substrate.

In microorganism selection, not only the wild-type microorganisms but also the hyperproducing mutants or recombinant microorganisms should be considered, since there is considerable progress in the cloning and the expression of xylanase genes in more suitable microorganisms for large-scale production.

Many properties of xylanases produced from various microbial sources are different in spite of the considerable overlap in the molecular biology and biochemistry of bacterial and fungal xylanases, as indicated by amino acid sequence homologies and structural and biochemical similarities. Indeed, many microorganisms produce several xylanases having different physicochemical properties as products of different genes. To illustrate, 1,4-β-D-endoxylanase molecular weight and isoelectric points are reported in ranges of 8 to 150 kDa and 3 to 10, respectively. Optimum pH values of fungal xylanases are acidic, whereas those of bacterial xylanases are neutral to basic. Many thermophilic bacteria, fungi, and archaea produce thermostable xylanases, which can resist high temperatures for prolonged periods, a very desirable property in many industrial applications. On the other hand, thermolabile xylanases produced by psycrophilic microorganisms facilitate xylan hydrolysis at low temperatures since their optimum temperature is about 10°C. So the optimum pH and temperature values of 1,4-β-D-endoxylanases are given in the range of 3 to 10 and 10 to 110°C, respectively, and their heat, cold, and alkaline stabilities are naturally different.

Fungal xylanases are generally produced together with cellulases, while bacterial xylanases are usually produced as cellulase-free. Cellulase-free production of xylanases, which are active at alkaline pH, make the bacterial xylanases more suitable for bleaching operations in the paper and pulp industry. However, it is possible to control fungal cellulase-free xylanase production by adjusting fermentation conditions such as the use of pure xylan as a carbon source, use of low nitrogen to carbon ratio in the fermentation medium, and/or selecting proper temperature, oxygen concentration, agitation rate, etc. However, careful analysis is required since no generalization is possible. For example, presence of cellulosic compounds may be essential for xylanase production by some fungal species. Therefore, deleting cellulose from the fermentation medium to prevent cellulase production can completely block xylanase production as well.

## Substrate Selection and Medium Optimization

Although constitutive production of xylanases is reported, the production of xylanolytic enzymes is generally controlled by induction and catabolite repression. Therefore, regardless of the cultivation method for the predetermined microorganism, the choice of carbon source and concentration is very important, since in most cases the carbon source functions as an inducer, too. Xylanase induction by xylan, various xylooligosaccharides, including xylobiose, xylotriose, acyl esters, and thioanalogs, and positional isomers of xylobiose are well documented.

In the case of induction by xylan, since it cannot enter the cells and signal the synthesis of the xylanases, according to an accepted xylanase biosynthesis regulation theory, low levels of xylan-degrading enzymes are produced constitutively and extracellularly so that they degrade xylan. Then, the low-molecular-weight soluble catabolites formed by xylan hydrolysis can enter the cell and induce xylanase production. Use of glucose as a main carbon source or as an additive causes severe catabolic repression in almost all microorganisms. The ultimate xylan hydrolysis end product, xylose, can induce or repress xylanase production in different microorganisms due to different control systems. Similarly, other easily metabolizable sugars such as fructose, lactose, maltose, sorbose, and cellobiose may also have either an inducing or repressing effect depending on the microorganism. The catabolic repression by simple carbohydrates affects xylanase yield in SmF much more than in SSF. Small xylooligosaccharides such as dimers are not always the best inducer system due to their rapid degradation in the cells to monomers which can cause catabolic repression to enzyme synthesis. Much higher yields of enzyme are obtained when the catabolic repression or hydrolysis of the inducer is avoided. This can be achieved by supplying the inducer at a very slow rate, by using synthetic analogs of natural inducers, or by using slowly metabolized inducers. The gratuitous inducers, such as thioanalogs of xylobiose or xylooligosaccharides, are metabolically inert and retain the capacity to interact with the cell enzyme synthesis. On the other hand, acyl esters of xylobiose or xylooligosaccharides are useful because they are slowly metabolized.

Many reports show better xylanase induction by using agricultural, forestry, and food-processing by-products rather than pure xylan. The most commonly used by-products include straws and brans of different cereals, corn hull and cobs, cassava and sugarcane bagasse, many different sawdusts, and fruit-processing, oil-processing, and coffee-processing residues. However, one should keep in mind that these lignocellulosic by-products may also induce other lignocellulosic enzymes, including cellulases, but pure xylan may selectively induce xylanase production. Pure xylan can be a good carbon source for selective xylanase production, but even traces of cellulose may induce cellulase production in some microorganisms. In some cases an insoluble xylan, rather than more soluble xylans such as arabinoxylan, may be a better inducer for xylanase production. Xylanase induction usually increases by increasing inducing-substrate concentration. These xylan-containing inducing substrates can be used in very high concentrations to enhance xylanase production in SSF, which is almost impossible in SmF. However using fed-batch systems instead of batch fermentations in the case of SmF may increase the concentration of substrate and ultimately the xylanase production.

Pretreatment of these hemicellulosic substrates, including alkaline washing, thermal pretreatment, and size reduction, increases the availability of xylan to the microorganisms, and as a result, xylanase production may increase severalfold. However, overly small particle size reduces xylanase production not only in SSF due to interference with aeration and respiration but also in SmF.

In addition to the carbon source, nitrogen, mineral, and trace elements are also added depending on the microorganism's need. As a nitrogen source, organic complex nitrogen substrates, such as yeast extract, peptone, or tryptone, inorganic nitrogen sources such as ammonium sulfate or urea, or in some cases high-protein containing hemicellulosic by-products such as soybean bagasse or corn steep powder can be used. The quantity of nitrogen and the nitrogen to carbon ratio should be adequate for growth and xylanase production, but organic nitrogen concentration should not be too high to induce protease production, which eventually decreases xylanase yield. In addition, the use of surfactants and natural zeolites as a source of various cations has been reported to enhance xylanase yields in many cases.

*Fermentation Conditions*

Similar to all other microbial fermentation processes, fermentation conditions, mainly temperature, pH, dissolved oxygen concentration, and agitation in SmF, and temperature, initial pH, initial substrate to moisture ratio, air circulation rate, and air moisture level in SSF, are important to enhance growth and xylanase production levels. Because the optimum fermentation conditions for microbial growth and xylanase production do not always coincide with each other, these variables should be optimized and carefully controlled during the fermentation. Cellulase coproduction, in many cases, is also a function of fermentation conditions.

Fungi require an acidic pH, but bacteria, especially *Bacillus* species, require neutral to basic pH for growth and xylanase production. Although aerobic organisms are primarily used for xylanase production, anaerobic bacteria, including *Clostridium* species and fungi such as *Neocallimastix* species, have also been reported to produce xylanases. Therefore, the airflow and agitation rates should be adjusted depending on the microorganism. The type of agitator and agitation rate should be selected carefully, especially for filamentous fungi since they are affected much more than bacteria and yeast. The shear and other mechanical forces produced by agitation can cause breakage of hyphae and change in morphology at high agitation rates. In SSF moist air is either circulated around or passed through the substrate on which microorganisms grow. SSF is generally performed under static conditions, but mixing may also be used.

*Application of Immobilized Cells*

The use of microorganisms that have been immobilized in support materials, such as natural and synthetic gels, fibers, and foams, for extracellular enzyme production has gained increasing interest, either for long-term repeated batch cultivation or for continuous systems. Severalfold increases in xylanase yields have been reported. The main disadvantage is the mass-transfer limitations, especially when insoluble and high-molecular-weight substrates are used. Naturally, the success of the process essentially depends on the nature of the carrier and the type of immobilization. Using carriers as thin films or attaching the cells on outside surfaces of membranes are often used to overcome this drawback.

## CONCLUSIONS

In summary, many different kinds of bacteria, fungi, and archaea have xylanolytic activities, and therefore, these microorganisms can be used for xylanase production. The choice of microorganism, fermentation technique, and conditions—especially the inducing carbon source—are the parameters affecting xylanase production efficiency. Depending mainly on the type of microorganism, substrate, downstream processing, and economic considerations, the fermentation technique can be submerged or solid-state. The use of immobilized microorganisms can also be a choice for long-term use of microorganisms in repeated batch or continuous fermentations with higher xylanase yields.

## SUGGESTED READINGS

Beg QK, M Kapoor, L Mahajan, and GS Hoondal (2001). Microbial xylanases and their industrial applications: A review. *Applied Microbiology and Biotechnology* 56:326-338.

Coughlan MP and GP Hazlewood (eds.) (1993). *Hemicelluloses and hemicellulases.* London: Portland Press.

Haltrich D, B Nidetzky, KD Kulbe, W Steiner, and S. Zupancic (1996). Production of fungal xylanases. *Bioresource Technology* 58:137-161.

Kulkarni N, A Shendye, and M Rao (1999). Molecular and biotechnological aspects of xylanases. *FEMS Microbiology Reviews* 23:411-456.

Pandey A, CR Soccol, and D Mitchell (2000). New developments in solid state fermentation: I. Bioprocesses and products. *Process Biochemistry* 35:1153-1169.

Sunna A and G Antranikian (1997). Xylanolytic enzymes from fungi and bacteria. *Critical Reviews in Biotechnology* 17:39-67.

# Xylanases: Properties and Applications

Lew Christov

## *INTRODUCTION*

The release of bleach-plant effluents with high absorbable organic halogen (AOX) levels into lakes, rivers, and oceans has become one of the major environmental problems for the pulp and paper industry in recent years. In response to environmental concerns and stringent emission standards, modifications of the production process at the pulping and bleaching stages have been developed. These include extending the cooking time for additional lignin removal, introduction of oxygen delignification as a pretreatment step, and elemental chlorine-free (ECF) and totally chlorine-free (TCF) bleaching with nonchlorine-based chemicals such as ozone and hydrogen peroxide. Another viable alternative is to introduce an enzyme prebleaching step. Over the past decade, a number of microbial enzymes have been assessed for their use in the pulp and paper industry. Among these, xylanases are gaining importance as biobleaching agents that can partially replace the use of hazardous chlorine-containing chemicals in the bleaching process. Although xylanases have been reported to find potential applications in the food and animal feed industry, their main use on a large scale is in the pulp and paper industry.

## *XYLAN STRUCTURE*

Xylan, next to cellulose, is the most abundant renewable polysaccharide in nature. It is a major component of plants and is located predominantly in the secondary cell walls of hardwoods and softwoods. The composition and structure of xylan are more complicated than those of cellulose and can vary quantitatively and qualitatively in various woody species. Whereas cellulose is present in all plants as a $\beta$-1,4-glucose polymer with a nonbranching structure, xylan is composed of $\beta$-1,4-linked xylose units forming a xylan backbone with a degree of polymerization (DP) of 150 to 200 and side chains connected to the backbone. The side-chain groups in xylan differ depending on the plant origin. The xylopyranose unit of the xylan main chain can be substituted at the C2 and/or C3 positions with acetic acid (at both C2 and C3 position in hardwoods), 4-*O*-methylglucuronic acid (at C2 position in both hardwoods and softwoods), and arabinose (at C3 position in softwoods). Arabinose may be further esterified by phenolic acids which cross-link xylan and lignin in the cell-wall matrix. In softwoods, every eight xylose residues are substituted with arabinose by α-1,3-glycosidic linkages, whereas the ratio of xylose to glucuronic acid is 5:1. In hardwoods, *O*-acetyl-4-*O*-methylglucuronoxylan is the main hemicellulose component, constituting 20 to 35 percent of the wood material. The degree of substitution of hardwood xylan with acetyl groups can vary; however, on average, every second xylose unit is acetylated.

During kraft pulping of wood chips, xylan is partially depolymerized, debranched, and solubilized in the cooking liquor. Subsequent losses of hemicellulose occur during the heating period of the kraft cook, whereby about 40 percent of xylan is lost and glucuronic acid is converted to hexenuronic acid by β-elimination reactions. By the end of the cook, 60 to 70 percent of the glucuronosyl and 10 percent of the arabinosyl substituents in softwood xylan are removed. Due to a pH drop in the pulping liquor caused by debranched acetyl residues toward the end of pulping, part of the dissolved xylan, lignin, and lignin-xylan complexes are reprecipitated back onto the fiber surface. The extent of this readsorption depends on the alkaline cooking conditions and the wood species; however, the reprecipitated xylan has a low molecular weight without side-chain groups and a high degree of crystallinity. For instance, half of the xylan content of pine kraft pulp is estimated to be relocated xylan, whereas up to 14 percent of birchwood xylan can be reprecipitated during kraft pulping.

During acid sulfite pulping, redeposition of xylans onto the fiber surface has not been observed. The possible reasons for this would be that the harsh cooking conditions and presence of acid-resistant residual acetyl and 4-*O*-methylglucuronic acid groups act as barriers against the adsorption and intercrystallization of xylan onto the cellulose micromolecules. Significant amounts of xylans are hydrolyzed and solubilized in the sulfite pulping process. For instance, in sulfite cooking of birch, only 45 percent of the original xylan remains in pulp after 20 min, and its original DP of 200 is reduced to less than 100. The bonds between the pentose units (arabinose and xylose) are hydrolyzed much more rapidly than the glycopyranosidic bonds. However, the glucuronic acid-xylose and xylose-acetic acid linkages are relatively more resistant to the acid hydrolysis conditions, and little cellulose is lost in the sulfite cook. The degradation products of the hemicellulose acid hydrolysis appear in the cooking liquor in the following approximate order: arabinose → galactose → xylose → mannose → glucose → acetic acid → glucuronic acid. In this order, glucose is derived mostly from the glucomannan rather than cellulose polymer. Thus, the residual xylan in sulfite pulps is less accessible because it is localized mainly in the secondary cell walls, although the xylan distribution across the cell wall is more uniform than in kraft pulps.

## XYLANASE PROPERTIES

Enzymatic hydrolysis of xylan to its monomers requires the use of several enzymes with different functions. These are classified in two groups, hydrolases and esterases, based on the nature of linkages that they can cleave. The glycosyl hydrolases are involved in the enzymatic hydrolysis of the glycosidic bonds of xylan. Of major importance is the endo-$\beta$-1,4-xylanases or 1,4-$\beta$-D-xylan xylanohydrolases (EC 3.2.1.8) that can randomly hydrolyze internal xylosidic linkages on the backbone of xylan polysaccharide. The main products formed from xylan hydrolysis by xylanase are xylobiose, xylotriose, and substituted xylooligosaccharides depending on the mode of action of the particular enzyme.

Xylanases can be classified structurally into two major groups, family 10 and family 11. Family 10 enzymes have a relatively high molecular weight, whereas family 11 xylanases are relatively low molecular weight with low or high pI values. The release of reducing sugars from pulp, however, has not been shown to correlate to bleachability or enzyme family. The enzyme-pulp interaction is dependent on substrate specificity and kinetic properties of the enzyme and can be influenced by pH, presence of xylan-binding domain, and ionic strength of protein and xylan molecules. Because xylan is negatively charged due to the presence of glucuronic acid side-chain groups, efficiency of binding of the enzyme to xylan is affected by the pH of the reaction and pI of the protein. For instance, if the pH is below the pI value, an enzyme can be completely bound to polysaccharides.

The xylanolytic enzyme systems of a variety of microorganisms have been extensively investigated. The optimization of fermentation techniques and isolation of more efficient microbial strains has led to a significant increase in the production rates of xylanase. Fungal systems are excellent xylanase producers, but they often cosecrete cellulases which can adversely affect pulp quality. One way of overcoming this is by using suitable separation methods to purify xylanases from contaminating cellulase activity. By applying appropriate screening methods and selection of growth conditions, it is possible to isolate naturally occurring microorganisms, which produce totally cellulase-free xylanases or contain negligible cellulase activity. Alternatively, genetically engineered organisms could be used to produce exclusively xylanase. Most xylanases studied are active in slightly acidic conditions (pH 4 to 6) and temperatures between 40 and 60°C. However, the current trend is to produce enzymes with improved thermostability and activity in alkaline conditions to fit operation conditions at mills.

## ENZYMATIC HYDROLYSIS OF XYLAN

Restrictions in the enzymatic removal of xylan from pulp have been assigned to retarded accessibility and chemical modification of residual hemicellulose. Accessibility problems arise from the fact that chemical pulping and bleaching apparently remove the more accessible portion of xylan from the cell walls, leaving the remaining part in locations that are less accessible to xylanase. It has been reported that prolonged incubation times were not as effective as a series of subsequent short treatments of pulp using xylanase, whereby about 50 percent of xylan could be removed. Xylan removal from pulp was improved when xylanase was supplemented with other hydrolyzing enzymes such as mannanase and endoglucanase. The endoglucanase treatment probably caused a partial hydrolysis and loosening of the cellulose structure, thereby increasing the hemicellulose accessibility to the synergistic action of xylanase and mannanase on pulp. The extent of xylan hydrolysis was also dependent on the substrate specificity of the particular enzyme used, as well as chemical composition and physical state of the xylan. Factors such as wood species and pulping method, inhibitory effect of residual pulping and bleaching chemicals in pulp, as well as degradation end products on xylanase efficiency, and the presence of xylan-lignin and xylan-cellulose bonds may also impact the extent of xylan hydrolysis.

## APPLICATIONS OF XYLANASES
## IN THE PULP AND PAPER INDUSTRY

### Biobleaching of Pulp with Xylanase

Pretreatment of kraft pulp with xylanase prior to bleaching can facilitate subsequent removal of lignin by bleaching chemicals, thereby reducing the demand for elemental chlorine or improving final paper brightness. A 25 percent reduction on average of the consumption of active chlorine can be achieved, which results in a decrease in the toxicity, color, chloride, and AOX levels of bleaching effluents. In the past decade, a significant research effort has been invested in the development of environmentally friendly enzyme-based bleaching technologies for the pulp and paper industry.

## Mechanisms of Biobleaching with Xylanase

A few hypotheses attempt to explain the phenomenon of xylanase-aided bleaching of pulp, although the exact mechanism is not completely understood. The initial model proposed suggested that xylanases attack and hydrolyze mainly xylan redeposited on the fiber surface, thereby enabling the bleaching chemicals better and smoother access to residual lignin. Pulps pretreated with dimethyl sulfoxide to specifically extract xylan showed no improvement in pulp bleachability. However, xylan-extracted pulps as well as pulps with low xylan content responded positively to xylanase pretreatment, indicating that xylan possibly exists in pulp in different forms, and the biobleaching effect induced by xylanases cannot be ascribed to enzymatic hydrolysis of reprecipitated xylan alone.

The second hypothesis suggests that xylanases can partly hydrolyze xylan that is involved in lignin-xylan complexes, thereby reducing the size of these complexes and improving their mobility and extractability from the cell walls. Indirect evidence does exist that lignin-carbohydrate bonds are formed during biosynthesis and aging of wood, as well as during kraft pulping, and that xylose is released as the main sugar component of isolated lignin-carbohydrate complexes. The biobleaching effect appeared to be accompanied by a decrease in the degree of polymerization of xylan and a slight reduction in xylan content without a notable solubilization of the polymer. Location of xylan within the cell-wall structure is of importance with respect to its accessibility to enzymes. It has been demonstrated that xylanase can solubilize lignin-xylan complexes from both the fiber surface and the inner fiber layers.

It has also been reported that xylan-chromophore associations can be generated during alkaline pulping which contribute to pulp color and brightness reversion of pulps. A direct brightening effect has been observed following xylanase pretreatment of pulp. This could be due to a direct removal of lignin fragments involved in lignin-xylan complexes and/or removal of xylan-derived chromophore structures. This hypothesis is supported by the recent findings that during the kraft cook the methylglucuronic acid of xylan can be modified to hexenuronic acid giving rise to double-bond chromophore-type formations.

Xylanases may also be able to disrupt to an extent the physical interlinking between xylan and cellulose within the fiber matrix, thereby improving the fiber swelling and generating macropores to facilitate lignin removal. The biobleaching effect observed with some hardwood sulfite pulps may also be caused by an improved pulp porosity. This suggestion is based on the fact that in acid sulfite pulps, in contrast to kraft pulps, xylan is not reprecipitated on the fiber surface but is largely entrapped across the fiber of the cell walls. The enzyme-mediated removal of xylan from the cell-wall capillaries may lead to the formation of larger pores, which enables an easier penetration of bleaching chemicals and subsequent removal of lignin.

It should be noted that the proposed mechanisms for xylanase-aided bleaching as described in this section are not mutually exclusive and more than one model can be involved depending on pulp type, on one side, and substrate specificity of xylanase to a specific xylan type in pulp, on another.

*Benefits from Biobleaching with Xylanase*

The benefits of using xylanases have been mostly the economic and environmental advantages which include

1. savings in bleaching chemicals;
2. increased throughput;
3. improved pulp properties such as brightness and strength properties (tear strength);
4. marketing advantage;
5. easy adaptation to different bleaching sequences with minimal investment costs; and
6. improved effluent with reduced AOX content.

Xylanases have been reported to reduce the kappa number of alkali-extracted pulps by two to four points, resulting in reduced chemical use following chemical bleaching. Greater savings of chlorine use have been achieved in biobleaching of hardwood kraft pulps (33 to 45 percent) as compared to softwood kraft pulps (20 to 26 percent). The xylanase-bleached pulps generally show increased viscosity due to the selective removal of the low-molecular-weight xylan. The strength properties of these pulps remain relatively unchanged and can be maintained at a desired level, especially in TCF bleaching. Another advantage of xylanase use is the corresponding reduction of the AOX load of bleach effluents due to decreased consumption of chlorine-containing bleach chemicals.

*Large-Scale Use of Xylanase*

Since biobleaching with xylanases was first reported in 1986, a number of mill trials in both Europe and North America have been conducted. The first industrial application of xylanases was carried out in Finland in 1991. In 1994, eighteen bleaching mills in Canada ran xylanase trials, and six are regular users of the enzyme to treat 750,000 tons of pulp representing 8 percent of Canada's bleached kraft pulp production.

The commercially available xylanase preparations most often reported to be applied on a large scale are of *Bacillus* and *Trichoderma* origin. However, strains of *Aureobasidium pullulans* and *Thermomyces lanuginosus* have also been used. There are certain requirements enzymes should fulfill to ensure success of enzyme bleaching:

1. stable at elevated temperatures (50 to 70°C);
2. active at neutral to alkaline pH conditions (pH 6 to 9);
3. resistant to inactivation and nonspecific binding to cellulose;
4. free of cellulase activity which is detrimental to viscosity, strength, and pulp yield;
5. high substrate specificity for pulp xylan; and
6. relatively low molecular weigh (<50 kDa) to avoid diffusional limitations.

The reasons for using xylanase vary from mill to mill depending on operating conditions and requirements. Most of the regular users of xylanases benefit from the increased pulp throughput, especially mills with ECF sequences where chlorine dioxide generators are of limited capacity, and from the marketing advantages associated with producing enzyme-bleached pulp. In TCF sequences, the motivation for xylanase use is improved final brightness and savings in bleaching chemicals without affecting strength properties.

Some problems have been encountered as well, associated mainly with corrosion of equipment, maintenance of residence time of xylanase treatment, pulp yield loss, and bleach-plant control. However, the xylanase bleaching technology at present is being further developed toward increasing the pH and temperature stability of xylanases, use of enzyme mixtures with supplementary hemicellulolytic accessory enzymes or enzymes with cooperative synergistic action to enhance xylanase efficiency, improving the competitiveness of xylanases with respect to enzyme price, and optimization of both ECF and TCF bleaching in conjunction with xylanases.

### *Xylan Removal from Dissolving Pulp*

Compared to other types of pulp, dissolving pulp (raw material for viscose rayon and other cellulose derivatives) contains less lignin and hemicellulose as a result of extensive pulping and bleaching. Although lignin is almost completely removed after bleaching, part of the hemicellulose (xylan) still remains in the pulp, causing problems at the later alkalization and spinning stages of the viscose process. Therefore, a more complete removal of residual xylan from dissolving pulp would facilitate its processing and would improve the quality of the final product. Using xylanase, restricted pentosan removal from bleached sulfite pulps (25 percent) and bleached kraft pulp (20 percent) have been reported. However, if more than one xylanase stage is used, as much as 50 percent of xylan in dissolving pulp could be removed.

### Other Applications of Xylanases

Xylanases have been reported to enhance interfiber bonding through fibrillation without reducing pulp viscosity. Xylanase-treated pulps have shown improved beatability and brightness stability. When applied together with cellulases, xylanases can improve the drainage rates of recycled fibers and can facilitate the release of toners from office waste and the following flotation and washing steps. Xylanases in combination with pectinases, cellulases, and other polysaccharidases have been used for enzymatic retting of flax and to soften and smooth surfaces of jute-cotton blended fabrics.

## CONCLUSIONS

Much progress has been made in understanding the basic mechanism of xylanase action on pulp. In addition, more robust and powerful genetically engineered enzymes have been designed. This would certainly broaden and strengthen the application potential of xylanases in various sectors of pulp and paper manufacture.

## SUGGESTED READINGS

Christov LP and BA Prior (1996). Repeated treatments with *Aureobasidium pullulans* hemicellulases and alkali enhance biobleaching of sulphite pulps. *Enzyme and Microbial Technology* 18:244-250.

Coughlan MP and GP Hazlewood (1993). β-1,4-D-Xylan-degrading enzyme systems: Biochemistry, molecular biology and applications. *Biotechnology and Applied Biochemistry* 17:259-289.

Fengel D and G Wegener (1984). *Wood: Chemistry, ultrastructure, reactions.* Berlin: Walter de Gruyter.

Tolan JS, D Olson, and RE Dines (1995). Survey of xylanase enzyme usage in bleaching in Canada. *Pulp and Paper Canada* 96:107-110.

Viikari L, A Kantelinen, J Sundquist, and M Linko (1994). Xylanases in bleaching: From an idea to the industry. *FEMS Microbiology Reviews* 13:335-350.
Viikari L, M Tenkanen, J Buchert, M Rättö, M Bailey, M Siika-aho, and M Linko (1993). Hemicellulases for industrial applications. In *Bioconversion of forest and agricultural plant residues,* JN Saddler (ed.). Wallingford, UK: CAB International, pp. 131-182.

# Modified Oligonucleotides

Adolfo M. Iribarren

## *INTRODUCTION*

Oligonucleotides (Figure III.31) are single-stranded oligomers of nucleo-side units linked together through phosphodiester bridges between a 3'-hydroxyl group of one monomer and the 5'-hydroxyl group of another. In particular, oligodeoxynucleotides can also be defined as short fragments of single-stranded DNA. During recent years, nucleic acid chemistry has generated an increasing degree of attention. Since Khorana first developed the synthesis of oligodeoxynucleotides, several improvements have been achieved. The most remarkable among these is the solid-phase synthesis strategy that made possible the complete automated preparation of long sequences as

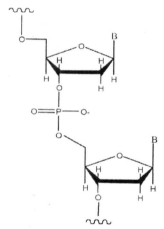

B: thymine, cytosine, adenine, guanine

FIGURE III.31. Oligonucleotide configuration

well as large amounts of natural and modified DNA fragments. These molecules offer a wide range of applications in fields such as biotechnology, molecular biology, and medicine for diagnosis and therapy.

Natural oligonucleotides have been extensively used for double-stranded DNA construction (synthetic genes), preparation of primers (used, for example, in sequencing or polymerase chain reaction [PCR] amplification), selection of DNA (hybridization probes or affinity purification), site-directed mutagenesis, selective inhibition of gene expression, and structural studies. However, the spectrum of applications can still be broadened by introducing chemical modifications into oligonucleotide structures.

## CONJUGATES

Conjugated oligonucleotides, resulting from the union with one or more molecules that confer particular properties, are one kind of useful analog. The coupled moieties can provide a particular reactivity, such as cross-linking with other nucleic acids or proteins (psoralen, alkylating groups, platinum complexes, disulfide bridges, which allow the generation of long-life hybrids and the study of protein-DNA interactions), or the cleavage of a target nucleic acid in a selective way (enzyme-linked, porphyrin complexes or iron-ethylene diamine tetraacetic acid [EDTA] complexes).

Other important conjugates are those that provide special intermolecular interactions such as intercalation (acridine, anthraquinone), enhanced cellular uptake (cholesterol, polylysine, peptides, etc.), and binding characteristics (biotin, digoxigenin). Conjugates are finding an increasing number of applications as diagnostic agents, mainly fluorescent hybridization probes (fluorescent, luminescent, chemiluminiscent tags), or labeled primers for PCR, which are also used in automated DNA sequencing.

## OLIGONUCLEOTIDE ANALOGS

Other examples of modified oligonucleotides are those that carry modifications in the nucleotide moiety. These alterations of the natural structure can be introduced in the base, sugar, or phosphate moieties and can confer increased stability in biological fluids. In these media (cellular culture media, serum, or cytoplasm), enzymes called nucleases (exo- and endonuclesases) rapidly degrade natural oligonucleotides. Therefore, these analogs are essential for in vivo applications, but the design of new modified oligonucleotides is a difficult task due to chemical, electronic, and steric concerns.

## Antisense Oligonucleotides

The field in which the research and development of new analogs has been most prolific is the antisense strategy. This approach is based on the ability of oligonucleotides to selectively inhibit gene expression of a target gene. In principle, the use of such compounds is very simple. It is necessary to synthesize an oligonucleotide carrying a base sequence complementary to that of a segment of the target mRNA coding for the protein for which expression is to be suppressed. This antisense oligonucleotide will recognize and bind to that mRNA, by Watson-Crick base pairing, thus selectively inhibiting gene expression. Today these compounds are considered to be a new drug generation.

Chemical modifications should confer appropriate antisense characteristics such as hybridization, resistance to nucleases, cellular uptake, selectivity, and, basically, good pharmacokinetic and pharmacodynamic properties.

So far, the most widely spread modification is thiophosphate (1, Figure III.32). However, this analog has some drawbacks, such as the formation of

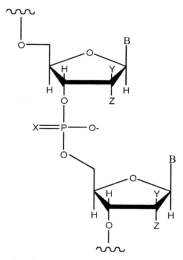

B: thymine, cytosine, adenine, guanine

1: X=S, Y=H, Z=H
2: X=O, Y=H, Z=O-Alkyl
3: X=O, Y=CH$_3$, Z=OH

FIGURE III.32. Antisense oligonucleotide configuration

diasteromeric mixtures during synthesis and the generation of nonspecific interactions with proteins. Numerous modifications have been proposed so far, but among them, 2'-*O*-alkyloligonucleotides (2, Figure III.31) seem to be the most promising. They form very stable hybrids with the complementary RNA and show a much better oral bioavailability. These derivatives are considered the second generation of antisense drugs.

The biological effects of oligonucleotides have been widely studied in vitro as well as in vivo, being the most representative fields the development of potential anticancer and antiviral drugs. Clinical trials in progress involve different targets such as antiviral drugs (human immunodeficiency virus [HIV-1] and hepatitis C [HCV]), inflammation and other immune disorders (intercellular adhesion molecule [ICAM-1]), and anticancer drugs (Bcl-2, PKCα, and c-Myc) among others. Finally, the application of modified oligonucleotides in the development of new therapeutic agents has been evidenced by Food and Drug Administration (FDA) approval of one antisense compound used to treat cytomegalovirus retinitis in AIDS patients.

### Ribozymes

An important improvement in antisense approaches can be achieved by using ribozymes that are RNA molecules, which catalytically cleave internucleotidic phosphate bonds of RNA substrates. The hammerhead ribozyme, originally found in plant viroids, is the simplest one. It can act intermolecularly *(trans)* and can be tailored to recognize by base complementarity different target sequences. These molecules provide a catalytic antisense mechanism and therefore are attractive molecules for the development of new drugs based on the gene therapy principle.

The design of resistant ribozymes becomes still more complex because proper folding of nucleic acid is needed in order to maintain catalytic activity. Several studies have shown that the presence of the 2'-hydroxyl group in specific positions of the catalytic core is essential for hydrolytic activity. One approach to overcome this problem is to use 2'-C-methyl nucleotides (3, Figure III.32), which, when substituted for a particular ribonucleotide, are expected to provide a 2'-hydroxyl group able to make similar interactions to those displayed by the natural moiety. When 2'-C-methyluridine was located in those positions where uridine 2'-hydroxyl was found to be essential, active ribozymes with increased stability to nucleases were obtained. Several experiments have already proven that ribozymes are effective gene expression inhibitors in vitro as well as in vivo.

## Aptamers

Similar considerations are applicable to the development of aptamers, which are RNA or DNA molecules individualized from a randomly synthesized library on the basis of a particular property. They are identified by repeated cycles of selection and amplification, using PCR technologies, called in vitro selection or systematic evolution of ligands by exponential enrichment (SELEX). Several sequences have been selected for a wide spectrum of functions. They can selectively recognize and strongly bind to proteins and small molecules, or they can promote catalytic reactions such as hydrolysis and ligation of nucleic acids or formation of peptide bonds, among others.

The characteristics of aptamers can be improved by chemical modification of selected sequences. There are two methods used to achieve this goal; one involves modification of the sequence after the selection procedure, and the other one, the use of modified triphosphates that are compatible with polymerases. In the first approach, different types of modifications can be assessed, but it is difficult to predict how they will modify the properties of the aptamer. The second method allows the selection of the proper structure, but only from unnatural monomers that can be enzymatically incorporated. Chemically modified aptamers have been selected, for example, against the platelet-derived growth factor (PDGF) α chain, vascular endothelial growth factor (VEGF), and thrombin, which evidenced the potentiality and feasibility of these strategies.

## Chimeric Oligonucleotides

Chimeric oligonucleotides constitute another interesting family of oligonucleotide analogs. These molecules are composed of different kinds of monomers that provide particular properties. Several examples are available: the use of normal DNA sequences flanked by modified ones, the use of different resistant modifications (i.e., one confers a region recognized by ribonuclease [RNase] H and the other improved thermal stability of the hybrid), and more recently, the use of DNA-modified RNA chimeras that have proved to be very active in homologous pairing reactions. This last strategy has enabled the correction of mutations (i.e., point mutation of the β-globin gene resulting in sickle-cell anemia) at a high frequency and has also found application in other biotechnological fields such as the in vivo manipulation of plant genes (for example, site-specific heritable mutations in maize genes were engineered by using chimeric oligonucleotides).

## DNA CHIPS

Finally, it is worth mentioning the recent development of probe arrays or DNA chips, which are promising and powerful tools in human genetics, diagnostic pathogen detection, and DNA molecular recognition. They consist of high-density arrays of oligonucleotides to which labeled test DNA is hybridized. Successful results have been obtained in the identification of mutations in some known disease genes and the determination of DNA polymorphisms on a large scale.

## CONCLUSIONS

Although the main uses of some modified oligonucleotides have been mentioned here, many others have not been described due to the vastness of the subject. Considering the accelerated growth of oligonucleotide applications observed so far, it is reasonable to expect that in the near future these molecules will play an even more important role in different fields related to biotechnology.

## SUGGESTED READINGS

Giles VG (2000). Antisense oligonucleotide technology: From EST to therapeutics. *Current Opinion in Molecular Therapeutics* 2(3):238-252.

Goodchild J (2000). Hammerhead ribozymes: Biochemical and chemical considerations. *Current Opinion in Molecular Therapeutics* 2(3):272-281.

Lai LW and YH Lien (2000). Therapeutic application of chimeric RNA/DNA oligonucleotide based gene therapy. *Expert Opinion Biological Therapy* 1(1): 41-47.

Lyer RP, A Roland, W Zhou, and K Ghosho (1999). Modified oligonucleotides–Synthesis, properties and applications. *Current Opinion in Molecular Therapeutics* 1(3):344-358.

Tillib SV and AD Mirzabekov (2001). Advances in the analysis of DNA sequence variations using oligonucleotide microchip technology. *Current Opinion in Biotechnology* 12(1):53-58.

Toulmé J-J (2000). Aptamers: Selected oligonucleotides for therapy. *Current Opinion in Molecular Therapeutics* 2(3):318-324.

# Organic Acids: Production and Application

## Citric Acid

Carlos Ricardo Soccol
Flávera C. Prado
Luciana P. S. Vandenberghe
Ashok Pandey

### INTRODUCTION

Historically, citric acid fermentation was the first fungal product of industrial importance. It was discovered by Wehmer in 1893 as a by-product of oxalic acid produced by a culture of *Penicillium glaucum* on sugar medium, but it was the work of Pierre Curie that opened up the way for successful industrial production of citric acid. In 1916, he observed that numerous strains of *Aspergillus niger* produced significant amounts of citric acid. Citric acid is widely distributed throughout nature, occurring in both plants and animals. It is one of the world's largest tonnage fermentation products, with an estimated annual production of about one million tons. Citric acid is a versatile and innocuous alimentary additive. It is accepted worldwide as GRAS (generally recognized as safe), approved by the Joint FAO/WHO Expert Committee on Food Additives. Table III.28 presents the main applications of citric acid. The food industry consumes about 70 percent of total citric acid production, followed by pharmaceutical industries (12 percent), and the remaining 18 percent is consumed by other industries. There is annual growth of 3.5 to 4.0 percent in demand/consumption rate of citric acid.

### RAW MATERIALS USED FOR CITRIC ACID PRODUCTION

Several raw materials such as hydrocarbons, starchy materials, and molasses have been employed as substrates for commercial production of citric acid. Generally, citric acid is produced by fermentation using inexpensive

TABLE III.28. Applications of citric acid

| Industry | Applications |
|---|---|
| Beverages | pH adjustment. Provides tartness and complements fruit and berry flavors. Increases the effectiveness of antimicrobial preservatives. |
| Wines and ciders | Prevents turbidity. Prevents browning in white wines. pH adjustment. |
| Soft drinks and syrups | Provides tartness. Stimulates natural fruit flavor. As acidulant in carbonated and sucrose-based beverages. |
| Jellies, jams, and preserves | pH adjustment. Acidulant. Provides the desired degree of tartness, tang, and flavor. |
| Dairy products | As emulsifier in ice creams and processed cheese. Acidifying agent in many cheese products and antioxidant. |
| Candies | Acts as acidulant. Provides tartness. Minimizes sucrose inversion. Produces dark color in hard candies. Prevents crystallization of sucrose. |
| Frozen fruit | Protects ascorbic acid by inactivating trace metals. Lowers pH to inactivate enzymes. |
| Pharmaceuticals | Effervescent in powders and tablets in combination with bicarbonates. Anticoagulant. Provides rapid dissolution of active ingredients. Acidulant in astringent formulation. |
| Cosmetics and toiletries | Buffering agent. pH adjustment. Antioxidant as a metallic-ion chelator. |
| Industrial applications | Buffer agent. Sequester metal ions. Neutralize bases. Used in nontoxic and biodegradable processes that meet current ecological and safety standards. |
| Metal cleaning | Removes metal oxides from surface of ferrous and nonferrous metals, for preoperational and operational cleaning of iron and copper oxides. |
| Others | Electroplating, metal cleaning, leather tanning, printing inks, bottle-washing compounds, floor cement, textiles, photographic reagents, concrete, plaster, refractories, adhesives, paper, polymers, waste treatment, etc. |

raw materials, including crude natural products such as starch hydrolysate, sugarcane broth, and molasses (sugarcane and beet). Due to its relatively low cost and high sugar content (40 to 55 percent), molasses is the most commonly used raw material, but beet molasses is preferred due to its lower content of trace metals, supplying better fermentation yields than cane molasses.

A variety of agroindustrial residues and by-products have also been studied for their potential to be used as substrates for citric acid production. A cost reduction on citric acid production possibly can be achieved by using such substrates. Table III.29 shows a wide variety of raw materials that have been used for citric acid production.

## MICROORGANISMS USED
## FOR CITRIC ACID PRODUCTION

Several microorganisms including fungi and bacteria such as *Arthrobacter paraffineus, Bacillus licheniformis, Corynebacterium* ssp., *Aspergillus niger, A. aculeatus, A. carbonarius, A. awamori, A. foetidus, A. fonsecaeus, A. phoenicis,* and *Penicillium janthinellum,* and yeasts such as *Candida tropicalis, C. oleophila, C. guilliermondii, C. citroformans, Hansenula anomala,* and *Yarrowia lipolytica* are capable of producing citric acid. Most of these, however, are not able to produce commercially acceptable yields. The fungus *A. niger* has remained the organism of choice for commercial production because it produces more citric acid per unit time. The main advantages of using *A. niger* are its ease of handling, its ability to ferment a variety of cheap raw materials, and high yields. In the production of citric acid using yeasts, generally there is simultaneous formation of isocitric acid.

Any increase in citric acid productivity would be of potential interest. With this in mind, attempts are continuously being made to improve the strains by mutagenesis and selection. The most frequently employed technique has been inducing mutations in parental strains using mutagens. Among mutagens, γ-radiation, ultraviolet (UV) radiation, and chemical mutagens are often used. To obtain hyperproducer strains, frequently UV treatment is combined with some chemical mutagens. The "single-spore technique" and the "passage method" are the principal methods of selecting strains. However, a serious limitation is the noncorrelation among the production of citric acid measured by different methods. Thus, a strain that produces good yields in solid-state or liquid-surface fermentation would not necessarily be a good producer in submerged fermentation. Another approach for strain improvement has been the parasexual cycle. Diploid strains display higher citric acid yields compared to their parent haploids, but they tend to be less stable. The protoplast fusion technique appears to be a promising tool to extend the range of genetic manipulation of *A. niger* with respect to citric acid production. It has produced fusant strains that have acid production capacities exceeding those of the parent strains.

TABLE III.29. Raw materials employed for citric acid production

| Fermentation type | Raw material | Strain | Citric acid production | Yield (percent) |
|---|---|---|---|---|
| SSF | Apple pomace | A. niger NRRL 567 | 883 g/kg[a] | – |
| SMF | Beet molasses | A.niger ATTC 9142 | 109 g/L | – |
| SMF | Black strap molasses | A. niger GCM 7 | 86g/L | – |
| SMF | Brewery wastes | A. niger ATTC 9142 | 19 g/L | 78.5 |
| SMF | Cane molasses | A. niger T 55 | – | 65 |
| SSF | Carob pod | A. niger ATCC 9142 | 264 g/kg | 60 |
| SMF | Carob pod extract | A. niger | 86 g/L | |
| SSF | Carrot waste | A. niger NRRL 2270 | 29 g/kg[a] | 36 |
| SSF | Cassava bagasse | A. niger LPB-21 | 347 g/kg[c] | 67 |
| SSF | Cellulose hydrolysate and sugarcane | A. niger | 29 g/kg | 44 |
| SMF | Coconut oil | C. lipolytica N-5704 | – | 99.6[b] |
| SSF | Coffee husk | A. niger CFTRI 30 | 150 g/kg[c] | – |
| SMF | Corn starch | A. niger IM-155 | – | 62 |
| SSF | Corncob | A. niger NRRL2001 | 250 g/kg | 50 |
| SMF | Date syrup | A. niger ATTC 9142 | – | 50 |
| SSF | Deoiled rice bran | A. niger CFTRI 30 | 92 g/kg | – |
| SMF | Glycerol | C. lipolytica N-5704 | – | 58.8[b] |
| SSF | Grape pomace | A. niger NRRL 567 | 600 g/kg[a] | – |
| SMF | Hydrolysate starch | A. niger UE-1 | 74 g/L | 49 |
| SSF | Kiwifruit peel | A. niger NRRL 567 | 100 g/kg[a] | – |
| SSF | Kumara (starch containing) | A. niger YANG n° 2 | 103 g/kg[c] | – |
| SSF | Mussel processing wastes (polyurethane foams) | A. niger | 300 g/kg | – |
| SMF | n-Paraffin | C. lipolytica N-5704 | – | 161[b] |
| SSF | Okara (soy residue) | A. niger | 51 g/kg[a] | 53 |
| SMF | Olive oil | C. lipolytica N-5704 | – | 119[b] |
| SSF | Orange waste | A. niger | 46 g/kg | – |
| SMF | Palm oil | C. lipolytica N-5704 | – | 155[b] |
| SSF | Pineapple waste | A. niger ACM 4942 | 194 g/kg[c] | 74 |
| SMF | Rapeseed oil | A. niger | – | 115[b] |
| SSF | Rice bran | A. niger CFTRI 30 | 127 g/kg | – |
| SMF | Soybean oil | Y. lipolytica A-101 | – | 63 |
| SMF | Soybean oil | C. lipolytica N-5704 | – | 115[b] |
| SSF | Sucrose (Sugarcane bagasse) | A. niger CFTRI 30 | 174 g/kg[b] | – |
| SSF | Sugarcane-pressmud and wheat bran (4:1) | A. niger CFTRI 30 | 116 g/kg | – |
| SSF | Wheat bran | A. niger CFTRI 30 | 85 g/kg | – |

| SMF | Wood hemicellulose | *A. niger IMI- 41874* | 27 g/L | 45[a] |
|---|---|---|---|---|
| SSC | Xylan and xylan hydrolysate | *A. niger YANG n⁰ 2* | 72 g/L | – |
| SSC | Yam bean starch | *A. niger YW-112* | – | 74[a] |

[a]Based on sugar consumed        SSF = solid-state fermentation
[b]Based on oils and fatty acids    SMF = submerged fermentation
[c]Based on dry matter              SSC = semi-solid culture

## CITRIC ACID PRODUCTION TECHNIQUES

Citric acid production by fermentation can be divided into three phases, which are preparation of inoculation and raw material, fermentation, and recovery of the product. Industrial citric fermentation can be carried out by three different methods: submerged fermentation (SmF), surface fermentation, and solid-state fermentation (SSF) (*koji* process).

### Submerged Fermentation

It is estimated that about 80 percent of world production of citric acid is obtained by submerged fermentation. The process employed on a large scale requires sophisticated installations and rigorous control. On the other hand, it presents several advantages such as higher productivity and yields, lower labor costs, and decreased contamination risk and labor consumption. Submerged fermentation can be carried out in batch, fed-batch, or continuous systems, although the batch mode is most frequently used. Different types of media employed demand pretreatment, addition of nutrients, and sterilization. After preparation, the medium is transferred into the fermentor and inoculated either by adding a suspension of spores with a surfactant in order to disperse them in the medium or a suspension of precultivated mycelia in which an inoculum size of 10 percent of fresh medium is generally required. The first two to three days are the most critical for the whole process, and the success of the process is determined by the metal ion contamination of the raw material used. Fermentation is normally concluded in 5 to 12 days depending on the process conditions.

Two types of fermentors are employed in submerged fermentation: conventional stirred tank fermentors and tower fermentors, although the latter is preferred due to the advantages it offers in price, size, and operation. Preferentially, fermentors are made of resistant materials such as high-grade steel because of the low pH level that develops during fermentation and the fact that citric acid is strongly corrosive. Also, fermentation requires provision of high dissolved oxygen tension, which makes an efficient aeration system necessary. Starting the process with low aeration in the phase of conidia germination and first mycelium growth is usually preferred because of economy.

### Surface Fermentation

Liquid-surface culture is the classic citric fermentation process and was the first industrial method of manufacture. It is still in use in small and medium-sized industries because it requires less effort in installation, operation, and energy cost. The process is carried out in a fermentation chamber in which trays are arranged in shelves. The culture solution is held in shallow trays with capacity of 0.4 to 1.2 m$^3$, and the fungus develops as a mycelial mat on the surface of the medium. The fermentation chambers are provided with effective air circulation, which passes over the surface to control humidity and temperature by evaporative cooling. This air is filtered through a bacteriological filter. The chambers should always be in aseptic conditions and should be conserved mainly during the first two days when spores germinate. Refined or crude sucrose and cane syrup or beet molasses are generally used as sources of carbon. The raw material is diluted to obtain 14 to 15 percent sugar, and pH is adjusted to 5.0 to 5.5. After sterilization and the addition of nutrients, the medium is transferred to trays. Inoculation is done by introducing spores into the system, either as a spore suspension or by mixing spores with the air blown over the tray surface. During fermentation, which is completed in 8 to 12 days, high amounts of heat are generated, presenting the need for high aeration rates to control the temperature and to supply air to the microorganism. After fermentation, the contents are separated into crude fermented fluid and mycelial mats, which are washed to remove the citric acid.

### Solid-State Fermentation

Solid-state fermentation, also known as the *koji* process, was first developed in Japan, where abundant raw materials such as fruit residues and rice bran are available. It is the simplest method for citric acid production and has been an alternative way to use agroindustrial residues. The solid substrate is moistened to about 70 percent moisture, depending on the substrate absorption capacity, and its initial pH is normally adjusted to 4.5 to 6.0. The temperature of incubation is about 28 to 30°C according to the microorganism used, and the process is completed within 90 hours under optimal conditions. The most commonly used organism in SSF is *A. niger*. However, there also have been reports with yeasts. The strains with large requirements of nitrogen and phosphorus are not ideal microorganisms for solid culture due to the lower diffusion rate of nutrients and metabolites occurring at lower water activity. In SSF, the presence of trace elements may not affect citric acid production as harmfully as it does in submerged fermentation, thus, substrate pretreatment is not required. Several types of fermentors have been used for citric acid production in SSF such as Erlenmeyer conical flasks, glass incubators, trays, rotating-drum bioreactors, packed-bed column bioreactors, single-layer packed-bed, multilayer packed-bed, etc. Classically, however, SSF has been carried out in trays, which facilitates aeration.

## FACTORS AFFECTING CITRIC ACID PRODUCTION

### Carbon Source

Citric acid accumulation is strongly influenced by the type and concentration of the carbon source. The presence of carbohydrates, which are rapidly taken up by microorganisms, has been found to be essential for good production of citric acid. Sucrose is the most favored carbon source, followed by glucose, fructose, and galactose. Glucose and fructose used together produce more acid than if used individually. Although sucrose is not taken up by the fungus, its hydrolysis has proven to be unnecessary because part of sucrose is broken down during sterilization of nutrient medium. In addition, the fungus possesses an extracellular mycelium-bound invertase, which is active under acidic conditions and is capable of hydrolyzing sucrose. Galactose contributes to a very slow growth of fungi and does not provide citric acid accumulation. Other sources of carbon such as cellulose, ethanol, sorbose, manitol, lactic acid, malic acid, and α-acetoglutaric acid allow limited growth and low production of citric acid. Starch, pentoses (xylose and arabinose), sorbitol, and pyruvic acid slow down growth of the fungus and provide minimum acid production. A maximal production rate is generally achieved in the range of 14 to 22 percent sugar. An initial sugar concentration of about 10 percent was reported as optimal for maltose, sucrose, mannose, and fructose, and 7.5 percent for glucose. No citric acid was produced at sugar concentrations of less than 2.5 percent. Studies have shown that initial glucose concentration affects both the rate of citric acid fermentation by *A. niger* and the morphology of the microorganism. Some critical factors such as cost and need for pretreatment should be considered for substrate selection.

### Phosphorus Source

Presence of phosphate in the medium strongly affects yield of citric acid. However, if the concentration of the metal ion is correctly maintained, the effect of phosphate is not so important. Low levels of phosphate have a positive effect in citric acid production, but the presence of excess phosphate leads to a decrease in fixation of carbon dioxide, increases the formation of certain sugar acids, and stimulates growth. Potassium dihydrogen phosphate has been reported to be the most suitable phosphorus source. Phosphorus at concentrations of 0.5 to 5.0 g/L is required by the fungus in a chemically defined medium for maximum production of citric acid.

### Nitrogen Source

Synthesis of citric acid is directly influenced by the concentration and nature of the nitrogen source. Nitrogen is generally supplied by salts such as urea, ammonium nitrate and sulfate, peptone, malt extract, etc. Urea has an absorbent effect, which assures pH control. Ammonium nitrate in higher amounts leads to the accumulation of oxalic acid, which is undesirable. Ammonium sulfate increases citric acid production without the formation of oxalic acid. Acidic ammonium compounds are preferred because their consumption leads to pH decrease, which is essential for citric acid fermentation. The concentration of the nitrogen source required for citric acid fermentation is generally between 0.1 to 0.4 g N/L. High nitrogen concentrations increase fungal growth and sugar consumption but decrease the amount of citric acid produced. Depending on the level of nitrogen in the medium at the start of fermentation, it is possible to produce either citric acid alone or a mixture of citric acid with other acids, such as gluconic acid.

Different microorganisms require different amounts of nitrogen and phosphorus in the medium. Strains with large requirements of N and P seem to be disfavored, due to the restriction of accessibility to the nutrients in the medium. The influence of the relationship between nitrogen and oxygen in citric acid production has also been studied. The production rate in the nitrogenous medium (0.01 g/L of ammonium nitrate) was 33 percent higher when oxygen was used instead of atmospheric air during the production phase. However, in the nonnitrogenous production medium, citric acid production was not influenced considerably when oxygen was used instead of air.

### Trace Elements

The presence of trace elements in raw materials, mainly in the submerged process, is the main problem in citric acid accumulation by *A. niger* because these elements can act as inhibitors and/or stimulants. High zinc levels maintain the fungus culture in the growth phase, which obstructs citric acid accumulation, while low zinc levels limit the growth of the fungus passing into the citric acid producing phase. Zinc favors the production of citric acid if added with potassium dihydrogen phosphate. The presence of a high level of manganese in the medium inhibits citric acid accumulation, increases cell growth, and decreases sugar consumption. Manganese deficiency represses anaerobic and tricarboxylic acid cycle enzymes with the exception of citrate synthetase, leading to overflow of citric acid as an end product of glycolysis. Even very low levels of manganese (about 1 ppm) are capable of reducing the yield of citric acid by 10 percent. Copper is capable of compensating for the effect of manganese in citric fermentation, perhaps through interference in manganese absorption by the cells. The presence of different copper concentrations in the pellet formation medium is very important in order to enhance a suitable structure, related to cellular physiology for citric acid production. Addition of iron decreases citric acid accumulation and has some effect on mycelial growth. Copper complements the ability of iron at an optimum level to enhance the biosynthesis of citric acid. Magnesium ion is required in the medium for fungus growth as well as for citric acid production. Optimal concentration of magnesium sulfate is in the range of 0.02 to 0.025 percent. A phosphate-free medium with manganese, iron, and zinc in high concentrations could cause the reduction of citric acid yields.

## *Lower Alcohols*

Lower alcohols added in pure material inhibit citric acid production but enhance production when added to crude carbohydrates. Methanol, ethanol, *n*-propanol, isopropanol, and methyl acetate neutralize the negative effect of metals in citric acid production, generally in amounts of about 1 to 5 percent. However, the optimal amount of methanol and ethanol depends upon the strain and the composition of the medium. Alcohols have been shown to principally act on membrane permeability in microorganisms by affecting phospholipid composition. They stimulate citric acid production by affecting growth and sporulation through action not only on cell permeability but also on space organization of the membrane or changes in lipid composition of the cell wall. Methanol is frequently used in citric fermentation in amounts that vary from 1 to 4 percent, but some research has shown that amounts up of 6 percent can yield high values of citric acid. Methanol is not assimilated by *A. niger* but helps in conditioning of mycelia without impairing their metabolism, and its presence might increase cell permeability to citrate.

## pH

The pH of a culture may change in response to microbial metabolic activities. The most obvious reason is the secretion of organic acids such as citric acid, which will cause pH decrease. Changes in pH kinetics also depend highly on the microorganism. With *Aspergillus* sp., *Penicillium* sp., and *Rhizopus* sp., pH can drop very quickly to less than 3.0. For other groups of fungi such as *Trichoderma, Sporotrichum,* and *Pleurotus* sp., pH is more stable between 4.0 and 5.0. The nature of the substrate also influences pH kinetics. A low initial pH, generally below 2.0, is of extreme importance for maximum production of citric acid and has the advantage of checking contamination and inhibiting oxalic acid formation. A pH about 3.0 could be optimum for fungus growth as well as for production of citric acid when used with a synthetic medium or pure carbon source, whereas a higher pH about 5.0 or 6.0 has been found to be optimum for citric acid production in molasses medium because some impurities of that material interfere with fungus germination and sometimes even with its development.

### Aeration

Because citric fermentation is an aerobic process, oxygen supply has a determinant effect on its production. Increased aeration rates lead to enhanced yields and reduced fermentation time. An interruption of aeration during batch fermentation will be quite harmful. Aeration should be performed through the medium during the whole fermentation process with the same intensity, although for economic reasons it is usually preferred to start with low aeration rates. The incorporation of oxygen together with atmospheric air in submerged fermentation results in increase of citric acid production but is economically unviable. However, it is possible to recirculate oxygen in the fermentor because the carbonic gas is removed from the process. High aeration rates lead to high amounts of foam, especially during the growth phase, so the addition of antifoaming agents and the construction of mechanical "defoamers" are required to tackle this problem. It has been reported that forced aeration in the beginning of fermentation in packed-bed reactors from solid-state fermentation allows high metabolic rates and, thus, high reactor productivities to be achieved. However, it is important to avoid the adverse effect of shear stress on the filamentous fungus, which may be caused by high airflow rates. Fungus mycelia immobilization by adsorption onto cellulose supports or into calcium alginate gel can reduce stress conditions on mycelia and decrease shear stress during operation conditions in conventional aerated or agitated bioreactors.

## PRODUCT RECOVERY

The two conventional processes for recovery of citric acid from fermented media are precipitation with calcium hydroxide slurry and extraction by solvent. In the precipitation method, acid is transformed into tricalcium citrate tetrahydrate that is lightly soluble. The precipitate is recovered by filtration and treated with sulfuric acid to obtain citric acid and to remove calcium in the form of calcium sulfate (gypsum). Then, citric acid solution is treated with active carbon and passed through cation and anion exchangers. Finally, the liquor is concentrated in vacuum crystallizers at 20 to 25°C, forming citric acid monohydrate. Anhydrous citric acid is obtained at crystallization temperatures higher than 36.5°C. The crystals are separated by centrifugation, and the drying is conducted at a temperature below 36.5°C for monohydrate product and above this for anhydrous product. Solvent extraction is another alternative to purify and crystallize citric acid. The mother liquor contains a small amount of impurities captured by the solvents. This method has the advantage of avoiding the use of calcium hydroxide and sulfuric acid, which are employed in high amounts, and the production of gypsum that presents elimination problems. Liquid-liquid extraction of citric acid has been found to be a promising alternative to the conventional process. Suitable extractants such as phosphorous-based, oxygen-containing, and amine-based extractants with functional groups effective for reversible complexation with acids should be used.

In recent years, some methods were developed to decrease the cost of the recovery, trying to overcome the drawbacks of the precipitation process, which have been responsible for the formation and disposal of enormous amounts of calcium sulfate, leading to pollution problems. Electrodialysis is an electrochemical separation process in which electrically charged membranes and electrical potential difference are used to separate ionic species from aqueous solutions. This technique is efficient in citric acid recuperation but is more expensive than current industrial-scale citric acid recovery processes. High costs of specific electromembranes and electric energy limit the electrodialysis applications to only high-value-added products. Many solid adsorbents have been considered for subsequent product recovery and used in batch fermentations. The advantage of a sorption method is simplification in the production flow sheet and technology. Citric acid production integrated with in situ product recovery may have the potential to increase the productivity and minimize process waste streams. An anion-exchange resin-packed column was attached to a fermentor for separation of citric acid from the fermentation broth. The broth was then returned to the fermentor and reused. This technique increases citric acid productivity and sugar conversion. Supported-liquid membrane is also being used to separate citric acid from fermented broth. The liquid membrane consists of an organic solution composed of trilaurylamine and a long-chain alcohol dissolved in a inert hydrocarbon solvent, which is immobilized in a microporous polypropylene support. Supported-liquid membranes offer some advantages such as overall recovery-cost reduction, lower energy consumption, higher separation factors in a single stage, ability to concentrate citric acid during separation, and smaller size of the complete separation plant. Different cross-linked copolymer polyacrylamide gels with variable amounts of cationic copolymer have been used to concentrate solutions of citric acid. Recovery of citric acid using this kind of gel is highly dependent on pH and on the percentage of fixed charges inside the gel. The advantages of using gels are that they have good absorption of ionic solutes and they are easily regenerated.

## SUGGESTED READINGS

Grewal HS and KL Kalra (1995). Fungal production of citric acid. *Biotechnology Advances* 13:209-234.

Kubicek CP and M Rohr (1986). Citric acid fermentation. *CRC Critical Reviews in Biotechnology* 3:331-373.

Pandey A, CR Soccol, JA Rodriguez-Leon, and P Nigam (2001). Production of organic acids by solid state fermentation. In *Solid-state fermentation in biotechnology—Fundamentals and applications*. New Delhi: Asiatech Publishers, Inc., pp. 113-126.

Röhr M, CP Kubicek, and J Kominek (1983). Citric acid. In *Biotechnology,* Volume 3, G Reed and HJ Rehm (eds.). Weiheim, Germany: Verlag Chemie, pp. 419-454.

Vandenberghe LPS, CR Soccol, A Pandey, and JM Lebeault (1999). Microbial production of citric acid. *Brazilian Archives of Biology and Technology* 42:263-276.

# Gallic Acid

## Rintu Banerjee

## INTRODUCTION

One of the important polyphenolic compounds present in plants is tannin, which is believed to occur in the vacuoles of intact plant cells, although some plants accumulate tannin in the bark and heartwood to protect them from unwanted microbial attack. Tannin is defined as water-soluble phenolic compounds with molecular weight ranging from 500 to 3,000 kDa. This compound also has properties to bind with the other macromolecules present in plant cells such as cellulose, proteins, gelatins, and pectins to form an insoluble complex.

## CLASSIFICATION OF TANNINS

Tannins can be broadly classified into two groups, hydrolyzable tannins and condensed tannins, as shown in Figure III.33 and Figure III.34. Hydrolyzable tannins consist of polyhydric alcohol esterified with gallic acid or derivatives of gallic acid. They can be further subdivided into gallotannins and ellagitannins. When hydrolyzed, gallotannin yields glucose and phenolic acid. Gallic acid is part of the core moiety of this group. On the other hand, when ellagitannin is hydrolyzed, it yields glucose and ellagic acid. Condensed tannins are made up of phenols of the flavone type and are often called flavolans because they are polymers of such flavan-3-ols as catechin or leucocyanidins. In contrast to the hydrolyzable tannins, sugar moiety is absent. A typical condensed tannin can be represented by the dimer procyanidin, to which the molecules of flavan can be added.

Hydrolyzable tannins can be cleaved by the enzymatic method. The enzyme responsible for this is called tannin acyl hydrolase, or tannase, which mainly acts on the ester and depside linkages in methyl gallate and *m*-digallic acid as shown in Figure III.35. Condensed tannin does not act by the enzyme tannase. There are some reports on the hydrolysis of condensed tannin, such as (−)epicatechin gallate and (−)epigallocatechin-3-gallate present in tea with the application of tannase.

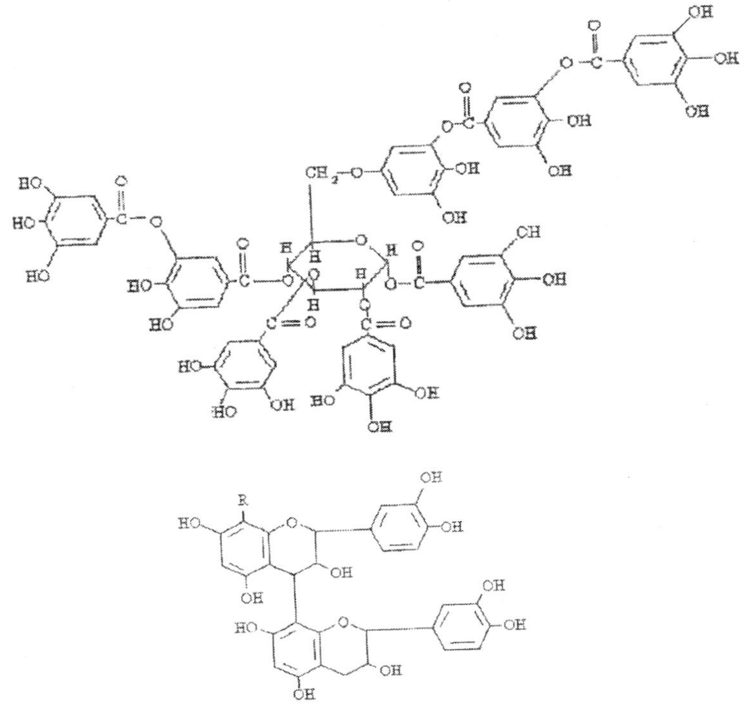

FIGURE III.33. Hydrolyzable tannin (top) and condensed tannin (bottom)

## PRODUCTION OF GALLIC ACID

Research has shown that tannase synthesis and gallic acid production are directly proportional. As more tannase is synthesized, more gallic acid is produced. Some organisms reported to produce tannin acyl hydrolase are *Aspergillus oryzae, A. niger, A. flavus, A. flaviceps, A. fumigatus, A. foetidus, A. japonicus, A. nidulans, A. pseudoflavus, A. parasiticus, A. tamarii, A. terreus, A. ustus, Penicillium chrysogenum, P. fellutanum, P. islandium, P. notatum, P. variable, Neurospora, Mucor prainii, Trichothecium roseum, Chaetomium globosum, Ascochyta boltshauseri, Bacillus pumilus, B. polymyxa* Q-47, *Klebsiella pneumoniae* Q-52, *Corynebacterium* sp., *Corynebacterium* Q-40, *Candida* sp., *Phycomyces blakesleeanus*, etc. *Rhizopus oryzae* RB13 NRRL 21498 and *Aspergillus foetidus* GMRB-013 MTCC 3557 are

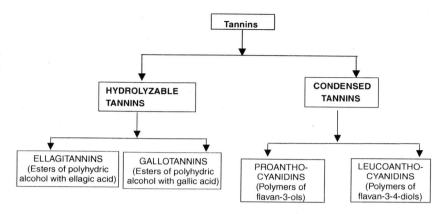

FIGURE III.34. Classification of tannins

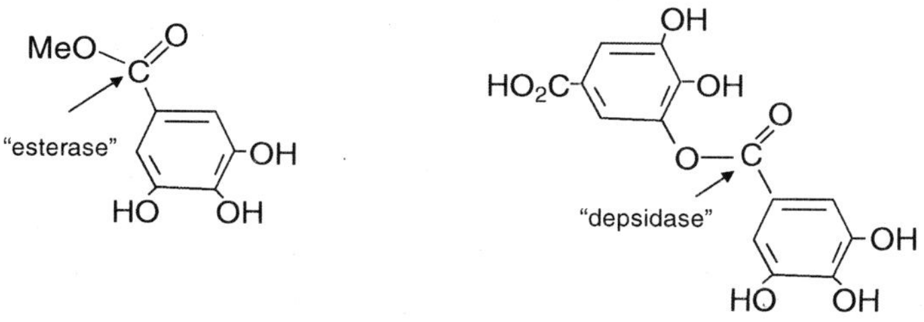

FIGURE III.35. Esterase and depsidase activities of tannase

two potent fungi isolated from the soil of the Indian Institute of Technology (IIT) Kharagpur campus. In addition to microorganisms, there are different sources of plant materials in which the tannin content of the raw materials varies from sample to sample. Important sources of hydrolyzable tannins are as follows:

- Gallotannin: Turkish tannin (*Quercus infectoria,* Fagaceae galls), Chinese tannin (*Rhus semialata,* Anacardiaceae galls), tara pods (*Caesalpinia spinosa,* Leguminosae), sumac leaves (*Rhus coriaria,* Anacardiaceae), staghorn sumac (*Rhus typhina,* Anacardiaceae)
- Ellagitannin: Myrobalan tannin (nuts of *Terminalia chebula*), algarobilla tannin (fruit pods of *Caesalpinia brevifolia*), divi-divi tannin (fruit pods of *Caesalpinia coriaria*), valonea tannin *(Quercus velonia,*

*Quercus aegilops),* oak bark tannin (bark of *Quercus* sp.), Garouille (root bark of *Quercus coccifera*), chestnut oak (bark of *Quercus prinus*), chestnut tannin (wood of the tree *Castanea sativa*).

- Condensed tannins: wattle tannin *(Acacia mollissimia),* quebracho tannin *(Schinopsis lorentzii),* cutch tannin *(Acacia catechu),* gambier tannin *(Uncaria gambier).*

Production of gallic acid with special emphasis on the optimization of extracellular tannase by pure substrate and pure culture, mixed substrate and pure culture, and mixed substrate and mixed culture techniques has been described. The fermentation conditions selected for these studies are submerged fermentation (SmF), solid-state fermentation (SSF), and modified solid-state fermentation (MSSF) methods. Agrorich residues such as myrobalan and gallo seed cover were used as the sole carbon sources. To meet the nutritional requirement of the organisms, modified Czapek-Dox medium was used where the carbon source was tannin-rich agro residues. Modified solid-state fermentation as developed in the author's laboratory gave the best result because some of the disadvantages of SSF could be easily overcome by the MSSF method of cultivation. When the three methods were compared as shown on Table III.30, maximum yield of gallic acid was 90.9 percent in the MSSF method of cultivation.

Microorganisms are highly dependent on environmental conditions for their growth, and the product yield is in turn dependent on the synthesis of the enzyme. The traditional approach is to change one control variable at a time while holding the rest constant. This method is inefficient in finding the true optimum condition, especially due to the probable interactions among the factors. Evolutionary Operation (EVOP), a multivariable search technique, could be applied very judiciously for studying bioprocesses. In

TABLE III.30. Comparison of different types of fermentation conditions

| SL. NO. | Parameters | SSF Range | SSF Optimum | SmF Range | SmF Optimum | MSSF Range | MSSF Optimum |
|---|---|---|---|---|---|---|---|
| 1 | Incubation period (h) | 24-96 | 72 | 24-96 | 48 | 24-96 | 72 |
| 2 | Substrate content | 0.5-4 | 2.0 | 2.5-20 | 10 | 5-40 | 20 |
| 3 | Initial pH | 3-6.5 | 4.5 | 3-6.5 | 5.0 | 3-6.5 | 4.5 |
| 4 | Temperature (°C) | 20-40 | 32 | 20-40 | 37 | 20-40 | 32 |
| 5 | Relative humidity (%) | 67-94 | 93 | | | 67-94 | 93 |
| 6 | Fermentation condition | Stationary | | Agitation | | Stationary | |
| 7 | Tannase activity (U/ml) | 18.87 | | 23.86 | | 32.76 | |
| 8 | Galic acid yield (%) | 30.48 | | 27.5 | | 90.9 | |

this methodology, the effects of two or three factors are studied together and the responses are analyzed statistically to arrive at the decision. The Evolutionary Operation technique has a clear-cut decision-making procedure, but in this process more than three variables are difficult to study. Considering the advantages of both of the methods, a new optimization technique, namely EVOP-Factorial design, has been developed to optimize the mixed culture process. These techniques were used for gallic acid production. It can be seen from Table III.31 that there was improvement in the yield of gallic acid, and the maximum yield recorded was 94.1 percent based on the total tannin content of the raw materials.

Extraction of gallic acid from fermented biomass in pure form is complex and needs careful investigation. A number of parameters influence the extraction process of gallic acid. The recovered gallic acid is analyzed by the melting-point method and thin-layer chromatography. Purity of recovered gallic acid is determined by a nuclear magnetic resonance (NMR) study.

## *PROPERTIES AND APPLICATIONS OF GALLIC ACID*

Gallic acid (3,4,5-trihydroxy benzoic acid) is a phenolic compound, which is sparingly soluble in cold water but is soluble in warm water (60°C). It is soluble in organic solvents such as ether, chloroform, and alcohol. Enzymatic hydrolysis has an advantage over the method of acid hydrolysis, the former being less energy intensive and less polluting. The major use of gallic acid is in pharmaceutical industries for the manufacture of trimethoprim (TMP), an antibacterial agent which is usually given along with sulfonamide. Together they have a broad spectrum of action. The consumption efficiency of gallic acid in the manufacture of trimethoprim is 4.8. Gallic acid is also used in enzymatic synthesis of gallic acid esters, e.g., propyl gallate, which is mainly used as an antioxidant in fats and oils, as well as in the manufacture of pyrogallol. Pyrogallol is used in staining fur, leather, and hair and also is used as photographic developer.

TABLE III.31. Coculture studies

| Parameters studied | Range | Optimum |
|---|---|---|
| Incubation period | 24-96 h | 48 h |
| Inoculum volume | 1-4 ml | 3 ml |
| Temperature | 25-40°C | 30°C |
| pH | 4-7 | 5 |
| Humidity | 70-90% | 80% |
| Gallic acid yield | | 94.1% |

## CONCLUSIONS

The degradation of hydrolyzable tannins and the correlated production of tannase have been well known for many years in fungal cultures, but the production by *Rhizopus oryzae* and *Aspergillus foetidus* were the first case in which a promising amount of bioconversion was observed. Gallic acid has numerous industrial applications, hence there are ample opportunities to work on biotechnological conversion of tannins to gallic acid.

## SUGGESTED READINGS

Haslam E, RD Haworth, and PF Knowles (1961). Gallotannins. I. Introduction and fractionation of tannase. *Journal of Chemical Society* 358:1829-1935.

Kar B, R Banerjee, and BC Bhattacharyya (1999). Microbial production of gallic acid by modified solid state fermentation. *Journal of Industrial Microbiology and Biotechnology* 23:173-177.

Lekha PK and BK Lonsane (1997). Production and application of tannin acyl hydrolase: State of the art. *Advances in Applied Microbiology* 44:215-260.

Pourrat GN, F Regerat, P Morvan, and A Pourrat (1987). Microbial production of gallic acid from *Rhus coriaria* L. *Biotechnology Letters* 9(10):731-734.

# Lactic Acid

Hwa-Won Ryu
Jong-Sun Yun
Young-Jung Wee

## *INTRODUCTION*

Lactic acid ($CH_3CHOHCOOH$, 2-hydroxypropionic acid) is a naturally occurring, chiral, and hydroxycarboxylic acid with a long history of use in the food industry. It was first discovered in sour milk by the Swedish chemist Scheele in 1780. Lactic acid is a versatile chemical, used as an acidulant, flavoring agent, and preservative in the food, pharmaceutical, leather, and textile industries, as well as for the production of principal chemicals. It can be polymerized to biodegradable polylactic acid and can be produced by biotechnological fermentation or chemical synthesis. It exists as two optical isomers, D(−)- and L(+)-lactic acid. The biotechnological fermentation of lactic acid has gradually received more interest in industrial applications due to the depletion of petroleum feedstocks and environmental problems, and has the advantage that by choosing a strain of lactic acid bacteria producing only one of the isomers, an optically pure product can be obtained, whereas chemical synthesis always results in a racemic mixture. It is also possible to use renewable feedstocks as substrates, such as starch and cellulose, during these fermentations.

Lactic acid is soluble in all proportions with water and exhibits a low volatility. Self-esterification often occurs in lactic acid solutions because of the hydroxyl and carboxyl functional groups. Although lactic acid is widely present in nature and has been produced as a by-product of many fermentation processes, it is not a large-volume produced chemical. Its worldwide production volume by 1999 had grown to approximately 80,000 tons/year. Lactic acid is thought of as a relatively mature fine chemical in that its use in only new applications, i.e., as a monomer in plastics or as an intermediate in the synthesis of high-volume oxygenated chemicals, would cause a significant increase in anticipated demand.

## PRODUCTION TECHNOLOGIES

### Microbial Synthesis

#### Microorganisms

In 1857, Pasteur first discovered that microorganisms caused the souring of milk. The presence of lactic acid bacteria in distilleries was noted in the 1860s and 1870s, and their growth characteristics were extensively investigated. Lactic acid bacteria consist of the Gram-positive genera: *Lactobacillus, Lactococcus, Enterococcus, Leuconostoc, Carnobacterium, Oenococcus, Pediococcus,* and *Streptococcus.* Strains of *Lactobacillus delbrueckii* have often been used for the commercial production of lactic acid. Currently, the strains used in industry are almost all proprietary, but it is believed that most of organisms used to belong to the genus *Lactobacillus.*

*Classification.* Lactic acid bacteria may be classified into two groups; homofermentative, which convert glucose almost quantitively to lactic acid, and heterofermentative, which ferment glucose to lactic acid, ethanol, acetic acid, and $CO_2$. Only the homofermentative microorganisms are currently found in industrial applications for lactic acid manufacturing. Homofermentative lactic acid bacteria are from the genera *Lactobacillus, Streptococcus,* and *Pediococcus* and are typically facultative anaerobes, but they are unable to synthesize adenosine triphosphate (ATP) by respiration. However, because lactic acid fermentations are carried out at high temperatures, low oxygen concentrations, high lactate concentrations, and low pH, severe contamination problems usually do not occur.

Homofermentative lactic acid bacteria catabolize glucose through glycolysis (Embden-Meyerhof pathway). As glycolysis results in only lactic acid as the end product of glucose metabolism, two lactic acid molecules are produced from each molecule of glucose, typically with a yield of more than 90 g lactic acid per 100 g glucose. Pentoses are also catabolized by some homofermentative microorganisms, with both acetic and lactic acid being the products of their metabolism. Microorganisms may produce L(+)-, D(−)-, or DL-lactic acid. The racemic DL-lactic acid could be formed by the action of two stereospecific lactate dehydrogenases or from one stereospecific dehydrogenase and a racemase.

#### Substrates and Nutrients

A number of different carbohydrates have been used, examined, or proposed for the manufacture of lactic acid by fermentation. The purest product is obtained when a pure sugar is fermented, resulting in lower purification costs. However, this is economically unfavorable, because pure sugars are expensive and lactic acid is a relatively cheap product. Raw materials for industrial lactic acid fermentations need to have desirable characteristics, such as a low cost, low levels of contaminants, a rapid fermentation rate, high lactic acid yields, little or no by-product formation, ability to be fermented with little or no pretreatment, and year-round availability. Crude feedstocks have traditionally been avoided because undesirable components in these substrates can cause separation problems in the recovery stage.

Glucose and maltose from hydrolyzed starch, whey-containing lactose, and sucrose from beet and cane sugar have been commercially used for lactic acid fermentation. Glucose from starchy materials is the most commonly used carbon source, and concentrated whey has been used without any other pretreatment. Molasses, a by-product of the sugar manufacturing process, is an efficient raw material for use in the fermentation industry, but its complex nature leads to difficulties in the recovery stages. Cellulosic materials such as corncobs, corn stalks, cotton seed hulls, waste paper, and woods have been also used. They consist mainly of hexoses, such as glucose, galactose, and mannose, and pentoses, such as xylose and arabinose, and need to be first hydrolyzed to monomers before they can be fermented. When using starch or cellulose as a carbon source, which also must be hydrolyzed before fermentation, the saccharification and fermentation steps can be achieved separately or simultaneously.

In addition to carbon sources, nitrogen sources, such as malt extract, corn-steep liquor, yeast extract, etc., are essential for fast and efficient lactic acid fermentation. Higher nutrient concentrations generally result in a positive effect on lactic acid fermentation. Some growth-enhancing substances in these nutrients, such as amino acids and vitamins, are labile to heat. Minimal amounts of nitrogen sources should be used in order to simplify the recovery process and reduce the production cost. Additional minerals are occasionally required when the carbon and nitrogen sources lack sufficient quantities.

Lactic acid bacteria are generally fastidious microorganisms and have complex nutrient requirements due to their limited ability to synthesize B vitamins and amino acids. Many growth stimulation factors have considerable effects on the fermentation rate. In many cases, mixtures of amino acids, peptides, and amino acid amides provide a characteristic increase in growth, the resulting growth rates being much higher than those obtained with free amino acids. Fatty acids also influence the growth of lactic acid bacteria, and phosphate is the most important salt required. Ammonium ions cannot serve as the sole nitrogen source, but they seem to have some influence on the metabolism of certain amino acids. The presence of minerals does not seem to be critical, and the natural content of complex media is in most cases sufficient.

*Fermentation Process*

Batch fermentation is a common method for industrial lactic acid production, but numerous investigations on continuous cultures as well as some fed-batch and repeated-batch fermentations exist. Batch fermentation is superior to continuous fermentation in all aspects except volumetric productivity. Repeated batch operations increase the lactic acid yield. If the substrate is expensive, the yield should be maximized, as in batch or repeated-batch operations, whereas the volumetric productivity should be maximized by continuous fermentation if investment costs are high. A high productivity is achieved by recycling the cells, resulting in a high cell mass without reducing the yield. Fermentation time is varied according to the selected strain but typically is one to two days for a 5 percent carbon source such as whey and two to six days for a 15 percent initial sugar such as glucose or sucrose. The productivities and yields of lactic acid after the fermentation stage are 1 to 3 g/L per h and 90 to 95 percent based on the initial sugar concentration, respectively. The yield of cell mass depends heavily on the amount of nitrogen sources used. The fermentation rate depends primarily on the temperature, pH, and concentration of carbon and nitrogen sources. Batch fermentations done with a controlled pH will proceed quickly at first. As the fermentation proceeds, the fermentation rate begins to slow because of the depletion of effective nutrients and the accumulation of lactic acid, with the undissociated or electroneutral form of lactic acid being more likely to inhibit the fermentation than lactate.

Lactic acid formed must be neutralized by the addition of salts such as calcium carbonate, calcium hydroxide, sodium hydroxide, and ammonium hydroxide. The neutralizing agent can be added in excess as slurry at the beginning of the fermentation or added intermittently during fermentation on the basis of the pH measurement. Calcium carbonate or calcium hydroxide is traditionally added to the fermentation broth to neutralize the lactic acid produced, giving calcium lactate, but the regeneration of lactic acid results in the production of large amounts of solid calcium sulfate. The broth containing calcium lactate is filtered to remove cells, carbon treated, evaporated, and acidified with sulfuric acid to convert the salt into lactic acid and insoluble calcium sulfate, which is removed by filtration. The filtrate is further purified by carbon treatment, ion exchange process, and evaporation to produce technical and food-grade lactic acid.

The recovery of lactic acid or lactate salts from the fermentation broth corresponds to a large portion of the total cost of manufacturing. Higher lactic acid concentrations and yields are achievable through the continuous removal of lactic acid using an in situ separation process such as extraction or electrodialysis. The extracting material must be biocompatible so as not to harm the microorganisms, and one way of achieving this is through aqueous two-phase systems, which provide good separation of lactic acid when combined with a tertiary amine. Recent developments in membrane-based separation and purification technologies, particularly in ultrafiltration and electrodialysis, have led to the foundation of new processes for lactic acid recovery. These processes lead to low-cost production of lactic acid, with a reduction in the amount of nutrient needed and without the problem of by-product formation. Electrodialysis can be used in two ways: as a pH controller producing the lactate anion, or in combination with sodium hydroxide to split the sodium lactate into sodium hydroxide and lactic acid. Desalting electrodialysis has been shown to require low quantities of energy to recover, purify, and concentrate lactate salts from crude fermentation broths. The recent developments in water-splitting electrodialysis with bipolar membranes enable the efficient production of protons and hydroxyl ions from water and can thus produce both an acid and a base from a salt solution. These advances have led to the development of proprietary technologies for lactic acid production from carbohydrates without producing salt or by-products.

### Chemical Synthesis

The chemical synthesis of lactic acid on a commercial scale began around 1963 in Japan and the United States. The chemical synthesis routes produce only a racemic lactic acid mixture, and commercial process is based on the hydrolysis of lactonitrile ($CH_3CHOHCN$), a by-product from acrylonitrile synthesis, by a strong acid. It involves base catalyzed addition of hydrogen cyanide (HCN) to acetaldehyde ($CH_3CHO$) to produce lactonitrile. This is a liquid-phase reaction that is followed by distillation, and the lactonitrile is then hydrolyzed to lactic acid using a concentrated strong acid, such as hydrochloric or sulfuric acid. This crude lactic acid is esterified with methanol, forming methyl lactate, which is then recovered and purified by distillation of the ester and hydrolyzed by water under acid catalysts to produce lactic acid. Further purification and concentration are achieved through steaming, carbon treatment, and ion exchange steps.

Another method for the chemical synthesis of lactic acid includes the continuous hydrolysis of lactonitrile in an aqueous sulfuric acid solution.

The resulting lactic acid is extracted with a solvent, such as isopropyl ether, and then recovered by back extraction with water. However, although these and other synthetic routes for lactic acid production have been developed, they are seen as economically and technically unfeasible processes.

## USES AND APPLICATIONS

Lactic acid is used in a wide range of food, cosmetic, pharmaceutical, and industrial applications (Table III.32). It is widely used in almost every segment of the food industry, where its products serve a wide range of functions: flavoring, pH regulation, improving microbial quality, and mineral fortification. Lactic acid is used extensively by the processed meat and poultry industry to give products an extended shelf life and enhanced flavor and to provide better control of food-borne pathogenic bacteria. It is also used in salads, dressings, and pickled vegetables that have a mild flavor, while maintaining microbial stability and safety, and is the preferred acidulant in delicately flavored soft drinks and fruit juices, giving rise to the mild acidity of juices and health and soft drinks.

Lactic acid and lactates are increasingly being used in many types of technical products and processes. Their main functions or properties make them useful as descaling agents, pH regulators/pH buffers, neutralizers, chiral intermediates, solvents, cleaning agents, slow acid release agents, metal-complexing agents, antimicrobial agents, and humectants. Natural lactic acid offers an excellent and safe solvent alternative—in a pure or a wipe solvent formulation—for many fine mechanical cleaning applications and for cleaning prior to the application of top coats. Its high solvency and specific solubility make it an excellent remover of polymers and resins. It is available in an enantiomeric purity higher than 98 percent and is suitable as a starting material in the synthesis of chiral products, e.g., herbicides or pharmaceuticals. Lactic acid is used as a monomer for polylactides, a new generation of biodegradable commodity plastics, and as a metal-complexing agent in Ni-plating processes because of its unique complexing constant for Ni. It offers better descaling properties than conventional organic descalers and is, therefore, used in many decalcification products such as cleaners for toilets, bathrooms, and coffee machines. Lactate esters can be used for degreasing and precision cleaning since they combine an excellent solvency for oils and oligomeric and polymeric stains with optimal environmental and toxicological properties.

Lactic acid offers natural products for use in cosmetic applications. With its multifunctionality, as a moisturizer and pH regulator, its humectancy, and antimicrobial nature, it is an ideally standard ingredient in the formula-

TABLE III.32. Applications of lactic acid and its derivatives

|  | Main functions and properties | Applications |
|---|---|---|
| Food | Flavoring | Meat and poultry products |
|  | pH regulation | Health and nutrition |
|  | Improving microbial quality | Pickled vegetables |
|  | Mineral fortification | Confectionery |
|  |  | Sugar-free products |
|  |  | Beverages |
|  |  | Dairy |
|  |  | Baked goods |
|  |  | Flavors |
| Industry | Descaling agents | Aerospace industry |
|  | pH regulators/pH buffers | Chemical industry |
|  | Neutralizers | Detergents |
|  | Chiral intermidiates | Metal industry |
|  | Solvents | Microelectronics industry |
|  | Cleaning agents | Paint and dye industries |
|  | Slow acid release agents |  |
|  | Metal-complexing agents |  |
|  | Antimicrobial agents |  |
|  | Humectants |  |
| Cosmetics | Moisturizers | Skin care |
|  | Skin rejuvenating agents | Toiletries |
|  | pH regulators | Antiperspirants |
|  | Skin-whitening agents | Oral care |
|  | Antiacne agents | Hair care |
|  | Humectants | Special skin care |
|  | Antitartar agents |  |
| Medical and Pharmaceutical | Electrolytes | Parenteral/IV solutions |
|  | Mineral sources | Dialysis solutions |
|  |  | Mineral preparations |
|  |  | Tabletting |
|  |  | Medical and pharmaceutical implants |

tion of a good base for cosmetic products. Every day the human body produces about 120 g of lactic acid. Lactic acid is also part of the NMF (natural moisturizing factor), which retains moisture in the skin. Being a natural ingredient and a natural constituent of the human body, lactic acid and lactates fit perfectly in today's trend toward natural and safer formulations and also possess special features as a skin-lightening and skin-rejuvenating chemical that make them very useful as active ingredients.

Lactic acid is also used in pharmaceutical and medical applications. It is commonly used as an electrolyte in many parenteral/IV solutions intended for fluid or electrolyte replenishment, such as Lactated Ringer's or Hartmann's solutions and in continuous ambulatory peritoneal dialysis (CAPD) solutions for nephric patients and in dialysis solutions for conventional artificial kidney machines. Furthermore, it is used in a wide variety of mineral preparations, tabletting, implantable medical devices, and pharmaceutical controlled drug-delivery systems.

It is also receiving a great deal of attention as a feedstock monomer for the manufacturing of polylactic acid (PLA) as a biodegradable commodity plastic. NatureWorks PLA, developed by Cargill Dow LLC, based in Minnetonka, Minnesota, will produce more than 300 million pounds (140,000 metric tons) of PLA annually. It will be the first commercially viable polymer produced from renewable resources that performs as good as or better than traditional polymers and is fully compostable in industrial and municipal compost facilities. Its future applications could include use in injection blow-molded bottles, foams, emulsions, and chemical intermediates. Furthermore, because lactic acid has an excellent reactivity that stems from it having both carboxylic and hydroxyl groups, it can undergo a variety of chemical conversions into potentially useful chemicals such as propylene oxide, propylene glycol, acrylic acid, 2,3-pentanedione, and lactate esters (Figure III.36).

## CONCLUSIONS

The opportunities for future growth in the application of lactic acid are classified into four categories: biodegradable polymers, oxygenated chemicals, green chemicals or solvents, and plant-growth regulators. PLA, the polymers of lactic acid, are biodegradable thermoplastics. These versatile yet biodegradable polymers are obtainable by copolymerization with other functional monomers, such as glycolides, caprolactones, and polyether polyols. The polymers are transparent, an important factor for packaging applications, and provide a good shelf life because they degrade slowly through hydrolysis, which can be controlled by adjusting their composition and molecular weight. They also have potential for use within a wide variety of consumer products, such as paper coatings, films, molded and foamed articles, and fibers.

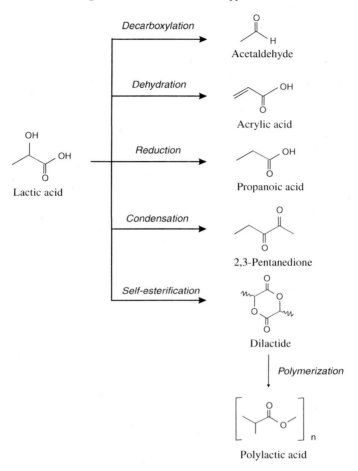

FIGURE III.36. Conversion pathways of lactic acid as an alternative feedstock of the petrochemical industry

## SUGGESTED READINGS

Datta R, SP Tsai, P Bonsignore, SH Moon, and JR Flank (1995). Technological and economic potential of poly(lactic acid) and lactic acid derivatives. *FEMS Microbiology Review* 16:221-231.

Varadarajan S and DJ Miller (1999). Catalytic upgrading of fermentation-derived organic acids. *Biotechnology Progress* 15:845-854.

VickRoy TB (1985). Lactic acid. In *Comprehensive biotechnology*, Volume 3, M Moo-Young (ed.). New York: Pergamon Press, pp. 761-776.

Wilke D (1999). Chemicals from biotechnology: Molecular plant genetics will challenge the chemical and fermentation industry. *Applied Microbiology Biotechnology* 52:135-145.

# Pigment Production

Kishor S. Wani
Bhushan S. Naphade
Bhushan L. Chaudhari
Sudhir B. Chincholkar

## INTRODUCTION

Since prehistoric times, pigments from animal, vegetable, and mineral sources were used for decorating tools, weapons, utensils, and cloths and for making pictures. Vegetative materials such as flowers, seeds, berries, nuts, bark, wood, and root plants served as materials of choice due to their frequent and easy availability. Most of these pigments were fugitive and soon faded when exposed to sunlight (being unsaturated). Exceptions were colors obtained from the madder root, the wood plant, or from the lac insect, which under not too unfavorable conditions sometimes lasted for centuries. Even the world famous paintings from the Ajanta Caves (India) have remained for several centuries.

Pigments are chemical substances that impart color to other materials. However, a pigment incorporated in paint could be defined as a powdered substance which, when mixed in the liquid vehicle, imparts color to a painted surface. Pigmentation occurs in nearly all living organisms. Almost all plants synthesize their own pigments, but animals may derive pigments from plant foods or synthesize them themselves. In plants, major pigments are the chlorophylls (green), carotenes (reddish orange to yellow), and the anthocyanins (red, blue, and violet). The red and yellow colors of autumn foliage are due to the exposure of anthocyanins after the decomposition of green chlorophyll pigments, which usually mask them.

The major animal pigments are the hemes (red) of blood hemoglobin, the carotenes, melanin (black and brown), and guanine (white and iridescent), wherein the latter three produce the surface coloration in most animals. In human beings, the degree of darkness of the skin, hair, and iris of the eye depends primarily on the amount of melanin present. The presence of hemoglobin and carotene in the blood contributes to skin color. The coloration may be caused by deposits of organic pigments in the tissues (as in human skin or in plant leaves), by optical effects of the refraction of light rays (as in mollusk shells and some butterfly wings and bird feathers), or by a combination of both. The pigmentation of many animals is adapted to their environment and aids in their survival. Pigments not only provide external coloration but also function in some physiological processes. In the retina of the eye, the pigment cells (of rods and cones) adjust or regulate the entering light. Among its other functions, carotene operates in the synthesis of vitamins and even chlorophyll.

## PLANT PIGMENTS

### Plant Pigments for Color and Nutrition

The pigments found in plants play important roles in plant metabolism and visual attraction in nature. Major plant pigments include carotenoids, anthocyanins and other flavonoids, betalains, and chlorophylls.

Plant pigments are important cues to humans and other herbivorous animals in helping identify plants, find plant parts such as fruit, leaves, stems, roots, or tubers, and determine stages of plant developments such as fruit ripeness. It was realized early in the twentieth century that many of these pigments play a positive role in human health. In 1919, Steenbock noted that yellow corn (*Zea mays* L.) and "yellow" vegetables [carrots (*Daucus carota* L.) and sweet potato (*Ipomoea batatas* L.)] eliminated the symptoms of vitamin A deficiency in rats. Since then, 40 carotenoids have been found to be vitamin A precursors. When provitamin carotenoids are consumed, they are enzymatically broken down to retinol (vitamin A).

Horticulturists have long studied plant pigments in vegetables, fruits, and ornamental crops because of their vital role in visual appeal. The orange and red vegetables (carrot, sweet potato, and tomato) have been listed as major sources of provitamin A carotenoids. Chemical and biotechnological approaches for the improvement of plant pigments are also encouraging.

### Modern Trends in Plant Pigment Production

In recent years, the demand for natural food colorants has increased due to adverse effects of synthetic colorants. Several food colorants such as anthocyanins and betalains are being produced in plant cell cultures and hairy root cultures at levels much higher than those in intact plants. In selected cell lines, carotenoids (carotenes and lycopenes) varied from 3 to 40 percent of that present in yellow-orange edible portions of carrot.

The high cost of saffron *Crocus sativus* L. (saffron plant) is due to the fact that the species grows only in specific geographic regions of the world and is labor intensive. About 150,000 flowers are required for obtaining 1 kg of saffron stigma. Direct production of stigmas in vitro has always been a challenging task for tissue culturists. Japanese scientists have cultured young stigmas and ovaries of saffron on Linsmeir and Skoog (LS) medium, which directly produced stigma-like structures (SLS) containing yellow pigments (crocin). Callus cultures raised on Murashige-Skoog (MS) tissue culture medium supplemented with 2,4-dichlorophenoxy acetic acid (2,4-D) and kinetin also produced red pigmentation, e.g., crocin and crocetins.

Internationally, the anthocyanin from grape is the most abundant source. However, anthocyanin from *Camellia japonica* and *Perilla* sp. is in great demand in Japan. Anthocyanins are stable at acidic pH. The acylation imparts greater stability and hence is preferred for food colors. Because of its increasing demand and GRAS (generally regarded as safe) status, a biotechnological method of production is currently being pursued.

Plant cell cultures appear to be an excellent source for anthocyanin production in view of the high productivity, ranging from 1 to 2 percent on dry weight basis of cells. A strain of *Euphorbia millii*, after 24 selections, accumulated about seven times higher amounts of anthocyanins.

Shikonin is a red-colored compound synthesized in cells of *Lithospermum erythrorhizon* from shikimic acid and isoprenoid pathways. By applying cell line selection, the pigment of shikonin from callus of *L. erythrorhizon* was increased by 12 percent on dry mass in cell cultures. Due to instability of production in cell cultures, recent approaches toward organ cultures, particularly transformed root (hairy root) cultures, are being explored.

### Production of Dyes from Traditional Plants

Recent changes in legislation on the use of some toxic synthetic dyestuffs and an increased preference by consumers for natural products have combined to reawaken an interest in dyes derived from crops. There is a growing consumer demand for naturally dyed textiles and nontoxic dyes for foodstuffs. Woad *(Isatis tinctoria),* Chinese woad *(Isatis indigotica),* madder *(Rubia tinctorum),* weld *(Reseda luteola),* and others are the dye plant species producing the primary colors, blue, red, and yellow.

The only source of blue pigment is woad indigo. In warmer climates, *Indigofera* yielded higher amounts of indigo. The roots of *Rubia tinctorum* (dyers madder, Rubiaceae), a perennial plant, produces a complex red dye. *Anthemis tinctoria* (yellow chamomile, Compositae) is a hardy perennial that produces a mass of foliage from which many yellow flowers emerge and which produces a deep yellow dye. *Reseda luteola* (weld, Resedaceae) is a perennial plant that produces a yellow dye in its stems, foliage, and flowers. *Reseda* species contain yellow flavonoids, mainly luteolin and apigenin but also at least three other components including quercetin. *Solidago canadensis* (goldenrod, Compositae), a common garden plant, is a tall perennial shrub that grows throughout the British Isles and produces a different yellow dye.

These dye plants have remained unimproved since 15,000 B.C. However, they possess great potential for improvement by classical breeding, selecting the best strains from progeny of crosses.

### Novel Sources for Natural Colorants

Recent reports provided a base for the availability of novel pigment sources. Extraction of fresh large cardamom pod husk with methanolic hydrochloric acid has yielded a mixture of two (deep pinkish red) pigments. Vitisin A and B and vitisidin A and B are four new anthocyanin pigments found in both red table wines and fortified wines in trace amounts and are thought to be formed in wines during maturation.

## MICROBIAL PIGMENTS

### Sources and Applications

In nature, a variety of microorganisms exhibit wide diversity in pigment production and have spectacular applications in the food, textile, and pharmaceutical industries (Table III.33). One of the leading microbial pigments is derived from *Janthinobacterium lividum* (bluish-purple color from wet silk thread). This bacterium was reported to produce large amounts of bluish-purple pigment violacein and deoxyviolacein on some media containing amino acids, such as Wakimoto medium. This pigment could be used to dye natural fibers such as silk, cotton, and wool as well as synthetic fibers such as nylon and vinylon; the shade depends on the material. The colorfastness of the dyed material could be about the same as that of materials dyed with vegetable dyes, but the color fades easily when the material is exposed to sunlight. Because the pigment can be produced in bulk quantity by culturing, these shortcomings could be overcome.

*Phaffia rhodozyma* is the only known yeast that produces astaxanthin, a red pigment having an application for fish feeding. *Flavobacterium multi-*

TABLE III.33. Pigment-producing microorganisms and their uses

| Name of organism | Pigment name and color | Uses |
|---|---|---|
| *Janthinobacterium lividum* | Mixture of violacein and deoxyviolacein (bluish purple) | For dyeing silk, cotton, wool, nylon, and vinyl fibers |
| *Flavobacterium multivorum* | Carotenoid (zeaxanthin) (yellow) | As a food colorant, in cosmetics, for coloring of legs, beaks, fat, flesh, and egg yolk of poultry |
| *Monascus purpureus* | Monascin and ankaflavin; rubropunctatin and monascorubin rubropunctamine and monascorubramine (yellow, orange, red) | As a food colorant in yogurt and others |
| *Haematococcus pluvialis* | Astaxanthin (red) | As animal feed, fish meal (salmonid pigmentation) |
| *Dunaliella salina* | Beta-carotene (yellow/orange) | Dietary supplement |
| *Cantharellus cinnabarinus* | Canthaxanthin (red) | Food and feed additives, in cosmetics and pharmaceuticals |
| *Chlorella pyrenoidosa* | Chlorophyll (deep emerald green) | As a food additive and in pharmaceuticals |
| *Spirulina* | Mixed carotenoid (phycocyanin) (deep blue green, red, and orange) | As a nutrient in pharmaceuticals |
| *Neospongiococcum excentricum* | Zeaxanthin (yellow reddish) | Colorant for poultry and fish |
| *Phaffia rhodozyma* | Carotenoid (astaxanthin) (red) | For coloring fish flesh and egg yolk |

*vorum* has been reported to produce a yellow-orange pigment, zeaxanthin, and the pigment-free cell mass is an ideal source of protein for poultry.

*Monascus* sp. is commonly employed for pigment production. A mutant strain, *Monascus* sp. B683M, obtained through ultraviolet (UV)-induced mutation of a locally isolated angkak strain, accumulated about 80 percent of the total pigments intracellularly. *Monascus purpureus* CCM 8112 has been successfully used in solid-state fermentation using natural cereal substrates such as rice, wheat, and puffed substrates. Pigment production depended on $a_w$ (moisture) and reducing sugar content in the substrate. *Haematococcus pluvialis* is a ubiquitous, unicellular green algae that produces the red carotenoid pigment, astaxanthin, when entering the resting or "haematocyst" stage, which are harvested, dewatered, and mechanically broken to improve the bioavailability of astaxanthin.

### Production

The steps involved in the pigment-production process are as follows:

- Selection of suitable species and strain for pigment production
- Optimization in terms of productivity and yield
- Development of cheap industrial media to support optimal microbial yield
- Identification and optimization of conditions for pigment accumulation
- Development of bioreactor designs, suitable for scale-up and for the mass cultivation of biomass
- Optimization of conditions in the bioreactor, downstream processing, and storage of the pigment
- Demonstration of the use of the pigment

The main hurdle to investigate new colorant sources is the cost to carry out the necessary toxicological tests, which requires a major investment. The Commission of European Communities has estimated the cost of food-additive assessment to be more than US$1 million for each compound.

Dependent upon the type of pigment producer, a medium of choice could be employed for its cultivation and maximum enhancement in pigmentation. Although the medium of choice differs for each individual microorganism, attempts have been made to use renewable carbon sources for the cultivation and pigment benefication of microorganisms. For instance, soy-soaking water, a wastewater of the industry from the soybean soaking phase, can be used for the cultivation of *M. purpureus*. In *Hypomyces* fungi, a 1 to 2 percent starch-containing syrup available from food industry waste is employed as a source of carbon. For astaxanthin, a red-colored pigment from *P. rhodozyma,* fermentation is performed in a fed-batch manner. The start wort has the following composition: (g/l) molasses 20, diammonium sulfate 0.6, diammonium hydrogenphosphate 0.8, and magnesium sulfate 0.125. The cultivation conditions are monitored as per requirement of the microorganism, and the process is optimized by the standardization of physico-chemical parameters.

## LEGISLATION INVOLVED IN THE USE
## OF MICROBIAL PIGMENTS

An official publication of the American Association of Feed Control Officials provides a list of microorganisms that the U.S. Food and Drug Administration (FDA) considers to be GRAS for use as food additives and for use in the production of food additives. The difference in number of permitted natural colors among countries arises from difference in emphasis, intent, and concern. In Europe, some colors are accepted that are not allowed in the United States. There is an even longer list of colorants approved in Japan that are not approved in the United States. Some are totally unknown to American product developers but have been used for many years in the Far East.

## PRESENT STATUS OF MICROBIAL PIGMENTS

Food coloration has been used for a long time; devoid of any nutritional value, this technological operation enables better food presentation. The development of products with an attractive appearance has always been an important goal in the food industry. There has been considerable interest worldwide in the development of food pigments from natural sources. Colorants from microbial species offer advantages because they are not subject to the vagaries of nature. Recent investigations made into new pigments are, for the most part, confidential. Commercialization of many of these pigments is increasing day by day. At present, the following microbial pigments are among those being commerically produced: *Monascus* (as lactopurpurin); astaxanthin (as AstaXin) of Igene Biotechnology Inc., Columbia, Maryland; CAROPHYLL Pink of Hoffmann-La Roche Ltd., Cambridge, Ontario; astaxanthin of Mera Pharmaceuticals Inc.; Beta-carotene of Parry Nutraceuticals, Parry Agro Industries Ltd.; *Spirulina* of New Ambadi Estates Pvt. Ltd., chlorella of Taiwan Chlorella Manufacturing Co. Ltd.

## CONCLUSIONS

A large global market exists for food colorants of about US$5 billion annually, of which synthetic colors enjoy a share of $4 billion, while only about $1 billion is expended for natural food colorants. However, there is an annual growth rate of 4 percent for natural food colorants compared to 2 to 3 percent for synthetic colorants. The potential market for astaxanthin pigments is approximately $200 million per year. Based on current production numbers and a more efficient means to produce natural astaxanthin, it is estimated that the natural material will cost 20 to 30 percent less than the synthetic material.

In Japan and European countries, the demand for synthetic colors has reduced. In the United States and much of the rest of the world, however, synthetic colors continue to grow annually. The current popularity of natural colorants is due to two factors. One is the public distrust of food additives in general, and the other is the perceived problem of safety with food colorants. In a nutshell, it seems that consumers make a close link between "health" and "natural" and believe that "natural is better." Due to this, it is expected that the demand for natural pigments will increase.

## SUGGESTED READINGS

Clement JS, TJ Mabry, H Wyler, and AS Dreiding (1994). Chemical review and evolutionary significance of the betalains. In *Carryophyllales: Volution and systematics*, HD Behnke and TJ Mabry (eds.). Berlin, Germany: Springer Verlag, pp. 247-261.

Pszczola DE (1998). Natural colours: Pigments of imagination. *Food Technology* 52:70-82.

Slugen D, SS Menta, and M Rosenberg (1998). Role of pH and $a_w$ for solid-state pigment cultivation of *Monascus purpureus* CCM 8112. Paper presented at the French Association for Development of Biotechnology and Bio-Industry (ADEBIO) symposium "*Monascus* Culture and Applications," July 8-10, Toulouse, France.

Sundara VR (1999). Natural food colors for commercial applications: A global perspective. In *Trends in food science and technology, Proceedings of technical sessions*. Mysore, India: Association of Food Scientists and Technologists (AFST) and Central Food Technological Research Institute (CFTRI), 5.5:146.

Wisgott U and K Bortlik (1996). Prospects for new natural food colorants. *Trends in Food Science and Technology* 7:298-302.

# Polyhydroxyalkanoate Production from Renewable Resources

Irene K. P. Tan

## INTRODUCTION

### Plastics: The Material

Plastic, with all its myriad properties and uses, is one of man's greatest inventions, taking into consideration all its positive features of inertness, lightweight, strength, imperviousness, and durability. Plastic has been used to make a wide spectrum of products, ranging from those that need to be durable to single-use disposables. Undeniably, such products have contributed significantly to modern lifestyles that include relatively easy and cheap transportation, high levels of sanitation, and consumer convenience. The euphoria did not last for long, however, as the negative impact of plastics on the natural environment was increasingly realized. To be fair, the material itself should not be considered the culprit, as it performs what for it is designed to. The problem lies largely in the indiscriminate disposal of synthetic plastics. Some of these disposable products, particularly those used in medical and sanitary applications (gloves, syringes, tubes, sanitary napkins, diapers, etc.), may have strong justification. Others such as packaging materials and cutleries seem frivolous in comparison. Nevertheless, they collectively contribute to environmental pollution, which has assumed global proportions because synthetic plastics are cheap and therefore widely utilized.

### The Problem

Synthetic plastics are not degradable and are not compatible with natural biogeochemical cycling of elements. They can not be composted with other organic solid wastes. Most disposed plastic materials end up in landfills where they take up precious space because they are also resistant to anaerobic decomposition. Incineration of plastics has been known to release toxic

653

compounds into the atmosphere. Animals have been trapped and killed by plastic bags and fishing lines and nets. Plastics are polymers of high molecular mass and are usually hydrophobic. If the undegraded material is allowed to accumulate in soil, e.g., when plastic products disintegrate into fine particles or powder (the molecular size and structure of the polymer do not change), this hydrophobicity would alter the physical and chemical nature of the soils, e.g., by reducing the water-holding capacity, which in turn would reduce the microbial population in the soil. As a result, soil quality deteriorates.

Synthetic plastics are made from petrochemicals at costs currently far below any alternative materials. However, stockpiles of fossil fuel are not infinite, therefore, petrochemicals are not renewable. If modern standards of health and living are to be maintained, then alternative materials to synthetic plastics must be developed, and they should have the following properties:

1. They should degrade readily and completely after disposal, and not leave toxic or hazardous intermediates in the natural environment.
2. They should be synthesized from renewable resources.
3. Such new materials should have properties and applications similar to synthetic plastics.

## PLASTIC DEGRADATION

With enforced legislation and increasing consumer demands for environmentally degradable plastic products, standards are drawn up, e.g., by ASTM (American Society for Testing and Materials) and ISO (International Organization for Standardization), to define the various forms of plastic degradation and to provide test protocols to determine the degradation. Plastics can degrade by various means:

1. *Photochemically:* Ultraviolet (UV) light energy breaks up some chemical bonds in the polymer.
2. *Chemically:* Chemical bonds are broken by oxidation in air or hydrolysis in water.
3. *Biochemically:* Chemical bonds are broken by enzymes.

Photodegradable and oxidizable polymers have some chemical bonds broken either by irradiation energy or oxygen. The polymer thus breaks down into oligomers, which, due to their simpler forms, may be more amenable to mineralization or cometabolization by microbes. However, these smaller molecules may also be recalcitrant in the natural environment and bring about different sets of problems such as toxicity, increased mobility and solubility, and biomagnification. One criticism questions the practicality of such polymers, because most products end up in landfills after disposal where the necessary light energy or oxygen is not available to initiate degradation.

Biodegradable polymers are defined as those whose chemical bonds are broken by microbial enzymes, which either mineralize the polymer or reduce it to intermediates that can be metabolized by microorganisms and plants. A significant advantage of biodegradable polymers is that they can be stored for longer periods between manufacture and usage. This is because biodegradable polymers require an environment of high microbial activities, such as that present in compost and landfills, in order to be degraded. Photodegradable and hydrolyzable polymers have to be stored properly, i.e., in the absence of light and moisture, if they are to retain their full functional properties at time of usage.

## BIOCOMPATIBILITY

Many biodegradable and hydrolyzable polymers have an additional positive feature of biocompatibility. This means that the polymer does not induce an adverse reaction from cells and tissues in contact with it, such as inflammation, tumor development, or tissue rejection. This property has immense applications in medical science, e.g., as tissue scaffoldings and surgical implants. If the material is both biocompatible and biodegradable, patients housing such products may not require additional surgery to have the inserts removed, thus reducing invasive procedures and trauma. This is an area in which the biggest growth of biodegradable and biocompatible polymers is envisaged, because the cost of such polymers is not the primary issue. However, in areas in which the need for biodegradable polymers is greatest, mainly in disposable plastic products, the cost of such polymers is the biggest deterrent to mass production and applications. Table III.34 shows some examples of environmentally degradable polymers with industrial potentials.

## POLYHYDROXYALKANOATES (PHAS)

PHA fulfills all the requirements desirable of an alternative material to conventional plastics:

1. It is a thermoplastic and has a wide range of chemical and material properties. Therefore, it can be used to make many types of products ranging from containers that require mechanical strength to impervious linings and adhesives.
2. It is biodegradable, nontoxic, and biocompatible.
3. The polymer is synthesized whole by bacteria and in plants. There is no need for additional chemical processes for polymerization.
4. It is produced from renewable resources, not dependent on petrochemicals.

PHA is a polyester produced naturally by many bacteria, usually as a carbon and energy storage material. It is composed of repeating units of 3-hydroxyalkanoic acids, each of which carries an aliphatic side-chain (R) (Figure III.37). The molecular weight of PHA ranges from $2 \times 10^5$ to $3 \times 10^6$. There are two main classes of PHA: the short-chain-length (scl) variety in which monomers are 4 to 5 carbon length, and the medium-chain-length (mcl) PHA in which monomers are 6 to 14 carbon length. The scl-PHA is typified by the well-known poly(3-hydroxybutyrate) (PHB), a homopolymer, and the poly(3-hydroxybutyrate-co-3-hydroxyvalerate) (PHBV) copolymer. The mcl-PHA are always heteropolymers, comprising, for example, 3-hydroxyhexanoate, 3-hydroxy octanoate, and 3-hydroxydecanoate monomers. The side chain (R) of mcl-PHA may be unsaturated. In the biosynthesis of PHB, two molecules of acetyl-CoA are condensed by the action of 3-ketothiolase to form acetoacetyl-CoA, which is reduced by an NADPH (nicotinamide adenine dihydrogen phosphate [reduced form])-dependent

TABLE III.34. Environmentally degradable polymers with industrial potential

| Polymer | Industrial use |
| --- | --- |
| Polyvinyl alcohol | Chemically synthesized, petrochemical feedstocks, hydrolyzable, allowed for food contact |
| Polycaprolactone | Chemically synthesized, petrochemical feedstocks, biodegradable, not suited for food contact |
| Polylactide | Monomers (lactic acid) made from renewable resources, polymerization by chemical processes, hydrolyzable, biocompatible, high potential in medical applications |
| Polyhydroxy-alkanoates | The whole polymer biosynthesized from renewable resources, biodegradable, biocompatible, mechanical strength, elastomeric, repel moisture, impervious to gas |
| Starch/cellulose-based composites | Natural products (starch/cellulose) blended with synthetics (petrochemicals), biodegradable but do not repel moisture, low cost gives it high potential for disposable products |

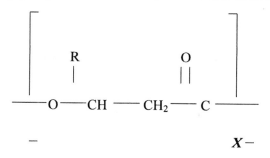

FIGURE III.37. General structure of a repeating unit of poly-3-hydroxyalkanoate. R = $-(CH_2)_n-CH_3$ where $n$ = 0 to 10 or more, $x$ = 4,000 to 20,000.

acetoacetyl-CoA reductase to form 3-hydroxybutyryl-CoA. The latter is added to the polymer chain by PHB synthase (polymerase). In the biosynthesis of the copolymer PHBV, the 3-hydroxyvalerate (3-HV) monomer could be formed directly from valeric acid or from a mixed substrate of glucose and propionic acid. In the latter case, acetyl-CoA and propionyl-CoA are first condensed to 3-ketovaleryl-CoA, then reduced to 3-hydroxyvaleryl-CoA and added to the polymer chain by PHB synthase. The scl-PHA are accumulated in large quantities in *Ralstonia eutropha* (formerly *Alcaligenes eutrophus*), *Azotobacter vinelandii*, *Alcaligenes latus,* and *Burkholderia cepacia* (formerly *Pseudomonas cepacia*).

The mcl-PHA are synthesized in bacteria that are different from those that synthesize the scl-PHA, because these two groups of bacteria have different sets of PHA-synthesizing enzymes. The mcl-PHA monomers are derived directly from the carbon substrate (alkanoic acids, alkanes, alkanols) or from intermediates arising from the beta-oxidation of long-chain carbon compounds, e.g., fatty acids. The mcl-PHA containing unsaturated monomers are derived from unsaturated carbon sources such as alkenes, fatty acids, and triglycerides. Only the fluorescent Pseudomonad group of bacteria is known to produce mcl-PHA, and the most commonly studied are *Pseudomonas oleovorans* and *P. putida*. Two PHA synthase genes are found in *P. oleovorans,* giving the bacteria the ability to incorporate a wide range of monomers to make a wide range of mcl-PHA.

In terms of material properties, PHB is highly crystalline and is, therefore, stiff and brittle. As such, the homopolymer has limited applications. Its copolymer, PHBV, however, is less crystalline, more flexible, and has a lower melting temperature $(T_m)$. Increasing the 3-hydroxyvalerate content in PHBV leads to increased toughness (elongation to break), lower $T_m$ and $T_g$ (glass transition temperature), and decreased stiffness and brittleness in the polymer. PHBV has been used to make bottles for personal-care products, disposable trays, and razor holders. The mcl-PHA are generally amorphous and elastomeric. Increasing chain length of the monomer leads to decreasing $T_g$ and $T_m$, with low or no crystallization. mcl-PHA occur as transparent films or as a sticky gel-like material, the latter being particular to those PHA with unsaturated carbon bonds. Cross-linking and binding with halogens are thus possible as a means of chemical modification. Potential applications would be lining and coating materials, adhesives, and controlled-release medium.

### Industrial Production of PHAs

The biggest drawback to mass production and applications of PHA is the cost of production. PHA is synthesized biologically, and currently the most viable factory is the bacterium. Biosynthesis and accumulation of PHA are triggered when the cells become stressed, e.g., by a deficiency in nitrogen or oxygen. The bacteria prepare for impending adverse conditions by synthesizing PHA as carbon and energy reserve. If we wish to exploit the bacteria as factories for PHA, we need to induce such adverse conditions, which may differ among different groups of bacteria producing different types of PHA. To maximize yield of PHA, cells should be harvested at peak PHA accumulation, i.e., before the intracellular PHA starts to be broken down as a source of food by the bacteria.

### Strategies to Counter High Production Costs of PHAs

#### Sources

In this era in which gene transfer has become almost a routine technology, producing recombinant microbes and transgenic plants appears to be the most likely route to maximize the yield of PHA from a producer organism. *Escherichia coli* has been successfully transformed with the operon for the synthesis of PHB, and it has potential as an industrial strain. Such novel organisms, however, do present challenges in terms of scaling-up production, a well-known one being genetic instability. Extra precautions and procedures may have to be incorporated into the bioprocess (e.g., addition of antibiotic into the fermentation medium) to maintain the integrity and expression of transformed microbes. Thus, the importance of screening for wild-type bacterial species and strains should not be overlooked nor underemphasized. In this respect, countries in the tropics, which have rich biodiversity, could be in a good position to tap their indigenous microbial resources and to link that to their natural renewable resources as feedstocks. In Malaysia, palm oil has been used as a sole carbon source to isolate and screen indigenous bacteria for the ability to synthesize mcl-PHA. Palm oil and its various components, such as fatty acids and glycerol, are readily available in Malaysia, and they are especially suited as feedstocks for the fermentation of mcl-PHA. Numerous studies have been conducted in producing scl-PHA copolymers in which some portions of the monomers are derived from nonnatural precursors such as 4-hydroxybutyric acid. Such copolymers possess improved material properties compared to the PHB homopolymer such as less brittleness and faster biodegradation. However, such copolymers are not totally synthesized from renewable resources. In comparison, mcl-PHA with different monomeric composition, giving it a range of material properties, is synthesized much more simply by using suitable microbes and suitable renewable precursors. A strategy for reducing production costs of mcl-PHA lies in obtaining bacterial strains that could metabolize triglycerides (vegetable oils or animal fats) directly and incorporate the range of fatty acids into the PHA.

There is much interest and ongoing effort to produce transgenic plants that carry the PHA-synthesizing genes to produce the polymer in large quantities. The rationale is that photosynthesizing plants would be the most efficient factory, with low maintenance requirements compared to microbial fermentation. One, however, should remember that once planted in the field, the crop would be subject to the vagaries of weather, soil quality, water and fertilizer supply, and pest control. Depending on where in the plant the PHA is synthesized, extraction and purification of the PHA would be no less difficult nor economical compared to PHA recovery from bacterial cells. A pertinent criticism questions the choice of planting crops for an industrial commodity such as plastics instead of as food to feed the world's ever-increasing human population, especially when arable land is at a premium and is decreasing in size.

## Substrates

The primary substrate to consider in terms of PHA fermentation is the carbon source. For economically viable fermentation, the primary feedstock should be renewable, readily available, and of considerable constant composition. The production cost of PHBV is high because glucose and propionic acid are used as carbon sources, and these are expensive because they are highly purified compounds and not bulk raw materials. Bulk or primary agricultural products such as sucrose, starch, and vegetable oils are much cheaper carbon substrates. Starch hydrolysates have been used by *R. eutro-*

*pha* and *Azotobacter chroococcum* to produce PHB, while vegetable oils and animal fats have been used by *Pseudomonas aeruginosa* and *P. resinovorans* to make mcl-PHA. *Pseudomonas oleovorans* and *P. putida* could not utilize oils directly because they do not produce lipase enzyme. However, they could convert fatty acids (if the oils are saponified) into mcl-PHA. Primary agricultural products may not be cheap, but they are renewable, and their diversified uses, e.g., as fermentation feedstocks, in addition to their primary use as food crop, would benefit the farmers and the countries that produce them. Attempts to utilize palm oil in Malaysia and sucrose in Brazil as feedstock for PHA fermentation should, therefore, be viewed positively as a means to integrate a renewable and readily available raw material with the industrial production of a highly desirable biodegradable plastic.

Effluents generated from farms and mills, e.g., molasses and whey, are often considered to be good and cheap sources of microbial nutrients because they have high concentrations of organic carbon, nitrogen, and trace elements. However, the composition of elements in effluents may be variable because the composition is influenced by many factors: slight changes in the processes that generate the effluents, the amount of sun, rain, and temperature during growth, maturation, and harvest of the crop. This variation in effluent composition may vary the yield as well as the quality of a microbial product. Using defined agricultural products such as sucrose and vegetable oil would produce a more predictable yield and quality. This is especially pertinent if the microbial product formed is influenced by the chemical composition of the feedstock, e.g., mcl-PHA. For these, the variable composition of effluents renders them unsuitable as feedstock. PHB, on the other hand, is not influenced by the chemical composition of the feedstock because the carbon substrate is first converted to acetyl-CoA, two of which will condense to form 3-hydroxybutyryl-CoA which is the monomeric building block of PHB. Thus, molasses and whey have individually been used as a primary carbon source by *A. vinelandii* and recombinant *E. coli,* respectively, to make PHB.

In addition to agricultural products, carbon dioxide, which is also a natural renewable resource, has been used as a carbon source. Successful utilization of $CO_2$ for PHA biosynthesis would be beneficial in this age of global warming. Autotrophic bacteria obtain energy for carbon dioxide fixation from hydrogen oxidation, e.g., *R. eutropha* has produced good yields of intracellular PHA by this method. The greatest challenge to advancing this technology is in maintaining a tight control on the gaseous composition in the bioreactor. Because $H_2$, $O_2$, and $CO_2$ are required for the autotrophic activities, this combination is also potentially highly combustible. Developments are ongoing to improve the bioprocess to reduce the hazard.

*Bioprocess Design*

The engineering aspect of scaling-up production of microbial PHA is important in improving yield. Because PHA is an intracellular granule and there is a limit to how much cells can enlarge physically to accommodate increasing amounts of PHA, it is reasonable to link high PHA yield to high cell density culture in the fermentation process. High cell density and high yields of PHBV are obtained from fed-batch (glucose and propionic acid) culture of recombinant *E. coli* and *R. eutropha*. Continuous cultures produced lower productivities due mainly to incomplete utilization of substrates. The PHA recovery and purification processes are important aspects to target in efforts to reduce production cost because they currently constitute half or more of the cost. PHAs are effectively extracted from cells by chlorinated solvents, such as chloroform, which solubilize the polyester. Then it is precipitated by methanol. This method is good for laboratory-scale studies because very pure polymers are obtained. However, it is too costly and environmentally unsound to be used on an industrial scale. Better recovery methods may replace hazardous extraction solvents with proteolytic enzymes, which digest the cells but not the PHA. Producing cells with fragile walls, which spontaneously burst to release the hydrophobic PHA, would be another option worth developing.

## CONCLUSIONS

Although the economic viability of producing bacterial PHA for bulk commodity applications remains challenging, it must be realized that the yardstick used, i.e., synthetic plastics, is not entirely comparable. One needs to incorporate the value of biodegradability of PHA and the benefits to the environment. In addition, the use of renewable resources to make PHA would remove the dependence on fossil fuel. Synthetic plastics have none of these attributes. Continued effort is needed to improve the technology of PHA production in all aspects: the producer organisms (both natural and recombinant), renewable feedstocks, and the bioprocess and recovery methods. It is envisaged that the cost of production will be reduced from its current amount, but one should not expect it to go as low as current production cost of synthetic plastics for all the reasons stated.

## SUGGESTED READINGS

Braunegg G, G Lefebvre, and KF Genser (1998). Polyhydroxyalkanoates, bio-polyesters from renewable resources: Physiological and engineering aspects. *Journal of Biotechnology* 65:127-161.

Choi J and SY Lee (1999). Factors affecting the economics of polyhydroxy-alkanoate production by bacterial fermentation. *Applied Microbiology and Biotechnology* 51:13-21.

Ishizaki A, K Tanaka, and N Taga (2001). Microbial production of poly-D-3-hydroxybutyrate from carbon dioxide. *Applied Microbiology and Biotechnology* 57:6-12.

Jendrossek D, A Schirmer, and HG Schlegel (1996). Biodegradation of poly-hydroxyalkanoic acids. *Applied Microbiology and Biotechnology* 46:451-463.

Poirier Y, C Nawrath, and C Somerville (1995). Production of polyhydroxy-alkanoates, a family of biodegradable plastics and elastomers in bacteria and plants. *Journal of Biotechnology* 13:142-150.

Steinbuchel A, E Hustede, M Liebergesell, U Pieper, A Timm, and H Valentin (1992). Molecular basis for biosynthesis and accumulation of polyhydroxy-alkanoic acids in bacteria. *FEMS Microbiology Review* 103:217-230.

# Pretreatment of Lignocellulosic Substrates

Poonam Nigam Singh
Tim Robinson
Dalel Singh

## INTRODUCTION

Lignocellulose is a compact, partly crystalline structure comprising the two most abundant polymers on earth: lignin and cellulose. Lignin is made by an oxidative coupling of three major $C_6$-$C_3$ phenypropanoid units, namely, syringyl alcohol, guaiacyl alcohol, and *p*-coumaryl alcohol. These are arranged in a random, irregular, three-dimensional network that provides strength and structure and is consequently very resistant to enzymatic degradation (Figure III.38).

Cellulose is made up of a linear polymer chain, which in turn consists of a series of hydroglucose units in glucan chains (Figure III.39). The hydroglucose units are held together by β-1-4 glycosidic linkages, producing a crystalline structure that can broken down more readily to monomeric sugars. Another major component of the lignocellulose structure is hemicel-

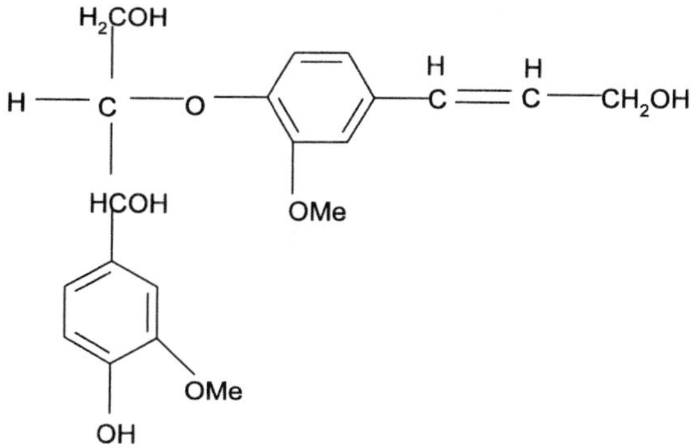

FIGURE III.38. Lignin structure

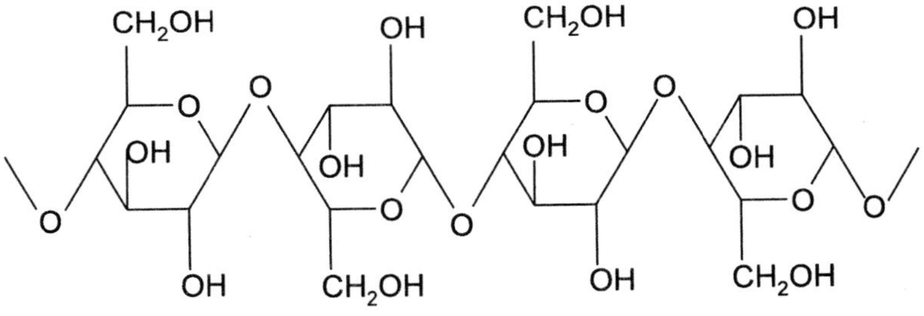

FIGURE III.39. Cellulose polymer chain

lulose, which is made up of various polysaccharides, namely, xylose, galactose, mannose, and arabinose. The function of hemicellulose has been proposed as a bonding agent between lignin and cellulose. Mannose can be used as a fermentable substrate by many yeasts, with more specific yeasts being able to utilize arabinose and xylose.

Lignocellulosic residues are an ideal energy source if the two components can be successfully separated or treated. Over 300 million tons of lignocellulose are produced annually worldwide. This renewable biomass has the potential to be used for the production of fuels, chemicals, animal feed, etc. Sometimes these agroindustrial residues are seen as waste and pose disposal problems for the associated industries. This can be solved through its utilization, turning a valueless waste into a valuable substrate for fermentation processes. The main components of lignocellulose and their occurrence in various agroindustrial residues are shown in Table III.35.

Because glucose can be readily fermented by most microorganisms, yielding a variety of products, it is very much in demand by the fermentation industries. Glucose as cellulose is present in large quantities in lignocellulosic residues, but its recovery from the lignocellulosic complex poses a problem. To make monomeric sugar utilization from these residues a viable option, various physical, chemical, and biological pretreatments have been explored (Table III.36).

## PHYSICAL PRETREATMENT

Mechanical and thermal methods exist to treat lignocellulose, but these methods tend to require a high-energy input which can increase the processing cost considerably. Product separation for fermentation purposes can also make physical pretreatments expensive.

TABLE III.35. Components of some lignocellulosic residues

| Lignocellulose residue | Lignin (%) | Cellulose (%) | Hemicellulose (%) |
|---|---|---|---|
| Corncobs | 15 | 45 | 35 |
| Maize straw | 13 | 32 | 28 |
| Oat straw | 18 | 49 | 25 |
| Rice straw | 17 | 35 | 25 |
| Spruce | 29 | 42 | 27 |
| Sugarcane bagasse | 14 | 33 | 22 |
| Wheat straw | 15 | 30 | 50 |

TABLE III.36. Pretreatment of lignocellulosic residues

| Pretreatment | Effect of pretreatment | Examples |
|---|---|---|
| Physical | Fine, highly decrystalized structure | Milling |
| | Increased pore size/hemicellulose hydrolysis | Steam explosion |
| | | Irradiation |
| | Depolymerization | |
| Chemical | Lignin/hemicellulose degradation | $NaOH$, $NH_3$, $H_2O_2$ |
| | | Peroxyformic acid, organosolvents |
| Biological | Lignin degradation | White-rot fungi (*Phanerochaete chrysosporium*, *Bjerkandera adusta*) |
| | | Specific bacteria |
| Enzymatic | Selective lignin/hemicellulose degradation | Lignin peroxidases (LiP, MnP, laccase) |

## *Steam Explosion*

One efficient physical pretreatment method is steam explosion, in which lignocellulosic biomass is pressurized with steam for a period of time followed by a rapid decompression, producing an explosive reaction that acts on the lignocellulose structure. This process is carried out at high pressure and high temperature (180 to 240°C) and breaks up the lignocellulose structure by blowing apart the three-dimensional lignin component, as well as causing the decomposition of some hemicellulose into uronic and acetic acids, which catalyzes the depolymerization of hemicellulose and lignin.

Once the lignin and cellulose components have been separated, efficient isolation of these components is required, which is a major constraint in this technology. It is, however, an essential and crucial part of the pretreatment or delignification process as, depending on the subsequent product, lignin needs to be fully removed. For example, if the cellulose will be used for high-quality paper or chemical production, then the quantity of lignin in the final product will affect its purity. Fractionation, separating the major components, can be carried out by solvent extraction.

Steam explosion as a pretreatment has been successfully carried out for ethanol production using agroindustrial residues such as rice and wheat straw. It has also been used for bioconversion of olive oil cake for the production of ethanol. Several other residues such as cassava bagasse, sugarcane bagasse, etc., have also been treated by steam explosion and then used for production of various other industrial products.

Steam explosion offers a variety of advantages for the pretreatment of lignocellulosic substrates because it allows increased susceptibility to cellulose-degrading enzymes. There are no recycling or environmental costs, unlike those associated with chemical treatments. In comparison to mechanical methods, such as milling, energy requirements are lower and can be reduced further through the use of more energy-efficient equipment.

If steam explosion is to be viable on an industrial scale, energy requirements need to be considered. Although this pretreatment is highly successful, it consumes large quantities of energy and subsequently has a high running cost. For example, the heat-insulating material of the explosion apparatus as well as the pressure and holding times should be optimized, improvements which may make this pretreatment more energy and economically efficient.

## CHEMICAL PRETREATMENT

Chemical pretreatments have been widely used to remove or degrade lignin content of lignocellulose. In paper and pulp industries, chemical pretreatments, such as alkali or acid hydrolysis, have commonly been employed to recover cellulose for paper production. These treatments tend to be expensive and are therefore not used for bioconversion purposes. Caustic swelling is a common chemical method that has the effect of increasing the surface area of the lignocellulose residue due to the swelling and disruption of lignin. Disadvantages of chemical pretreatments for lignin removal include the need for corrosion-resistant apparatus, an effective washing strategy, and the capability for the safe disposal of used chemicals.

## Hydrogen Peroxide ($H_2O_2$)

Hydrogen peroxide ($H_2O_2$) is used as a pretreatment for lignocellulosic residues at operational temperatures of $\geq 100°C$ in alkaline solution. In paper and pulp industries it is used for bleaching and delignification purposes (to improve the brightness of pulp as it reacts with colored carbonyl-containing structures in the lignin structure). Decomposition of $H_2O_2$ in alkaline conditions is rapid, and as a consequence more reactive radicals, such as hydroxyl radicals ($HO^{\cdot}$) and superoxide anions ($O_2^{\cdot -}$), are produced, which are responsible for lignin degradation. However, the $H_2O_2$ treatment process is expensive. It becomes particularly unstable in the presence of certain transition metals, e.g., Mn, Fe, and Cu, at high temperatures, necessitating the addition of chelants to reduce the rate of decomposition. Delignification by this process on a large scale can, therefore, be costly. Current research has focused on reducing energy requirements of this process, and working temperatures have been reduced by over 50 percent, with 82 percent and 88 percent lignin dissolution occurring at temperatures of 40 and 70°C, respectively, in 2 percent $H_2O_2$ (pH 11.5).

## Organosolvents

The pretreatment of lignocellulosics with organosolvents involves the use of an aqueous solvent such as ethanol, butanol, phenol, etc., in the presence of a catalyst. This hydrolyzes lignin bonds as well as lignin-carbohydrate bonds, but many of the carbohydrate bonds in the hemicellulose component are also broken. Lignin is dissolved as a result of the action of the solvent, and cellulose remains in solid form.

The use of organosolvents for lignin removal is an attractive process because solvents can be recovered and recycled. It also has the advantage of being able to separate lignin from the solid cellulose with the hemicellulose hydrolysate found in liquid form.

## Ozone

Ozone has restricted use as a pretreatment for lignocellulosic substrates because it not only attacks the lignin molecule but also degrades the cellulose component. Hydroxyl radicals are formed during ozonation, and although lignin is attacked more rapidly, the cellulose is also targeted when the protective layer of lignin has been removed. It also has the effect of disrupting the association between carbohydrate polymers and lignin, yielding a residue that is more susceptible to attack by cellulases. Due to this unspecific nature, ozonation is more widely used as a pretreatment for the pulping industry.

### Peroxyformic Acid

Peroxyformic acid (PFA) is generated in situ by mixing formic acid with hydrogen peroxide. The lignocellulosic material is added to it and cooked at 80°C for three hours. The formation of PFA causes the production of electrophilic $HO^+$ ions, which react with the lignin. The next stage involves an increase in the reaction temperature for a period of time, and it is in this stage that most delignification occurs. At these higher temperatures, the cellulose component may be detrimentally affected. The third and final stage of the treatment is designed to degrade any remaining lignin. This pretreatment is known as the Milox process, derived from "mileu pure oxidative pulping."

## BIOLOGICAL PRETREATMENT

White-rot fungi and certain bacteria have been commonly used for biological pretreatments of lignocellulosics. Although lignin removal through lignin degradation is possible using biological methods, it is, however, unselective, as lignin is degraded only to obtain the more readily metabolized cellulose and/or hemicellulose.

### White-Rot Fungi

Due to their ability to degrade lignin as well as the polysaccharides found in cellulose and hemicellulose, white-rot fungi have the potential not only to act as a biological pretreatment, but also to degrade all the major components of lignocellulose to yield a valuable product. Although lignin can be degraded by these microorganisms, the enzymes responsible are produced only when other widely available substrates are unavailable. The purpose of lignin degradation by white-rot fungi is to allow better access to the cellulose and hemicellulose components.

Three main enzymes are thought to be involved in ligninolytic degradation, namely, lignin peroxidase (LiP), manganese peroxidase (MnP), and laccase. LiP has the ability to take an electron from the lignin molecule to create a cation radical, which then initiates an oxidative reaction that results in the oxygenation and depolymerization of the lignin. MnP oxidizes Mn (II) to Mn (III), which has the ability to diffuse into the lignin structure and initiate the oxidation process. Laccase is a phenol oxidase that differs from peroxidases in that it does not require hydrogen peroxide to directly attack lignocellulose.

White-rot fungi such as *Phanerochaete chrysosporium, Trametes versicolor,* and *Bjerkandera adusta* have the ability to degrade lignin and can be used as an effective biological pretreatment (Table III.37). This is a cheap and effective method of delignification. As fungi grow on these lignocellulose residues, they utilize the polysaccharides after lignin degradation in order to grow and reproduce. This, in turn, has the effect of increasing the nutritional value of the lignocellulose substrates that are generally low. After fermentation, this may be used as an animal feed or soil fertilizer. This process is mostly carried out under solid-state fermentation (SSF) conditions.

Recent work has concentrated on trying to make biological treatments more selective through the use of genetically manipulated fungi with cellulase-promoting enzymes inactivated. This allows lignin degradation without affecting the cellulose component of the complex. Disadvantages of using mutant fungi include their high dependence on an external carbon source and an increase in hemicellulose degradation. This is true of *Sporotrichum pulverulentum* mutants.

Some processes have focused on directly converting lignocellulosic residues to single-cell protein (SCP). In a method known as the Institut Armand-Frappier (IAF) process, a *Chaetomium cellulolyticum* mutant and *Pleurotus sajor-caju,* as well as strains of *Aspergillus* and *Penicillium* spp., are used. This cocultivation of fungi has the ability to utilize cellulose and hemicellulose, after lignin degradation, for SCP production. In this case, there is no need for any other pretreatment method, as together these fungi

TABLE III.37. White-rot fungi as biological pretreatment for lignocellulosic residues

| White-rot fungi | Lignocellulose substrate | Product |
|---|---|---|
| *Bjerkandera adusta* | Wood chips | Delignification for pulp refining |
| *Cyathus stercoreus* | Rice straw<br>Maize straw | Improve nutritional quality |
| *Pleurotus ostreatus*<br>*Trametes versicolor* | Wheat straw | Animal feed |
| *Trametes versicolor* | Kraft pulp | Delignification and bleaching |
| *Trametes versicolor* | Lignocellulosic hydrolysates | Peroxidase and laccase for delignification prior to ethanol fermentation |

are capable of separating lignocellulose into its individual components. The cellulose obtained may also be used for paper production or as SCP for animal or human feed.

Biological pretreatments require a long time period in comparison to other tried and tested physical and chemical methods. A period of two to five weeks may be required for sufficient delignification. The direct application of ligninolytic enzymes has also been investigated in order to reduce the length of the treatment period, but the direct use of enzymes for delignification is expensive and suffers from poor enzyme activity on the lignocellulose material.

## CONCLUSIONS

Lignocellulose residues in the form of agricultural wastes have the potential to be converted to glucose and from this to various chemicals, feeds, and fuels. Due to the highly recalcitrant nature of lignocellulose, especially the lignin component, pretreatments are a necessary step in the bioconversion process.

A wide variety of pretreatments are currently available, with steam and organosolvent treatments being the most effective. As physical and chemical methods are currently more selective in their lignin degradation and require only a short treatment period, they tend to be more widely used in industry. Biological treatments, through genetic manipulation, may also prove to be an effective and cheap alternative in the future, if this technology can be refined to make it more competitive with the effective physical and chemical treatments.

## SUGGESTED READINGS

Grayson M (ed.) (1980). *Microbial enzymes and bioconversions.* London: Academic Press.

Martin AM (ed.) (1998). *Bioconversion of waste materials to industrial products,* Second edition. London: Blackie Academic and Professional.

Rose AH (ed.) (1984). Fuels from biomass. In *Recycling, fuel and resource recovery: Economic and environmental factors.* New York: John Wiley and Sons.

# Recycling Agricultural By-Products and Residues for Animal Feeding

## Z. G. Weinberg

### INTRODUCTION

Agricultural by-products are obtained from food processing, surplus fruits and vegetables, or animal excreta. Examples include hulls of various nuts; apple, grape, and tomato pomace; beet and citrus pulp; cotton seeds; bakery waste; various brans; whey, fruit, and vegetable refuse; and broiler litter. These by-products can be utilized by ruminants for their feed sources. The digestive system of ruminants includes the reticulorumen, in which intensive fermentation activity of rumen microorganisms takes place and enables ruminants to utilize fibrous materials that are indigestible to monogastrics. Thus, ruminants do not compete with other animals for their feed sources, and they can utilize many by-products efficiently. These by-products can serve as excellent feed ingredients for cattle, for their fiber and energy contents and also for their nonprotein nitrogen (NPN) contents that are converted by the rumen microflora to energy and true protein which are available to the animal.

Many products currently used routinely for animal feeding are actually by-products that result from the processing of some agricultural primary products, and their value may even be equal to that of the primary product. In general, feeds for ruminants are categorized as concentrates, which are high in energy and protein, and roughage which is high in fibers. Examples in this context include cottonseed meal, from the cotton lint and oil industries, and soybean and sunflower meals, which are high in fiber and protein; hulls and bran from various cereal sources, which are used mainly for their fibers; and fishmeal and slaughterhouse wastes, which are good protein sources.

Agricultural by-products are usually cheap, but in many cases they are seasonal. During the season they might be produced in amounts too high to be used on the farm. Because of their high moisture, carbohydrate, and nitrogen contents, they are very perishable and spoil rapidly; therefore, they cannot be stored in their raw form for long periods. Accumulation of such materials might create serious environmental problems. For example, seepage from moist materials might pollute water sources because of its high BOD (biological oxygen demand) values, and large piles of rotting materials might emit noxious odors and attract undesirable insects and rodents, which might transmit diseases. In moldy materials, mycotoxins might be produced that present a serious health hazard to both humans and animals.

Thus, recycling of by-products for animal feeding presents two benefits: a supply of inexpensive, highly nutritional feed and reduction of environmental pollution. Because of their susceptibility to spoilage, by-products must be preserved in order to enable their use beyond the harvest season. The preservation technology should be economically appropriate to the value of the by-products. In principle, the preservation of food products may involve any technology that inhibits the activity of spoilage factors, microorganisms in particular. The main technologies that are used in the food industry are application of heat, cooling and freezing, dehydration, use of preservatives, and fermentation. However, most of these are not economical for the preservation of agricultural by-products for animal feeding.

Forage crops are preserved by either of two methods: hay making, which is based on field drying, and ensiling, which is based on lactic acid fermentation under anaerobic conditions. Hay making is restricted to thin plants that can be spread widely in the field, and it requires that no rain falls during drying. Therefore, ensiling is more applicable to most by-products that are moist and whose morphology does not allow fast drying. Ensiling is based on spontaneous solid-state fermentation under anaerobic conditions, whereby epiphytic lactic acid bacteria convert water-soluble carbohydrates into organic acids, mainly lactic acid. As a result, the pH decreases and the biomass is preserved. Successful ensiling requires an appropriate chemical and microbiological composition: the dry matter (DM) content should be 30 to 45 percent (depending on the crop), the content of soluble sugars—which serve as substrate for fermentation—should be at least 3 to 5 percent of the DM, and the crop should have a low buffering capacity (which indicates the resistance to pH change). The correct composition of the crop should encourage the development of lactic acid bacteria when anaerobic conditions are established within the silage. If the crop is too moist and its buffering capacity is too high, the resulting silage will be of poor quality and preservation losses will increase. On the other hand, if the crop is too dry, fermentation will be slow and losses will result as well.

In many cases the composition of agricultural by-products is not suitable for ensiling by regular technology, and the resulting "silage" might spoil rapidly and lose much of its value. Therefore, special solutions for ensiling by-products should be developed according to their specific properties. The following sections summarize the research on and the experience in using some by-products. This description can form the basis of guidelines for handling other similar by-products.

## CROP RESIDUES

The vegetative biomass of some crops may weigh as much as the harvested grains, and it could serve as roughage for ruminants because of its high fiber content. In many cases, when the grain is harvested, the crop residue has lower nutritional value for ruminants, because at that stage of maturity the high level of lignification blocks the utilization of structural carbohydrates as an energy source. Utilization of crop residues can be made more efficient by culture and management practices, such as selection of the crop variety and the stage of maturity at harvest. An example is the use of dual-purpose sorghum for food and feed, which is the practice in some parts of Africa. Some sorghum varieties remain nonsenescent during the grain harvest, therefore, their biomass still retains high digestibility for ruminants at this point. If the grains are harvested at a later stage, the biomass can be treated chemically (by alkaline) to improve its digestibility. In addition, it is possible to improve the nutritional value of various straws that have high indigestible lignocellulose contents, by enriching them with protein through solid-state fermentation with suitable fungi (e.g., *Aspergillus niger*). Solid-state fermentation can be accomplished simply, on aerated trays, and this might also be appropriate for underdeveloped areas. It is possible to combine aerobic solid-state fermentation and ensiling of straw: cell-wall hydrolyzing enzymes (cellulases and xylanases) which are produced during the solid-state fermentation improve the straw digestibility and supply soluble carbohydrates necessary for the ensiling fermentation.

Ensiling of the crop residues offers advantages over grazing for the following reasons: reduced field losses, improved palatability, and flexibility of use. In the semiarid tropics of Africa, preservation of crop residues of acceptable quality ensures a forage supply for the dry season, which might have an enormous impact on smallholder cattle owners. Their small dairy farms, which own only a few cows, cannot afford expensive ensiling facilities, but they could use ensiling in individual plastic bags (10 to 20 kg). If the residues are low in sugars, molasses might be added to enhance the ensiling fermentation.

Potato vines are yet another example of a crop residue. The vines are a potentially attractive by-product for feeding ruminants, because of their low fiber content and high crude protein and carbohydrate contents. In the usual practice the vines are killed with herbicides prior to harvest, at a cost of $85 to $125/ha in the United States, in order to toughen the potato skins. Unfortunately, the dead vines may harbor various potato diseases and other vectors in the field which might infect the succeeding crop. Therefore, harvesting of the vines could not only yield feed value but also reduce herbicide and pesticide use in potato production. However, preservation of the vines by ensiling poses two major problems: their DM content is too low, so they do not wilt easily, and they are contaminated with soil. To overcome these problems, in one study the vines were mixed with alfalfa hay, barley grains, or whole-crop maize. Thus, a DM content appropriate for ensiling was approached, the excess soil was diluted, and the resulting silage was of acceptable quality (Table III.38). The mixed silages were also more resistant to aerobic spoilage than the vine-only silages. Ensiling two different crops together to enhance silage quality can be done if their harvesting seasons coincide and if it is possible to mix them properly.

In a different study, cassava tops were ensiled with or without molasses. The ensiling process resulted in a significant decrease in cyanide content; molasses enhanced the ensiling fermentation.

## *BY-PRODUCTS*

### *Citrus Peels*

Citrus peels are an example of a seasonal moist by-product. The peels are a by-product of the citrus juice and concentrates industry, and they are abundant during the picking season. Citrus peels have a high nutritional value and can be used as fodder. They are especially high in water-soluble carbohydrates and pectin (Table III.39) and, therefore, serve as an excellent energy source. However, the peels are very moist and harbor high yeast populations, therefore they spoil rapidly. The peels exude much seepage with a very high BOD value—higher than that of domestic sewage. If the peels accumulate they become an environmental nuisance.

TABLE III.38. Composition of silages containing potato vines

| Treatment | Dry matter % | pH | Crude protein % | Lactic acid % | Acetic acid % |
|---|---|---|---|---|---|
| Vines alone | 11-16 | 5.5-5.9 | 12-18 | 0-4 | 8-10 |
| +Alfalfa | 29-34 | 4.9-5.1 | 17-20 | 4-6 | 3-5 |
| +Barley | 29-32 | 4.0-4.1 | 17-18 | 6-7 | 1 |
| +Corn (1:1) | 24-26 | 4.2-4.7 | 15-17 | 6 | 2-4 |

TABLE III.39. Composition of citrus peels

| Parameter | Fresh | Silage |
|---|---|---|
| % Dry matter | 13-21 | 14-16 |
| pH | 4.3-4.8 | 3.3-3.5 |
| Water-soluble carbohydrates | 18-34 | 5-10 |
| Crude protein | 5-7 | |
| Crude fiber | 11-13 | |
| Ash | 2.5-5 | |
| Pectin | 9-18 | |
| Lactic acid | 3 | |
| Acetic acid | 3 | |
| Ethanol | 14-16 | |
| Lactobacilli | $10^5$-$10^7$ | $10^6$-$10^8$ |
| Yeasts | $10^4$-$10^6$ | $10^4$-$10^7$ |
| BOD of seepage (mg $O_2$/l) | | 58,600 |

*Note:* Chemical contents are expressed as percentages of DM; microbiological data are in $\log_{10}$ CFU/g.

In some places the peels are treated with a calcium salt, to open up the pectin structure to facilitate water removal, and are then pressed, thermally dehydrated, and pelletized. In Brazil, where both peels and sugarcane bagasse are abundant, the dry bagasse serves as fuel for the drying ovens. Drying reduces shipment volumes and costs. However, in many places fuel costs are too high compared to the value of the peels, and drying is not economical. In such cases, an alternative method for preservation of the peels is ensiling. In experiments in which the peels were ensiled without any prior treatment, fermentation was wild and ensiling losses were very high (30 percent of DM), as were seepage volumes. The resulting silages had exceptionally high ethanol contents (around 15 percent of the DM), which led to the conclusion that high yeast populations were the main spoiling factor. This was confirmed by high yeast counts (Table III.39). In order to improve the preservation of the peels by ensiling, means to inhibit the yeasts had to be applied: blanching at 80°C or treatment with 0.05 percent K-sorbate reduced DM losses to less than 10 percent. However, these treatments were too expensive compared to the price of the peels ($10 to $15 per ton in Israel). Therefore, in practice, the peels are simply mixed and ensiled in piles along with broiler litter, which is dry and has a composition that complements that of the peels.

*Broiler Litter*

Poultry manure is a by-product from the poultry industry and can be used in feedstuffs for ruminants, although it has some limitations. In practice, feeding with the manure depends on its nutritional value and on the levels of negative factors such as pathogens, drug residues, and heavy metals. Broiler litter is of higher nutritional quality than that of layer manure because it is collected more often and has a lower mineral content. Broiler litter is composed of bedding material (straw or wood shavings), excreta, wasted feed, and feathers. It contains (on a DM basis) 30 percent crude protein (half of which is true protein), 15 percent ash (minerals), and 15 percent crude fiber. Its metabolic energy content for cattle is about 2,200 kcal/g. The litter produced by broilers amounts to about 25 percent of the fodder consumed plus 10 percent of the bedding. Because of the recent problems associated with feeding forage of animal origin (such as mad cow disease), it is recommended that the litter be fed only to growing heifers and beef steers, and not to lactating cows.

To ensure its safety, the litter should be processed before use to eliminate pathogenic microorganisms and drug residues. Several technologies are available for dealing with the litter: fumigation, thermal pasteurization, and ensiling. In Israel, the thermal process includes raising the moisture content of the litter to 40 percent, after which the material is transferred into large chambers into which air is pumped. This initiates intensive aerobic microbiological activity, and the temperature within the litter rises to 70°C. It is possible to control the temperature increase by manipulating the moisture content and the airflow into the chambers. The litter is kept at 70°C for three days, after which it is considered safe. The cattle in Israel are vaccinated against botulism, and this is no longer a concern with regard to litter feeding.

Ensiling involves raising the moisture content of the litter to about 50 percent, applying some consolidation, and sealing with polyethylene sheeting for six weeks. Thanks to its high nitrogen and ash contents, the litter has a very high buffering capacity (which means that it is resistant to pH decrease), but, nevertheless, ensiling results in a decrease in pH to about 5.5. It is possible to mix the litter with a complementary ingredient which would enhance the ensiling process and improve the nutritional quality of the final product. For example, it is common in Israel to mix broiler litter with citrus peels at a 1:1 ratio (on a wet-weight basis). The peels, rich in water-soluble carbohydrates, bring the pH down to 5.0, as compared to 5.4 when the litter is ensiled alone. Similarly, it is possible to mix the litter with such materials as potato residues or to add molasses as a source of fermentable carbohydrates, where citrus peels are not available.

## Whey and Dairy By-Products

Whey is a by-product of the cheese industry and contains, on a DM basis, about 13 percent crude protein, 10 percent minerals, and more than 75 percent lactose. Its DM digestibility for cattle is over 80 percent, therefore, it can serve as an excellent energy and protein source for the animals. If not used, it becomes a serious environmental pollutant. It is possible to feed whey in several forms, e.g., as liquid or as whey-protein concentrate. It is also possible to add whey to forage crops during silage making; it is a good source of fermentable lactose and of lactic acid bacteria, and therefore improves the ensiling process.

Dairy products that are returned after the sell-by date has passed can also be fed to cattle. Preliminary experiments in our laboratory indicate that liquid milk and cottage cheese can be successfully ensiled together with straw, which absorbs the excess of moisture. The combination of milk and straw ensiles readily, thanks to the lactose in the milk. The combination with the cottage cheese had to be enhanced with molasses to ensure adequate sugars for the fermentation.

## CONCLUSIONS

The variety of by-products that can be utilized for cattle feed is very large. Each by-product has unique properties, according to which an appropriate preservation technology should be chosen to ensure safe use and prolonged shelf life of the resulting material. The benefits from utilizing by-products for animal feeding arise from both their nutritional value and the alleviation of the environmental load. The utilization of by-products might be especially important in poor areas where forage is scarce.

## SUGGESTED READINGS

Ashbell G, T Kipnis, M Titterton, Y Hen, A Azrieli, and ZG Weinberg (2001). Examination of a technology for silage making in plastic bags. *Animal Feed Silage and Technology* 91:213-222.

Ashbell G, G Pahlow, B Dinter, and ZG Weinberg (1987). Dynamics of orange peel fermentation during ensilage. *Journal of Applied Bacteriology* 63:275-279.

Ashbell G, ZG Weinberg, and Y Hen (1995). Studies of quality parameters of variety ensiled broiler litter. *Animal Feed Silage and Technology* 52:271-278.

Huber JT (ed.) (1980). *Upgrading residues and by-products for animals.* Boca Raton, FL: CRC Press, Inc.

Yang X, HZ Chen, HL Gao, and ZH Li (2001). Bioconversion of corn straw by coupling ensiling and solid-state fermentation. *Bioresource Technology* 78(3):277-280.

# Solid-State Fermentation for Bioconversion of Biomass

## Design of Bioreactors for Solid-State Fermentation

Matt Hardin

### *INTRODUCTION*

A number of distinct reactor designs exist for solid-state fermentation (SSF). This variety reflects the diversity of organisms that have been used in SSF and the general lack of knowledge in the SSF field that could allow an optimum design to be selected and developed in the same way that the stirred, aerated vessel became the standard for most submerged-culture techniques.

The design and operation of SSF reactors is still very much an art, and extensive trials are almost invariably required for any new SSF process. This chapter introduces the basic design considerations of SSF reactors and then explains how different reactor designs have met these considerations. It is not an exhaustive analysis of fermentor design, nor does it cover modeling of fermentations.

### *DESIGN CONSIDERATIONS*

Bioreactors perform two major roles: containment and environmental control. Containment includes prevention of contamination of the fermentation by environmental organisms, as well as prevention of contamination of the environment by the fermentation organism. Environmental control includes maintenance of optimal or close to optimal conditions for productivity, as well as maintenance of homogeneity within the vessel for uniform productivity. In addition, bioreactors can facilitate and even participate in other aspects of processing, including substrate preparation, sterilization, loading, unloading, and product extraction.

### Temperature Control

Temperature is the limiting design consideration for most SSF systems. A high amount of metabolic heat is produced by organisms during growth. Because solid particles do not conduct heat very well and forced convective heat transfer within the bed is severely limited, the temperature of SSF cultures often increases to levels incompatible with growth.

On a lab scale, temperature control is relatively simple, as a large surface area to volume ratio facilitates free convection of heat conducted from the substrate bed to the walls of the reactor. As the scale increases, this mechanism of heat transfer rapidly becomes inadequate. On a larger scale, the forced addition of air is usually necessary to allow evaporative cooling of the substrate. This method of cooling, although effective, results in a loss of water from the system. In some cases, this water is replaced as a by-product of metabolism. In many cases, however, it is not, and the result is a gradual drying of the substrate. Some form of moisture control is then required. Methods used include water sprays and the alternate use of humidified and dry air.

Another serious issue for temperature control in SSF operations is the formation of gradients within the substrate bed. This is can be become a serious issue in unmixed reators and limits the effectiveness of trays and static packed-bed reactors. Radial mixing in rotating drums is generally adequate to prevent radial gradients, although evidence suggests that axial temperature and moisture gradients can form in large-scale rotating drums. These gradients prevent the production of a uniform product and reduce the overall effectiveness of the reactor.

### Shear

The most commonly grown organisms for SSF are the filamentous fungi, particularly of *Rhizopus, Aspergillus, Trichoderma,* and *Penicillium* species. These fungi grow by production of hyphae, which often bind together into compact tufts known as mycelia, and reproduce by producing spores on the ends of aerial hyphae (known as conidiophores). Mycelia and conidiophores are quite fragile structures and are easily crushed or broken. This means that the shear imposed on the organisms by mixing could impair growth and reproduction and limit spore production.

To date, there has been no work done quantifying the effect of shear on fungi during mixing. Observations as to the effect of shear are limited to direct observation of damaged hyphae after fermentation. This makes it difficult to weigh the detrimental effects of shear against the requirements for good mixing.

## *REACTOR TYPES*

### *Trays*

Trays are by far the most common type of reactor used in SSF. The technology for tray reactors is quite old and is still used to produce traditional SSF products such as tempe, as well as more modern products, e.g., antibiotics and industrial enzymes. Trays are a simple design consisting of a flat tray (often perforated) upon which the substrate is evenly spread up to a depth of 40 mm (Figure III.40). The substrate is left unmixed or is infrequently manually mixed. Air of a controlled temperature and humidity is circulated around the tray, allowing temperature control and aeration.

Trays are limited by heat and mass transfer and can develop large internal temperature and gas concentration gradients at greater depths than about 40 mm. This limits scale-up of tray fermentations to the addition of more trays. Although this is a simple method, the associated labor costs rapidly make large-scale operation with trays uneconomical. Automation of all the different steps of tray fermentations is extremely difficult. Hence, the labor intensiveness of trays means that their use is suited only to countries where labor costs are low.

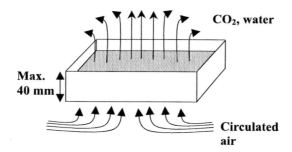

FIGURE III.40. Typical tray bioreactor. Air is circulated around the tray and through the perforated base. Water and $CO_2$ are driven off by convective heating through the top of the bed. Substrate bed depths greater than 40 mm result in temperature and gas concentration gradients within the bed.

## Packed Beds

Packed-bed bioreactors consist of substrate packed into a column, with air blown through from one end to the other. The most commonly used orientation is a vertical column, with the substrate supported on a perforated base plate and the air passing upward from the bottom, although other configurations have been used (Figure III.41). Packed beds have been used on a lab and pilot scale to produce products as diverse as ethanol, oxytetracycline, biopesticides, cellulase, and aflatoxin.

There are various mechanisms for heat transfer within packed beds. Within the bed there is radial and axial heat conduction, and axial convection and evaporation associated with the airflow. From the outer surfaces of the bed there is conduction across the bioreactor wall, and convection of heat away from the wall by the surrounding air or by cooling water if the bed is jacketed. The design and operation of the packed bed determine which of these phenomena dominate heat removal. Large-scale bioreactors would typically be quite wide, making the contribution of radial heat conduction negligible. Such bioreactors would require high aeration rates, and therefore axial convection and evaporative cooling would be quite important.

Because static packed-bed bioreactors are not mixed, it is not practical to use dry air to promote evaporation, since this would very quickly dry out the bottom of the column. Therefore, the air blown into packed beds is typically almost saturated. However, the temperature of the air increases with height,

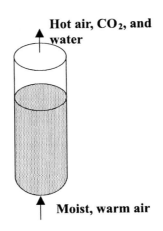

**Hot air, CO$_2$, and water**

**Moist, warm air**

FIGURE III.41. Typical packed-bed bioreactor. Cooling is mainly by forced axial convection and evaporation. There is also a degree of radial convection depending on the scale of the vessel.

and this increases the air's water-holding capacity, causing some evaporation to occur in packed beds, even when the aeration air is saturated when it enters the column. Control of fermentation parameters is limited to manipulating the flow rate and temperature of the inlet air, and the flow rate and temperature of the cooling water running through the water jacket or cooling plates if these are present.

Even with axial convection and evaporation, heat removal can be a problem. As the air removes heat from the substrate by convective cooling, it warms as it rises through the column, and therefore cools the substrate bed less effectively with height. As a result, an axial temperature gradient is established, with the highest temperature at the very top of the column. Although both oxygen and temperature gradients arise in packed-bed bioreactors, if the aeration rate satisfies the heat removal requirements, then it will easily satisfy the oxygen supply requirements. Despite these gradients, forced aeration gives better heat removal than that found in tray fermentations.

The most advanced static packed-bed design to date contains vertical internal heat transfer plates spaced at 50 mm intervals running the length of the reactor in order to alleviate the heat transfer problems commonly encountered with static packed-bed bioreactors. Cooling water is circulated through the plates. This design uses the internal heat transfer plates to promote heat transfer in the horizontal direction.

Another important phenomenon in static packed-bed bioreactors is the pressure drop through the column, which can affect the ability of the process air to pass through the column. As the fungus grows on the surface of the substrate particles, it grows into the interparticle voids, restricting airflow. At high biomass densities, the fungus can occupy up to 34 percent of the space between substrate particles, reducing the relative permeability of the bed to around 1 percent of the original value. The increasing pressure drop can actually be used as an online measure of growth.

The high pressure drops obtained in static packed beds has consequences for airflow. The energy requirements for aeration depend directly on the pressure drop, and if the inlet pressure is not increased, then the rate of flow of air through the column will decrease as the pressure drop increases. High pressure drops also increase the likelihood of channeling occurring. This is undesirable, since most of the air will flow through the channel and relatively little will reach the other parts of the bed. In a related phenomenon, shrinkage of the bed late in fermentation can allow air to pass between the bed and the wall, which results in oxygen transport within the bed being limited to diffusion. Pressure drops can be minimized by agitating the substrate, but this cannot be done where such agitation would have deleterious effects on the fermentation.

Other operability considerations include filling and emptying of the reactor. Filling is typically not a problem. The substrate can be dropped through the top, using a solids-conveying device. Removal is potentially more of a problem, especially if it is desired to harvest an undisturbed bound substrate cake, such as might be required for production of a fermented food. Packed beds can be mounted on a pulley system so that the substrate will drop out the bottom when the reactor is raised. Other options may be to hinge the column along a vertical plane so that it can split open, or hinge the base plate so that it can drop open at harvest time.

Packed beds are a good alternative to trays for shear-sensitive fermentation processes. Given that there will always be some SSF processes for which mixing is undesirable, packed-bed bioreactors will always have a place in SSF, despite their problems with overheating at the air-outlet end. Compared to trays, the advantages of packed beds include a dramatic decrease in the temperature and gas concentration gradients through the substrate bed, improved use of space, and simplification of downstream processing, as many processes can be performed in situ, such as drying, air stripping of ethanol, and solvent extraction of antibiotics.

### Fluidized Beds

Air-solid fluidized beds (ASFBs) are vertical columns through which air is blown upward through the perforated base plate at a sufficient velocity to fluidize the substrate bed. A breaker may be placed just above the base plate to break up agglomerates, which, due to their large size, settle to the bottom of the bioreactor. The column must be taller than the unfluidized bed to allow for bed expansion, which takes place upon fluidization. At the top of the column a space is required for disengagement of the solids from the air. A mechanical separator may be placed here to facilitate separation (Figure III.42). Kikkoman Corporation constructed an air-solid fluidized-bed bioreactor of 8,000 liter working volume in 1975 and used the system for production of enzymes by *Aspergillus sojae* on wheat bran. Despite the successful operation of this reactor, with higher yields obtained compared to static-bed SSF, there are very few other examples of use of air-solid fluidized beds for SSF.

Although heat transfer in air-solid fluidized-bed bioreactors has not been addressed, convection and evaporation will be quite effective due to the high airflow rates required to fluidize the substrate. It may not even be necessary to use dry air, since convective cooling alone may be sufficient to remove the waste metabolic heat. The substrate bed will be quite well mixed, and

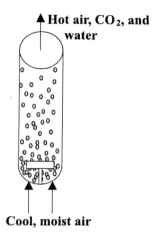

**Hot air, $CO_2$, and water**

**Cool, moist air**

FIGURE III.42. Typical fluidized-bed bioreactor. The breaker at the bottom is to prevent particle agglomeration. Cooling is mainly by forced convection by the high-velocity fluidizing air.

the mixing action should be relatively gentle when compared to mixing by mechanical agitators.

Good mixing means that there should be minimal gradients within the reactor. Any changes made with the aeration air should be able to control the conditions within the reactor. It is also relatively easy to supply additives such as water, nutrient solutions, or even dilute acids or alkalis for pH control. Operating expenses for this reactor are likely to be quite high, although this might be compensated by higher yields.

Obviously, fluidization will happen only if the substrate particles have suitable properties. For example if the substrate is too sticky, then it will tend to agglomerate and the bed will not fluidize. In addition, variations among particles in the substrate bed could lead to segregation of particles according to size and shape. Therefore, this type of bioreactor is not suitable for all SSF processes.

Air-solid fluidized beds have a high degree of operability compared to other SSF bioreactors. It should be possible to sterilize the substrate in place, although problems may occur if the substrate becomes sticky during the cooking process. If desired, it is also possible to dry the substrate in the bioreactor when the fermentation is complete, simply by switching from moist to dry air.

## Drums

There are three basic types of drum designs for SSF (Figure III.43):

1. *Rotating drums*—horizontal drums are partially filled with substrate. Air is blown through the headspace, and mixing is provided by the rotation of the drum around its central axis. The drum may contain internal lifters (baffles) to enhance the mixing action caused by the rotation.
2. *Stirred horizontal drums*—these have many similarities with rotating drums, but typically the body of the bioreactor does not move. Mixing action is provided by paddles or screws mounted on a central rotating shaft. Air is blown through the bioreactor headspace.
3. *Rocking-drum bioreactors*—the substrate bed is held between two concentric perforated cylinders. Air is blown through from the central cylinder to the outside. The outer cylinder rotates back and forth to provide some mixing action. These have yet to see industrial use and are not described in detail in this section.

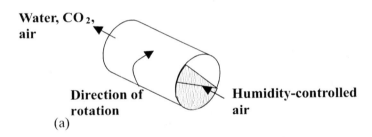

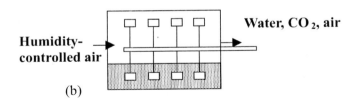

FIGURE III.43. Typical drum bioreactors: (a) rotating drum, (b) stirred drum. These reactors, while superficially different, demonstrate similar characteristics of high shear and good mixing, and they use a mixture of evaporative cooling and conduction through the vessel walls for cooling. Cooling depends on the scale of the vessel, with convection of the walls of the vessel dominating at small scales and evaporative cooling becoming more prominent as scale increases.

The main advantages of drums lie in their good heat and mass transfer and their homogeneity. They are not suitable for shear-sensitive organisms. A large variety of products have been produced in these studies, including animal feed, antibiotics, and spores for blue cheese production. Large rotating drums have also been used to compost municipal solid waste.

Drum bioreactors can be conceptually divided into three subsystems. The first of these phases is the substrate bed, which consists of both the moist substrate particles, to which the microbe is attached, and the interparticle gas phase. The second subsystem is the gas headspace above the bed. The third subsystem is the bioreactor wall. Heat generated by the microbe within the substrate bed can be transferred by evaporation or convection to the headspace air, or by conduction to the bioreactor wall. The bioreactor wall is cooled by convection to either the headspace gases or the surrounding atmosphere. The dominant cooling phenomenon in a rotating-drum bioreactor (RDB) depends on the surface area to volume ratio of the reactor. At a laboratory scale, the major heat removal mechanism is transfer through the wall of the reactor due to the relatively large surface area to volume ratio. As reactor volume increases, heat removal by evaporation becomes the major factor.

The variables that are most readily controlled during the fermentation are the flow rate, temperature, and humidity of the inlet air and the drum rotation rate. Because the bed is mixed, dry air can be used to promote evaporation, as long as water is replenished by spraying or misting it onto the substrate.

An increase in rotation speed facilitates mass and heat transfer between the substrate and the gas phase and improves homogeneity. Optimal mixing in rotating drums occurs with fill depths of approximately 30 percent. Once the process has commenced, the fill depth is typically not altered by additions or removals in batch systems, although it may decrease due to consumption of the solids by the microbe. In practice, rotation rates of 2 to 3 rpm are most common, although values as low as three revolutions per day and as high as 40 to 50 rpm have been reported.

Rotating-drum bioreactors can be used in continuous-flow operations. To promote the flow of solids, either the central axis may be inclined or the baffles can be designed to push solids along the drum. Baffles improve mixing and heat and mass transfer, although they have not been extensively used in SSF applications

Stirred horizontal drums have the additional consideration of mixer design. The agitation device must provide adequate mixing without damaging the substrate. If it is poorly designed, there is potential for substrate to be squashed between the agitator and the drum wall. The positive mixing action of the agitator will give much better mixing at low rpm than an unbaffled rotating drum, in which slumping flow behavior occurs. Other related operability considerations include the ease of cleaning the mixing device and its susceptibility to mechanical fatigue.

Little mention is made in the literature of filling depths for stirred drums, although active stirring should permit greater fill depths than those used in RDBs. From a design perspective, the static drum eases additions to the substrate during the fermentation and greatly simplifies the attachment of instruments.

Stirred horizontal drums are ideally suited to continuous operation, using the augers to push the substrate through the reactor or using either a rotating internal coil or a helical ribbon to stir and drive the substrate through the reactor in plug flow.

The temperature, humidity, and flow rate of the inlet air can be manipulated. Varying the proportion of wet to dry air is the preferred method of controlling evaporation as opposed to alternating between wet and dry air. This method gave a greater yield of biomass and finer temperature control compared to the system in which variation of airflow rate was used as the control variable. Although the use of dry air tends to dry the substrate, water can be dripped into the inner cylinder and allowed to permeate into the substrate bed.

## CONCLUSIONS

A thorough understanding of the requirements for the optimal growth conditions for organisms in SSF is required before a reactor design can be chosen. Choice of reactor will need to be followed by further work optimizing the design and operating conditions. The wide variety of basic designs, although daunting, allows the reactor to be tailored to the process. Poor definition of actual design constraints makes SSF a challenging field to in which to work; however there are an expanding number of applications, and this situation should lead to a deeper knowledge of SSF processes and better reactor design and operating techniques.

## SUGGESTED READINGS

Hardin MT and DA Mitchell (1998). Recent developments in the design, operation and modeling of bioreactors for solid-state fermentation. In *Recent research developments in fermentation and bioengineering,* F Kaowai and K Sasaki (eds.), Volume 1. Trivandrum, India: Research Signpost, pp. 205-222.

Mitchell DA, BK Lonsane, A Durand, R Renauad, S Almanza, J Maratray, C Desgranges, PS Crooke, K Hong, GW Malaney, and RD Tanner (1992). Reactor design. In *Solid substrate cultivation*, HW Doelle, DA Mitchell, and CE Rolz (eds.). London: Elsevier Ltd., pp. 115-139.

Pandey A (1992). Recent process developments in solid-state fermentations. *Process Biochemistry* 27:109-117.

# Engineering Aspects of Solid-State Fermentation

Mario Fernández-Fernández
Ricardo Pérez-Correa
Eduardo Agosin

## *INTRODUCTION*

Solid-state fermentation (SSF) systems are microbiological processes in which growth and product formation are carried out inside a solid medium, generally porous, in the absence of excess water. They comprise four interacting phases: a gas phase, a solid insoluble support, a liquid phase containing dissolved substrates and products, and a biotic phase formed by the microorganisms.

Although several works have been reported using yeasts and bacteria in SSF, filamentous fungi are by their nature the most adapted to this kind of environment. This is due to their specific capacity to colonize the interparticle spaces of the solid matrix that sustains them and to their ability to grow well at water activities under 0.99.

Given the inherent complexity of scaling-up heterogeneous solid-substrate reactors, SSF has not been developed at the same technological level as submerged fermentation (SmF) processes. In addition, efficient operation of SSF bioreactors is hampered by the lack of reliable and affordable devices to measure relevant operating variables inside the fermenting bed (such as pH, water content, dissolved oxygen, biomass, and substrate concentration). Furthermore, the metabolic heat generation and the slow heat transfer inside the bed cause a temperature rise difficult to regulate. However, several advantages over SmF have been identified for SSF processes, including higher productivities, low-cost substrates, and differential gene expression. In spite of these advantages, the state of the art in SSF technology is profitable only in small-scale processes associated with products of high added value, such as those of biopharmaceutical origin (antibiotics, drugs, enzymes, and organic acids). In our opinion, SSF technology can be significantly improved if the latest developments in process modeling, instrumentation, and control are incorporated into the design and operation of SSF bioreactors. Hence, the scope of applicability of SSF processing will be widened extensively, particularly in large-scale production.

## BIOREACTORS AND MODELING

Design of bioreactors and modeling are very important issues related to SSF. Therefore, they are discussed separately in the chapters "Design of Bioreactors for Solid-State Fermentation" and "Modeling in Solid-State Fermentation."

## STANDARD INSTRUMENTATION

### Temperature

Any SSF control system should include several temperature measurements to monitor the bed temperature distribution and to measure inlet and outlet air temperature so that energy and water balances are kept under control. Several inexpensive temperature sensors are commercially available, thermocouples (TCs) being the most widely used within industrial environments. Their low cost, wide measuring range, and fast and linear response explain their popularity among process engineers; however, thermocouples show poor precision and accuracy.

Although our experience indicates that thermocouple performance in SSF can be significantly improved if they are calibrated frequently, other temperature sensors are superior. Specifically, resistance temperature detectors (RTDs) are better suited for SSF processing needs. These devices are stable, precise, respond fast, and do not need periodic calibration, although they are more expensive and fragile than thermocouples.

### Bed Water Content

Bed water content is a key variable in SSF processing and should be kept tightly regulated, especially during the exponential growth phase. Although the humidity of the fermenting substrate can be measured offline easily with an infrared radiation (IR) balance device, it is rather difficult to measure it online. None of the methods commonly used to measure the water content of solid samples have gained wide acceptance in the SSF field. Conductivity-based devices (those in which an electric current circulates through the solid sample) are too sensitive to the electrodes/sample contact area and the apparent density of the sample. However, if properly calibrated and compensated, these devices may be useful to measure the solid water content in static packed-bed reactors.

Other commercially available humidity-measuring devices such as infrared or neutron radiation sensors are not only expensive but also impractical to use in SSF reactors and provide information regarding only the solid's surface. More promising are those based on the emission of radio frequency fields or on time domain reflectometry (TDR), since they provide a representative value of the water content in the three-dimensional zone covered by the electrodes.

### Air Relative Humidity

Some bed-temperature control strategies need inlet air-humidity manipulation. Furthermore, to control the water content of the fermenting bed, water balances are generally determined. Both operations require continuously measuring the humidity of the inlet and outlet airstreams. Consequently, most of the SSF bioreactor designs include one or more air relative-humidity sensors. Traditionally, the relative humidity (RH) in an airstream was measured using both the dry- and wet-bulb temperature. Although simple, this method is not precise, it presents a slow response time, and care should be taken to avoid drying of the wet bulb. Today, relative humidity is measured with electrochemical devices based on thin-film hygroscopic capacitive cells. It is worth noting that the precision of these devices severely decays near saturation; usually high-quality humidity sensors show a precision of ±0.1 percent for RH < 95 percent and ±1 percent for RH > 95 percent.

### Gas-Flow Rate

Several methods exist for measuring gas-flow rates, depending if it is volumetric or massic. Differential pressure producers (DPP), such as Pitot tubes, Venturi tubes, or orifice plates, are commonly used to measure volumetric flow rates; they are reliable and simple, and their precision ranges from 0.8 percent to 5 percent. DPP require a differential pressure transducer to transmit the measurement signal to the control system. In addition, their precision is severely reduced at low flow rates and their operating costs are high due to the energy loss. Other less expensive sensors are usually preferred, such as rotating devices (turbine anemometers) or hot-wire anemometers. Positive displacement devices are recommended when accurate and high-precision measurements are needed. For mass flow rate measurements the same volumetric devices can be used, although pressure and temperature compensation must be included. Alternatively, mass flow rate can be directly measured with high precision within a wider measurement range using Coriolis force-based devices such as vibration tubes.

## Off-Gas Analysis

Continuous monitoring of $CO_2$ and $O_2$ concentrations in the exhaust gas stream of SSF bioreactors is required to assess the physiological state and respiration rate of the culture. Usually, measurements of $CO_2$ and $O_2$ are used to compute online derived variables such as carbon dioxide production rate (CPR) and oxygen consumption rate (OCR), which are easier to interpret. In turn, CPR and OCR can be used to compute the respiratory quotient (RQ) and to estimate online the specific biomass growth rate, allowing an easy assessment of the bioreactor operation.

Off-gas analysis can be performed by gas chromatography (GC) or by specific gas analyzers. In both cases, care must be taken to keep the flow rate regulated and to dry the air sample before entering the instrument, in order to obtain meaningful results. GC is sometimes preferred over specific gas analyzers, since many compounds, in addition to $CO_2$ and $O_2$, can be monitored with the same instrument and over a wider range of values. On the other hand, gas analyzers are more precise and provide faster response (few seconds compared to the several minutes that a GC measurement can take). These devices make use of chemical or physical properties, such as paramagnetism or infrared absorption, which characterize the gases measured. Paramagnetic analyzers, available for $CO_2$ and $O_2$, are probably the most effective. Although expensive, they are very precise, do not require periodic calibration, present low interference with other gases, and last long. These instruments exploit the property of some gases being magnetized when they are exposed to a magnetic field. $CO_2$ can also be measured reliably with infrared instruments, which are precise and have a long lifetime, although they are expensive and need occasional calibration. Infrared analyzers use the capacity that $CO_2$ has to absorb infrared radiations within a characteristic spectrum. Electrochemical analyzers are commonly used to measure $O_2$ concentrations, since they are inexpensive and provide good precision; however, the measuring cell must be changed periodically.

## Pressure

Filamentous growth of fungi causes the substrate to become more and more compact during fermentation, limiting $CO_2$ and $O_2$ transfer between the gas and the fermenting bed. In addition, removal of the metabolic heat becomes even more difficult under this condition. Hence, detecting excessive bed compactness is a major concern in operating static or periodically agitated packed-bed SSF bioreactors. This effect can be assessed online by monitoring the pressure drop through the solid bed. Bourdon tubes are widely used pressure sensors. They are simple, inexpensive, and reliable, although they are not fast and precise instruments. On the other hand, piezoelectric sensors can be used to measure pressure within a wider range, their response time is extremely short, and they are insensitive to temperature. Differential pressure sensors comprise two oil-filled chambers, which are connected internally to a rod and externally to high- and low-pressure measuring devices. When a difference of pressure is sensed the rod is displaced in the chambers, producing a signal.

## ADVANCED INSTRUMENTATION

### Soft Sensors

Soft sensors are mathematical procedures employing process models and secondary measurements to provide an online estimation of a variable of interest. The technique is widely applied in SmF for indirect measurements of specific consumption or production rates, yields, concentrations, and heat loads. In SSF, it has been mainly applied at an experimental level for biomass concentration, bed water content, and heat load estimations.

### Mass Spectrometry

Mass spectrometers (MS) are very flexible instruments that have been extensively used in submerged fermentation for online gas analyses. The operation principle of a mass spectrometer is related to the production of charged ions through high-vacuum ionization. Then, ions are classified according to their electrical charge to atomic mass ratio and their detectability. The instrument also comprises software that compares and quantifies the measured spectra based on specialized libraries. Mass spectrometers provide more precise, more reliable, and faster measurements (around ten compounds in few seconds) than gas chromatographs. However, MS instruments are more expensive, with high maintenance costs, and require specialized personnel to operate them.

### Infrared Spectroscopy

Infrared spectrometers apply infrared radiation to the sample of interest, affecting all but its diatomic molecules; IR interacts with the natural vibration and rotation modes of the affected molecules. When the frequency of the incident radiation coincides with the frequency of any natural mode of some of the components, partial absorption of the incident radiation occurs.

The spectrum of this absorption uniquely identifies and quantifies the molecules in the sample. The IR spectrum ranges from 12,500 per cm to 10 per cm or in terms of frequency from 0.8 µm to 1,000 µm, though the region of interest for analytical purposes is divided into two: the near infrared (NIR), from 12,500 to 4,000 per cm (0.8 µm to 2.5 µm), and the medium infrared (MIR), from 4,000 per cm to 670 per cm (2.5 µm to 15 µm). IR spectroscopy is a very attractive analytical technique since it is fast, nondestructive, and flexible. Its calibration is time consuming though, and effective mathematical tools should be applied. It is routinely used in a wide range of industries, including food, pharmaceutical, textile, cosmetics, or polymers. Several components can be measured simultaneously with IR instruments, and in the particular case of SSF processes, it has been used to measure biomass, water content, carbon, and nitrogen.

### Biosensors

Biosensors are compact and highly specific analytical instruments that comprise biological sensing components such as tissues, cells, enzymes, organelles, membranes, or antibodies. The sensing component can be coupled to a potentiometer, amperometer, optical device, calorimeter, conductimeter, or any device able to produce a measurable signal (transducer). The main advantage of biosensors is at the same time their main limitation: given that they can identify and quantify components with high specificity, to measure the complete range of components of interest in fermentation processes, many instruments are required. To the best of our knowledge, this type of instrument has not been evaluated in SSF so far.

## PROCESS CONTROL

SSF processes usually last for several days, and during this period the microorganism environment—temperature, water availability, nutrient concentration, etc.—should be tightly regulated to achieve the expected production yields and product quality. This regulation requires process control or automation techniques, which may be applied at increasing levels of complexity:

- *Monitoring,* the simplest level, demands that the operator of the system has real-time access to the process measurements. This requires corrective actions, based on past experience, to compensate for any observed deviation of the measurements from prespecified values. In these cases, it is convenient to use statistical process control (SPC) techniques to distinguish between a true measurement deviation and natural process noise.

- *Supervision* is a higher level of automation, in which measurements are processed in real time to generate more useful information (oxygen uptake rate [OUR], CPR, etc.), so that process operators can take more appropriate corrective actions.
- In *automatic control,* such corrective actions are not taken by human operators, but rather by microprocessor-based devices, such as programmable logic controllers (PLC), data acquisition systems (DAS), or computers.
- There are even more sophisticated automation systems, in which the corrective actions taken by control devices are also supervised (by process engineers or other computers) in order to avoid operational problems or to achieve optimal performance.

The main components of an automatic control system (control or feedback loop, see Figure III.44) are the measuring device, the decision device, and the final control device. The *measuring device* (sensor, instrument) senses the process variable and sends this information to a *decision device* (controller). Here, the measured value is compared to a preestablished reference (set point). If these values differ, the controller sends a signal to the *final control device* (actuator) so that corrective action can be taken. Today the decision device is a computer- or microprocessor-based system, with the control law (or algorithm) programmed into it. An actuator is any device that can be operated remotely in order to alter a process input variable such as airflow rate or heat input.

### *Control Algorithms*

The simplest algorithm available is the On/Off control, and it is widely used in all kinds of processes, from home appliances to complex industrial

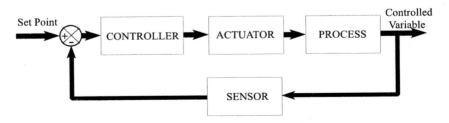

FIGURE III.44. Outline of an automatic control system

facilities. On/Off controllers generate a binary output signal so that the actuator can operate at only two possible states. The switching between the two states is triggered when the measured value crosses a defined threshold, i.e., when the error (difference between the measured and required values) changes sign. To control the amplitude of oscillation of the measured value, the switching speed can be altered using a transition zone or "differential band." Although effective, inexpensive, and simple, the On/Off algorithm is not appropriate to control critical variables that should be kept close to the required value (set point) or when oscillations are deleterious to the process.

PID controllers can be found in almost all industrial installations because they are the first choice when a smooth control action is required. They produce an output signal that is a linear combination of the error (**P**roportional action), the integral of the error over time (**I**ntegral action), and the time derivative of the error (**D**erivative action). The selection of "weights" in this linear combination is called "tuning," and many control textbooks provide tuning rules. If the process presents a complex dynamic behavior, PID tuning may be time consuming or demand periodic human supervision. In some extreme cases, PID can completely fail to provide the expected performance.

Expert control algorithms make use of "If . . . Then . . . Else" rules to incorporate the knowledge of operators and engineers, so that corrective actions can be taken automatically. Expert control has shown to be effective in emulating successful manual operation, emergencies, process start-ups, and shut-downs. In addition, they may prove useful when the process is poorly instrumented or when it presents a complex dynamic behavior. They are difficult to develop though, and other advanced algorithms may perform better.

When a process model is used to compute the control actions according to some optimum criterion, we talk about model-based control algorithms. These models are usually linear with fixed parameters, and the optimization can include constraints on inputs, outputs, or any process variable. In addition, the control algorithm may include more manipulated variables than controlled variables, so that the design of the control strategy becomes much simpler. If the process dynamic is highly nonlinear, then better performances can be achieved if a nonlinear model is used in the optimization problem. However, the mathematical problem gets much more complicated and efficient optimization routines are required to solve it. Adaptive controllers may be a good option, especially if the process exhibits variable time delays or moderate nonlinear dynamic behavior. Here, an algorithm that estimates model parameters online is associated with a control law so that its parameters or "weights" are tuned online without human supervision. Model-based controllers are difficult to develop, operate, and maintain, and they should be used only when PID controls fail.

### *Control Strategies*

Temperature regulation in SSF processes is difficult on one hand, given the limited capacity of the solid substrate to dissipate the metabolic heat, and on the other hand, this regulation is critical because most microorganisms of interest in SSF processing can tolerate a relatively narrow range of temperature. Therefore, no SSF bioreactor can operate without an efficient temperature-control system. This explains why it is the most studied and developed area in SSF automation. Several devices, strategies, and control algorithms have been designed and tested from laboratory to industrial-scale production.

In practice, the solid bed can be cooled by three mechanisms: conduction, using cool surfaces such as reactor walls; convection, forcing cool air through the solid; or evaporative cooling, forcing dry air through the solid. Often these mechanisms are enhanced by continuous or periodic bed agitation. In laboratory-scale static-bed SSF reactors (less than 100 cc volume) the surface to volume ratio is large enough for conduction to provide very effective cooling. In these cases, usually the reactor (column) is placed inside a thermoregulated bath. For larger reactors, heat removal through walls can be significantly enhanced by bed agitation, so that reactors up to 2 m$^3$ can be appropriately cooled. However, agitation is not generally applicable since the growth rate of some microorganisms will slow down or stop completely. Alternatively, a large-scale static SSF bioreactor can be cooled effectively by placing extended cool surfaces inside its bed, although these may complicate its design and operation. Conduction cooling is also applicable to tray bioreactors. At industrial-scale production, the trays are located inside a controlled atmosphere camera, where the environmental air is cooler than the solid layers. An even more effective cooling can be achieved by direct tray cooling. Here, the trays are formed by two parallel plates separated by a gap, which is used for circulating cooling fluid. On/Off controls perform well in conduction cooling of small bioreactors. PID, expert control, or model-based control (using an energy balance) may be necessary for pilot or industrial-scale bioreactors.

When continuous agitation of the solid bed causes an undesirable reduction in the biomass growth rate or when conduction cooling plus agitation does not remove enough heat, convection cooling may be combined effectively with periodic agitation to achieve good temperature regulation. Here, for example, convection cooling can be used to regulate the average (or maximum) bed temperature, while agitation can be applied when the temperature gradient surpasses some predefined threshold. However, in many practical cases, convection plus agitation cooling is not enough to cool large-scale bioreactors. In these cases, it has been shown that conduction plus convection with agitation cannot remove more than 50 percent of the metabolic heat. The other 50 percent must be removed by evaporative cooling. Partially saturated air should be forced through the solid bed, where the evaporation rate, and consequently the cooling rate, can be regulated by manipulating the inlet air humidity. This evaporation causes bed drying, so the temperature control should be coupled with a water-content bed control. Evaporative cooling can also be used in tray bioreactors, where the environmental air is kept under saturation. The dynamic response of the process and the control configuration can become very complicated when evaporative cooling is used, resulting in highly interactive loops, long delay times, and strong nonlinearities. Therefore, advanced control techniques such as expert control or model-based control are usually required to achieve optimum bioreactor performance.

Although not as difficult, bed humidity control is as critical for bioreactor performance as temperature control. On one hand, an excess of water content severely reduces the oxygen transfer through the biofilm, causing a reduction in the growth rate. On the other hand, growth may be limited if not enough water is available for the microorganism. Obviously, water-content control will be unavoidable if evaporative cooling is used; however, it has been shown that even if saturated air is fed into the reactor, some degree of bed drying will occur. The bed humidity can be easily adjusted by periodic addition of fresh water plus agitation for homogenization. However, the lack of appropriate online water-content sensors makes this adjustment rather difficult. Most of the time, measurements of periodically taken samples will be enough to keep the water content under control. However, if the evaporation rate is high, model-based techniques (using a water balance) should by applied to obtain an online estimation of the water content, so that the exact amount of required water will be added at the right time.

It has been experimentally verified that homogeneous growth in static beds can be achieved if a high level of aeration is applied. However, high aeration rates may be expensive or cause too much bed drying. Therefore, by regulating either the $CO_2$ or the $O_2$ concentration of the outlet gas, the optimum aeration rate can be established. This regulation is rather simple, and good results can be obtained by switching between different aeration rates or by using PID control coupled with a modulated-valve or variable-speed blower.

## CONCLUSIONS

It is disappointing to see that only a small fraction of the large number of SSF processes that have been successfully developed on the laboratory scale are able to reach industrial production. This fact is partially explained by the extreme difficulty involved in SSF automation. To simplify the scaling-up of economically competitive SSF technology, these bioreactors should be operated optimally and should be flexible, so that many different micro-organisms can grow in them. Even though a control system may work well at a laboratory or pilot scale for a given reactor type, it is not a trivial task to make the same control system for the same reactor type work on an industrial scale. From an automation point of view, the main limitations of large-scale SSF bioreactors are

- lack of affordable and reliable instrumentation to monitor the state of the culture in the solid bed,
- heterogeneity of the cultivation in static or partially agitated reactors,
- slow dynamic response (large time constants and long time delays),
- nonlinear and time-varying dynamic behavior, and
- strong interaction between the temperature and water-content control loops.

Despite these limitations, many industrial facilities worldwide success-fully operate SSF processes, although some of them produce relatively small quantities of high-added-value products that do not require large-scale bio-reactors. In other cases, the bioreactors do not operate optimally, or bioreactors that are not easily adaptable for different processes are used. We believe that in the near future flexible and optimum-performance large-scale SSF bioreactors will be designed, built, and operate successfully, although more engineering research is needed. These reactors will use low-cost and reliable instruments, specially designed for solid-substrate cultures, and sophisticated control strategies that will include advanced control techniques such as expert and model-based control.

## SUGGESTED READINGS

Henson MA and DE Seborg (1996). *Nonlinear process control.* Upper Saddle River, NJ: Prentice-Hall ECS.

Liptak GB (2000). *Instrument engineers handbook,* Volume 1, *Process Measurement,* Third edition. Boca Raton, FL: CRC Press.

Mitchell DA, DM Stuart, and RD Tanner (1999). Solid-state fermentation—Microbial growth kinetics. In *The encyclopedia of bioprocess technology: Fermentation, biocatalysis and bioseparation,* Volume 5, MC Flickinger and SW Drew (eds.). New York: John Wiley, pp. 2407-2429.

Ogunnaike BA and WH Ray (1994). *Process dynamics, modeling, and control.* New York: Oxford University Press.

Pérez-Correa JR and E Agosin (1999). Solid substrate fermentation—Automation. In *The encyclopedia of bioprocess technology: Fermentation, biocatalysis and bioseparation,* Volume 5, MC Flickinger and SW Drew (eds.). New York: John Wiley, pp. 2429-2446.

Suryanarayan S and K Mazumdar (2000). *Solid state fermentation.* Bangalore, India: World Intellectual Property Organization, PCT WO 00/29544.

# General Aspects of Solid-State Fermentation

Ashok Pandey
Febe Francis
Abdulhameed Sabu
Carlos Ricardo Soccol

## *INTRODUCTION*

Solid-state (substrate) fermentation (SSF) is generally defined as the growth of the microorganism on (moist) solid material in absence or near absence of free water. SSF is comparatively an older technology in relation to submerged fermentation (SmF), which is being pursued as a "high-technology" application. SSF has its origins in food fermentation, particularly with cheese making in Asia, bread making in Egypt, and *koji* process in China for the production of soy sauce. During the last part of the nineteenth century and early twentieth century, SSF reemerged as a technology for the treatment of solid organic wastes. In the meantime, SmF established itself as a major technology. SSF has recently gained fresh attention due to some major advantages it offers, especially in the utilization of agroindustrial residues and pollution prevention.

The process of SSF may be briefly described as follows: the moistened solids are mixed with an inoculum (seed) and placed within a bioreactor (fermentor) to form a "solid-substrate bed." This bed may be viewed as a gas-liquid-solid mixture in which an aqueous phase is intimately associated with a solid surface in various states of sorption and is in contact with a gas phase continuous with the external gaseous environment. Some of the water may be tightly bound to solid surfaces, some are less tightly bound, and some may exist in a free state within the capillary regions of the solid. This can vary with the moisture content of the solid. The gas-liquid interface so formed provides a boundary for mass and heat transfer. The microorganisms grow on the particle surfaces and may penetrate into the solid substrate and extend into the interparticle spaces. Most processes are aerobic, and the microorganism obtains air from the interparticle air space. The major carbon (energy) sources are usually carbohydrates and are often macromolecules, such as starch or cellulose. Microbes secrete hydrolytic enzymes into the substrate particle that release soluble sugars from the polymers.

These soluble sugars diffuse to the surface of the particle, where they are taken up by the microbes and converted to new biomass. These reactions are exothermic, and growth of the microorganism releases waste metabolic heat, which is directly proportional to the metabolic activities of the microorganism. Removal of this heat occurs through the mechanisms of conduction, convection, and evaporation.

In comparison to SmF, which generally employs less-complex carbon sources, solid substances provide mixed substrates of high-molecular-weight carbon compounds, which can bring about induction, inhibition, or repression mechanisms in microbial metabolism. This unique property of SSF provides a selective environment at low moistures for mycelial organisms that produce a variety of extracellular enzymes, surface bound or free, and that can grow at high nutrient concentrations near solid surfaces.

## CHARACTERISTICS OF SSF

In SSF, microorganisms and substrates are static and water usage is limited, which results in generation of lesser quantities of liquid effluent. Because the physical nature of the fermentation mash is solid, the volume is also smaller. In SSF, aeration is achieved by diffusion.

## ADVANTAGES AND DISADVANTAGES OF SSF

SSF has a marked advantage over SmF in terms of productivity, concentration of the products, and effluent generation. The various advantages of SSF are as follows:

- Higher product titres
- Low capital and recurring expenditures
- Lower wastewater output
- Reduced energy requirement
- Absence of foam formation
- Simple and highly reproducible
- Simpler fermentation media
- Less fermentation space
- Absence of rigorous control of fermentation parameters
- Easier aeration
- Economical to use even on smaller scale
- Easier control of contaminants
- Applicability of using fermented solids directly

- Storage of dried fermented matter
- Lower cost of downstream processing

In spite of the aforementioned advantages, there are a few limitations of the SSF technique in comparison to the SmF technique:

- Heat buildup
- Occasional bacterial and fungal contamination
- Limitation of microbial types that can be used
- Need for use of indirect methods for biomass estimation
- Difficult control of moisture content of the medium
- Extensive pretreatment which may be expensive
- Need for production of large-spore inoculum
- pH control during fermentation is almost impossible
- Higher power requirement for continuous agitation
- Limited knowledge on engineering and development aspects
- Nonavailability of well-defined scale-up criteria

### FACTORS THAT INFLUENCE SSF

In SSF, factors are generally considered to be independent, although this is not the case. Numerous factors, as well as their interactions, guide the fermentation in a specific path, but only those factors that have a decisive role in the development of the SSF process are usually analyzed. These factors have an impact on strain selection, design and characteristics of the medium of fermentation, substrate conditioning, control criteria, and design of reactors.

#### Biological Factors

Biological factors influence the behavior of the microbial species in SSF. Based upon the type of microorganism used, SSF processes are classified as *natural* (indigenous) SSF and *pure-culture* SSF. Composting and ensiling are two typical natural SSF processes. Pure-culture SSF is generally used industrially for targeted products.

Selection of a suitable strain is one of the most important criteria in SSF. Microorganisms are screened for their capability to produce commercially acceptable yields of targeted products, amount of by-products, and their nature of growth and proliferation on the substrate. Selection of substrate for SSF process depends on factors related to cost and availability. Solid substrate has a dual role in SSF, as a nutrient reserve as well as the support to which the cells anchor. Tropical agroindustrial residues offer numerous advantages in this respect.

## Inoculum Size

The size of inoculum determines biomass production in the solid medium. Too low or too high a density of biomass is often undesirable in enzyme production, and an optimum level is often observed specific to the product. At the laboratory scale, spores from agar slants are used for inoculation. At industrial levels, the preparation of spore suspension in itself has a separate entity. Use of moldy substrates for inoculation is also practiced.

## Physicochemical Factors

Physicochemical factors govern the various transport processes and thereby the growth and product formation by the microbes.

### Carbon Source and C:N Ratio

Carbon source represents the energy source available for the growth and propagation of the microorganism. Carbon forms the principal component of cellular biomass (40 to 60 percent). Thus, any medium formulation invites significant considerations on carbon source. The yield of a product in kinetic studies is generally based on the consumption of the carbon source $(Y_{x/s})$.

Nitrogen determines growth and protein synthesis as a component of amino acids and nucleic acids. It amounts to 3 to 12 percent of the biomass. The relationship between the mass of carbon and nitrogen (C:N) is crucial for a particular process to obtain a specified product, especially if it is nongrowth associated. Supplementation of organic and inorganic nitrogen compounds is often found to enhance enzyme production in SSF.

### Temperature

Biological processes are characterized by the fact that they are developed in a relatively narrow range of temperature. The significance of temperature in the development of a biological process is such that it could determine the effects of protein denaturation, enzymatic inhibition, promotion or suppression of the production of a particular metabolite, or cell viability and death. The classification of microorganisms into psychrophiles, mesophiles, and thermophiles points to the limitation of using a particular strain of microorganism for a process defined by temperature.

Fermentation processes are generally developed for mesophilic strains (30 to 45°C). Recent trends are to develop processes with thermophilic strains, as it could allow solving problems of heat evolution to some extent. Rise in temperature due to exothermic characteristics of SSF poses the main difficulty in process scale up, and temperature control is quite difficult in SSF as compared to SmF. This is because the solid substrates lack homogeneity in the reactor which results in the existence of temperature gradients. The nonhomogenous nature also makes heat exchange difficult.

*Moisture and Water Activity* ($a_w$)

Viable cells are characterized by a moisture content of 70 to 80 percent, and thus water availability becomes a deciding factor in the synthesis of new cells. Moisture as a factor is associated in the definition of SSF. In a monolayer region at the surface, water is tightly bound to the solid surface. In a multilayer region beyond the surface monolayer, water is less tightly bound in additional layers at progressively decreasing energy levels. Beyond this, free water exists in a region of capillary condensation. The water activity of the medium is considered to be the fundamental parameter for mass transfer of water and solutes across the cell membrane. The control of this parameter can be used to control and modify the metabolic activity of the microorganism. Water activity *($a_w$)* is defined as the relative humidity of gaseous atmosphere in equilibrium with the substrate. Pure water has $a_w = 1.0$, and $a_w$ decreases with the addition of solutes. It has been established that the moisture of the solid matrix must be higher than 70 percent for the growth of bacteria. Yeast has a preferential range of 60 to 70 percent, and fungi have a range as wide as 20 to 70 percent.

*pH*

Every microorganism has a pH range for its growth and activity, with an optimum value falling in this range. The growth and proliferation of microbes on the substrate brings about a change in pH. Therefore, pH control becomes a problem as the process is being scaled up, as a pH gradient gets established in the reactor, owing to the heterogeneous nature of the substrate. Lack of proper equipment for the measurement and control of pH is a drawback in SSF. Interestingly, some agroindustrial residues have a distinct advantage of having a buffering capacity that is generally not observed on other solid matrices.

*Aeration and Agitation*

Aeration and agitation play a determinant role in SSF due to two funda-mental aspects:

1. Supply of oxygen to the aerobic process
2. Control of heat and mass transfer in the heterogeneous system

SSF has a distinction over SmF in this respect. It is not necessary to have a mechanism for the dissolution of oxygen in the liquid phase prior to its use for metabolism. Only the mass transfer from the bulk air to the cellular inte-rior limits uptake of oxygen. Therefore, lower aeration levels are sufficient for SSF as compared to SmF.

*Particle Size of Substrate*

Particle size determines several factors through which a heterogeneous system is characterized. Of these, void fraction ($\varepsilon$) and form factor ($\varphi_s$) are important. Void fraction is found to vary as fermentation proceeds. Particu-larly in SSF using filamentous fungal strains, growth of mycelium is found to diminish $\varepsilon$. $\varphi_s$ determines the availability of surface area for the growth of the organism. $\varphi_s$ may be improved by various pretreatment measures such as milling, pelletizing, etc.

## SUBSTRATES FOR SSF

Cost and availability are the chief factors governing the choice of sub-strate for SSF. An ideal substrate provides all the necessary nutrients for the growth and propagation of the microbes. Pretreatment of substrates are of-ten a necessity, for proper access and anchorage of the organism on them. Research on the selection of suitable substrates has mainly centered on trop-ical agroindustrial crops and residues. These include crops such as cassava, soybean, sugar beet, sweet potato, potato, and sweet sorghum; crop residues such as bran and straw of wheat and rice, sugarcane bagasse; residues of the coffee processing industry such as coffee pulp and coffee husk; residues of fruit processing industries such as pomace of apple and grape, pineapple and banana wastes, and spent grains; and residues of oil processing mills such as coconut oil cake, soybean cake, peanut cake, canola meal, and palm oil waste. Many processes have been developed that utilize these as raw ma-terials for the production of bulk chemicals and valuable products such as ethanol, single-cell proteins (SCP), mushrooms, enzymes, organic acid, and biologically active secondary metabolites. SSF also offers distinct advantage in detoxification and degradation of such residues.

## CONCLUSIONS

Recent developments in the area of fermentation and bioprocess technology have proved the feasibility of adopting solid-state fermentation as a tool for commercial processes development. However, several factors need to be looked at extensively to develop solid-state fermentation that is equally sophisticated to liquid fermentation. Hopefully in the coming years this will be achieved as the result of extensive global efforts.

## SUGGESTED READINGS

Pandey A (1992). Recent process developments in solid-state fermentation. *Process Biochemistry* 27(2):109-117.

Pandey A (ed.) (1994). *Solid state fermentation.* New Delhi: Wiley Eastern Limited.

Pandey A (guest ed.) (1996). *Solid state fermentation.* Special Issue of the *Journal of Scientific and Industrial Research* 55(5/6):311-482.

Pandey A (ed.) (1998). *Advances in biotechnology.* New Delhi: Educational Publishers and Distributors.

Pandey A, CR Soccol, JAR Leon, and P Nigam (2001). *Solid-state fermentation in biotechnology.* New Delhi: Asiatech Publishers Inc.

Pandey A, CR Soccol, and DA Mitchell (2000). New developments in solid-state fermentation: I. Bioprocesses and products. *Process Biochemistry* 35(10):1153-1169.

# Modeling in Solid-State Fermentation

David A. Mitchell
Oscar F. von Meien
Nadia Krieger

## *INTRODUCTION*

Mathematical models are useful tools for understanding and optimizing solid-state fermentation (SSF) processes. They can describe either overall bioreactor performance or particle-scale phenomena. This chapter uses case studies of both model types to explore the overall structure of models and the structure of their key equations, in order to illustrate the general principles of modeling of SSF.

## *BIOREACTOR MODELS*

Although there are currently no reports of the use of models to design large-scale SSF bioreactors, models must be used in the future if the efficiency of large-scale SSF bioreactors is to be improved. This section outlines the basic features of SSF bioreactor models in the context of a case study of a model for an intermittently mixed, forcefully aerated bioreactor that was proposed by von Meien and Mitchell in 2002. During most of the fermentation the bed remains static, and therefore during these periods the bioreactor performs identically with a packed-bed bioreactor. However, provision is made for brief intermittent mixing events. The case study bioreactor might appear as in Figure III.45.

Typically it is appropriate to recognize up to three phases: the substrate bed, the headspace air, and the wall (Figure III.45). In the case study, the headspace and wall are ignored and the bed is divided into separate air and solid phases. A model must describe heat and mass transfer within and between these phases and the interaction of these processes with microbial growth (Figure III.46). Furthermore, it must describe how the key process variables change over time and how the direction and rate of these changes are affected by the operating variables. In the case study, the available operating variables are the flow rate, temperature, and humidity of the inlet air and the intensity, frequency, and duration of mixing events. The key process

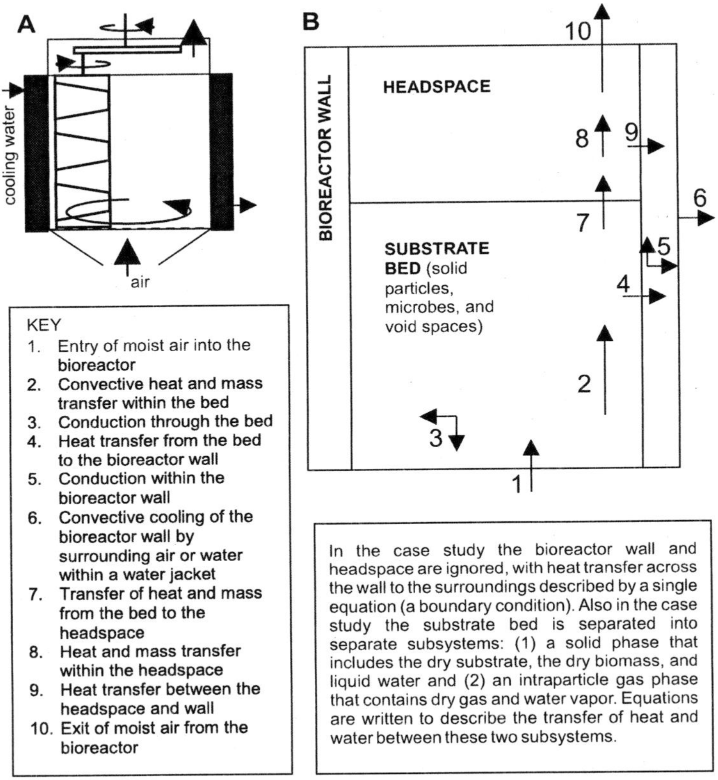
A
cooling water
air
B
BIOREACTOR WALL
HEADSPACE
SUBSTRATE BED (solid particles, microbes, and void spaces)
1
2
3
4
5
6
7
8
9
10
KEY
1. Entry of moist air into the bioreactor
2. Convective heat and mass transfer within the bed
3. Conduction through the bed
4. Heat transfer from the bed to the bioreactor wall
5. Conduction within the bioreactor wall
6. Convective cooling of the bioreactor wall by surrounding air or water within a water jacket
7. Transfer of heat and mass from the bed to the headspace
8. Heat and mass transfer within the headspace
9. Heat transfer between the headspace and wall
10. Exit of moist air from the bioreactor
In the case study the bioreactor wall and headspace are ignored, with heat transfer across the wall to the surroundings described by a single equation (a boundary condition). Also in the case study the substrate bed is separated into separate subsystems: (1) a solid phase that includes the dry substrate, the dry biomass, and liquid water and (2) an intraparticle gas phase that contains dry gas and water vapor. Equations are written to describe the transfer of heat and water between these two subsystems.

FIGURE III.45. (A) An SSF bioreactor and (B) the subsystems and processes within a bioreactor that are typically incorporated into mathematical models. Note that the number of phases recognized, their physical orientation and relative spatial arrangement, and the processes included in the model depend on the bioreactor type and the degree of sophistication of the model.

variables are those that have the most influence on growth and can be most directly influenced by the manner in which the bioreactor is operated, namely, the temperature and water activity of the bed. Inclusion of intraparticle nutrient and $O_2$ concentrations would require the description of intraparticle diffusion processes, greatly complicating the model. Therefore, the kinetic equations are typically empirical equations in which the parameters are expressed as empirical functions of the temperature and water activity, as is done in the present case study.

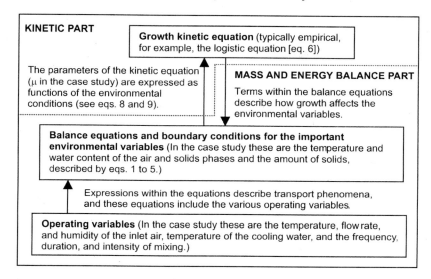

FIGURE III.46. The general structure of bioreactor models showing how they have kinetic, and mass and energy balance parts

The key equations for the periods of static operation in the case study are shown in Table III.40. Mixing is modeled by triggering mixing events when the humidity of the outlet air falls below a set point. During the mixing event the water content and temperature of the bed are brought back to their initial values and the biomass is redistributed uniformly throughout the bed. Each event is presumed to take 15 minutes during which there is no growth, with the resumption of growth immediately after static operation is resumed.

In equation (1) the second term on the left hand side (LHS) describes convective flow of water vapor in the gas phase. The term on the right hand side (RHS) describes the exchange of water between the gas and the moist solids. Equation (2) also contains this term, although with opposite sign, as well as a term for metabolic water production. In equation (3) the second term on the LHS describes convective heat removal, while the RHS describes heat transfer between the solid and gas phases. The heat transfer term appears as the first term on the RHS of equation (4), with the last two terms on the RHS describing the heat removed from the solid by evaporation and the release of metabolic heat. Equations (5) and (6) describe growth and the consumption of dry solids, respectively. Empirical equations, which are not shown, are used to describe the water sorption isotherm of the sub-

TABLE III.40. Mass and energy balances and kinetic equations in the bioreactor model of von Meien and Mitchell

| Description and equation | Eq. |
|---|---|
| Water balance within the gas phase | |
| $$\varepsilon \cdot \rho_g \frac{\partial \varphi_g}{\partial t} + G \frac{\partial \varphi}{\partial z} = K'a\left(\varphi_s - \varphi_s^*\right)$$ | (1) |
| Water balance within the solid phase | |
| $$\frac{\partial\left(S\varphi_s\right)}{\partial t} = -K'a\left(\varphi_s - \varphi_s^*\right) + Y_{WB}\left(S\frac{\partial b}{\partial t} + b\frac{\partial S}{\partial t}\right)$$ | (2) |
| Energy balance within the gas phase | |
| $$\varepsilon \rho_g \left(C_{Pg} + \varphi_g C_{Pv}\right)\frac{\partial T_g}{\partial t} + \left(C_{Pg} + \varphi_g C_{Pv}\right)G\frac{\partial T_g}{\partial z} = -ha\left(T_g - T_s\right)$$ | (3) |
| Energy balance within the solid phase | |
| $$S\left(C_{Ps} + \varphi_s C_{Pw}\right)\frac{\partial T_s}{\partial t} = ha\left(T_g - T_s\right) - \lambda K'a\left(\varphi_s - \varphi_s^*\right) + Y_Q\left(S\frac{\partial b}{\partial t} + \frac{\partial S}{\partial t}\right)$$ | (4) |
| Growth of the biomass | |
| $$\frac{\partial b}{\partial t} = \mu b\left(1 - \frac{b}{b_m}\right)$$ | (5) |
| Consumption of the dry solids | |
| $$\frac{\partial S}{\partial t} = Y_{SB}\left(S\frac{\partial b}{\partial t} + b\frac{\partial S}{\partial t}\right)$$ | (6) |

*Source:* Adapted from von Meien and Mitchell, 2002.
*Note:* $t$ = time, $\varepsilon$ = void fraction, $\rho_g$ = density of the gas phase, $\varphi_g$ = water content of the gas phase, $G$ = flow rate of gas through the bed, $z$ = axial coordinate, $K'a$ = overall mass transfer coefficient, $\varphi_s$ = true water content of the solid phase, $\varphi_s^*$ = water content the solid phase would have if it were in temperature and moisture equilibrium with the gas phase, $b$ = biomass concentration, $\mu$ = specific growth rate constant, $S$ = dry solid concentration (sum of dry biomass plus dry residual substrate), $C_{Pg}, C_{Pv}, C_{Ps}, C_{Pw}$ = heat capacities of the dry gas, water vapor, dry solids, and liquid water, ha = overall heat transfer coefficient, $T_g, T_s$ = temperatures of the gas phase and solid phases, $\lambda$ = enthalpy of evaporation of water, $Y_{WB}, Y_Q$ = yields of water and heat from growth, $Y_{SB}$ = the change in dry solids per kilogram of biomass produced.

strate and the dependence of the specific growth rate constant in equation (5) on the water activity and temperature.

Solution of the model requires specification of the initial and boundary conditions and the values of the various parameters. Some of these will depend on the substrate and the microorganism and must be determined in independent experiments. Parameters such as heat and mass transfer coefficients must be expressed as functions of various operating variables, such as the airflow rate. After numerical integration, the model predicts how the key process variables change throughout the fermentation as a function of both time and position within the bed. For example, simulations made with the case study model suggest that if the bioreactor is operated without the humidity-based control scheme, then growth will quickly become limited by low water contents in the majority of the bioreactor (Figure III.47). On the other hand, if the humidity-based control scheme is used, then the importance of water limitation can be greatly reduced, and temperature limitation becomes important, because the strategy of mixing infrequently cannot prevent high temperatures from being reached at the top of the bed when the bed is static for long periods.

Although detailed predictions are not shown here, such a model can be used to explore the best strategy for design and operation in terms of the flow rate, temperature, and water content of the inlet air, the relative humidity set point, and the bed height.

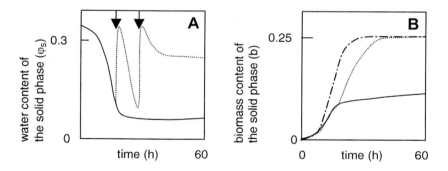

FIGURE III.47. Typical fermentation profiles predicted by the case study model. (A) Substrate water content ($\varphi_s$, kg water per kg dry solids) at midheight of the bed in the absence (——) and presence ($\cdots$) of the humidity-based control scheme. The arrows indicate the mixing events. (B) Predicted profiles of the volume-weighted dry biomass content (b, kg biomass per kg dry solids) in the absence (——) and in the presence ($\cdots$) of the humidity-based control scheme. The logisitic equation with $\mu = \mu_{opt}$ is shown for comparison (– · –).

## MODELS OF PARTICLE-SCALE PHENOMENA

Models of particle-scale phenomena can provide insights into how the intraparticle processes affect growth within SSF systems. Intraparticle processes include the diffusion of $O_2$ and nutrients through the particle, with simultaneous uptake by the microorganisms; the diffusion of enzymes and their action within the substrate; the extension of the biomass above the surface; and the shrinkage of the residual substrate particle. The case study of the model proposed by Rajagopalan and Modak in 1985 that is presented here describes the system shown in Figure III.48. It represents a wet biofilm of constant density growing on a spherical particle of constant size surrounded by a gas phase of constant composition. The particle contains starch as the carbon and energy source.

The model equations are summarized in Table III.41. Enzyme release is described by an empirical equation (not shown). To simplify the model, it is assumed that the enzyme, glucoamylase, is liberated into the substrate at the biofilm/particle boundary and cannot cross this boundary into the biofilm. Equation (7) represents Fickian diffusion of the enzyme in a spherical geometry. Starch hydrolysis is assumed to follow Michaelis-Menten kinetics as shown in equation (8). On the RHS of equation (9) the first term describes the liberation of glucose from starch by the enzyme and the second term the diffusion of this glucose through the particle. Once this glucose enters the biofilm it both diffuses within the biofilm, represented by the first term on the RHS of equation (10), and is consumed by the cells, represented by the second term on the RHS of equation (10). Oxygen also diffuses within the biofilm and is taken up by the cells, represented by the two terms on the RHS of equation (11). Growth and therefore growth-related activities such as nutrient and $O_2$ uptake are assumed to be simultaneously limited by $O_2$ and glucose. In both equations (10) and (11), the first term on the RHS describes diffusion within the biofilm and the second term describes the uptake of the particular component. Equation (12) is a calculation, by integration across the biomass layer, of the total amount of growth within the biofilm. The overall amount of biomass is then used to calculate the overall particle radius *(R)* in equation (13), noting that the biomass forms a spherical shell starting at the particle/biomass boundary at $R_i$.

This model suggests that $O_2$ limitation can be expected within biofilms. During periods of rapid growth all the $O_2$ is consumed by outer parts of the biofilm, leaving inner parts without $O_2$, particularly during periods of rapid growth (Figure III.47). Limitation of supply of glucose to the biofilm is less important, tending to occur only in the outer regions of the biofilm, and only becoming important when the starch within the substrate particle is ex-

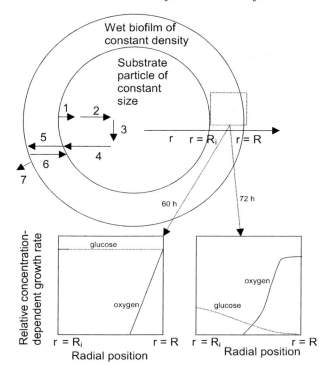

FIGURE III.48. Diagrammatic representation of the system modeled by the single-particle mass transfer model of Rajagopalan and Modak and predictions, made at two different times during the fermentation, of the extents to which glucose and oxygen concentrations limit the specific growth rate. *Note:* (1) release of glucoamylase; (2) diffusion of glucoamylase; (3) hydrolysis of starch; (4) diffusion of glucose within the substrate; (5) diffusion of glucose within the biofilm with simultaneous uptake; (6) diffusion of oxygen within the biofilm with simultaneous uptake; (7) expansion of the biofilm due to growth. (*Source:* Adapted from Rajagopalan and Modak, 1995.)

hausted, thereby limiting the supply of glucose from the substrate to the biomass.

Such a biofilm of constant density as modeled in this case study might be expected for a biofilm of a unicellular organism or a fungus growing totally or largely within a surface-liquid film. However, it is also possible to describe concentration profiles of biomass above the surface, such as might be expected for growth of fungal hyphae into the void spaces between parti-

TABLE III.41. Equations of the single-particle mass transfer model of Rajago-palan and Modak

| Description and equation | Eq. |
|---|---|

Diffusion of glucamylase within the substrate particle

$$\frac{\partial C_E^s}{\partial t} = \frac{D_E^s}{r^2} \frac{\partial}{\partial r}\left(r^2 \frac{\partial C_E^f}{\partial r}\right) \tag{7}$$

Hydrolysis of starch within the substrate particle

$$\frac{\partial C_S^s}{\partial t} = -K_{cat} C_E^s \left(\frac{C_S^s}{K_S + C_S^s}\right) \tag{8}$$

Production of glucose and glucose diffusion within the substrate particle

$$\frac{\partial C_G^s}{\partial t} = K_{cat} C_E^s \left(\frac{C_S^s}{K_S + C_S^s}\right) + \frac{D_G^s}{r^2} \frac{\partial}{\partial r}\left(r^2 \frac{\partial C_G^s}{\partial r}\right) \tag{9}$$

Diffusion of glucose into the biofilm and consumption by the microorganism

$$\frac{\partial C_G^f}{\partial t} = \frac{D_G^f}{r^2} \frac{\partial}{\partial r}\left(r^2 \frac{\partial C_G^f}{\partial r}\right) - \mu_m \rho_x Y_{GX} \left(\frac{C_{O2}^f}{K_{O2} + C_{O2}^f}\right)\left(\frac{C_G^f}{K_G + C_G^f}\right) \tag{10}$$

Diffusion of $O_2$ into the biofilm and consumption by the microorganism

$$\frac{\partial C_{O2}^f}{\partial t} = \frac{D_{O2}^f}{r^2} \frac{\partial}{\partial r}\left(r^2 \frac{\partial C_{O2}^f}{\partial r}\right) - \mu_m \rho_x Y_{O2X} \left(\frac{C_{O2}^f}{K_{O2} + C_{O2}^f}\right)\left(\frac{C_G^f}{K_G + C_G^f}\right) \tag{11}$$

Overall growth of the biomass within the biofilm

$$\frac{dX}{dt} = \int_{R_i}^{R} \mu_m \rho_x \left(\frac{C_{O2}^f}{K_{O2} + C_{O2}^f}\right)\left(\frac{C_G^f}{K_G + C_G^f}\right) 4\pi r^2 \, dr \tag{12}$$

Overall radius of the particle

$$R = \sqrt[3]{\frac{3X}{4\pi\rho_x} + R_i^3} \tag{13}$$

*Source:* Adapted from Rajagopalan and Modak, 1995.
*Note:* $t$ = time, $r$ = radial position in the particle, $K_{cat}$ = catalytic rate constant, $K_S$ = Michaelis-Menten constant for starch, $\mu_m$ = maximum specific growth rate, $\rho_x$ = the density of the biomass, $Y_{O2X}$ and $Y_{GX}$ = stoichiometric coefficients for $O_2$ and glucose, respectively. $C$ represents a concentration and $D$ a diffusivity where the superscripts $s$ and $f$ represent the subsystem, being substrate and film, respectively, and the subscripts $S$, $G$, $E$, and $O2$ represent starch, glucose, enzyme, and oxygen, respectively.

cles. In this case it is necessary to describe the movement of glucose within the mycelium to the tips of the aerial hyphae, since it is here that the growth process occurs. The rate of diffusion depends on the hyphal concentration, since the glucose can diffuse only within the hyphae and not through the air. Note also that the case study treats only a single particle, with growth of the biofilm not being spatially restricted by surrounding particles. Growth within the complex three-dimensional particle arrangement that exists within a solid-substrate bed deserves attention in the future.

## CONCLUSIONS

The case studies show how mathematical models can give insights into what controls growth in SSF systems. At the macroscale in the intermittently stirred, forcefully aerated bioreactor, high temperatures become important soon after a mixing event and control the growth rate for long periods, but low water activities become of major importance just before a mixing event. At the scale of individual particles, $O_2$ can be limiting in the inner part of the biofilm for much of the time, while glucose limitation becomes of importance only near the end of the fermentation, and then only in the outer parts of the biofilm.

It is easy to see how models can be used as tools to optimize and understand SSF systems. Bioreactor models can be used to investigate how the various operating parameters should be manipulated to optimize bioreactor performance. Particle models can show how growth can be limited by intraparticle diffusion processes. An understanding of this helps to avoid futile attempts to manipulate the bioreactor operating variables in order to improve a process that is limited by intraparticle processes.

Current models are still highly simplified representations of the system, which does limit their predictive power. Many improvements are necessary, including the development of better equations to describe how variations in temperature and water activity influence growth, as well as the effects of shear forces in agitated beds on growth. With increased computing power in the future, it may become appropriate to include intraparticle processes in bioreactor models, allowing a more direct evaluation of the relative importance of macroscale and particle-scale processes in limiting growth. There is also an urgent need to validate current models experimentally, modifying them if necessary. Once these improvements are made, mathematical models will become indispensable tools in the establishment of commercial SSF processes.

## SUGGESTED READINGS

Mitchell DA, M Berovic, and N Krieger (2000). Biochemical engineering aspects of solid-state bioprocessing. *Advances in Biochemical Engineering/Biotechnology* 68:61-138.

Rajagopalan S and JM Modak (1995). Evaluation of relative growth limitation due to depletion of glucose and oxygen during fungal growth on a spherical solid particle. *Chemical Engineering Science* 50:803-811.

von Meien OF and DA Mitchell (2002). A two-phase model for water and heat transfer within an intermittently-mixed solid-state fermentation bioreactor with forced aeration. *Biotechnology and Bioengineering* 79:416-428.

# Xylitol Production from Hemicellulosic Substrates

Poonam Nigam Singh
Tim Robinson
Dalel Singh

## INTRODUCTION

Xylitol ($C_5H_{12}O_5$) is naturally occurring sugar polyalcohol, obtained as a result of xylose metabolism (Figure III.49). It occurs naturally in low concentrations in fruit and vegetables and is also generated through metabolism of carbohydrates in animals and humans. Concentrations of xylitol in the blood range from 0.03 to 0.06 mg/100 ml. Xylitol is recognized as a suitable substitute for conventional sugars, with its sweetness comparable to sucrose, and is of higher sweetening power than other polyols such as sorbitol and mannitol. It has one-third fewer calories than sucrose and commands a US$28 million market in the areas of special dietary foods, toothpastes, and chewing gums. Xylitol dose not require insulin for regulation of its metabolism and thus is seen as a suitable sugar alternative for diabetics. The metabolism of xylitol does not involve glucose-6-phosphate dehydrogenase, which also makes it an ideal sweetener for those who are deficient in this enzyme.

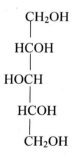

FIGURE III.49. Xylitol structure

Xylitol possesses anticarcinogenic properties and is seen as beneficial with regard to dental care and hygiene. It is not degraded by *Streptococcus mutans*, a naturally occurring microorganism present in the buccal cavity, and so prevents the formation of acids that attack tooth enamel. Xylitol also promotes enamel remineralization by reversing small lesions, due to its favorable interaction with saliva, inducing increases in calcium ions and phosphate.

The molecular structure of xylitol prevents the browning of foods such as that caused by the Maillard reaction. It is, therefore, an ideal additive for foods that are processed at high temperatures. Xylitol cannot be fermented by yeasts, so it can be used in syrups and soft drinks with no need for pasteurization or the addition of preservatives to increase shelf life. Xylitol is, therefore, of great interest to the food and pharmaceutical industries, as well as oral health care authorities.

## PRODUCTION OF XYLITOL

The main materials used for the production of xylitol are the wood component of birch and beach trees, as well as other plant structural tissues such as wheat and flax straw, corn stalks, cotton seed, sugarcane bagasse, peanut hulls, and wood pulp. Each of these substrates contains sufficient quantities of xylans (11 to 35 percent), which are hydrolyzed yielding D-xylose, L-arabinose, D-mannose, and D-galactose. The predominant component of the xylan breakdown is D-xylose (80 to 85 percent). It is this pentose sugar that is widely utilized as the starting material required for xylitol production. Utilization of hemicellulose for xylitol production does not produce waste gas, as in paper industries, and the waste dreg that is produced as a by-product can be used as fuel or for compost.

### Chemical Production

Xylitol can be produced by reduction of D-xylose. In this process, xylans are converted to xylose by hydrolysis and then to xylitol by hydrogenation. The xylitol is then purified and crystallized. The critical step in this procedure is the purification of xylose from the acid hydrolysate.

On an industrial scale, hydrolysis of the hemicellulose component of, for example, birch wood or beech wood is required, followed by an extraction phase using methanol to produce D-xylose. Hydrogenation of xylose with $Ni/Al_2O_3$ is needed for D-xylitol synthesis, with a series of purification and separation steps needed for the removal of by-products. The yield of xylitol from xylans is only 50 to 60 percent, and so the production of xylitol by chemical means is expensive. With separation and purification steps also adding to costs, other methods of xylitol production have been explored for efficient and cost-effective production.

## Microbial Production

Xylitol can also be produced by biotechnological process such as through the use of microorganisms and/or enzymes. Unlike chemical production, biotechnological methods require very little xylose purification, which reduces the complexity and cost of the process. Although hemicellulosic materials are abundant and widespread, they are difficult to ferment. Only a few microorganisms have been reported that are capable of xylitol production to a satisfactory level. Xylitol production is dependent on fermentation parameters such as pH, inoculum and substrate concentrations, etc.

### Yeasts

Only a few selected yeasts are capable of producing xylitol through the fermentation of xylose. Some examples include *Candida* sp., *C. boidinii, C. guilliermondii, C. pelliculosa, C. shehatae, C. tropicalis, Pachysolen tannophilus,* etc. *Candida* sp., however, generally utilize glucose in the presence of xylose and glucose mixtures, due to the repression of the enzymes responsible for xylose degradation. It is only after complete glucose degradation that xylose-metabolizing enzymes are produced, which as a consequence results in a lag period before xylitol production can occur. This has the effect of increasing production time and also has a detrimental influence on ultimate product yield. Ethanol production through glucose utilization can also occur and may inhibit or reduce cell proliferation. Induction of xylose metabolism and the removal of ethanol may be beneficial in increasing fermentation yields.

Yeasts such as *Candida* sp. and *P. tannophilus* are capable of producing xylitol in an amount that can exceed 15 percent of the initial D-xylose concentration. Mutant strains of *C. tropicalis* have also been shown to produce xylitol almost quantitatively from D-xylose. *Saccharomyces* sp. have been tested for their ability to produce xylitol from D-xylose. Some strains were shown to produce similar amounts of xylitol as *Candida* spp. (10 to 15 percent) but were unable to utilize the xylose as efficiently or effectively. Recombinant strains of *Saccharomyces* sp. have also been employed with varying degrees of success.

*Bacteria*

Xylitol production has been reported by several bacteria such as *Coryne-bacterium* sp., *Enterobacter liquefaciens,* and *Mycobacterium.* Bacterial cells can be used to transform D-xylose to xylitol with a 70 percent yield being produced by *Mycobacterium smegmatis.* Cells can either be washed or immobilized. Xylitol can also be produced using D-xylose with commercial D-xylose isomerase from *Bacillus coagulans* and immobilized *M. smegmatis.*

*Enzymatic*

The enzymatic method of xylitol production allows product formation using free enzymes on a continuous basis. An ultrafiltration membrane in such a setup allows the efficient reuse of biocatalysts and enzymes during substrate recycling, with NADP(H) (nicotinamide adenine dihydrogen phosphate) also being retained. *Candida pelliculosa,* coupled with the oxioreductase system of a methanogen capable of recycling NADP(H), has been used successfully with a 90 percent conversion of xylitol. Feasibility of xylitol production by enzymatic processes requires strict optimization of conditions, as well as an adequate downstream processing system for enzyme recovery.

## XYLITOL PRODUCTION PATHWAYS

In general, D-xylose can be isomerized to D-xylulose by xylose isomerase, or can be reduced to xylitol by xylase reductase in the presence of NADPH or NADH. Xylitol produced can be dehydrogenated to D-xylulose by xylitol dehydrogenase in the presence of $NADP^+$ or $NAD^+$, which are produced as a product of the previous reaction.

As mentioned previously, small amounts of xylitol are produced in the human body, namely the liver. Again, this is an NADP-linked dehydrogenase reaction, with L-xylulose as the starting component. Xylitol is produced as a metabolite of the glucuronate-xylulase pathway.

In microorganisms, xylitol is formed as a result of D-xylose metabolism. This can occur in two ways: D-xylose can be converted to xylitol by NADPH-dependent aldedhyde reductase, or D-xylose may be initially isomerized to D-xylose by D-xylose isomerase and can then be reduced to xylitol by NADH-dependent xylitol dehydrogenase.

The oxioreductase pathway with xylitol as an intermediate has been reported to be the most common pathway for D-xylose conversion to xylitol. Such oxioreductive pathways have been found in yeasts such as *Candida pulcherrima, C. utilis, Rhodotorula,* and *Pichia albertensis*. The production pathways for the fungus *Petromyces albertensis* can be seen in Figure III.50. In the first pathway:

1. D-xylose is directly reduced to xylitol using NADH.
2. An alternative pathway is that D-xylose is isomerized to D-xylulose and then reduced to xylitol, again using NADH. Where pathways have been found and understood in other microorganisms, NADPH has been shown to serve as a reductant. For example, NADPH serves as a reductant for D-xylose conversion to D-xylitol by the enzyme aldoreductase in *Rhodotorula gracilis*.
3. Alternatively, NADH and NADPH have been reported to be used as cofactors for D-xylose reductase. This is evident in *Pachysolen tannophilus*. D-xylulose acccumulates in the fermentation medium and is then phosphorylated by D-xylulokinase and enters the pentose-phosphate pathway, yielding ethanol as a by-product.

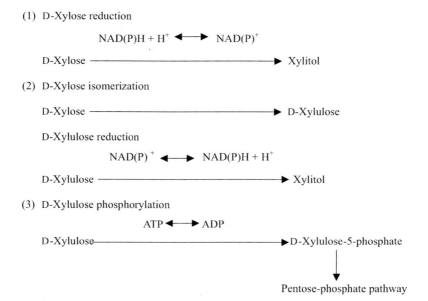

(1)  D-Xylose reduction

$$NAD(P)H + H^+ \longleftrightarrow NAD(P)^+$$

D-Xylose $\longrightarrow$ Xylitol

(2)  D-Xylose isomerization

D-Xylose $\longrightarrow$ D-Xylulose

D-Xylulose reduction

$$NAD(P)^+ \longleftrightarrow NAD(P)H + H^+$$

D-Xylulose $\longrightarrow$ Xylitol

(3)  D-Xylulose phosphorylation

$$ATP \longleftrightarrow ADP$$

D-Xylulose $\longrightarrow$ D-Xylulose-5-phosphate

$\downarrow$

Pentose-phosphate pathway

FIGURE III.50. Pathways for the conversion of xylose to xylitol in *Petromyces albertensis*

## OPTIMIZING XYLITOL PRODUCTION

### Aeration

Oxygen is required by many yeasts to facilitate sugar uptake, while stimulating sugar transport in others. Xylitol production is directly coupled with the growth of biomass and is strongly influenced by oxygen consumption. Therefore, aeration of the medium enhances xylose conversion to xylitol. Sufficient aeration of the fermenting medium is required in order to achieve adequate cell growth for xylitol production. However, because xylitol is produced under anoxic conditions, continuous high-level aeration would lead to the production of D-xylulose by dehydrogenation.

Xylitol production under near-anaerobic or semi-anaerobic conditions is also possible. Reduced aeration has been explored to attempt to increase xylose metabolism, although this is hampered by lack of understanding concerning aeration rates and has not always led to an increase in xylitol production.

Current research is examining the possibility of using yeasts for xylitol production under anaerobic conditions. Theoretically, fermenting hemicellulose substrates under anaerobic parameters can produce high quantities of xylitol. This requires feeding the microorganism a secondary carbon source to fuel NADPH for the regeneration and production of xylitol. Reduced xylose concentrations are, therefore, required for cell growth, with more being available for xylitol formation.

### Nitrogen

In yeasts such as *Saccharomyces cerevisiae,* the pentose-phosphate pathway is regulated by nitrogen. Ammonium salts have also been found to stimulate the oxidative pentose-phosphate pathway. In *P. tannophilus,* addition of ammonium salts stimulates growth as the presence of NADH normally inhibits D-glucose-phosphate dehydrogenase. Ammonium salts decrease the intracellular level of NADPH, depressing D-glucose-phosphate dehydrogenase, thereby increasing the oxidative pentose pathway activity.

Quantities of xylitol can be as much as doubled by the addition of an organic nitrogen source. This is due to a stimulated increase in the level of the enzyme xylitol dehydrogenase. The addition of ammonium acetate and yeast extract, for example, has been shown to have this effect on *C. shehatae.* In contrast, research concerning polyol formation by *Pichia,* has shown that low nitrogen levels are more suited for obtaining high yields.

## Xylose Concentration

The addition of a high concentration of xylose tends to produce an increase in xylitol production rates and yields. However, this is very much dependent on the ability of the microorganism to tolerate this initial high sugar concentration and subsequent higher osmotic pressure. Research has suggested that the interaction between D-xylose concentration and the lower aeration rate is related to cell concentration. Therefore, at a lower D-xylose concentration and aeration level, the cell concentration is reduced, with xyliyol production being possible in the early phase of cultivation. By reducing aeration to the fermentation at an early stage, xylose metabolism can be induced with a reduction in lag time.

Cell growth and xylitol yields have also been shown to be adversely affected by high levels of xylose. Product inhibition has also been noted in some strains such as *Petromyces albertensis,* with an early and rapid production of xylitol being a disadvantage, unless the product is removed on a continual basis.

## Nonxylose Sugars

Glucose has been shown to inhibit D-xylose utilization, especially in *Candida* sp. and *Schizosaccharomyces.* These microorganisms preferentially metabolize glucose in the presence of xylose and glucose mixtures. This is due to the inhibition of xylose-degrading enzymes in the presence of high levels of glucose. A lag period exists between the time taken for glucose metabolism to occur and the subsequent stimulation of xlyose-degrading enzymes. Inhibition, rather than inactivation or repression, is suggested as a possible mechanism for the microorganisms' inability to utilize xylose in the presence of high concentrations of glucose. The lag period in xylitol fermentation increases production time and reduces product yields. This is because much of the energy obtained as a result of substrate utilization is used for cell growth and enzyme production. A substantial reduction in this lag period will be of great benefit to industry.

The effectiveness of other sugars such as arabinose, galactose, glucose, and mannose for xylitol production has also been investigated. It was found that these sugars were rapidly fermented and utilized exclusively for growth and ethanol production.

## *Methanol*

Addition of methanol has been shown to produce a slight increase in xylitol yield. A possible reason for this could be methanol oxidation, yielding NADH, which in turn would enhance D-xylose and D-xylulose reduction.

## CONCLUSIONS

Although xylitol is present in small quantities in fruits and vegetables, it is economically unfeasible to recover it from these sources. Xylitol production by chemical means has been proven to be too expensive, due to the essential purification and separation steps. Even after these processes, only a relatively small yield in relation to the energy invested is produced (50 to 60 percent).

Many biotechnological processes using microorganisms have been shown to be very effective in producing yields of 90 percent and more. The use of hemicellulose for fermentation means that xyltiol can potentially be produced all over the globe, with the actual production process creating jobs and wealth as well as associated industries, such as crop cultivation for fermentation material. Rapidly growing crops such as eucalyptus trees can be totally replaced in a few years and can provide a renewable source of hemicellulosic material for xylitol production.

Although xylitol production by biological processes has been shown to be effective and economical, for adequate industrial-scale production, greater understanding of aeration supply, product inhibition, and the reduction of the lag period between glucose and xylose metabolism is required. Yeasts are effective at producing large amounts xylitol, with the potential yields being further increased through the use of recombinant microorganisms.

## SUGGESTED READINGS

Nigam P and D Singh (1995). Process for fermentative production of xylitol—A sugar substitute. *Process Biochemistry* 30:117-124.

Singh D, P Kumari, and JS Dahiya (1990). Xylitol production from sugar cane baggase by fermentation. In *Modernisation of the Indian sugar industry,* JK Gehlawat (ed.). New Delhi: Arnold Publishers, pp. 292-303.

Thonart P, X Gomez, J Didelez, and M Paquot (1974). Biotechnological conversion of xylose to xylitol by *Paschysolen tannophilus*. In *Anaerobic digestion and carbohydrate analysis of waste,* GL Ferrera, MP Ferranti, and H Naveau (eds.). New York: Commission of the European Communities, pp. 429-431.

Touster O (1974). The metabolism of polyols. In *Sugars in nutrition*, HL Sipple and KW McNutt (eds.). New York: Commission of the European Communities, pp. 229-232.

# Index